# Register Now
## to

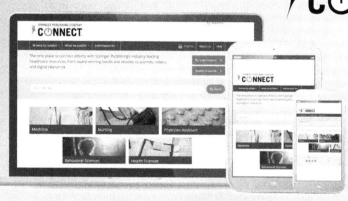

Your print purchase of *Multicultural Perspectives in Working With Families, Fourth Edition,* **includes online access to the contents of your book**—increasing accessibility, portability, and searchability!

### Access today at:

http://connect.springerpub.com/content/book/978-0-8261-5415-6
or scan the QR code at the right with your smartphone
and enter the access code below.

## GLBV2S0E

*Scan here for quick access.*

If you are experiencing problems accessing the digital component of this product, please contact our customer service department at cs@springerpub.com

The online access with your print purchase is available at the publisher's discretion and may be removed at any time without notice.

**Publisher's Note:** New and used products purchased from third-party sellers are not guaranteed for quality, authenticity, or access to any included digital components.

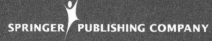

View all our products at springerpub.com

**Elaine P. Congress**, DSW, LCSW, is associate dean and professor at Fordham University Graduate School of Social Service. She has authored 10 books on cultural diversity, immigrants, health, and ethics including two editions of *Social Work with Immigrants and Refugees* and her recent book on *Health and Social Work*. This book is the fourth edition of her book *Multicultural Perspectives in Working With Families*. Several of her books have been translated into Korean. She created the *culturagram*, a family assessment tool that has been widely used in professional work with immigrants, refugees, children, older people, indigenous peoples, survivors of family violence, and those with health problems. More information about her culturagram and work with immigrants can be found in these podcasts: http://socialworkpodcast.com/2008/12/visual-assessment-tools-culturagram.html and http://www.socialworkpodcast.com/2009/02/social-work-with-immigrants-and.html. Most recently, she developed the Intersectional Design Tool to promote better understanding of clients and their families.

Dr. Congress has presented locally at conferences in New York City; nationally at conferences in Orlando, Atlanta, Washington, Philadelphia, Saratoga, and Boston; and at international conferences in Guelph, Canada, London, Amsterdam, Tempere, Finland, Munich, Seoul, and Adelaide. At the United Nations, Dr. Congress represents the International Federation of Social Workers, participates as the vice chair of the NGO Committee on Mental Health, recording secretary of the NGO Committee on the Rights of Indigenous Peoples, and also is a member of the NGO Committee on Migration and the NGO Committee on the Status of Women. A former president of NYC National Association of Social Workers and currently on the board of NASAW Pioneers, she now serves on the Governing Council of the American Public Health Association and on the boards of the International Council on Psychology (ICP) and the Manhattan Psychological Association. She has received awards from the National Association of Social Workers, American Public Health Association, the Latino Social Work Coalition, the Hispanic Mental Health Professionals, and the NYS Social Work Education Association. Dr. Congress has a master's of rts in teaching from Yale, a master's of science in social work from Columbia University, a master's of arts in psychology from the New School of Social Research, and a doctorate in social welfare from the City University of New York.

**Manny John González**, PhD, earned his MSW degree from New York University and his PhD from Adelphi University. He is an associate professor and program coordinator of the doctoral program at the Phyllis and Harvey Sandler School of Social Work at Florida Atlantic University in Boca Raton, Florida. Prior to his current appointment at Florida Atlantic University, he held tenured faculty positions at the Silberman School of Social Work at Hunter College, The Graduate Center of the City University of New York, and Fordham University Graduate School of Social Service. Dr. González's research and scholarship interests include mental health/mental illness, the application of developmental and psychodynamic theories to clinical practice, psychological and physical well-being among Hispanic immigrants, the psychodynamics of fathering and fatherhood, doctoral education and clinical research using qualitative and quantitative methods. He has taught graduate courses at the MSW and PhD levels in clinical practice, relational psychotherapy, group therapy, psychopathology, evidence-based mental health practice, translational science, research proposal development, contemporary psychodynamic theories, and social work education. Dr. González has published numerous articles and chapters on mental health practice with immigrants and refugees, clinical practice with Hispanics, urban children, evidence-based practice, clinical social work practice, and interprofessional collaboration. His book credits (co-edited) include *Mental Health Care of New Hispanic Immigrants: Innovations in Contemporary Clinical Practice* and *Multicultural Perspectives in Social Work Practice With Families* (Springer Publishing Company). Dr. González was awarded the Hunter College Presidential Award for Excellence in Teaching in 2016. He has practiced as a clinician for over 33 years specializing in community mental health—and maintained a private practice in psychodynamic psychotherapy and clinical supervision in Brooklyn Heights, New York, until his arrival at Florida Atlantic University in 2017.

# Multicultural Perspectives in Working With Families

## A Handbook for the Helping Professions

**FOURTH EDITION**

*Elaine P. Congress, DSW, LCSW*
*Manny John González, PhD*

EDITORS

SPRINGER PUBLISHING COMPANY

Copyright © 2021 Springer Publishing Company, LLC
All rights reserved.
First Springer Publishing edition 1997; subsequent editions 2005, 2013.

No part of this publication may be reproduced, stored in a retrieval system, or transmitted in any form or by any means, electronic, mechanical, photocopying, recording, or otherwise, without the prior permission of Springer Publishing Company, LLC, or authorization through payment of the appropriate fees to the Copyright Clearance Center, Inc., 222 Rosewood Drive, Danvers, MA 01923, 978-750-8400, fax 978-646-8600, info@copyright.com or on the Web at www.copyright.com.

Springer Publishing Company, LLC
11 West 42nd Street, New York, NY 10036
www.springerpub.com
connect.springerpub.com/

*Acquisitions Editor*: Kate Dimock
*Compositor*: Exeter Premedia Services Private Ltd.

*ISBN*: 978-0-8261-5414-9
*ebook ISBN*: 978-0-8261-5415-6
*DOI*: 10.1891/9780826154149

**Qualified instructors may request supplements by emailing textbook@springerpub.com**

19 20 21 22 / 5 4 3 2 1

The author and the publisher of this Work have made every effort to use sources believed to be reliable to provide information that is accurate and compatible with the standards generally accepted at the time of publication. The author and publisher shall not be liable for any special, consequential, or exemplary damages resulting, in whole or in part, from the readers' use of, or reliance on, the information contained in this book. The publisher has no responsibility for the persistence or accuracy of URLs for external or third-party Internet websites referred to in this publication and does not guarantee that any content on such websites is, or will remain, accurate or appropriate.

**LCCN: 2020000625**

Contact us to receive discount rates on bulk purchases.
We can also customize our books to meet your needs.
For more information please contact: sales@springerpub.com

Elaine P. Congress: 0000-0002-4043-6146
Manny John González: 0000-0001-6729-2616

*Publisher's Note*: **New and used products purchased from third-party sellers are not guaranteed for quality, authenticity, or access to any included digital components.**

Printed in the United States of America.

This book is dedicated to all the social workers and psychologists who work with people from many different cultures and backgrounds.

*In memory of our dear friend and colleague Dr. Carmen Ortiz Hendricks whose dedication, commitment, and wisdom in working with clients and students from different backgrounds was outstanding. Dr. Ortiz Hendricks was the former Dean at Wurzweiler School of Social Work, Yeshiva University—and is the author of Chapter 8, Multicultural Triangle of the Child, Family, and the School: Culturally Competent Approaches.*

Elaine P. Congress and Manny John González

*In memory of Dr. Gladys María González-Ramos—friend, colleague, and sister. Her clinical and research contribution in the areas of mental health, delivery of care to Hispanic children and families, and Hispanic mothers' cultural child-rearing values was outstanding—and her examination of the clinical social worker's role in health care, interdisciplinary team training, and the provision of psychosocial treatment to persons with Parkinson's disease and their caregivers was absolutely ground-breaking. While the essence of Dr. González-Ramos's work will continue to thrive, she will always be missed.*

Manny John González

# Contents

*Contributors* ix
*Foreword* Joseph G. Ponterotto, PhD *xiii*
*Foreword* Mo Yee Lee, PhD *xv*
*Preface* *xvii*
*Acknowledgments* *xxv*

## PART I: OVERVIEW

1. Using the *Culturagram* and an Intersectional Approach in Practice With Culturally Diverse Families  3
   Elaine P. Congress and Winnie W. Kung

2. Practice With Multiracial Individuals and Families  27
   Jennie Park-Taylor, Alea Holman, and Steven Carter

3. Transracial Adoption and Transracial Socialization: Clinical Implications and Recommendations  39
   Jason D. Reynolds (Taewon Choi) and Hannah M. Wing

4. *The DSM-5* From a Multicultural Perspective  55
   Betty Garcia and Zsuzsanna Monika Feher

5. Evidence-Based Practice With Ethnically Diverse Clients  69
   Manny John González

## PART II: ADMINISTRATIVE AND LEGAL PERSPECTIVES

6. Managing Agencies for Multicultural Services  83
   Manoj Pardasani and Lauri Goldkind

7. Legal Issues in Practice With Immigrants and Refugees  101
   Fernando Chang-Muy

## PART III: LIFE CYCLE PERSPECTIVES

8. The Multicultural Triangle of the Child, the Family, and the School: Culturally Competent Approaches  117
   Carmen Ortiz Hendricks (deceased) and Manny John González

9. Cross-Cultural Perspectives on Working With Adolescents  137
   Daniel Kaplin and Uwe P. Gielen

10. Working With Culturally Diverse Older Adults  153
    Janna Heyman and Linda White-Ryan

## PART IV: PRACTICE WITH INDIVIDUALS AND FAMILIES FROM DIFFERENT RACIAL/ETHNIC BACKGROUNDS AND GENDER ORIENTATION

11. Practice With African American Families    *169*
    *Samuel R. Aymer*

12. Practice With Hispanic Individuals and Families    *181*
    *Manny John González and Gregory Acevedo*

13. Practice With Asian Immigrant Families and Intergenerational Issues    *195*
    *Grace S. Kim and Julie M. AhnAllen*

14. Practice With Native American Families    *209*
    *Hilary N. Weaver*

15. Practice With Arab American Families    *227*
    *Wahiba Abu-Ras and Sameena Azhar*

16. Practice With Lesbian, Gay, Bisexual, and Transgender People and Their Families    *251*
    *Gerald P. Mallon*

## PART V: PHYSICAL AND MENTAL HEALTH ISSUES WITH MULTICULTURAL FAMILIES

17. Health Beliefs, Care, and Access of Individuals and Families From Diverse Backgrounds    *279*
    *Elaine P. Congress*

18. Spirituality and Culturally Diverse Families: The Intersection of Culture, Religion, and Spirituality    *295*
    *Zulema E. Suárez and Edith A. Lewis*

19. HIV/AIDS and Latinx Families: Practice Considerations    *315*
    *Claudia Lucia Moreno*

20. Substance Abuse    *333*
    *Linda White-Ryan and Janna Heyman*

21. Practice With Immigrant Victims of Domestic Violence    *347*
    *Patricia Brownell, Zsuzsanna Monika Feher, and Denise Gosselin*

22. Culture, Intersectionality, and Suicide    *385*
    *Dana Alonzo and Robin Edward Gearing*

## PART VI ETHICAL ISSUES AND FUTURE DIRECTIONS

23. Ethical Issues and Future Directions    *421*
    *Elaine P. Congress*

*Index*    *433*

# Contributors

**Wahiba Abu-Ras, PhD, MSW, MPA,** Professor, Adelphi University, School of Social Work, Garden City, New York

**Gregory Acevedo, PhD,** Associate Professor, Fordham University Graduate School of Social Service, New York, New York

**Julie M. AhnAllen, PhD,** Associate Director of Diversity and Inclusion, Director of Training, Boston College University Counseling Services, Boston, Massachusetts

**Dana Alonzo, PhD,** Associate Professor, Graduate School of Social Service, Fordham University, New York, New York

**Samuel R. Aymer, PhD,** Chair, Clinical Practice Method, Associate Professor, Silberman School of Social Work, Hunter College, New York, New York

**Sameena Azhar, PhD, LCSW, MPH,** Assistant Professor, Fordham University Graduate School of Social Service, New York, New York

**Patricia Brownell, PhD,** Associate Professor Emerita of Social Service, Fordham University, New York, New York

**Steven Carter, MSEd,** PhD Student, Counseling Psychology, Fordham University, New York, New York

**Fernando Chang-Muy, MA, JD,** Thomas O'Boyle Lecturer in Law, University of Pennsylvania School of Law, Philadelphia, Pennsylvania

**Elaine P. Congress, DSW, LCSW,** Professor and Associate Dean, Fordham University Graduate School of Social Service, New York, New York

**Zsuzsanna Monika Feher, MA,** Clinical Psychology (APA Accredited) Doctoral Student, Chicago School of Professional Psychology, Los Angeles, California

**Betty Garcia, PhD,** Professor Emerita, Department of Social Work Education, California State University, Fresno, Fresno, California

**Robin Edward Gearing, PhD, LCSW,** Professor and Director, Center for Mental Health Research and Innovation in Treatment Engagement and Service (MH-RITES Center), University of Houston, Graduate College of Social Work, Houston, Texas

## CONTRIBUTORS

**Uwe P. Gielen, PhD,** Executive Director, Institute for International and Cross-Cultural Psychology, Department of Psychology, St. Francis College, Brooklyn, New York

**Lauri Goldkind, PhD, LMSW,** Associate Professor, Graduate School of Social Service, Fordham University, New York, New York

**Manny John González, PhD,** Associate Professor and Program Coordinator of the Doctoral Program, Phyllis and Harvey Sandler School of Social Work, Florida Atlantic University, Boca Raton, Florida

**Denise Gosselin, MSW,** Fordham University Graduate School of Social Service, New York, New York

**Janna Heyman, PhD, LMSW,** Professor and Endowed Chair Henry C. Ravazzin Center on Aging and Intergenerational Studies, Fordham University, Graduate School of Social Service, New York, New York

**Alea Holman, PhD,** Assistant Professor, School Psychology Program, Division of Psychological and Educational Services, Graduate School of Education, Fordham University, New York, New York

**Daniel Kaplin, PhD,** Associate Professor, Graduate School of Social Service, Fordham University, New York, New York

**Grace S. Kim, PhD,** Clinical Associate Professor, Department of Counseling Psychology and Applied Human Development, Boston University Wheelock College of Education and Human Development, Boston, Massachusetts

**Winnie W. Kung, PhD,** Associate Professor, Graduate School of Social Service, Fordham University, New York, New York

**Edith A. Lewis, PhD,** Professor Emerita of Social Work and Women's Studies, University of Michigan School of Social Work, Ann Arbor, Michigan

**Gerald P. Mallon, PhD, DSW,** Julian Lathrop Professor of Child Welfare and Associate Dean of Research and Scholarship, Silberman School of Social Work at Hunter College, New York, New York

**Claudia Lucia Moreno, PhD,** Fordham University, Faculty Trainer HASA Program and Private Therapist, New York, New York

**Carmen Ortiz Hendricks, PhD,**[‡] Dean Emeritus and Professor, Wurtzweiler School of Social Work, Yeshiva University, New York, New York

---

[‡] Deceased

**Manoj Pardasani, PhD, LCSW, ACS,** Associate Provost, Hunter College, The City University of New York, New York, New York

**Jennie Park-Taylor, PhD,** Associate Professor, Counseling Psychology Program, Fordham University, New York, New York

**Jason D. Reynolds (Taewon Choi), PhD,** Assistant Professor, Counseling Psychology PhD Program, Department of Professional Psychology and Family Therapy, Seton Hall University, South Orange, New Jersey

**Zulema E. Suárez, LGSW, ACSW, PhD,** Core Faculty, School of Public Service Leadership, Department of Social Work, Capella University

**Hilary N. Weaver, PhD, DSW,** Professor, School of Social Work, University of Buffalo, Buffalo, New York

**Linda White-Ryan, PhD, LCSW, RN, CASAC,** Assistant Dean, Graduate School of Social Service, Fordham University, New York, New York

**Hannah M. Wing, BA,** Doctoral Student, Counseling Psychology Department, Division of Psychological and Educational Services, Fordham University, New York, New York

# Foreword

Though there are many multicultural-focused books in the counseling, social work, and psychology professions, only a handful can be considered "classic" contributions to the helping professions. One measure of "classic" is that the readership, interest, and citation counts propel a book beyond a second or third edition. The series of editions of *Multicultural Perspectives in Working With Families: A Handbook for the Helping Professions* can now be considered a classic contribution to the mental health field. In this newest fourth edition, Professors Elaine P. Congress and Manny John González have gathered a diverse and interdisciplinary group of gifted authors, clinicians, and researchers to provide the latest comprehensive updates on assisting culturally diverse families and communities with a host of psychological and mental health issues. In a historical period where the United States, and many parts of the world, are mired in sociopolitical division, ethnic and immigration tensions, and religious, gendered, and social-class animosities, never has a new book on assisting culturally diverse families been so timely and important. Let me be fairly direct here: This newest edition of *Multicultural Perspectives in Working With Families* is a must read for any mental health professional, student, administrator, or policy advocate.

As a counseling psychologist and mental health counselor I have been guilty of often sticking to the literature in only these two specialty areas. In reading the broad and diverse topics in this new edition of *Multicultural Perspectives in Working With Families*, with applied and practical chapters written by social workers, family therapists, counseling psychologists, an immigration attorney, and cross-cultural psychologists, my eyes were opened to a wider array of theory, best ethical practices, and practical tools to help me in my multicultural practice, teaching, and research. In fact, I now believe that without an interdisciplinary knowledge base across the various helping professions, including legal and policy knowledge, one cannot align with truly best practices in their professional work. Fortunately, for our interrelated mental health specialties, this new edition of *Multicultural Perspectives in Working With Families* provides the comprehensive knowledge base we all need to markedly advance our multicultural clinical competence.

I want to highlight some of the particular strengths and innovations in this fourth edition. First, in reading the diverse chapters, it becomes immediately clear that not only are the authors up-to-date on the research, best practice, and ethics literature, but they also collectively have a breadth and depth of clinical experience with culturally diverse clients and families that shines through in the writing. As a practicing psychologist, I see these authors as exemplary role models for my own clinical work.

Second, research and experience in the last decade have led to an emphasis on our multiple identities and the intersection of these identities in our daily "lived experience." In this new edition of *Multicultural Perspectives in Working*

*With Families*, intersectionality across its many identities is embedded throughout the chapters. Among these identities and their intersections that growing numbers of families and individuals navigate, are race, ethnicity, religion, social class, gender identity and sexual orientation, and adoptee status, among others. Impressively, the editors and authors of this text have addressed this layered complexity in an accessible and comprehensive fashion.

A third strength of this new edition is the family and lifespan coverage of the material. Naturally there is an anchoring focus on families, and there is also adequate attention given to diverse developmental cohorts including children, adolescents, adults, and our older populations. As we contemplate the growth of multiracial couples and families on one hand, and the large baby boomer generation now entering their later years, this birth to death coverage is a notable strength of the text. Fourth, the breadth of coverage is both fascinating and impressive, including state-of-the-art chapters on multiracial families, transracial adoption, and African American, Hispanic, Asian immigrant, Native American, Arab, and LGBT families.

It is difficult to separate our general health from our mental health, and this new edition of *Multicultural Perspectives in Working With Families* includes a fifth strength, which is a comprehensive discussion of this intersection, including treatment issues related to substance abuse, HIV and AIDS, family violence, and suicide—all human experiences that transcend race, ethnicity, and culture. A sixth unique feature of this newest edition is detailed coverage of selected and timely topics, knowledge of which is critical to culturally competent services. These topics include the use and limits of relying on the *DSM-5* in cultural contexts, up-to-date coverage of evidence-based multicultural practice, working with multicultural service agencies, emergent legal and ethical issues, and the centrality of understanding the role of spirituality in many of our culturally diverse families. A final strength of this volume, and a strength in previous editions, is the accessible and clinically practical strategies infused throughout the text. The case vignettes, case studies, culturagrams, and other practical and visual tools are of immense value to both the student and seasoned multicultural clinician. In reading the chapters, I at times felt as though I was in individual supervision, learning from master clinicians. This fourth edition of *Multicultural Perspectives in Working With Families: A Handbook for the Helping Professions* is an extraordinary contribution to the mental health and human services professions. I wish you a good read!

*Joseph G. Ponterotto, PhD*
Professor of Counseling Psychology
Coordinator, School and Mental Health Counseling Programs
Graduate School of Education, Fordham University
Fellow of the American Psychological Association
Counseling Psychologist and Mental Health Counseling in
Private Practice

# Foreword

*Multicultural Perspectives in Working With Families: A Handbook for the Helping Professions* has been a classic reference for social workers and other helping professionals since 1995 when the first edition of the book was published. Recognizing the diversity of families and that social work and other helping professionals must be able to understand cultural differences among and within families for effective and respectful treatment, this book significantly contributes to promoting cultural competence and cultural humility in professional practice with families from diverse backgrounds.

Another important contribution is that this book locates family at the center of treatment as opposed to individually focused treatment approaches. The focus on family resonates with the pivotal and primary role of family throughout different life stages in a person's life for many cultures. The fourth edition of this book further highlights the increasing complexities and changing nature and demographics in U.S. families. A simplistic understanding of families based on cultural and ethnic differences inevitably discards influences of other aspects of identity on a person's experience. U.S. families also look quite different now than two decades ago and are becoming much more global.

The inclusion of an intersectional approach, an expansive view of family, and the addition of new chapters addressing these changes make this book a dynamic reference that effectively responds to the forever changing and evolving nature of families.

*Mo Yee Lee, PhD*
Professor, College of Social Work, The Ohio State University
Editor, *Journal of Ethnic & Cultural Diversity in Social Work*

# Preface

*Multicultural Perspectives in Working With Families, Fourth Edition,* differs greatly from earlier versions because of two main changes. The first is the adoption of an intersectional approach in working with families. Over the years I have become increasingly aware of the multiple factors that can be used to describe a person. While culture and ethnicity are certainly important, socioeconomic class, education, gender, age, religion, immigration status, and sexual orientation influence how an individual interacts with others in their environment and also how others interact with this person. The chapters in this book all reflect this intersectional approach.

As in earlier editions of this text, culture is used as an umbrella term that includes ethnicity, race, national origin, and religion (Lum, 2010). Although religion and race are often subsumed under culture, class is not. The practitioner must also consider the socioeconomic class of the family in order to avoid inaccurate generalizations. Many families that have recently migrated to the United States and/or have been frequently the victims of racism and discrimination often have limited income. Clinicians must always be aware of what financial resources are available to the family. Other relevant factors in assessing families of diverse cultural backgrounds include: degree of acculturation, poverty, history of oppression, language and the arts, racism and prejudice, sociopolitical factors, child-rearing practices, religious practices, family structure, values and attitudes specific to life, and help-seeking behaviors (Lum, 2004). The authors in this book have addressed many of these issues in their chapters.

Another major change in the fourth edition is that four chapters have been written by psychologists. These chapters are Chapter 2, Practice With Multiracial Individuals and Families, by Jennie Park-Taylor, PhD, Associate Professor, Fordham School of Education, Alea Holman, PhD, Assistant Professor, Fordham School of Education, and Steven Carter, MSEd, PhD student, Fordham University; Chapter 3, Transracial Adoption and Transracial Socialization: Clinical Implications and Recommendations, by Jason D. Reynolds (Taewon Choi), PhD, Counseling Psychology, PhD program, Department of Professional Psychology and Family Therapy, Seton Hall University and Hannah M. Wing, BA, Doctoral Student, Fordham University; Chapter 9, Cross Cultural Perspectives in Working With Adolescents by Daniel Kaplan, PhD, Associate Professor, Fordham Univeristy, and Uwe Gielen, PhD Professor and Executive Director, Institute for International and Cross-Cultural Psychology, St. Francis College; and Chapter 13, Practice With Asian Immigrant Families by Grace Kim, PhD, Clinical Associate Professor at Boston University and Julie M. Ahn/Allen Since both social workers and psychologists frequently work with families from many different backgrounds, it was important to have chapters written by both helping professions in this new edition.

This edition of *Multicultural Perspectives in Working With Families* addresses cutting-edge issues in the assessment and treatment of families from diverse cultural backgrounds. These chapters are not all-inclusive, but rather focus on some of the most important, emerging issues in multicultural practice with families. A new edition always includes "something old and something new." The old of previous editions has been significantly revised to include current knowledge and research to help practitioners work more effectively with culturally diverse families. Also, many of the case vignettes and discussions have been revised. A third of the chapters are completely new, such as Chapter 2, Practice With Multiracial Individuals by Jeannie Park-Taylor, Alea Holman, and Steven Carter; Chapter 3, Transracial Adoption and Transracial Socialization by Jason D. Reynolds (Taewon Choi) and Hannah Wing; Chapter 4 titled *The DSM-5 From a Multicultural Perspective* by Betty Garcia and Zsusanna Monika Feher; and Chapter 17, Health Beliefs, Care, and Access of Individiuals and Families From Diverse Backgrounds by Elaine P. Congress, one of the editors of this book.

Both micro and macro perspectives are important in working with culturally diverse families. Working with families with an intersectional lens involves an understanding of the environment including the community where families live as well as the larger social political factors affecting families. Micro assessment of families occurs simultaneously with the beginning of treatment. A good assessment should include an understanding of family boundaries, rules, roles, and structure. The Olson self-report assessment tool (Olson, Russell, & Sprenkle, 1989) looked at a family's reactions to situational stress in terms of flexibility and cohesion. The Beavers model (Beavers & Hampson, 1993) and the McMaster model (Epstein, Bishop, Ryan, Miller, & Keitner, 1993) have been used in assessing family functioning. The ecomap (Hartman & Laird, 1983) looked at the relationship of the family to external resources, while the genogram (McGoldrick, Gerson, & Schallenberg, 1999) helps the practitioner learn more about family relationships, both current and past. The child welfare field has adopted several ways to assess families (Child Welfare Information Gateway, 2019)

An important focus involves assessing risk and protective factors (training. cfsrportal.acf.hhs.gov/section-2-understanding-child-welfare-system/2984). In recent years there has been much attention paid to the effects of trauma, especially on children (Adverse Childhood Experiences, 2019) and families affected by child abuse, domestic violence, physical abuse, sexual abuse, substance abuse, mental illness, divorce, and incarceration are seen to be most at risk.

Existing family assessment instruments never focused much on understanding the cultural background of the family. This led to the development of the *culturagram* (Congress, 1994) and its revision (Congress, 2002, 2008). The first chapter in the book looks at the culturagram as an assessment and treatment planning modality. The authors, Congress and Kung, use clinical examples from their extensive teaching and practice experience to illustrate different parts of the culturagram and how it can be used in assessment. There was a need to expand the culturagram to include a more intersectional approach. Thus for the first time a draft of the Intersectional Design Tool is presented in the chapter to further our understanding of families from diverse backgrounds.

As we began to work on this book we became very aware of how much families have changed since the first edition appeared in 1995. Over the last 20 years families have become much smaller. The average American family only has 1.9 children (which is below the "replacement rate" of about 2.1 children; Krogstad, 2019). Over a quarter of families are single parented usually by mothers and most women work outside the home (Grall, 2018). Traditional nuclear families are very diminished and many families are extended. Also there are many families with two parents of the same gender with adopted or biological children through fertilization. There are also transgender parents and children. As many as 6 million American children and adults have an LGBT parent and are more likely to be racial and ethnic minorities. An estimated 39% of same-sex couples with children under age 18 at home are non-White, as are half of their children. States with the highest proportions of same-sex couples raising biological, adopted, or stepchildren include Mississippi (26%), Wyoming (25%), Alaska (23%), Idaho (22%), and Montana (22%). LGBT individuals and same-sex couples raising children face greater economic challenges than non-LGBT counterparts. Single LGBT adults raising children are three times more likely than comparable non-LGBT individuals to report household incomes near the poverty threshold (Gates, 2013). Many immigrant families are mixed in that some have legal status as citizens or green card holders while others are undocumented. The current social political climate has led to much stress for families who are separated or live with the fear of being separated. These chapters are not all-inclusive, but rather focus on some of the most important, emerging issues in multicultural practice with families. This edition captures the three emerging elements in cross-cultural practice that must be incorporated into the effective psychosocial treatment of ethnic cultural groups: the client's worldview, language, and religion (González, 2002), as well as socioeconomic class, education, and immigration status.

This book is based on the belief that one should not regard families only on having one culture and ethnicity. Two of the new chapters focus on two increasing types of multicultural families one in which the birth parents are from different ethnic backgrounds (Chapter 2) and another chapter that focuses on a growing phenomenon of transracial adoptions (Chapter 3).

There has been much concern in how and if the *DSM-5* is applied accurately in assessing families from different cultures and socioeconomic classes. There has been some evidence that often people from different cultural groups and poorer socioeconomic classes are given more severe psychiatric diagnoses. The fourth edition includes a chapter (Chapter 4) on this topic and also emphasizes the importance of skilled interpreters as an important way to increase the likelihood of accurate diagnosis.

What treatment methods are the most effective in working with culturally diverse families? Evidence to support the use of different treatment modalities is viewed as paramount in the delivery of social services (Gambrill, 2010). In Chapter 5, Dr. González looks at evidence-based practice that supports the use of specific interventions with multicultural families. Culturally adapted cognitive–behavioral therapy is highlighted as an exemplar of evidence-based treatment for ethnically and racially diverse patient populations.

Most people seek help because of family problems and are seen in family service or mental health agencies. No matter how skilled the clinician is, if agency context is not considered, then family engagement, assessment, and intervention may not be successful. Green (1999), for example, has noted that multicultural skills and knowledge are not just for individual providers of psychosocial care. Human service organizations—the social systems in which most providers of care are employed—must also deliver culturally competent clinical services. In Chapter 6, Drs. Pardasani and Goldkind present new ideas about how practitioners and administrators can "manage for diversity competence" within the workplace. They suggest that agency leaders must continually assess their cultural competence at all levels—boards of directors, administrators, staff, policies, and programs. They raise concerns about microaggressions that occur in the workplace and how they can be addressed.

The second section of the book focuses on work with families from diverse backgrounds across the life cycle. School is the primary place where children from very different cultures interact and learn. In Chapter 8, one of the editors of this book Dr. Manny González has updated the chapter by the late Dr. Ortiz Hendricks. In this chapter the multicultural triangle of child, family, and school is identified. Social workers and psychologists need to understand the different, sometimes conflicting, cultures in order to work effectively with children and their families within the school system. An important starting point is an assessment of a clinician's own cultural backgrounds.

Adolescence is often a challenging time for adolescents around the world. In Chapter 9, Drs. Kaplan and Gielen write about cross cultural understanding of adolescents and their families. Understanding of trends and assessment and understanding of adolescents and their role in the family are the subjects of this chapter.

Older people are increasing in the United States as the number of Americans aged 65 and older is *projected to nearly double* from 52 million in 2018 to 95 million by 2060. The older population is becoming *more racially and ethnically diverse*. In Chapter 10, Drs. Heyman and White Ryan point out important issues in family work with older people from diverse cultural backgrounds. This chapter looks at health disparities among diverse older populations, important assessment issues, service utilization, and treatment approaches with older people and their families. The need for clinicians to understand and work within the cultural background of older clients and their families is illustrated through a case vignette.

This book also includes chapters on different racial/ethnic/cultural groups.

In Chapter 11 on Practice With African American Families, Dr. Aymer addresses the historical background of African Americans in the United States and the racism they encounter. The importance of adopting an Afrocentric framework, the use of language, spirituality, family relationships, and conceptions of mental health are all addressed in this chapter.

In Chapter 12, Dr. González, the co-editor of this book, and Dr. Acevedo look at clinical issues in working with Latino families. Since Hispanics/Latinos are the minority population showing the largest increase in numbers in the United States, this new chapter is particularly timely. The authors look at the diversity of national backgrounds of Hispanics, as well as important cultural characteristics of Hispanics such as *simpatía, personalismo, familismo, confianza respeto*, and the gender roles of *marianismo* and *machismo*. The importance of religion and spirituality for many Hispanics/Latinos is stressed. This new chapter concludes with strategies to use in clinical work with this expanding population.

The number of Asian American families is rapidly increasing and, in Chapter 13, Drs. Kim and AhnAllen look at clinical assessment and treatment issues that have an impact on work with Asian families. The authors address timely issues such as intergenerational conflict, challenges in working with Asian American families, and culturally responsive interventions.

Native American families are again the focus of a chapter in this book. As many of the Native Americans have been decimated over the centuries because of disease and war and are now often invisible in cities, the number of American Indians in the United States constitute only about 1% of the total population. In Chapter 14, Dr. Hilary Weaver, Associate Dean and Professor at the University of Buffalo and also a Lakota social work educator, examines how trauma and oppression have negatively impacted the economic, social, and psychological well-being of American Indians. Understanding the importance of the medicine wheel—mind, body, spirit, and heart—to Native American families increases clinicians' ability to provide culturally sensitive services to these families.

The fourth edition of *Multicultural Perspectives* in Working With Families again has a chapter on Arab American families. This chapter written by Dr. Samena Azhar looks at this growing U.S. immigrant group that is misunderstood, especially post–9/11. Practitioners will learn more about the differences among Arab countries and the religious backgrounds of Arabs, their psychosocial needs, attitudes toward mental health, family relationships, and treatment issues.

In Chapter 16, Dr. Mallon addresses issues that gay and lesbian people face within their families. The psychosocial needs and risks of gay and lesbian people, clinical issues in working with gay and lesbian people, and recommendations for working with this population are addressed.

In Chapter 18, Drs. Suárez and Lewis describe the role of spirituality in culturally diverse families. Major religious trends in the United States, as well as the differences between religion and spirituality, are outlined. This chapter focuses on the interrelationship between cultural and religious views and the effects they have on psychological and interpersonal behavior. Implications for practice with culturally diverse families who recognize their religious beliefs and spirituality conclude the chapter.

Many culturally diverse families have members with differing status ranging from citizen to "green card holder" and "undocumented." Chapter 7, by Fernando Chang-Muy, a law professor at University of Pennsylvania and my co-author of *Social Work With Immigrants and Refugees: Legal Issues, Clinical Skills and Advocacy*, serves to demystify the confusing complex legal status of clients that we serve. This chapter presents relevant immigration policies and laws with a specific focus on three newcomer populations—women, children, and refugees. Ways in which social workers and others in the helping professions can work with lawyers in advocating for the rights of immigrant clients and families are discussed.

The fourth edition of *Multicultural Perspectives in Working With Families* now includes a new chapter on health. This chapter is written by this editor, who, along with Janna C. Heyman, was also the editor of *Health and Social Work: Practice, Policy, and Research*, published by Springer Publishing Company in 2019. Assessment of health issues especially for immigrants, as well as access for healthcare are addressed in Chapter 17.

Although HIV/AIDS is more treatable now than a decade ago, the effects of HIV/AIDS for both infected individuals and their families are devastating. In Chapter 19, Dr. Moreno looks at the stigma and treatment issues for the Latinx community*, especially women and LGBT individuals. The chapter concludes

---

*Latinx* refers to Latino and Latino individuals and the use of this term is becoming increasingly widespread. It is used in several chapters of this book, either on its own or interchangeably with Latino/Latina and Hispanic.

with a discussion of interventions that have been especially helpful in working with Latinos and their families who have been affected by HIV/AIDS.

While the previous edition looked at a specific treatment intervention that is used with problem drinkers and their families, in Chapter 20, Drs. Linda White-Ryan who is also a registered nurse and Janna Heyman adopt an intersectional perspective to look at substance abuse and how it affects clients and their families.

Domestic violence presents special problems in families from culturally diverse backgrounds. Chapter 21 by Drs. Patricia Brownell, Zsuzsanna Monika Feher, and Denise Gossein discusses the unique needs and challenges that many culturally diverse women who have been abused encounter first in acknowledging the need for help, as well as in seeking and securing services. Special difficulties for nondocumented women, as well as issues specific to Latino battered women, Asian battered women, and Southeast Asian women are discussed. Different types of treatment interventions as well as policies that affect the identification and treatment of battered women from diverse cultural and socioeconomic backgrounds conclude this chapter.

Latinos are the fastest growing ethnic group in the United States and by mid-century 25% of adolescents will be of Hispanic background. A growing concern is the increasing number of suicide attempts by adolescent Latinas. Chapter 22 by Drs. Alonzo and Gearing describes strategies for prevention and intervention in Latina adolescents and their families. Treatment interventions are illustrated through a case vignette.

The final chapter of the book by Dr. Congress looks at ethical issues. Families in the United States as well as around the world are changing and current trends will be discussed. At this time there are many new ethical challenges brought about by technology in our work. This chapter looks at how both last year the National Association of Social Workers, the primary social work organization, approved a new code of ethics that provides current standards for ethical practice with the use of technology. This chapter addresses some of these issues and the dilemmas they present, especially for clients from many different cultural and socioeconomic backgrounds. Both social work and psychology address this similarly.

In closing, we hope that you will find this book interesting and helpful in working with diverse families. While Dr. Congress and Dr. González were the primary architects of this book, each of the social workers and psychologists who contributed chapters focused very well on important themes affecting families. We also want to thank our editor Kate Dimock who encouraged and guided us in writing this fourth edition. Also, we greatly appreciate the support that Mindy Chen in the early stages and then Mehak Massand in the final stages provided us in writing the book. And finally, last but certainly not least, we thank two very able research assistants, Abigail Asper, MSW, who worked so diligently in the beginning and then Wendy Perello who helped so much during the final stages of preparing this book for publication.

*Elaine P. Congress, MSSW, DSW*
*Manny John González, MSW, PhD*

# REFERENCES

Adverse Childhood Experiences. (2019, April 2). Retrieved from https://www.cdc.gov/violenceprevention/childabuseandneglect/aces/fastfact.html

Beavers, W. R., & Hampson, R. B. (1993). Measuring family competence: The Beavers systems model. In F. Walsh (Ed.), *Normal family processes* (2nd ed.). New York, NY: Guilford Press.

Child Welfare Information Gateway. (2019). *Family Assessment.* Retrieved from https://training.cfsrportal.acf.hhs.gov/section-2-understanding-child-welfare-system/3026

Congress, E. (1994). The use of culturagrams to assess and empower culturally diverse families. *Families in Society, 75*(9), 531–540. doi:10.1177/104438949407500901

Congress, E. (2002). Using culturagrams with culturally diverse families. In A. Roberts & G. Greene (Eds.), *Social work desk reference* (pp. 57–61). New York, NY: Oxford University Press.

Congress, E. (2008). Using the culturagram with culturally diverse families. In A. Roberts & G. Greene (Eds.), *Social work desk reference* (2nd ed., pp. 57–61). New York, NY: Oxford University Press.

Epstein, N. B., Bishop, D. S., Ryan, C., Miller, I., & Keitner, G. (1993). The McMaster model view of health family functioning. In F. Walsh (Ed.), *Normal family processes* (pp. 138–160). New York, NY: Guilford Press.

Gambrill, E. (2010). Evidence-informed practice: Antidote to propaganda in the helping professions? *Research on social work practice.* Thousand Oaks, CA: Sage.

Gates, G. J. (2013, February). *LGBT parenting in the United States.* Retrieved from https://williamsinstitute.law.ucla.edu/research/census-lgbt-demographics-studies/lgbt-parenting-in-the-united-states/

González, M. J. (2002). Mental health intervention with Hispanic immigrants: Understanding the influence of client's worldview, language and religion. *Journal of Immigrant and Refugee Services, 1*(1), 81–92. doi:10.1300/J191v01n01_07

Grall, T. (2020, January). *Custodial mothers and fathers and their child support: 2015, United States Census Report.* Retrieved from https://www.census.gov/content/dam/Census/library/publications/2020/demo/p60-262.pdf

Green, J. (1999). *Cultural awareness in the human services: A multi-ethnic approach* (3rd ed.). Boston, MA: Allyn and Bacon.

Hartman, A., & Laird, J. (1983) *Family oriented treatment.* New York, NY: Basic Books.

Krogstad, J. (2019). *5 facts about the modern American family.* Washington, DC: Pew Research Center. Retrieved from https://www.pewresearch.org/fact-tank/2014/04/30/5-facts-about-the-modern-american-family

Lum, D. (2004). *Social work practice and people of color* (5th ed.). Belmont, CA: Brooks-Cole.

Lum, D. (2010). *Culturally competent practice: A framework for understanding* (4th ed.). Belmont, CA: Brooks/Cole.

McGoldrick, M., Gerson, R., & Schallenber, S. (1999). *Genograms: Assessment and intervention.* New York, NY: W.W. Norton.

Olson, D. H., Russell, C. S., & Sprenkle, D. H. (Eds.). (1989). *Circumplex model: Systemic assessment and treatment of families.* New York, NY: Haworth Press.

# Acknowledgments

We want to thank Kate Dimock for guiding us every step of the way in publishing this fourth edition of *Multicultural Perspectives in Working With Families*. Also, we are so appreciative of Mehak Massand, for helping to organize and lead us to the completion of our book, and of Kris Parrish, who assisted us with the final copyediting. We hope readers will find this book both interesting and informative.

We want to especially thank our two very knowledgeable and efficient research assistants, Abigail Asper and Wendy Perello, whose hard work, organizational and technological skills helped make the fourth edition of *Multicultural Perspectives in Working With Families* possible.

# Part I

Overview

# 1

# Using the Culturagram and an Intersectional Approach in Practice With Culturally Diverse Families

ELAINE P. CONGRESS AND WINNIE W. KUNG

## INTRODUCTION

The United States is becoming increasingly culturally diverse. It is estimated that by the year 2049 less than half (49.7%) of the population will be non-Hispanic Caucasian (Frey, 2014). While the number of foreign-born people is 13% at the national level, in large metropolitan areas, such as New York City, as many as 37% of its residents are foreign-born (Batalova, Batalova, Blizzard, & Bolter, 2020; New York City Mayor's Office of Immigrant Affairs, 2018). Additionally, approximately 38% of the U.S. population, aged 5 years and older, speak a language other than English at home, with Spanish being the most common other language (U.S. Census Bureau, 2015). In large urban areas such as New York City, one in every two people speak a language other than English at home (New York City Department of City Planning, 2017).

From the beginning of the profession, social workers have stressed the importance of respect for clients from diverse backgrounds (Addams, 1911). In the most recent Code of Ethics, social workers are advised to understand cultural differences among clients, to demonstrate competence in working with people from different cultures, and to work against discrimination based on immigration status (National Association of Social Workers [NASW], 2018). The *culturagram*, a family assessment instrument discussed in this chapter as well as in the previous editions of *Multicultural Perspectives in Working With Families*, grew out of the recognition that families are becoming increasingly culturally diverse and that social workers must be able to understand cultural differences among and within families.

When attempting to understand diverse families, it is important to assess the family within its cultural context. Considering a family only in terms of a generic cultural identity, however, may lead to overgeneralization and stereotyping (Congress, 2008b). A Puerto Rican family that has lived in the United States for 40 years is very different from a Mexican family that emigrated last month, although both families are Hispanic. A Chinese family that emigrated to the United States in the early 20th century is very different from a Tibetan refugee family that has recently been relocated. Even two families from the same country and region can be very different.

Understanding cultural and ethnic differences, however, only provides a partial view of understanding and working with families. An intersectional approach stresses the importance of considering different aspects that contribute to a person's identity. The current NASW Code of Ethics stresses the importance of adopting an intersectional approach in addition to understanding the effect of culture and ethnicity (NASW, 2018).

> Social workers should obtain education about and seek to understand the nature of social diversity and oppression with respect to race, ethnicity, national origin, color, sex, sexual orientation, gender identity or expression, age, marital status, political belief, religion, immigration status, and mental or physical ability. (NASW Code of Ethics 1.05 c)

This is very apparent when providing social work services to people from different cultures and ethnicities. Even within the same ethnic group, there are many other differences that can affect our work; for example, a member of an Asian Indian family that is well educated and from a high socioeconomic status is very different from a member of a poor family. While social workers often work with clients who are of lower socioeconomic background, this is not always the case. To help understand this within-group diversity, an intersectional analysis is helpful and is discussed more in depth and applied to case examples later in the chapter.

## THE *CULTURAGRAM*

While traditional family assessment tools such as the ecomap (Hartman & Laird, 1983) and genogram (McGoldrick, Gerson, & Petry, 2008) are useful tools in assessing the family, they do not address the important role of culture in understanding the family. The culturagram was first developed (Congress, 1994, 1997) and revised (Congress, 2002, 2008b) to help in understanding the role of culture in families. This tool has been used to promote culturally competent practice (Lum, 2010) and in work with battered women (Brownell & Congress, 1998), children (Webb, 1996), the elderly (Brownell, 1997; Brownell & Fenly, 2008), immigrant families (Congress, 2004a), and families with health problems (Congress, 2004b; Congress, 2018). Most recently, the culturagram has been used to work with Indigenous peoples (Congress & Ellington, 2018; Ellington & Roy, 2018), and

# 1. USING THE CULTURAGRAM AND AN INTERSECTIONAL APPROACH 5

there has been initial discussion about its possible use with those with late onset of visual disabilities (L. van de Meibel, personal communication, April 29, 2019).

The culturagram, a family assessment tool, serves to individualize culturally diverse families (Congress, 1994, 2002, 2008b). Completing a culturagram on a family can help a clinician develop a better understanding of the sociocultural context of the family, which can shed light on appropriate interventions to take with the family. Revised in 2008, the culturagram examines the following 10 areas (Figure 1.1):

1. Reasons for relocation
2. Legal status
3. Time in the community
4. Language spoken at home and in the community
5. Health beliefs and access
6. Impact of trauma and crisis events
7. Contact with cultural and religious institutions, holidays and special events, food and clothing
8. Oppression and discrimination, bias and racism
9. Values about education and work
10. Values about family structure—power, hierarchy, rules, subsystems, and boundaries

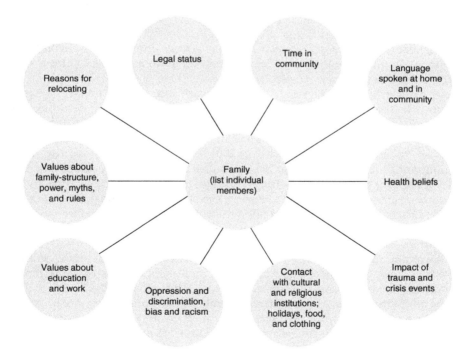

Figure 1.1 *Depiction of a culturagram assessment tool.*

Source: Reproduced from Chang-Muy, F., & Congress, E. (Eds.). (2016). *Social work with immigrants and refugees: Legal issues, clinical skills, and advocacy* (2nd ed., p. 75). New York, NY: Springer Publishing Company.

## Reasons for Relocation

Reasons for relocating to the United States vary among families. Many families come because of economic opportunities in the United States, while others relocate because of political and religious discrimination, and social unrest in their countries of origin. For some, it is possible to return home again. They often travel back and forth for holidays and special occasions and may ultimately move back to their countries of origin. Being able to maintain continuous close social ties with families of origin and other acquaintances in their native countries reduces the sense of uprootedness that families experience in migrating. Such close contacts also facilitate families, especially younger members, to maintain their cultural heritage and identity. The cultural gap between the generations in these immigrant families may be diminished as a result. For those who know they can never go home again, the sense of isolation and the need for a greater social network in this new land becomes more poignant. The social worker can encourage them to actively reach out to their ethnic communities. Modern means of communication such as email, WhatsApp, Facebook, and Skype have made it possible for immigrants to maintain contact with relatives who still live in their countries of origin.

In contrast to earlier immigration patterns, current immigrants come as families or parts of families (Lum, 2010). Some exceptions include undocumented immigrants from Fuzhou in southern China (Kwong, 1997), and South Asians from India and Pakistan, who frequently come as single persons. Many want to marry within their ethnic group, and "mail-order brides" are not an uncommon phenomenon (Loiselle-Leonard, 2001). Because immigrant brides have to adjust to new roles within their families and adapt to a different culture and geographic location, their stresses are enormous (Liao, 2006).

In cases where the marriage does not work out, these women may feel trapped in this foreign land with no social support. Some may even have to endure domestic violence since the prospect of making it outside of the home in the United States is so dim and the shame of going back to their home countries so unbearable (Loiselle-Leonard, 2001). They feel trapped because their immigrant procedures have not been completed, and they fear deportation if they leave their husbands. Fortunately, changes in immigration laws allow some battered women without legal status to stay (Violence Against Women Act, 2019). This has brought relief and hope to many oppressed immigrant women. However, depending on the current political wind, this guarantee could become precarious.

A common assumption is that most migrants come to large urban centers like New York, Chicago, or Los Angeles. An increasing number of immigrants, however, relocate to rural and suburban areas. After arrival in the United States some migrants move again, often from a rural to a more urban area, due to dwindling economic opportunities. Internal migration involves additional challenges for migrants who must establish a new social network and adjust to a new location as well.

## Legal Status

The legal status of a family may have an effect on both individuals and the family as a whole. In the same family, there may be members who are citizens, those who are "green card holders" with the legal right to remain in the United States and proceed toward citizenship, and those who are undocumented without legal status. Chang-Muy's chapter "Legal Issues in Practice With Immigrants and Refugees" in this book explains in greater detail different immigrant statuses. If family members are undocumented and fear deportation, the family may become secretive and socially isolated. Latency-age children and adolescents will be discouraged from developing peer relationships because of the fear of others learning about their status. Using the family systems lens, the external boundaries of these families may become more rigid and, within these families, a corresponding trend toward more diffuse internal boundaries leading to greater enmeshment. The family may resist seeking necessary social and health services lest they be deported. There was increased anxiety about this after the World Trade Center attack and even more so in recent years when the immigration issue became a heated political debate with more imminent threat of deportation.

Some undocumented immigrants come to this country on their own, leaving behind their families and support system. An example is the influx of immigrants from Fuzhou, southern China, in the 1990s (Kwong, 1997). These immigrants have experienced enormous hardship, handicapped by the language barrier and the enormous economic burden of having had to repay the smuggling debts to come to this country (Kwong, 2002). Moreover, the lack of medical benefits makes life even harder when they have health or mental health problems (Kwong, 2002). A social worker working with this population in Chinatown in New York City revealed that, perhaps due to social isolation and enormous stress, many individuals suffering from schizophrenia displayed a revolving-door phenomenon, going in and out of hospitals after brief psychiatric treatments. The relapse rate was as frequent as four times a year.

A more recent influx of refugees from Central America has raised enormous concern in the United States. The higher rate of migration is due to the unstable social condition in those countries partly due to economic hardship, and partly from powerful gangs threatening people's lives and livelihood. Some came without legal documents as refugees and wanted to seek asylum, and some came to join their relatives who are legal residents of the United States. The receptivity in this country and communities could make life easier or harder for these immigrants.

### Length of Time in the Community

The length of time living in the community may differ for individual family members. Usually family members who arrived earlier are more assimilated than other members. A recent phenomenon involves mothers from Guatemala or South America first immigrating to the United States and then sending for their children. These circumstances can certainly impact individual and family development. Not only does the disruption of the primary caregiver at a critical period affect the child's development, the subsequent reunion at an older age in this country could also cause some adjustment problems for the family, which is often manifested as the child's behavioral problems at school (Patel, Clarke, Eltareb, Macciomei, & Wickham, 2016). Sciarra (1999) suggested that the issues these families face include resentment by the children over the parents' earlier "abandonment," the conflict between loyalty toward the reunited parents and the interim caregiver from whom the child is now forced to separate, inadequate parental authority and leadership, and the different level of acculturation between the parent and the child. Sciarra (1999) found that techniques such as reframing the intergenerational conflicts as intercultural issues and stating the treatment goal as working toward biculturalism were helpful.

The problems faced by other immigrant families are the exact opposite of these reunited families. These have been called the "astronaut families" (Irving, Benjamin, & Tsang, 1999). Because of the political instability in Taiwan and Hong Kong in the past couple of decades, many Chinese families migrated to the United States, Canada, and Australia. However, such moves often meant an economic loss to these families since the breadwinner, usually the father, experienced diminished income in his career as his professional qualifications and experiences overseas are often not recognized in the host country. Many families opt to have the children and the mother migrate first, while the father "shuttles" back and forth to join the family periodically. Not only does it pose challenges to the marital relationship, sometimes resulting in affairs and marital breakdown, it also jeopardizes the father–children relationship. These are high prices to pay for migration.

## Language

Language is the vital medium through which families communicate. Often families may use their own native language at home, but use English in contact with the outside community. Sometimes children may prefer English as they see knowledge of this language as most helpful for survival in their newly adopted country. This may lead to conflict within the family. A very real communication problem may develop when the parents speak no English and the children only minimally speak their native tongue. Another key factor affecting family communication is that members relocate at different ages. As children attend American schools and develop peer relationships, they often pick up the new language and culture more quickly than their parents. This may lead to shifts in the power structure of the family as the parents' limited English competency can erode their authority (Hendricks, 2013; Hong, 1989). In some situations, the children may assume the role of interpreter and cultural broker for the family, and sometimes even the leadership role since they have better knowledge about community resources. This may be especially difficult for cultures in which the generational hierarchy within the family is important (Tamura & Lau, 1992).

One of the challenges in the work of bilingual social workers with a bilingual family is that they have to decide which language to adopt and when. Caution should be taken to ensure that the worker does not appear to be "siding" with either the English or the native speaker. For families in which the children can understand but not speak the native language, it is important for the bilingual worker to speak mostly in the native tongue even when talking to the children to indicate that the language is respectable and to show respect to the parents (Hong, 1989). When an interpreter is needed, care must be taken if the worker decides to use a family member as interpreter to ensure that they do not avoid or distort sensitive messages. For example, social workers must ensure that the interpreting family member does not avoid explorations of suicidal ideations when they do not feel comfortable asking the questions and believe that suicide would not happen (Hong, 1989). Discussion with an external interpreter before meeting with the family is also helpful to ensure that the interpreter understands the major thrust of the session (Hadziabdic & Hjelm, 2013).

## Health Beliefs and Access

Families from different cultures have varying beliefs about health, disease, and treatment (Congress, 2004b, 2018; Congress & Lyons, 1992). Many medical anthropologists have contended that individuals' cultural beliefs influence the way they perceive the etiology of an illness, interpret the symptoms, and act on the symptoms (Cheng, 2001; Kleinman, 1980; Tseng, 2001). Individuals' and families' health beliefs, which include their perception of their susceptibility, the seriousness of the consequence of an illness, and the benefit of medical intervention, affect their readiness to use preventive health services and to seek actual help when a family member faces an ailment (Hsu & Gallinagh, 2001; Rosenstock, 1990). Families' reactions to an illness can affect the course, outcome, and level of incapacitation of an illness and the families' adjustment to it (Lescano, Brown, & Lima, 2009). For example, a delay in seeking treatment for HIV/AIDS because of stigma could lead to more devastating and lasting impact on the family through transmission of the illness to other family members.

There are differences between immigrant and refugee groups in how they understand mental illness (Bemak & Chung, 2000). Among many Asians, mental illness is seen as the result of malingering bad thoughts, lack of willpower, and personality weakness (Kleinman & Hall-Clifford, 2009; Narikiyo & Kameoka, 1992; Suan & Tyler, 1990; Sue & Morishima, 1982). Hence, self-control and solving one's own problems are culturally valued, and seeking help from mental health professionals is often delayed or avoided (Boey, 1999; Sue, Cheng, Saad, & Chu, 2012; Zhang, Snowden, & Sue, 1998). Given Asian Americans' tendency to somatize emotional distress, emphasize the physical expression of one's distressed state (Kleinman, 1980; Kung & Lu, 2008; Yang, Cho, & Kleinman, 2008; Zhang et al., 1998), or subscribe to the holistic mind–body–spirit conceptualization, they are likely to turn to physicians, herbalists, acupuncturists, fortune tellers, or ministers for help instead of mental health professionals (Kung, 2001; Kung & Lu, 2008; Sue, Nakamura, Chung, & Yee-Bradbury, 1994). Some Hispanics may rely on botanicas or spiritualists as the first and sometimes the only attempt to dealing with health or mental health problems (Congress, 2004a). The intense stigma attached to mental illness in some cultures also poses barriers to seeking mental health service (Kung, 2004; Kung & Lu, 2008). Some of these impediments to help seeking among Asians include the attribution of psychiatric problems to hereditary causes, interpreted as "genetic taints" and "bad seeds" (Kung, 2003; Pearson, 1993; Sue & Morishima, 1982). Because of the sociocentric nature of the Asian culture (Triandis, 1989), families are concerned about the loss of face and avoid reaching out for help beyond the immediate family, thus overburdening the family (Kung, 2001; Sue & Morishima, 1982; Sue, Sue, Neville, & Smith, 2020). Hispanics may seek to avoid the label of "loco" because of the stigma connected with this designation (Congress, 2018).

In the face of physical illness, many immigrants prefer to use healthcare methods other than traditional Western/European medical care involving diagnosis, pharmacology, x-rays, and surgery (Congress, 2018). The social worker who wishes to understand families must study their unique healthcare beliefs (Congress, 2013).

Immigrants, especially those who are undocumented, may have limited access to ongoing healthcare (Derose, Escarce, & Lurie, 2007; Goldman, Smith, & Sood, 2006). Denied access to regular healthcare and prevention, many immigrants are forced to rely only on emergency care. The Health Care Reform Act (NILC, April 2010) did not greatly expand healthcare coverage to immigrants as it denied healthcare to undocumented immigrants and limited healthcare even for those immigrants who had legal status to remain in the United States. Some states, however, have chosen to provide Medicaid and Children's Health Insurance Program (CHIP) benefits to children and pregnant women. Even those who are entitled to receive healthcare could be denied access to needed care due to the lack of bilingual service providers serving the monolingual citizens who are non-English speakers (Kung, 2004).

## Crisis Events

Many immigrants have experienced multiple traumas in their homelands, in transit, and in their current situation. Often, these traumas can affect the mental health of immigrants and refugees detrimentally (Pumariega, Rothe, & Pumariega, 2005).

Families can encounter developmental crises as well as "bolts from the blue" crises (Congress & Kung, 2013). Developmental crises may occur when a family moves from one life stage to another. Stages in the life cycle for culturally diverse families may be quite different from those for traditional Caucasian middle-class families. For example, for many culturally diverse families, the "launching children" stage may not occur at all, as single and even married children may continue to live in close proximity to the parents (Pew Research Center, 2016). This may be especially true for Hispanics and Asian American families (Snowden, 2007). If separation is forced, this developmental task might become traumatic.

Families also deal with unexpected events and crises in different ways. During the 9/11 attack on the World Trade Center, people from more than 80 countries of origin died (Lum, 2010). There has also been concern that many victims, especially those who were undocumented, were never acknowledged and their families often were not able to secure the assistance that others received. A family's reaction to crisis events is often related to its cultural values. The death or injury of the male head of household may be a major crisis for an immigrant family that highly values the role of the father as a provider. While rape is certainly a major crisis for any family, the rape of a teenage girl may be especially traumatic for a family that highly values virginity. Furthermore, corporal punishment which may be a rather common disciplinary approach in some immigrant families may cause them to be accused of child abuse and become involved with child protective agencies and the legal system. A referral to child protective services is perceived as a crisis to many families and especially so for those who interpret court-ordered counseling upon disciplining a child as an outrageous punishment—a crisis that evokes tremendous anger and shame (Waldman, 1999).

Different beliefs about the treatment of physical ailments may result in different approaches to remedy these problems. Some approaches may result in parents being accused of abuse or neglect. For example, methods such as coining or cupping administered by parents to help relieve the child's bodily pain may leave scars that may be misinterpreted as child abuse (Vitale & Prashad, 2017). Some parents may refuse to have their children take medication or have immunizations because of possible side effects or because of their health beliefs, and as a result, in some states they may be accused of child neglect (Parasidis & Opel, 2017). The consequences of such refusal for vaccination are seen as contributing to the recent measles epidemic in some communities.

## Holidays and Special Events, Contact With Cultural and Religious Institutions, Food, and Dress

Each family has particular holidays and special events. Some events mark transitions from one developmental stage to another, for example, a christening, a *bar mitzvah*, a wedding, or a funeral. It is important for the social worker to learn the cultural significance of these events, as they are indicative of what families see as major transition points in their lives. Some ethnic families have their own high holidays, such as the Lunar New Year, which is often considered as important to many Asian families as Thanksgiving to many native-born Americans, if not more so. It is worth encouraging immigrant families to celebrate their own important holidays to help them uphold their tradition and to strengthen their cultural identity. Special foods may be associated with the celebration of these holidays.

Contact with cultural institutions often provides support to an immigrant family. Family members may use cultural institutions differently. For example, a father may belong to a social club, the mother may attend a church where her native language is spoken, while the adolescent children may refuse to participate in either because they identify more with the American culture. Religious faith may provide much support to culturally diverse families, and the clinician will want to explore their contact with formal religious institutions. Some clansmen's associations are common among Asian Americans, often providing important support to immigrant families. For example, they provide significant financial support for new Chinese immigrants from Fuzhou in New York City (Kwong, 1997). The support among business owners is also found to be an important factor accounting for the successes among many Korean American businesses (Park, 1997). The social worker should be aware of these resources so as to help families tap into them. Most Asian clansmen's groups, however, do not provide assistance or support on psychosocial issues due to the lack of knowledge about mental health issues and fear of stigma by many of these immigrant groups.

## Oppression and Discrimination, Bias, and Racism

Many immigrants have experienced oppression in their native countries, which has led to their departure from their homelands and immigration to the United States. Some of them enter the United States as refugees because of the extent of social, political, physical, and emotional discrimination and threats they experienced in their countries of origin, while others apply for asylum status after their arrival here because they fear a return to their homelands.

Other immigrants, however, may have been the majority population in their home country and thus never experienced prejudice until their arrival in the United States. In the United States, they may be the victims of discrimination and racism based on linguistic, cultural, and racial differences. The current U.S.

policies on undocumented immigrants further serve to separate and discriminate this newcomer population from other Americans. Social workers should be sensitive to the needs of this vulnerable group within their immediate environments, such as bullying of these immigrant groups in school or discrimination in work settings. Support from family members and sympathetic community organizations for these groups should be rallied, and advocacy through consciousness raising can also be part of social workers' roles to prevent and reduce discrimination and oppression.

After review of previous versions of the culturagram and feedback about the instrument, this area was added in 2008 as an important aspect in understanding the immigrant families' experience.

## Values About Education and Work

All families have differing values about work and education, and culture is an important influence on such values. Social workers must explore what these values are in order to understand the family. Economic and social differences between the country of origin and the United States can affect immigrant families. For example, employment in a low-status position may be very denigrating to the male breadwinner in some cultures. It may be especially traumatic for the immigrant family when the father cannot find work or is engaged in work of a menial nature. This is often a result of the individual's professional qualifications and experience in their native land not being recognized in this country. Such a downward move in the socioeconomic hierarchy often induces additional stress and challenges for many immigrant families.

Sometimes a conflict in values arises due to competing desires of family members. An example of this occurred when an adolescent child was accepted with a full scholarship to a prestigious university miles away from home. While the family had always believed in the importance of education, the parents believed that the family needed to stay together and did not want to have their only child leave home, even to pursue education.

Another example of such value conflict occurs when latency-age children attend large schools far from their ethnic communities and begin to develop peer relationships apart from their families. For immigrant families that come from backgrounds in which education has been minimal and localized, and where young children were expected to work and care for younger siblings, the American school system with its focus on individual academic achievement and peer relationships may seem alien. Some cultures value education differently for different genders. In the past, many Hispanic girls dropped out of school because academic attainment for girls is not highly valued compared with boys, but this may be changing as more Latinos in general continue in school (Jackson, 2013; Krogstad, 2016). Nonetheless, Latino girls still have major responsibilities in taking care of the household and younger siblings. They often find little or no time left to attend to their academic demands after school and thus have a harder time keeping up with academic work, and may eventually drop out from school.

Furthermore, immigrant children who have experienced a history of individual or family oppression may feel very isolated and lonely in their new academic environments, which is made worse when actual bullying by peers and discrimination by insensitive school personnel take place.

## Values About Family Structure—Power, Hierarchy, Rules, Subsystems, and Boundaries

Each family has its unique structure, beliefs about power relationships, rules, boundaries within and outside the family, and significance of certain familial relationships. The clinician should explore the individual family's characteristics and also needs to understand them in the context of the family's cultural background. Some families may have particular beliefs about male–female relationships, especially within marriage. Families that promote a male-dominant hierarchical family structure may encounter challenges in American society with its stated preference for more egalitarian gender relationships. This may result in conflict and an increase in domestic violence among minority families (Erez & Globokar, 2009). Traditionally gendered roles within the family also exert significant impact on the family, especially when circumstances change after migration. For example, in some cultures, women are expected to take care of internal familial affairs, including household chores and child care, while men are expected to work outside and be income earners. However, changes in the socioeconomic status of the family after migration may necessitate both spouses to work outside of the home. If the role of domestic caretaker continues to be rigidly assigned only to women, they may become overburdened. In situations in which the woman is able to find a job while the man is unemployed and the family lacks flexibility in their role adaptation, conflict, blame, and burden in the family may become so enormous that it may threaten the survival of the family unit.

Not only is gender hierarchy much affected by cultural norms, so is generational hierarchy. More traditional cultures tend to ascribe much higher authority and respect to the older generation, and in some cultures, parental authority can be rather absolute (Tamura & Lau, 1992). Clinicians should recognize such inherent cultural differences, and sometimes mediate between the generations. They have to navigate cautiously: They should show respect to the family's culture on the one hand, but tactfully facilitate communication across the generations on the other hand, in order to ease the tension and conflict. Through careful mediation, it is hoped that views from both sides can be heard and considered in the final decision-making. However, sometimes the social worker may have to accept that some cultures do dictate that senior members have the ultimate power in decision-making after the views of the younger generation are articulated, unless it is a violation of the basic human rights of the latter.

Finally, families from different cultures may place varying emphasis on family subsystems. In Western culture, the spousal subsystem is considered the bedrock of the family (Minuchin, 1974). In some cultures, though, the primary unit is the parental subsystem, emphasizing the co-parenting role between the spouses (Connell, 2010). In some cultures, such as the traditional Chinese culture, the parent–child subsystem (both the father–son and mother–son dyads) and even the relationship among brothers are considered more important than the spousal relationship (Tamura & Lau, 1992). Further, the parental subsystem could also be much more inclusive than only the biological parents—for example, not only are grandparents, aunts, and uncles important partners in the parental subsystem, but the godparents' role could also be very significant in Hispanic families (McGoldrick, Giordano, & Garcia-Preto, 2005). Clinicians should be conscious of cultural values and practices so as not to leave out important system players who could be valuable resources to the family.

Whether the boundary within a family or within a subsystem is considered appropriate or overly diffuse is also very cultural (Connell, 2010). For example, in some Asian cultures, since the future care of the aging mother is dependent on the son, and the mother–son bond is usually close, a mother is often seen as being intrusive in the son's marital relationship and is sometimes domineering toward the daughter-in-law (Berg & Jaya, 1993). For some Asian families, to have the child to sleep with the parents till the age of 8 or 10 is considered a very normal practice, and it does not necessarily indicate marital dysfunction or enmeshment between parent and child (Berg & Jaya, 1993). Social workers have to avoid judgmental attitudes toward families who have different cultural values from their own.

As stated previously, learning about the cultural norms and values of individuals and families and their unique immigration experiences is only the first step. The clinician also needs to consider other aspects of an individual's identity such as race, ethnicity, religion, nationality, immigration status, ability/disability, socioeconomic status, health status, education, occupation, and sexual orientation that affect how the individual self identifies. Each person is a member of many communities and many cultures. In this sense, each of us is "multicultural." It is important to note that these social categories carry with them varying levels of power, or lack thereof. Such dimensions further intersect and overlap with each other, and with the culture and ethnic groups to which individuals belong. For individuals who fall into multiple minority statuses, oppression is further aggregated (Crenshaw, 1989; Dill & Zinn, 1994). To expand our understanding, an intersectional design tool (IDT) was developed and is presented here in Figure 1.2.

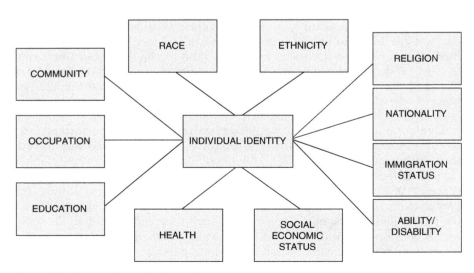

Figure 1.2 *Intersectional design tool.*

*Source:* Elaine P. Congress (2017).

# 1. USING THE CULTURAGRAM AND AN INTERSECTIONAL APPROACH 15

In the two case vignettes that follow both the culturagram and the IDT will be used to promote greater understanding of clients and families from diverse backgrounds.

## CASE VIGNETTES

Mrs. Maria Sanchez, 32 years old, contacted a family service agency in her community because she was having increasing conflicts with her 12-year-old son, José, who had begun to cut school and stay out late at night. She also reported that she had a 9-year-old daughter, Maritza, who was "an angel." Maritza was very quiet, never wanted to socialize with other children, and instead preferred to stay at home with her mother helping her with household chores. Maria indicated the source of much conflict was that José believed he did not have to respect Manuel, Maria's current partner, as the latter was not his real father. José complained that his mother and stepfather were "dumb" because they did not speak English. José felt it was very important to learn English as soon as possible since several students at school had made fun of his accent. He felt that his parents did not understand how difficult his school experience was as he believed that teachers favored lighter-skinned Latinos. José had much darker skin than his mother, his mother's partner, or his half-sister Maritza. The recent holidays had been especially difficult as José had disappeared during the New Year's weekend. Mrs. Sanchez was Catholic but did not go to church because she could not understand in the masses which were in English.

At 20, Maria had moved to the United States from Puerto Rico with her first husband José Sr. The two were very poor in Puerto Rico and had heard there were better job opportunities here. When José Jr. was an infant, José Sr. had made a visit back to Puerto Rico and never returned. Shortly afterward, Maria met Manuel, who had come to New York from Guatemala. After she became pregnant with Maritza, they began to live together. Manuel indicated that he was very fearful of returning to Guatemala, as several people in his village had been killed in political conflicts. Because Manuel was undocumented, he had been able to find only occasional day work. He was embarrassed that Maria had been forced to apply for the government's Supplemental Nutritional Assistance Program (SNAP). Maria received minimum wages as a home care worker. She was very close to her mother, Gladys, who had come to live with the family 9 years ago. Gladys had urged Maria to seek help from a spiritualist to help her with her family problems before she went to the neighborhood social work agency to ask for help. Manuel has no relatives in New York City, but he has several friends at the social club in his neighborhood.

Not only does the culturagram and IDT facilitate the social worker in assessing families from different cultural backgrounds, they also give directions for appropriate interventions. After completing the culturagram (see Figure 1.1) and IDT (see Figure 1.2), the social worker was better able to understand the Sanchez family, assess their needs, and begin to plan for treatment (see Figure 1.3). She noted that Manuel's undocumented status was a source of continual stress in this family. She referred Manuel to a free legal service that provided help for undocumented persons to secure legal status. She also explored their religious affiliation and found that although the family subscribed to the Catholic faith, they had not attended church since they came to this country, because they could not find a church with Spanish-speaking masses. The worker helped the family find a Catholic church in the neighborhood that has a weekly mass in Spanish and a large proportion of Hispanic parishioners. The church later became a support network for the family as Maria and Maritza became involved with the women's and children's groups at the church.

The social worker recognized some kind of communication problem across the generations. While José and Maritza are bilingual, they often speak English

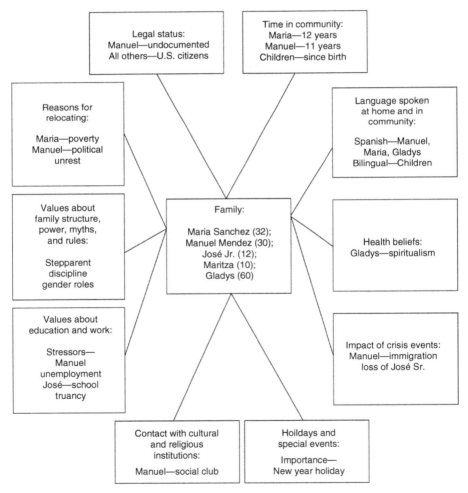

Figure 1.3 *Culturagram and IDT applied to the Sanchez's case example.*

Note: The previous version of the culturagram appeared in Congress (2008a) and the IDT was first presented at CSWE APM (2017).

at home, which for the most part Maria and Manuel do not understand. The adults communicated with each other and the children in Spanish. Maria and Manuel sometimes wanted to practice their English with the children, but the latter, especially José, were rather impatient with their parents' broken English. In any case, communication was limited to basic information exchange and rule setting. The social worker encouraged the couple to study English in a free English as a secondary language (ESL) adult education program in their neighborhood. The bilingual worker, however, was careful to speak in Spanish when seeing the couple and especially during family sessions so as to subtly convey respect for the language to the children. When she had individual sessions with the children, she used English since they were better able to express themselves.

Due to language barriers, José occasionally had to act as interpreter on behalf of the family, for instance, when the family had to deal with the Social Security department or with his grandmother's medical doctors during a serious illness that involved hospitalization. José was sometimes resentful toward these familial obligations as it took away time from being with his peers. He also felt that all his mother and stepfather wanted was to ask him to help out in the family and to impose rules on him without ever caring about his needs. The worker reframed his responsibility for the family as having an honorable task as cultural broker, but recognized his need for appropriate autonomy. While the worker worked toward the therapeutic goal of empowering the parents, especially the mother, to assert control over José, she also acted as a mediator to help the parents understand José's need to gain more age-appropriate independence.

Within the school, José reported that he had often been the subject of bias and discrimination. The clinician working with this family might want to contact the school to learn more about their policies and programs in helping students from different cultural backgrounds.

Maritza's social withdrawal was also explored. It was found that Maritza wanted to stay home to do the household chores as this was expected of her as a girl. She noted that her family did not think it appropriate that men in the family (her father Manuel and her brother José) help out with household chores. She wished to spare her mother from additional chores after a hard day's work outside, and to lighten her grandmother's load because of her frail health. As a result, she sacrificed her playtime with peers and stayed home to take care of the house. The social worker tactfully invited Manuel to be more involved in domestic duties on days that he did not have to work and reframed it as his way of showing his love for the family through such sacrifice. Maritza was also encouraged to attend activities at the church and after-school programs so as to socialize more with her peers.

Being a racial minority, coming from lower socioeconomic background and being immigrants to the United States, Maria's family is in a position of having very little power, and even experiences oppression (e.g., José being bullied by his peers). In addition to the social worker's role of providing counseling in promoting better understanding and communication within the family, and helping each member to meet their own needs, it was important to help them to navigate around the systems in order to gain access to needed resources. For this family, it included assistance to Manuel in applying for legal status, locating free adult

ESL classes for Maria and Manuel, and finding a Spanish-speaking church for the family.

The following is another case vignette about an immigrant family.

> Ping is a 44-year-old Chinese woman who was referred for counseling at a family service center in Chinatown by the psychiatrist who was treating her husband for his mental illness. At the intake interview, she revealed to the social worker that she suffered from nervousness, frequent palpitations of the heart, difficulty breathing, and insomnia as she was faced with her husband's frequent temper tantrums. She often felt "caught in the middle" in her relationships with her in-laws over the care of her husband and her two children aged 18 and 16.
>
> Ping came from a poor rural area in southern China. She immigrated to the United States 20 years ago as part of an arranged marriage to a man whose family had successfully immigrated to this country. The marriage was an explicit arrangement in which the groom's family found a wife for a son with mental health issues, and the bride's family could gain American citizenship. The client's motive for marrying was a filial willingness to better her family's prospects.
>
> The client worked in restaurants in Chinatown when she first came to the United States but eventually became fully preoccupied with the care of her husband and their two children. The husband has been diagnosed with schizophrenia, and three years ago contracted HIV through prostitutes. The couple has not been sleeping together for over 10 years, and the client did not react strongly to this. It was when the husband began a regimen of anti-viral drug treatment for his HIV that his mental health seriously deteriorated. The erratic and paranoid behavior that followed affected the son who became prone to violent outbursts. Neither the husband nor the son admitted to any mental health or emotional problems, and the extended family was opposed to the client's efforts to seek help outside of the traditional and familial channels. Ping persisted, however, and eventually was able to gain access to a range of services including psychiatric care for her husband, and counseling help for herself. The family was very poor as Ping and her children receive public assistance and her husband Supplemental Security Income (SSI). Since the amount of public assistance she received was very low, she occasionally supplemented her income by day work in a Chinese restaurant where she knew the owner.
>
> By the time the client arrived at the agency, there had been an amelioration of her husband's symptoms, though caring for him still left her drained. The young daughter lived separately with her paternal grandparents and had been doing reasonably well. The client's major concern from the outset was the fear that her son would "get into trouble with the police." Because of his developmental disability, the son was receiving vocational training with other individuals with mental or physical disabilities, whom he found threatening. Ping feared that he would succumb to bad influences if she could not find him a suitable employment. He also did some "volunteer work"

in a small grocery store owned by one of Ping's friends and had been active in a martial arts group. Over the course of several sessions, it gradually became clear to the social worker that the client sometimes threatened to withhold affection from her son, then left the apartment and stayed with her in-laws and her daughter. This was her way of obtaining compliance and good behavior from the son. The son, in response, however, became more insistent and even violent in an effort to secure his mother's attention.

Another major issue was that Ping is so preoccupied with her care-giving roles that she rarely thought about her own needs and self-care. It was, however, also a reality that she played a very vital role in her family, which was sustained by the social and cultural presuppositions of her marriage. One of the few areas where the client found time for herself was in her life of faith. She was a Buddhist and spent several hours in the temple each Sunday, where some kind of small group sharing and support was often available. The client's cultural understanding of "help-seeking" seemed to have caused her to look up to the helping professionals as the experts, thereby relinquishing her own initiative and input in the counseling process. Due to the fragmentation of services, the need to respond to many agencies on behalf of her family was itself a significant stressor for Ping, especially with her limited English proficiency.

Using the culturagram and IDT, the worker was able to gain a more comprehensive understanding of Ping and her family's situation. First, through exploration of the reason for relocation, it was clear that at the outset the client agreed to enter into a very difficult situation with an arranged marriage to a person with mental illness. Her obligation to stay in the marriage to facilitate her family of origin to migrate to the United States could be a pressure in addition to the usual migration stress experienced by new immigrants. The worker came to an appreciation of the importance of the cultural value of filial piety to the client and her obligation to her family of origin as well as her family of procreation. The worker understood and respected the centrality of family in the Chinese culture. However, the worker was able to help the client to strike a balance in taking care of herself and her family by highlighting the fact that if she were not in a state of well-being, she was in no shape to perform her familial roles adequately. In this reframing, the worker started where the client was, fully accepting her cultural obligation to her family.

Although Ping had migrated to the United States two decades ago, because of her language barrier her contact and support in the community were very limited. The worker took note of the client's Buddhist faith and the support she obtained from it spiritually and through social support at the temple. The client was encouraged to maintain regular visits there. Due to the limited social support the client had, the worker also referred her to a support group at the counseling agency for relatives of patients with a mental illness. The worker also encouraged Ping to enroll in ESL adult classes to improve her English so as to increase her mobility in the city beyond the Chinese community. It should be noted here that many entitlement agencies, health, mental health, and social services are in extreme shortage of bilingual staff to provide services to minorities with limited or no English proficiency. This is indeed discrimination. Various agencies and organizations were involved with the family, including Social Security, Medicaid and mental healthcare for her husband, vocational training and counseling for her son, individual and group counseling for the client, and an Asian community center with adult education programs of ESL for the client. The worker had to do a lot of advocacy and case management functions on behalf of the client and her family in order to attain the needed services. Ping's family's situation was similar to that of Maria in that, given the family's racial minority status, lower socioeconomic background, immigrant status, and the disability of Ping's husband and son, the family had little power to obtain adequate resources to sustain their well-being. Thus, the social worker's assistance to navigate the systems and to advocate on their behalf to attain needed services could not be overstated.

In the helping process, the worker also realized the deferential stance that Ping often took in relating to him. From an empowerment and strengths-based approach he emphasized the fact that the client knew herself and her family best and thus elicited her input in the counseling process. Conscientious effort was made by the worker to formulate the treatment goals together with Ping throughout. She gradually responded and became more active in the helping process. The client was indeed a very strong and resilient person; her strengths were often reflected back to her by the worker.

As Ping indicated, her family had a lot of resistance in seeking external help for her husband's mental health and health problems. Delayed help-seeking especially for mental health issues is a rather common phenomenon among Asian Americans since problems are expected to be resolved within the family. The reluctance is partly due to the strong stigma attached to mental illness in many Asian cultures. It was fortunate that the client persisted in her effort to seek external help and eventually was hooked up with various services through the help of the worker. The worker complimented the client's willingness to seek help, and assured her that sharing difficulties with the worker ("an outsider") about her family was an active and positive way to help herself and her family instead of a betrayal to her family. Continual family psychoeducation about the nature of mental illness and its course was necessary to help the family to stay in treatment and ameliorate the shame and stigma attached to mental illness.

It is important to note that within the Chinese culture, the parenting role is given greater importance compared to the spousal role. Hence, when Ping chose to focus her concern on her children instead of her husband, it was important that the worker went along with it. Also, the extended family was of great importance in the Chinese culture, and given the circumstance, the client did not want to alienate this source of support. The worker suggested to the client some strategic ways to interact with the son so as to reduce the negative vicious cycle of mutual escalation. He also helped the client to ameliorate the frequent conflicts with her in-laws.

In the Chinese culture, work is given very high value (Yang et al., 2014). Thus, to be able to find some kind of job for Ping's son is important to her and her family. The worker also noted the informal resources the client was able to rally for the son to engage him in productive activities. The volunteer opportunity at the local grocery store and the martial arts group are important resources available in the Chinese community from which the son can benefit.

The preceding discussions help to clarify how the culturagram and IDT can be used not only to assess the family, but also to help plan pertinent interventions. The culturagram has been seen as an essential tool in helping social workers provide more effective services with families from many different cultures. It enables the practitioner to gain a more longitudinal understanding of immigrant families. As Drachman (1992) stresses, in working with immigrants, it is important to understand not only their current situation but also what they experienced in their homelands and in transit. The culturagram helps the worker to understand the multiple physical and emotional traumas immigrants may have encountered in their countries of origin, their transit to the United States, and in their current environment and thus plan appropriate interventions. The introduction of an intersectional perspective also helps the social worker to understand the multiple groupings that an individual or a family may belong to and how such groups, when they intersect, may affect clients' self-identity and power within the social structure, and what may be necessary to ensure that they have adequate resources to attain and sustain their well-being.

## REFERENCES

Addams, J. (1911). *Twenty years at Hull-House*. New York, NY: Macmillan.

Batalova, J. B. J., & Alperin, E. (2018, August 1). Immigrants in the U.S. states with the fastest-growing foreign-born populations. Retrieved from https://www.migrationpolicy.org/article/immigrants-us-states-fastest-growing-foreign-born-populations

Bemak, F. P., & Chung, R. C. (2000). Psychological intervention with immigrants and refugees. In J. F. Aponte & J. Wohl (Eds.), *Psychological intervention and cultural diversity* (2nd ed., pp. 200–213). Needham Heights, MA: Allyn & Bacon.

Berg, I. K., & Jaya, A. (1993). Different and same: Family therapy with Asian-American families. *Journal of Marital and Family Therapy, 19,* 31–38. doi:10.1111/j.1752-0606.1993.tb00963.x

Boey, K. W. (1999). Help-seeking preference of college students in urban China after the implementation of the "open-door" policy. *International Journal of Social Psychiatry, 45*(2), 104–116. doi:10.1177/002076409904500203

Brownell, P. (1997). The application of the culturagram in cross-cultural practice with elder abuse victims. *Journal of Elder Abuse and Neglect, 9*(2), 19–33. doi:10.1300/J084v09n02_03

Brownell, P., & Congress, E. (1998). Application of the culturagram to assess and empower culturally and ethnically diverse battered women. In A. Roberts (Ed.), *Battered women and their families: Intervention and treatment strategies* (pp. 387–404). New York, NY: Springer Publishing Company.

Brownell, P., & Fenly, R. C. (2008). Older adult immigrants in the United States: Issues and services. In F. Chang-Muy & E. Congress (Eds.), *Social work with immigrants and refugees: Legal issues, clinical skills, and advocacy* (pp. 277–307). New York, NY: Springer Publishing Company.

Cheng, A. T. A. (2001). Case definition and culture: Are people all the same? *British Journal of Psychiatry, 179,* 1–3. doi:10.1192/bjp.179.1.1

Congress, E. (1997). Using the *culturagram* to assess and empower cultural diverse families. In E. Congress (Ed.), *Multicultural perspectives in working with families* (pp. 3–16). New York, NY: Springer Publishing Company.

Congress, E. (2002). Using *culturagrams* with culturally diverse families. In A. Roberts & G. Greene (Eds.), *Social work desk reference* (pp. 57–61). New York, NY: Oxford University Press.

Congress, E. (2004a). Cultural and ethnic issues in working with culturally diverse patients and their families: Use of the *culturagram* to promote cultural competency in health care settings. *Social Work in Health Care, 39*(3/4), 249–262. doi:10.1300/J010v39n03_03

Congress, E. (2004b). Crisis intervention and diversity: Emphasis on a Mexican immigrant family's acculturation conflicts. In R. Dorfman, P. Meyer, & M. Morgan (Eds.), *Paradigms of clinical social work* (Vol. 3, Emphasis on diversity, pp. 125–144). New York, NY: Brunner-Routledge.

Congress, E. (2008a). Using the culturagram with culturally diverse families. In A. Roberts & G. Greene (Eds.), *Social work desk reference* (2nd ed., pp. 57–61). New York, NY: Oxford University Press.

Congress, E. (2008b). The *culturagram*. In A. Roberts & G. Greene (Eds.), *Social work desk reference* (2nd ed., pp. 57–61). New York, NY: Oxford University Press.

Congress, E. (2013). Immigrants and health care. In Public Health Social Work Section of the American Public Health Association (Ed.), *Handbook for public health social work* (103–121). New York, NY: Springer Publishing Company.

Congress, E. (2018) Immigrant health. In J. Heyman & E. Congress (Eds.), *Health and social work: Practice, policy, and* research. New York, NY: Springer Publishing Company.

Congress, E. & Ellington, L. (2018). Using the culturagram with indigenous people: A tool for accessing indigenous culture and migraton, IACCP conference, July 4, Guelph, Canada.

Congress, E. P., & Kung, W. W. (2013). Using the culturagram to access and empower culturally diverse families. In E. P. Congress & M. Gonzales (Eds.), *Multicultural perspectives in working with families* (3rd ed., pp. 1–20). New York, NY: Springer Publishing Company.

Congress, E., & Lyons, B. (1992). Cultural differences in health beliefs: Implications for social work practice in health care settings. *Journal of Social Work Practice in Health Care, 17*(3), 81–96. doi:10.1300/J010v17n03_06

Connell, C. (2010) Multicultural perspective and considerations within structural family therapy: The premises of structure, subsystem and boundaries. *Journal of Marriage and Family, 72*, 420–439. doi:10.1111/j.1741-3737.2010.00711.x

Crenshaw, K. (1989). Demarginalizing the intersection of race and sex: A Black feminist critique of antidiscrimination doctrine, feminist theory and antiracist politics. *University of Chicago Legal Forum, 1989*, 139–167.

Derose, K. P., Escarce, J. J., & Lurie, N. (2007). Immigrants and health care: Source of vulnerability. *Health Affairs, 26*(5), 1258–1268. doi:10.1377/hlthaff.26.5.1258

Dill, B. T., & Zinn, M. B. (Eds.). (1994). *Women of color in U.S. society*. Philadelphia, PA: Temple University Press.

Drachman, D. (1992). A stage of migration framework for service to immigrant populations. *Social Work, 37*, 68–72.

Ellington, L. & Roy, P. (2018). Le culturagramme: outil d'exploration culturelle et migratoire pour mieux comprendre les realites vecues par la clientele autochotone en travail social. Retrieved from http://revueintervention.org/numeros-en-ligne/148/le-culturagramme-outil-dexploration-culturelle-et-migratoire-pour-mieux

Erez, E. & Globokar, J. (2009). Compounding vulnerabilities: The impact of immigration status and circumstances on battered immigrant women. *Sociology of Crime, Law & Deviance, 30*, 129–145. doi:10.1108/S1521-6136(2009)0000013011

Frey, W. (2014). *Diversity explosion: How new racial demographics are remaking America*. Washington, DC: Brookings Institution Press.

Goldman, D. P., Smith, J. P., & Sood, N. (2006). Immigrants and the cost of medical care. *Health Affairs, 25*(6), 1700–1711. doi:10.1377/hlthaff.25.6.1700

Hadziabdic, E., & Hjelm, K. (2013). Working with interpreters; Practical advice for use of an interpreter in health care. *International Journal of Evidence Based Health Care, 11*(1), 1744–1609. doi:10.1111/1744-1609.12005

Hartman, A., & Laird, J. (1983). *Family-oriented social work practice*. New York, NY: Free Press.

Hendricks, C. O. (2013). The multicultural triangle of the child, family, and school: Culturally competent approaches. In E. Congress & M. Gonzalez (Eds.), *Multicultural perspectives in working with families* (3rd ed., pp. 57–73). New York, NY: Springer Publishing Company.

HispanicAd. (2014). Hispanic millenniums: Living at home, delaying marriage, and focusing on college (INSIGHT). HispanicAd.com.

Hong, G. K. (1989). Application of cultural and environmental issues in family therapy with immigrant Chinese Americans. *Journal of Strategic and Systemic Therapies*, 8(bonus), 14–21. doi:10.1521/jsst.1989.8.bonus.14

Hsu, H. Y., & Gallinagh, R. (2001). The relationships between health beliefs and utilization of free health examinations in older people living in a community setting in Taiwan. *Journal of Advanced Nursing*, 35(6), 864–873. doi:10.1046/j.1365-2648.2001.01924.x

Irving, H. H., Benjamin, M., & Tsang, A. K. T. (1999). Hong Kong satellite children in Canada: An exploratory study of their experience. *Hong Kong Journal of Social Work*, 33(1–2), 1–21. doi:10.1142/S0219246299000029

Jackson, M. (2013). Fact sheet: The states of Latinas in the United States. Retrieved from https://www.americanprogress.org/issues/race/reports/2013/11/07/79167/fact-sheet-the-state-of-latinas-in-the-united-states/

Kleinman, A. M. (1980). *Patients and healers in the context of culture*. Berkeley, CA: University of California Press.

Kleinman, A., & Hall-Clifford, R. (2009). Stigma: A social, cultural and moral process. *Journal of Epidemiology and Community Health*, 63(6), 418–419. doi:10.1136/jech.2008.084277

Krogstad, J. (2016). 5 facts about Latinos and education. Retrieved from https://www.pewresearch.org/fact-tank/2016/07/28/5-facts-about-latinos-and-education/

Kung, W. W. (2001). Consideration of cultural factors in working with Chinese American families with a mentally ill patient. *Families in Society: The Journal of Contemporary Human Services*, 82(1), 97–107. doi:10.1606/1044-3894.221

Kung, W. W. (2003). The illness, stigma, culture, or immigration? Burdens on Chinese American caregivers of patients with schizophrenia. *Families in Society: The Journal of Contemporary Human Services*, 84, 547–557. doi:10.1606/1044-3894.140

Kung, W. W. (2004). Cultural and practical barriers to seeking mental health treatment for Chinese Americans. *Journal of Community Psychology*, 32(1), 27–43. doi:10.1002/jcop.10077

Kung, W. W. & Lu, P.-C. (2008). How symptom manifestations affect help seeking for mental health problems among Chinese Americans. *Journal of Nervous and Mental Disease*, 196(1), 45–54. doi:10.1097/NMD.0b013e31815fa4f9

Kwong, P. (1997). Manufacturing ethnicity. *Critique of Anthropology*, 17(4), 365–387. doi:10.1177/0308275X9701700404

Kwong, P. (2002). Forbidden workers and the U.S. labor movement: Fuzhounese in New York City. *Critical Asian Studies*, 34(1), 69–88. doi:10.1080/146727102760166608

Lescano, C., Brown, L., & Lima, L. (2009). Cultural factors and family-based HIV prevention intervention for Latino youth. *Journal of Pediatric Psychology* 34(10), 1041–1052. doi:10.1093/jpepsy/jsn146

Liao, M. S. (2006). Domestic violence among Asian Indian immigrant women: Risk factors, acculturation, and intervention. *Women and Therapy*, 29(1–2), 23–39. doi:10.1300/J015v29n01_02

Loiselle-Leonard, M. (2001). Arranged marriage, dowry and migration: A risky combination for Hindu women. *Canadian Social Work Review*, 18(2), 305–319.

Lum, D. (2010). *Culturally competent practice: A framework for understanding diverse groups and justice issues [Paperback]* (5th ed.). Belmont, CA: Brooks-Cole-Thomson.

McGoldrick, M., Gerson, J., & Petry, S. (2008). *Genograms: Assessment and intervention*. New York, NY: W. W. Norton.

McGoldrick, M., Giordano, J., & Garcia-Preto, N. (Eds.). (2005). *Ethnicity and family therapy* (3rd ed.). New York, NY: Guilford Press.

Minuchin, S. (1974). *Families and family therapy*. Cambridge, MA: Harvard University Press.

Narikiyo, T., & Kameoka, V. (1992). Attributions of mental illness and judgments about help seeking among Japanese-American and White American students. *Journal of Counseling Psychology, 39*(3), 363–369. doi:10.1037/0022-0167.39.3.363

National Association of Social Workers. (2018). *Code of ethics*. Washington, DC: NASW Press.

New York City Mayor's Office of Immigrant Affairs. (2018). State of our immigrant city. Retrieved from https://www1.nyc.gov/site/immigrants/about/press-releases/03-19-2018.page

New York City Department of City Planning. (2017). *Top language spoken at home: Universe population 5 years and over*. 2011–2015 American Community Survey Public Use Microdata 5-Year Sample New York City and Boroughs.

Parasidis, E., & Opel, D. J. (2017). Parental refusal of childhood vaccines and medical neglect laws. *American Journal of Public Health, 107*, 68–71. doi:10.2105/AJPH.2016.303500

Park, K. (1997). *The Korean American dream: Immigrants and small business in New York City*. Ithaca, NY: Cornell University Press.

Patel, S. G., Clarke, A. V., Eltareb, F., Macciomei, E. E., & Wickham, R. E. (2016). Newcomer immigrant adolescents: A mixed-methods examination of family stressors and school outcomes. *School Psychology Quarterly, 31*(2), 163–180. doi:10.1037/spq0000140

Pearson, V. (1993). Families in China: An undervalued resource for mental health. *Journal of Family Therapy, 15*, 163–185. doi:10.1111/j.1467-6427.1993.00752.x

Pumariega, A. J., Rothe, E., & Pumariega, J. B. (2005). Mental health of immigrants and refugees. *Community Mental Health Journal, 41*(5), 581–597. doi:10.1007/s10597-005-6363-1

Rosenstock, I. M. (1990). The health belief model: Explaining health behavior through expectancies. In K. Glanz & F. M. Lewis (Eds.), *Health behavior and health education: Theory, research, and practice* (pp. 39–62). San Francisco, CA: Jossey-Bass.

Sciarra, D. T. (1999). Intrafamilial separations in the immigrant family: Implications for cross-cultural counseling. *Journal of Multicultural Counseling and Development, 27*, 31–41. doi:10.1002/j.2161-1912.1999.tb00210.x

Snowden, L. (2007). Explaining mental health treatment disparities: Ethnic and cultural differences in family involvement. *Culture, Medicine, and Psychiatry: New York, 31*(3), 389–402. doi:10.1007/s11013-007-9057-z

Suan, L. V., & Tyler, J. D. (1990). Mental health values and preference for mental health resources of Japanese-American and Caucasian-American students. *Professional Psychology: Research & Practice, 21*(4), 291–296. doi:10.1037/0735-7028.21.4.291

Sue, S., Cheng, J. K. Y., Saad, C. S., & Chu, J. P. (2012). Asian American mental health: A call to action. *American Psychologist, 67*(7), 532–544. doi:10.1037/a0028900

Sue, S., & Morishima, J. K. (1982). *The mental health of Asian Americans*. San Francisco, CA: Jossey-Bass Publishers.

Sue, S., Nakamura, C. Y., Chung, R. C.-Y., & Yee-Bradbury, C. (1994). Mental health research on Asian Americans. *Journal of Community Psychology, 22*, 61–67. doi:10.1002/1520-6629(199404)22:2<61::AID-JCOP2290220203>3.0.CO;2-T

Sue, D. W., Sue, D., Neville, H. A., & Smith, L. (2020). *Counseling the culturally different: Theory and practice*. New York, NY: Wiley.

Tamura, T., & Lau, A. (1992). Connectedness versus separateness: Applicability of family therapy to Japanese families. *Family Process, 31*(4), 319–340. doi:10.1111/j.1545-5300.1992.00319.x

Triandis, H. C. (1989). The self and social behavior in differing cultural contexts. *Psychological Review, 96*, 508–520. doi:10.1037/0033-295X.96.3.506

Tseng, W.-S. (2001). *Handbook of cultural psychiatry*. San Diego, CA: Academic Press.

US Census Bureau. (2015). Census Bureau reports at least 350 languages Spoken in U.S. homes. Retrieved from https://www.census.gov/newsroom/press-releases/2015/cb15-185.html

Violence Against Women Act of 2019, H.R. 1585, 116th Cong. (2019).

Vitale, S., & Prashad, T. (2017). Cultural awareness: Coining and cupping. *International Archives Nursing Health Care, 3*, 080. doi:10.23937/2469-5823/1510080

Waldman, F. (1999). Violence or discipline? Working with multicultural court-ordered clients. *Journal of Marital and Family Therapy, 25*, 503–516. doi:10.1111/j.1752-0606.1999.tb00265.x

Webb, N. (1996). *Social work practice with children*. New York, NY: Guilford Press.

Yang, L. H., Chen, F. P., Sia, K. J., Lam, J., Lam, K., Ngo, H., . . . Good, B. (2014). "What matters most:" A cultural mechanism moderating structural vulnerability and moral experience of mental illness stigma. *Social Science & Medicine, 103*, 84–93. doi:10.1016/j.socscimed.2013.09.009

Yang, L. H., Cho, S. H., & Kleinman, A. (2008). Stigma of mental illness. Retrieved from https://www.sciencedirect.com/science/article/pii/B9780123739605000472?via=ihub

Zhang, A. Y., Snowden, L. R., & Sue, S. (1998). Differences between Asian and White Americans' help seeking and utilization patterns in the Los Angeles area. *Journal of Community Psychology, 26*(4), 317–326. doi:10.1002/(SICI)1520-6629(199807)26:4<317::AID-JCOP2>3.0.CO;2-Q

# 2

# Practice With Multiracial Individuals and Families

JENNIE PARK-TAYLOR, ALEA HOLMAN, AND STEVEN CARTER

## INTRODUCTION

Multiracial individuals are at the forefront of the country's significant demographic changes, yet, despite robust growth over the past several decades, the multiracial population has only recently been fully acknowledged by the U.S. Census Bureau and thus only officially accounted for in recent years. Prior to 2000, individuals responding to the U.S. Census surveys were forced to identify with only one discrete racial group, which yielded population estimates that essentially hid the multiracial population. The option to select more than one race only started in the year 2000, and this change resulted in a significant increased accounting of the multiracial population (Parker, Horowitz, Morin, & Lopez, 2015). In 2013, the U.S. Census Bureau found that 9 million Americans self-identified with two or more races, up by 32%, since the last census. Furthermore, between the years of 2000 and 2010, the multiracial Asian and White populations increased by 87% and the multiracial Black and White populations more than doubled. It is estimated that by 2060, the projected number of individuals in the United States who identify as multiracial is expected to reach 26 million from 9.6 million now, an approximate 171% increase, which is more than any other racial group (U.S. Census Bureau, 2014). Although the recent rise in the multiracial population is an outcome of the change in the census survey, it is also the direct result of changes made to anti-miscegenation laws that legally enforced racial segregation at the level of marriage and intimate relationships.

On July 1 at 2 a.m., in 1958, less than a century after the Emancipation Proclamation that ended slavery, a sheriff entered the home of Mildred and Richard Loving, a married interracial couple, and forced them out of their beds and into jail (History.com Editors, 2017). Richard, who was a White man, and Mildred, who was a Black woman, were both tried and convicted of violating the state's interracial marriage laws. They were given the option to spend a year in prison or leave the state of Virginia for 25 years. This encouraged the couple to move to Washington, D.C., where their marriage was legal. However, upon visiting relatives in another state 5 years later, they were again arrested for traveling together as an interracial couple. After this incident, Mildred pursued legal action with the help of the American Civil Liberties Union (ACLU) resulting in the landmark 1967 case *Loving vs. Virginia*. The U.S. Supreme Court ruled against the "anti-miscegenation" statute, finding it unconstitutional under the 14th Amendment ultimately ending state laws banning interracial marriage. Since the *Loving vs. Virginia* case, interracial marriages increased from 150,000 in 1960 to over a million in 1990. In terms of current estimates of interracial marriages, nearly 75% were between Whites and non-Blacks, with the remaining percentage of interracial marriages between Blacks and Whites (U.S. Census Bureau, 2014).

Despite the elimination of some legal barriers to interracial relationships, interracial couples continue to experience discrimination, inappropriate comments, and rejection based on their relationship status (Guzman & Nishina, 2017; Kroeger & Williams, 2011; Nash, 1997; Rosenthal & Starks, 2015; Toledo, 2016; van der Walt & Basson, 2015). The degree of scrutiny experienced by an interracial couple, however, can be moderated by factors such as the couple's socioeconomic status, educational background, and the geographic area in which they live (Nash, 1997). Furthermore, the levels of stress experienced by interracial couples may be much higher if they are facing rejection across multiple ecologies such as within their family environments as well as within broader communities, such as within friendships (Nash, 1997). Indeed, for individuals in interracial relationships, stigma experienced from friends has been found to be the most harmful (Rosenthal & Starks, 2015). Quantitative analyses from the study showed that stigma from friends was associated with lower levels of commitment, trust, love, and sexual communication, and attributed this higher level of harm compared to family stigma because, as adults, the individuals may feel a closer relationship with their friends compared to family members (Rosenthal & Starks, 2015). Even adolescents who are in interracial relationships endorse that they are less likely to exhibit public displays of affection compared to their intra-racial couple counterparts, due to fear of discrimination (Vaquera & Kao, 2005). Along with negotiating how to cope with external pressures related to their status as an interracial couple, monoracial adults in an interracial union also face challenges when they bear children, who are multiracial.

## MONORACIAL PARENTS OF MULTIRACIAL CHILDREN

Decades of developmental research suggest that parenting and family processes play important roles in youth development and have been linked to overall youth well-being (Bamaca, Umana-Taylor, Shin, & Alfaro, 2005; Bronfenbrenner, 1986). Interracial couples often have to negotiate their parenting practices due to cultural differences in childrearing and may also adjust their parenting styles to protect their children from discrimination (Blanco, Bares, & Delva, 2013). For interracial couples, a significant aspect of parenting is racial socialization, which is the process of providing children with an understanding of how race impacts identity, group relationships, and social systems (Thornton, Chatters, Taylor, & Allen, 1990). Several studies assessed the impact of racial socialization provided by monoracial parents of multiracial children (Csizmadia, Rollins, & Kaneakua, 2014; Rollins & Hunter, 2013; Snyder, 2012; Stone & Dolbin-MacNab, 2017). Although racial socialization is important for all children, regardless of their race, monoracial parents of multiracial children face unique challenges engaging in this process. Rollins and Hunter (2013) found that mothers of biracial parents engage in different forms of racial socialization—promotive, protective, and passive—with promotive and protective parents able to instill a greater sense of self in their children and help prepare them for possible experiences of discrimination later in life.

The process of providing racial socialization can be difficult, and although parents may feel helpless or inadequate (Blanco et al., 2013), there are several factors that have been found to influence racial socialization (Anderson & Stevenson, 2019; Blanco et al., 2013; Csizmadia et al., 2014; Stone & Dolbin-MacNab, 2017). Factors such as geographic location, parental race and age, and how parents view their child's race impact the frequency of racial socialization practices (Csizmadia et al., 2014). For example, families in urban communities discuss race-related issues more frequently than parents in rural areas, older White parents may be less comfortable discussing race in general and therefore do not discuss it with their children, and parents who identified their children as White have conversations about the child's heritage less frequently than parents who identify the child as a minority race or biracial (Csizmadia et al., 2014). Some monoracial White mothers of multiracial youth, who have never dealt with issues of race until they have a biracial child, may feel ill equipped to help their children negotiate their minority racial identity or understand their unique experiences as multiracial individuals (Blanco et al., 2013; Crawford & Alaggia, 2008). However, apart from fixed factors such as parental race and location and parental lack of racial socialization experiences, researchers have found that experiences such as participating in family events (Blanco et al., 2013), creating a biracial family identity (Stone & Dolbin-MacNab, 2017), and having open communication about racially stressful experiences (Anderson & Stevenson, 2019) are forms of racial socialization that can have positive impacts on mental health and can protect against future experiences of discrimination. The multiracial offspring of interracial couples experience the world differently than their parents. In the following section, we briefly highlight the research that focuses on the experiences of multiracial individuals.

## EXPERIENCES OF MULTIRACIAL INDIVIDUALS

With over 6 million individuals identifying with more than one race in the 2000 Census, multiracial individuals represent one of the fastest growing minority groups in the country (Shih & Sanchez, 2009). In fact, it is estimated that by 2050, 20% of Americans will identify as multiracial (Farley, 2001). Unfortunately, literature focused on multiracial individuals lags behind research on underrepresented minority groups due to the historical lack of recognition of mixed race individuals (Fisher, Reynolds, Hsu, Barnes, & Tyler, 2014). Indeed, early conceptualizations about racial group categorizations favored placing or forcing individuals into discrete racial groups with early researchers utilizing a one-drop rule to categorize individuals of mixed racial backgrounds into one specific minority group (Fernandez, 1996). More recently, there is a movement toward utilizing "multiracial" to describe individuals of mixed racial backgrounds (Fisher et al., 2014). Furthermore, instead of seeing multiracial individuals as either falling into a monoracial or biracial identity paradigm, a recent study recommends a multidimensional view of racial identity for multiracial individuals, whereby they "choose" their identity based on what is structurally available to them (Rockquemore & Brunsma, 2002). According to these authors, the two major factors that influence the racial identity negotiations for multiracial individuals are social networks and appearances.

In terms of appearances, many multiracial individuals, who have one White parent and whose skin color is lighter and similar to the skin tone of White Europeans, may "pass" as White and choose to identify as White due to colorism (associating whiteness or lighter skin with attractiveness and privilege), social groups, and family upbringing (Harris, 2018). Individuals' reasons to pass for White may vary due to their other minority racial group memberships and personal factors. However, Harris (2018) states that, "to deny an aspect of one's identity is a challenging decision that can be psychologically detrimental if not thoughtfully and consciously considered" (p. 2083). Indeed, experiences, attitudes, and characteristics differ based on multiracial individuals' racial makeup and how their racial subgroups are viewed by society. For example, in a recent study, authors found that 69% of multiracial individuals who have a Black background are likely to report that society views them as Black and also report that their attitudes and behaviors are often more aligned with the Black community (Parker et al., 2015). Multiracial individuals who identify as both Asian and White and those who identify as Native American and White are more likely to feel connected to Whites compared to other Asians (Parker et al., 2015). In the following section, we discuss the racial identity development of multiracial individuals and the microaggressions these individuals experience in their everyday life.

## MULTIRACIAL IDENTITY DEVELOPMENT AND MICROAGGRESSIONS

Racial identity development may be a significant focus when counseling multiracial individuals, due to its relation to many factors that contribute to an individual's mental health (Charmaraman, Quach, Woo, & Erkut, 2014; Fisher, Zapolski, Sheehan, & Barnes-Najor, 2017; Villegas-Gold & Tran, 2018). The history of multiracial identity development is limited compared to racial identity theories of monoracial groups. The first proposed theory of biracial identity was developed by Stonequist (1937), in which he claimed that an individual of two identities is the "marginal man," who is part of both worlds but belongs to neither. This theory posed a negative view of biracial identity, where the individual was destined to be filled with internal conflict. Several decades later, Gibbs (1987) returned to the concept of marginality in the identity development of biracial adolescents and also included treatment strategies regarding the integration of both ethnic identities and the development of self-esteem in the adolescent.

Inspired by Cross's (1971) model of African American racial identity development and view of reference group orientation (Cross, 1987), Poston (1990) developed a positive view of multiracial identity that deviated from the deficit models created by Stonequist (1937) and Gibbs (1987). In this theory,

Poston (1990) proposed five stages of racial identity development that describe this development in a healthy way, which integrates the complex cultural, social, and personal factors that are a part of identifying with multiple racial groups. The five stages are Personal Identity, Choice of Group Categorization, Enmeshment/Denial, Appreciation, and Integration (Poston, 1990). The stages begin in childhood when the individual has an identity that is not based on a specific racial group but is rather based on self-esteem and self-worth learned from the family. Societal pressure then forces the individual to choose one ethnic group to identify with. This experience then leads to confusion, guilt, and self-hate due to choosing only one group that is not representative of the individual as a whole. Ultimately, through the support of parents and/or community, the individual is able to appreciate their multiple identities and learn about all of their heritages and cultures. Lastly, through this appreciation, the individual is able to develop a secure, integrated identity. Embracing all ethnic identities may not come until the individual is into adulthood due to the life experience necessary to move through the previous stages.

Two other theories of multiracial identity development have presented a more fluid and less linear depiction of multiracial identity development (Root, 1990), and an ecological perspective of this racial group's identity development by focusing on factors such as peer culture, cultural knowledge, and physical appearance (Renn, 2008). Though valuable, the life span approach posed by Poston (1990) may be more valuable for clinical purposes as it addresses the conflicts and individual experiences during this stage of development. As the study of multiracial individuals became more prevalent, researchers began to analyze how certain forms of discrimination impacted multiracial individuals' identity development, as well as their overall mental health (Franco, Katz, & O'Brien, 2015; Lusk, Taylor, Nanney, & Austin, 2010; Townsend, Fryberg, Wilkins, & Markus, 2012). One form of discrimination that has been under-researched among the multiracial population is the experience of microaggressions.

Sue et al. (2007) defined racial microaggressions as "brief, everyday exchanges that send denigrating messages to people of color because they belong to a racial minority group" (p. 273). While recent research has explored the impact of racial microaggressions (Liu et al., 2019; Sue et al., 2019), minimal attention has been given to the multiracial population. One of the first studies of multiracial microaggressions was conducted by Johnston and Nadal (2010), where they provided an initial conceptualization of multiracial microaggressions, which would include a new taxonomy of microaggressions specific to multiracial individuals. This taxonomy was developed based on Root's (2003) study of the experience of multiracial individuals and included five multiracial microaggression categories: (a) *exclusion or isolation*, (b) *exoticization and objectification*, (c) *assumption of monoracial or mistaken identity*, (d) *denial of multiracial reality*, and (e) *pathologizing of identity and experiences* (Johnston & Nadal, 2010). In addition to conducting a mixed-methods study to learn more about how multiracial microaggressions compared to monoracial microaggressions (Nadal et al., 2011), Nadal, Sriken, Davidoff, Wong, and McLean (2013) also conducted a qualitative study to discover the impact of microaggressions within families. From this analysis emerged five domains of within-family microaggressions experienced by multiracial individuals: (a) *isolation within the family*, (b) *favoritism within the family*, (c) *questioning of authenticity*, (d) *denial of multiracial identity* and experiences by monoracial family members, and (e) *feelings about not learning about family heritage or culture* (Nadal et al., 2013). Aligned with the taxonomy developed by Johnston and Nadal (2010), a recent qualitative study found that multiracial individuals experience microaggressions related to denial of a multiracial reality, assumption of a monoracial identity, and being not monoracial enough to "fit in" (Harris, 2017). Although additional research is necessary to understand if the multiracial microaggression taxonomy is applicable on a larger scale, it is clear that multiracial individuals experience racial microaggressions and that these experiences impact their identity negotiations. The following case vignette and case discussion highlight the multitude of factors that can influence the identity development of multiracial individuals.

## CASE VIGNETTE

Johanna Smith is a multiracial 17-year-old cisgender girl who was referred for counseling at a community mental health clinic for panic attacks, generalized anxiety, and difficulty sleeping. She was recently hospitalized for a panic attack, which she and her father assumed was a cardiac emergency. Although this was Johanna's first panic attack, she has been experiencing elevated levels of anxiety and sleep issues since she was 12 years old.

Johanna's mother, Nirvana Anderson, is a cisgender White woman, who grew up in San Francisco, California, in the late 1960s to "hippie parents." Nirvana is the only child of Josh and Stella Anderson. After Josh decided to follow his dream of joining a small folk band, he left Stella to raise Nirvana. Stella worked multiple part-time jobs to care for Nirvana and raised her on her own. Nirvana met her husband, Johanna's father, Kyle Smith, while living and working near Cal Berkeley. Kyle was a computer engineering student at Berkeley when he met Nirvana at the coffee shop where she worked. Kyle is a cisgender African American man, who grew up in a tight-knit extended family in Atlanta, Georgia. His mother was a part-time social worker and a homemaker, his father was a mechanical engineer for Delta Airlines, and his two younger sisters are elementary school teachers and married with two children each. Kyle was raised Methodist and his family are all extremely devoted to and active in the church. When he first introduced Nirvana to his family, they were cautiously open to meeting and getting to know her. However, after several very heated political and religious arguments over family holidays during the first year of their marriage, the family ties between Nirvana and Kyle's family have been tenuous at best.

Although Nirvana and Kyle were very much in love at first, their relationship became increasingly conflictual over time. They argued frequently about how to raise Johanna with Nirvana favoring home schooling and opposed to organized religion and structured activities, and Kyle in favor of traditional schooling and enrichment experience for Johanna. They also argued about how to talk to Johanna about racism and other forms of discrimination and had difficulty talking about these subjects with each other in general. While Nirvana felt very strongly that Johanna should know about gender and LGBT discrimination, she minimized the importance of talking to her about racism because she said, "Johanna is not going to experience racism, she looks

White, just like the girl next door." Although Kyle was not very comfortable talking about racism with Johanna himself, he enlisted his younger sisters, his mother, and his aunts to talk to Johanna about a few instances of racism and microaggressions she experienced in school. When Johanna was 14, her parents divorced and, based on custody agreements, she spent every other weekend and part of the week with her father and every other weekend and part of the week with her mother. Transitioning from each house was extremely difficult and straining for Johanna because each household seemed like a different world with distinct rules. At her mother's house, she avoided talking about attending religious services with her dad and his family, her cool AP teacher, and her excitement about going to a 4-year college right after high school, but instead talked about cooking and her recent romantic feelings for a girl from her class. On the other hand, at her father's house, although she felt like she could talk about being a straight "A" student and her aspirations for college, she felt extremely hesitant to share her bisexual identity with her father and her father's side of the family.

## Working With Multiracial Individuals and Families: The Case of Johanna

Multiracial families or families where at least one member has a different racial heritage than the other members is an expanding population in the United States (Wehrly, Kenney, & Kenney, 1999). The scope of multiracial practice has been broadened to incorporate multiracial individuals of all racial backgrounds, interracial couples, and multiracial families (Wehrly et al., 1999). In the case of Johanna, whose biological mother is White and biological father is Black, there are several important clinical implications when working either individually with Johanna or when working with Johanna and her family. In the following section, we provide some clinical considerations through an examination of the case of Johanna.

## Racial Identity and Experiences of Racism and Colorism

Individuals within a multiracial family unit may be at different stages of racial identity development, and these differences may result in conflicting perceptions regarding the salience of race and racism and may also influence reactions to incidences of racism. Furthermore, members in a multiracial family will have distinct experiences of privilege and access on the one hand and prejudice and racism on the other hand based on differences in their phenotypic racial features and their skin tone.

In the case of Johanna, both her mother and father demonstrate a strong discomfort in discussing issues of race and racism with her reflecting that they may be at earlier stages of racial identity development. Although Johanna's mother prefers to focus on Johanna's other oppressed identities (e.g., gender identity and sexual orientation identity), she minimizes the importance of race and points out Johanna's ability to "pass" as White, like "the girl next door" as the reasons she believes Johanna will not experience racism. Unfortunately, her mother's comments reflect an inability to provide Johanna with the racial socialization she may need to navigate her multiracial identity in a racialized world (Csizmadia et al., 2014) and fail to acknowledge the complex and confusing experience associated with "passing" (Harris, 2018). Johanna's father's discomfort discussing race and racism with Johanna leads him to seek the support of his family members, who may or may not be able to provide Johanna with the racial socialization discussions she needs. Clinicians need to remember that monoracial minority parents or relatives may be able to discuss racism and colorism from the point of view of a monoracial minority individual but may not fully understand or know how best to support a multiracial child's experience (Crawford & Alaggia, 2008).

If a therapist were to work with Johanna and her parents, the therapist would need to encourage Johanna's parents to develop a level of understanding, appreciation, and acceptance of each partner's cultural and racial identity. In the case of Johanna, this understanding between her parents seems to be lacking and so the counselor would need to assist each person in gaining perspective and insight into how one's cultural values and racial identities influence the relationship dynamics in terms of feelings, behaviors, and conflict. The counselor must be open to learning and using culturally competent skills to help each partner understand the need for different cultural frameworks when working with each person (Anderson & Stevenson, 2019).

In multiracial families, parents may be unaware that children feel a lack of support due to differences in racial identities among family members. This seems to be true in the case of Johanna, where she clearly is split in terms of what parts of her identity and experience she feels comfortable disclosing to each parent. For Johanna's family, parent educational counseling can help her parents learn healthy racial socialization, which can help them feel comfortable talking about the consequences of racial oppression with Johanna (Anderson & Stevenson, 2019). In addition, an intersectional lens may be useful when mental health professionals help multiracial families, like Johanna's, develop and negotiate their multiple and intersecting identities across contexts and over time (DePouw, 2018).

## Multiracial Individuals/Families and Intersectionality

In addition to negotiating their multiracial identity and coping with the social stigmatization and discrimination that sometimes accompany their membership in multiple racial groups, multiracial individuals' social experiences are also impacted by their intersecting social identities (Shih & Sanchez, 2009). Indeed, to understand the implications of racism for multiracial individuals, one needs to appreciate the ways in which race intersects with other oppressed identities across contexts and time (Gillborn, 2015). Crenshaw's original conceptualization of intersectionality (1990) is a useful framework through which to understand the experiences of multiracial individuals. Intersectionality reminds us to resist the pull to generalize experiences of multiracial individuals and calls us to explore intragroup differences in lived experience and positionality (DePouw, 2018). Furthermore, as DePouw (2018) suggests, an intersectional lens coupled with a critical race perspective may be helpful for White monoracial parents of multiracial children as a way to both understand and resist the complex and insidious ways in which a racism interferes with the healthy identity development of multiracial individuals and families.

The case of Johanna highlights the intersecting and powerfully dynamic nature of identity within multiracial families. First off, Johanna has a White mother and a Black father, and this particular union is associated with negative stereotypes that are steeped in historically rooted taboos and fears about interracial relationships between Black men and White women (Romano, 2003). Negative attitudes towards interracial Black and White couples continue to be stronger than negative attitudes toward White and non-Black couples, which may have an impact on Johanna. Furthermore, if Johanna's parents are uncomfortable talking about their own experiences of discrimination as an interracial couple, they may leave Johanna with few tools to help her navigate her future romantic relationships with individuals of other races.

In addition to Johanna's multiracial background, she is also actively negotiating many other important social identities. She has identified as bisexual and disclosed this to her mother but not to her father. She also demonstrates some affiliation with her religious identity when with her father and his family, and this identity may or may not come into conflict with her sexual orientation identity. She is also navigating the different cultural messages she receives from her mother and her father regarding aspirations for higher education and career strivings. Johanna's inability to be fully real with either of her parents may result in what Nadal and his colleagues found to be true of other multiracial individuals, which is a sense of isolation within one's own family as well as a feeling of inauthenticity about oneself (Nadal et al., 2013).

### Therapists' Competence Working With Multiracial Individuals and Families

Clinicians must be aware and knowledgeable of the stages of racial identity development (Poston, 1990) when working with multiracial individuals because it is important that during each stage, the client is given the space to openly explore and ultimately work to move from an external view of their ethnicity or culture to a more internal perspective. For instance, the counselor serves a facilitative role during the stage of enmeshment/denial when the individual will likely be experiencing negative feelings toward themselves (Poston, 1990). Possibly most importantly, when working with these individuals, a therapist should be mindful of their own biases toward ethnic groups and cultures, remembering to always remain curious of the individuals' understanding rather than imposing their own predetermined ideas. Counselors working with these groups must be aware of their own biases and assumptions about interracial dating in addition to being willing to gain new knowledge and a new scope of understanding the unique individual's cultural values and worldview. In addition to this, the counselor needs to understand how those unique cultural differences shape the relationship dynamic (Blanco et al., 2013).

Practitioners and therapists should also be aware of the challenges faced by parents of biracial youth in order to adequately assess potential problems in communication or child–parent relationships (Blanco et al., 2013). Providing parents of children with psychoeducation regarding the challenges a child may face can, in terms of ethnic identity development, be a useful intervention. Sharing research findings that show the tendency for biracial youth to feel unsupported and distanced from parents (especially mothers) in addition to explaining the limitations of that research can be useful as well. Therapists can look at communication patterns while also normalizing difficulties faced in the experience as a monoracial parent of a multiracial child (Blanco et al., 2013).

## Discussion Questions

1. What are your impressions of the messages Johanna is receiving from each of her parents about what it means to be a multiracial, bisexual, and religious young woman?
2. How might you work with Johanna to help address her mental health concerns in the context of her split living arrangements with her mother and father?
3. What are some family therapy or systemic approaches that may facilitate a positive change in Johanna's environment?

## REFERENCES

Anderson, R. E., & Stevenson, H. C. (2019). RECASTing racial stress and trauma: Theorizing the healing potential of racial socialization in families. *American Psychologist, 74*, 63–75. doi:10.1037/amp0000392

Bamaca, M. Y., Umana-Taylor, A. J., Shin, N., & Alfaro, E. C. (2005). Latino adolescents' perception of parenting behaviors and self-esteem: Examining the role of neighborhood risk. *Family Relations, 54*, 621–632. doi:10.1111/j.1741-3729.2005.00346.x

Blanco, E. I. L., Bares, C. B., & Delva, J. (2013). Parenting, family processes, relationships, and parental support in multiracial and multiethnic families: An exploratory study of youth perceptions. *Family Relations, 62*, 125–139. doi:10.1111/j.1741-3729.2012.00751.x

Bronfenbrenner, U. (1986). Ecology of the family as a context for human development: Research perspectives. *Developmental Psychology, 22*, 723–742. doi:10.1037/0012-1649.22.6.723

Charmaraman, L., Quach, A., Woo, M., & Erkut, S. (2014). How researchers studied multiracial populations? A content and methodological review of 20 years of research. *Cultural Diversity and Ethnic Minority Psychology, 20*, 336–352. doi:10.1037/a0035437

Crawford, S. E., & Alaggia, R. (2008). The best of both worlds? Family influences on mixed race youth identity development. *Qualitative Social Work: Research and Practice. 7*, 81–98. doi:10.1177/1473325007086417

Crenshaw, K. (1990). Mapping the margins: Intersectionality, identity politics, and violence against women of color. *Stanford Law Review, 43*, 1241. doi:10.2307/1229039

Cross, W. E. (1971). The Negro-to-Black conversion experience: Toward a psychology of Black liberation. *Black World, 20*, 13–27.

Cross, W. E. (1987). A two-factor theory of Black identity: Implications for the study of identity development in minority children. In J. S. Phinney & M. J. Rotherham (Eds.), *Children's ethnic socialization: Pluralism and development* (pp. 117–133). Newbury Park, CA: Sage.

Csizmadia, A., Rollins, A., & Kaneakua, J. P. (2014). Ethnic–racial socialization and its correlates in families of Black–White biracial children. *Family Relations, 63*(2), 259–270. doi:10.1111/fare.12062

DePouw, C. (2018). Intersectionality and critical race parenting. *International Journal of Qualitative Studies in Education, 31*(1), 55–69. doi:10.1080/09518398.2017.1379620

Farley, R. (2001). *Identifying with multiple races. Report 01-491*. Ann Arbor, MI: University of Michigan, Population Studies Center.

Fernandez, C. A. (1996). Government classification of multiracial/multiethnic people. In M. P. Root (Ed.), *The multiracial experience: Racial borders as the new frontier* (pp. 15–36). Thousand Oaks, CA: Sage.

Fisher, S., Reynolds, J. L., Hsu, W., Barnes, J., & Tyler, K. (2014). Examining multiracial youth in context: Ethnic identity development and mental health outcomes. *Journal of Youth Adolescence, 43*, 1688–1699. doi:10.1007/s10964-014-0163-2

Fisher, S., Zapolski, T. C., Sheehan, C., & Barnes-Najor, J. (2017). Pathway of protection: Ethnic identity, self-esteem, and substance use among multiracial youth. *Addictive behaviors, 72*, 27–32. doi:10.1016/j.addbeh.2017.03.003

Franco, M. G., Katz, R., & O'Brien, K. M. (2015). Forbidden identities: A qualitative examination of racial identity invalidation for Black/White biracial individuals. *International Journal of Intercultural Relations, 50*, 96–109. doi:10.1016/j.ijintrel.2015.12.004

Gibbs, J. T. (1987). Identity and marginality: Issues in the treatment of biracial adolescents. *American Journal of Orthopsychiatry, 57*(2), 265–278. doi:10.1111/j.1939-0025.1987.tb03537.x

Gillborn, D. (2015). Intersectionality, critical race theory, and the primacy of racism: Race, class, gender, and disability in education. *Qualitative Inquiry, 21*(3), 277–287. doi:10.1177/1077800414557827

Guzman, N. S., & Nishina, A. (2017). 50 Years of loving: Interracial romantic relationships and recommendations for future research. *Journal of Family Theory & Review, 9*, 557–571. doi:10.1111/jftr.12215

Harris, J. C. (2017). Multiracial college students' experiences with multiracial microaggressions. *Race Ethnicity and Education, 20*(4), 429–445. doi:10.1080/13613324.2016.1248836

Harris, K. L. (2018). Biracial American colorism: Passing for White. *American Behavioral Scientist, 62*(14), 2072–2086. doi:10.1177/0002764218810747

History.com Editors. (2017). *Loving v. Virginia*. Retrieved from https://www.history.com/topics/civil-rights-movement/loving-v-virginia

Johnston, M. P., & Nadal, K. L. (2010). Multiracial microaggressions: Exposing monoracism in everyday life and clinical practice. In D. W. Sue (Ed.), *Microaggressions and marginality: Manifestation, dynamics, and impact* (pp. 123–144). New York, NY: Wiley & Sons.

Kroeger, R. A., & Williams, K. (2011). Consequences of Black exceptionalism? Interracial unions with Blacks, depressive symptoms, and relationship satisfaction. *The Sociological Quarterly, 52*(3), 400–420. doi:10.1111/j.1533-8525.2011.01212.x

Liu, W. M., Liu, R. Z., Garrison, Y. L., Kim, J. Y. C., Chan, L., Ho, Y., & Yeung, C. W. (2019). Racial trauma, microaggressions, and becoming racially innocuous: The role of acculturation and White supremacist ideology. *American Psychologist, 74*(1), 143. doi:10.1037/amp0000368

Lusk, E., Taylor, M., Nanney, J., & Austin, C. (2010). Biracial identity and its relation to self-esteem and depression in mixed Black/White biracial individuals. *Journal of Ethnic & Cultural Diversity in Social Work, 19*(2), 109–126. doi:10.1080/15313201003771783

Nadal, K. L., Sriken, J., Davidoff, K. C., Wong, Y., & McLean, K. (2013). Microaggressions within families: Experiences of multiracial people. *Family Relations, 62*(1), 190–201. doi:10.1111/j.1741-3729.2012.00752.x

Nadal, K. L., Wong, Y., Griffin, K., Sriken, J., Vargas, V., Wideman, M., & Kolawole, A. (2011). Microaggressions and the multiracial experience. *International Journal of Humanities and Social Sciences, 1*(7), 36–44.

Nash, R. D. (1997). *Coping with interracial dating*. New York, NY: Rosen.

Parker, K., Horowitz, J. M., Morin, R., & Lopez, M. H. (2015). *Multiracial in America: Proud, diverse and growing numbers*. Retrieved from https://www.pewsocialtrends.org/2015/06/11/multiracial-in-america

Poston, W. C. (1990). The biracial identity development model: A needed addition. *Journal of Counseling & Development, 69*(2), 152–155. doi:10.1002/j.1556-6676.1990.tb01477.x

Renn, K. A. (2008). Research on biracial and multiracial identity development: Overview and synthesis. *New Directions for Student Services, 2008*(123), 13–21. doi:10.1002/ss.282

Rockquemore, K. A., & Brunsma, D. L. (2002). Socially embedded identities: Theories, typologies and process of racial identity among Black/White biracials. *The Sociological Quarterly, 43*, 335–356. doi:10.1111/j.1533-8525.2002.tb00052.x

Rollins, A., & Hunter, A. G. (2013). Racial socialization of biracial youth: Maternal messages and approaches to address discrimination. *Family Relations, 62*(1), 140–153. doi:10.1111/j.1741-3729.2012.00748.x

Romano, R. (2003). *Race mixing: Black-White marriage in postwar America*. Cambridge, MA: Harvard University Press.

Root, M. P. (1990). Resolving "other" status: Identity development of biracial individuals. *Women & Therapy, 9*(1–2), 185–205. doi:10.1300/J015v09n01_11

Root, M. P. (2003). Issues and experiences of racially mixed people. In M. P. P. Root & M. Kelly (Eds.), *The multiracial child resource book: Living complex identities* (pp. 132–134). Seattle, WA: Mavin Foundation.

Rosenthal, L., & Starks, T. J. (2015). Relationship stigma and relationship outcomes in interracial and same-sex relationships: Examination of sources and buffers. *Journal of Family Psychology, 29*(6), 818–830. doi:10.1037/fam0000116

Shih, M., & Sanchez, D. T. (2009). When race becomes even more complex: Toward understanding the landscape of multiracial identity and experiences. *Journal of Social Issues, 65*(1), 1–11. doi:10.1111/j.1540-4560.2008.01584.x

Snyder, C. R. (2012). Racial socialization in cross-racial families. *Journal of Black Psychology, 38*(2), 228–253. doi:10.1177/0095798411416457

Stone, D. J., & Dolbin-MacNab, M. (2017). Racial socialization practices of White mothers raising Black–White biracial children. *Contemporary Family Therapy, 39*(2), 97–111. doi:10.1007/s10591-017-9406-1

Stonequist, E. V. (1937). *The marginal man: A study in personality and culture conflict*. New York, NY: Scribner/Simon & Schuster.

Sue, D. W., Capodilupo, C. M., Torino, G. C., Bucceri, J. M., Holder, A. M. B., Nadal, K. L., & Esquilin, M. (2007). Racial microaggressions in everyday life: Implications for clinical practice. *American Psychologist, 62*(4), 271–286. doi:10.1037/0003-066X.62.4.271

Sue, D. W., Alsaidi, S., Awad, M. N., Glaeser, E., Calle, C. Z., & Mendez, N. (2019). Disarming racial microaggressions: Microintervention strategies for targets, White allies, and bystanders. *American Psychologist, 74*(1), 128. doi:10.1037/amp0000296

Thornton, M. C., Chatters, L. M., Taylor, R. J., & Allen, W. R. (1990). Sociodemographic and environmental correlates of racial socialization by Black parents. *Child Development, 61*, 401–409. doi:10.1111/1467-8624.ep5878989

Toledo, E. M. (2016). When loving is not enough. *California Law Review, 104*(3), 769. doi:10.15779/Z38VC4G

Townsend, S. S., Fryberg, S. A., Wilkins, C. L., & Markus, H. R. (2012). Being mixed: Who claims a biracial identity? *Cultural Diversity and Ethnic Minority Psychology, 18*(1), 91. doi:10.1037/a0026845

U.S. Census Bureau. (2014). *Table 10. Projections of the Population by Sex, Hispanic Origin, and Race for the United States: 2015 to 2060* (NP2014-T10). Retrieved from https://www.census.gov/data/tables/2014/demo/popproj/2014-summary-tables.html

van der Walt, A., & Basson, P. (2015). The lived experience of discrimination of White women in committed interracial relationships with Black men. *Indo-Pacific Journal of Phenomenology, 15*(2), 1. doi:10.1080/20797222.2015.1101834

Vaquera, E., & Kao, G. (2005). Private and public displays of affection among interracial and intraracial adolescent couples. *Social Science Quarterly, 86*(2), 484–508. doi:10.1111/j.0038-4941.2005.00314.x

Villegas-Gold, R., & Tran, A. G. (2018). Socialization and well-being in multiracial individuals: A moderated mediation model of racial ambiguity and identity. *Journal of Counseling Psychology, 65*(4), 413. doi:10.1037/cou0000277

Wehrly, B., Kenney, K. R., & Kenney, M.E. (1999). *Counseling multiracial families*. Thousand Oaks, CA: SAGE Publications.

# 3

# Transracial Adoption and Transracial Socialization: Clinical Implications and Recommendations

Jason D. Reynolds (Taewon Choi) and Hannah M. Wing

## INTRODUCTION

The history of transracial adoption has deep roots in the United States, dating back to the 1850s with the domestic adoption of Indigenous and Native American children by White families (Engel, Phillips, & DellaCava, 2012). In the 1950s, the domestic adoption of African American children as well as the international adoption of Korean children by White families became more prevalent in America (Davis, 2011; Kim, 2010). The practice of transracial adoption triggered a debate between supporters and detractors of mixed-race families (Barn, 2013)—both because antimiscegenation laws legally prevented mixed-race marriage until 1967 and because many in the African American community, including Black social workers, objected to the adoption of Black children by White parents. Critical discourse on domestic adoption practices and the colonization of children of color via international adoption is ongoing, as adoption represents part of the larger narrative of historical oppression and institutionalized discrimination of communities of color domestically and internationally (Kim, 2010; Lee, 2007). The prevalence, continuation, and long-term outcomes of transracial adoption remain controversial.

Considerable research over the past two decades has explored a variety of factors related to domestic and international transracial adoption. Extant adoption research exists on identity development of transracial adoptees (Reynolds, Ponterotto, & Lecker, 2016), adoption microaggressions (Baden, 2016; Garber & Grotevant, 2015), names and identity for transracial adoptees (Reynolds, Ponterotto, Park-Taylor, & Takooshian, 2017), authenticity for transracial adoptees

(Reynolds, Kim, & Ponterotto, 2019), and racial, ethnic, and cultural socialization of adoptees (Barn, 2013; Kim, Reichwald, & Lee, 2013; Langrehr, 2014; Mohanty, 2015). Despite this wide-ranging research, adoption itself is still largely unexplored. More research is needed to better understand the adoption triad (i.e., adoptee, birth family, adoptive family) and provide clinical information for practitioners working with adoptees and their families.

This chapter seeks to provide clinicians and practitioners with a brief history of domestic and international transracial adoption practices, knowledge about transracial socialization patterns (i.e., racial, ethnic, and cultural) and their long-term effects, and the clinical implications of working with transracially adopted individuals. In addition, a case vignette and discussion questions are provided at the end of the chapter.

## HISTORY AND CONTEXT OF TRANSRACIAL DOMESTIC AND INTERCOUNTRY ADOPTION

Contemporary adoption nomenclature categorizes adoptions by whether or not the child and adoptive parents share the same race and country of origin. Same-race adoption refers to someone who is adopted by a family of the same race (Arnold, Braje, Kawahara, & Shuman, 2016). Transracial adoption refers to an individual who is adopted by a family of a different race. Adoptions in which children are placed with families within their country of origin are termed domestic adoptions, whereas children placed with families in another country are designated as intercountry or international adoptions (the two terms will be used interchangeably in this chapter). The vast majority of intercountry adoptions involve children from Eastern countries adopted by parents living in Western countries (Ma, 2017). This chapter focuses on transracial adoption within or to the United States and discusses prevalent adoption trends. While there are commonalities in transracial adoption across the globe, each adoption experience varies according to racial demographics and the dynamics of the society.

## CONTEXT OF TRANSRACIAL ADOPTION

The United States has been the recipient of hundreds of thousands of transracial intercountry adoptees since 1970 (Selman, 2002). In 85% of international adoptions (Vandivere, Malm, & Radel, 2009) and 40% of all U.S. adoptions, domestic and international, the child was adopted into a family of a different race (Donaldson Adoption Institute, 2011). Because most of these adoptive parents are White, transracial adoption is considered the most visible form of adoption, given the mismatch in racial appearance between the parents and child (Arnold et al., 2016).

## DOMESTIC ADOPTION OF CHILDREN OF COLOR

### Adoption of Native American Children

There is a long history of transracial domestic adoption of Native American children in the United States. Indigenous children were forcibly removed from their families and placed in boarding schools between the 1850s and 1940s. Engel et al. (2012) reported that these "Indian orphanages" ostensibly addressed the large number of Indigenous children supposedly without parents. These "orphanages" served to assimilate Native American children into mainstream White culture, stripping them of their Indigenous languages and cultural heritage (Engel et al., 2012).

The 1960s and 1970s saw the Indian Child Welfare Crisis, as Native American children were regularly separated from their parents and communities (Jacobs, 2013). Under the influence of the Indian Adoption Project, from 1958 to 1967, the transracial adoption of Indigenous children was actively encouraged. It was developed collaboratively by the Federal Bureau of Indian Affairs and the largest adoption agency in the United States at the time, the Child Welfare League of America (Engel et al., 2012). Although the program was controversial, 35% (approximately 700) of adopted Native American children were placed with non-Indigenous families, almost exclusively White, in Eastern and Midwestern states (Engel et al., 2012).

Tribal nations protested the Indian Adoption Project. The Indian Child Welfare Act (ICWA) of 1978, a direct result of tribal advocacy efforts, gave tribes jurisdiction over children living on reservations (Engel et al., 2012). Intended to remedy the culturally genocidal impact of federally sanctioned forced removals of Native American children (Roemer, 2019; Sweeney & Pollack, 2017), the ICWA provided tribes with more rights in navigating the child welfare system and promoted cultural preservation of Indigenous families (Barnes, Constantine Brown, & McCarty-Caplan, 2019). The ICWA encouraged the adoption of Indigenous children by family members or even members of other tribal nations (Engel et al., 2012). Adoption by non-Native American parents was considered a last resort, as it was feared that Indigenous children would lose their culture entirely (Sweeney & Pollack, 2017). However, in an effort to reduce delays in the placement of children, the U.S. government passed the 1994 Multiethnic Placement Act, which enforced colorblind adoption policies (Engel et al., 2012). Despite dismay among Indigenous nations, placement into White families became increasingly common (Sweeney & Pollack, 2017). Interestingly, given the federal recognition of tribal nations, adoption of Native American children by non-Indigenous families could be considered intercountry adoption.

## Adoption of African American Children

The 1950s saw a rise in the number of Black children being adopted, which coincided with a decrease of "healthy" White infants available for adoption and an increase in White parents' desire to adopt (Davis, 2011). However, the adoption of children of color, particularly Black children by White parents, was viewed by some as "cultural genocide" (McRoy & Griffin, 2012). In 1972, the National Association of Black Social Workers (NABSW) issued a statement, advocating that Black children be placed with Black families to facilitate cultural identity development (NABSW, 2013). Yet, after the 1994 Multiethnic Placement Act was passed, there was an increase in transracial adoptions in which Black children were placed with White families (Sweeney & Pollack, 2017).

While domestic transracial adoption rates have increased over the years, Black children are the least likely to be adopted, particularly by White parents, compared to their Asian and Latinx counterparts (Kreider & Lofquist, 2014; Spence, 2013). As a result, Black children continue to be overrepresented in the U.S. child welfare system (McRoy & Griffin, 2012) and remain in foster care longer than any other adoptee group (U.S. Department of Health and Human Services [DHHS], 2015). Despite this, Raleigh (2016) reported that White parents tend to prefer privately adopting biracial Black infants domestically or from Africa or the Caribbean, reflecting the belief that biracial children and international adoptees will assimilate better into White culture.

## INTERCOUNTRY AND INTERNATIONAL ADOPTION

For almost 50 years, the United States has been the main "receiving" country for transracial intercountry adoptees (U.S. Department of State—Bureau of Consular Affairs, 2017). The majority of international adoptions are transracial in nature (Arnold et al., 2016). Most of these intercountry adoptees, more than 200,000 collectively, are from Asia (Selman, 2009). In the late 2000s and early 2010s, the top "sending" countries were China, Ethiopia, Russia, South Korea, Ukraine, and Guatemala (U.S. Department of State—Bureau of Consular Affairs, 2017). This account of intercountry adoption focuses on transracial adoption patterns for the main sending countries to the United States.

### East, Southeast, and South Asian Intercountry Adoptees

In the 21st century, the majority of intercountry transracial adoptees have come from Asia (Selman, 2009). Before this, Korea was the main sending country to the United States from the 1950s through the 1980s (Selman, 2002). Between 1999 and 2016, more than 100,000 children were adopted by families in the United States from China, South Korea, India, the Philippines, Vietnam, and Cambodia, with the majority (more than 78,000) from China (U.S. Department of State—Bureau of Consular Affairs, 2017). India (5,946) and Vietnam (5,621) were the two highest sending countries from South and Southeast Asia from 1999 to 2017.

#### Korean Adoptees

Adoption of Korean children by White Americans began in the 1950s as a direct result of American involvement in the Korean War. Between 1953 and 2007, more than 100,000 children from South Korea were placed with families in the United States (Evan B. Donaldson Institute, 2009; Kim, 2010). In the earlier years of the Korean War, some Korean children were informally "adopted" by American soldiers and later brought to the United States. However, after the 1956 Holt Adoption Program made it possible for American families to adopt Korean children without traveling to Korea, hundreds of children were adopted annually in the 1960s, and thousands in the 1970s (Oh, 2012). The majority of those children were orphans or biracial children who were not accepted in Korean society due to cultural stigma and lack of support for single mothers and children born out of wedlock (Kim, 2010; Lee, 2003; Oh, 2012). While originally viewed as refugees, by 1961, Korean adoptees were deemed "exemplary immigrants," because of their perceived assimilative qualities (Oh, 2012, p. 36). The peak of Korean adoption was in the mid-1980s: More than 6,000 children were adopted in 1984 and 1985 (Selman, 2002). In recent years, Korean transracial adoptions in the United States have declined, in part due to adoptee-led organizations' concerns about inadequate socialization (Lee, 2007).

## Chinese Adoptees

China became a main sending country as a result of the nation's One Child Policy (Selman, 2002). In 1979, China implemented laws limiting most couples in the country to having one child and imposed strict punishments for violations (Hesketh, Lu, & Xing, 2005). The strong preference for boys meant "undesired" girls were abandoned (Hesketh et al., 2005; Selman, 2015). Many were placed in orphanages, and some were subsequently adopted (Dowling & Brown, 2009). In 1992, China began allowing foreigners to adopt Chinese children, and by 1995, China had become the predominant source for intercountry adoption (Selman, 2002). Between 1992 and 2017, approximately 80,000 Chinese adoptees were placed in the United States. The peak years for adoptions from China were the early 2000s, with the highest number in 2005, when almost 8,000 children from China were adopted into the United States (U.S. Department of State—Bureau of Consular Affairs, 2017). From 1995 to 2017, China has almost consistently been the top sending country of children adopted into families in the United States (U.S. Department of State–Bureau of Consular Affairs, 2017). In the past decade, with changes in the countries' policies, there have been increasing rates of domestic adoption in China and Korea (Davis, 2011).

## Central and South American Intercountry Adoptees

As contraception and abortion were being legalized in the United States and the number of adoptees from Asia was declining after the Korean and Vietnam wars, the rates of intercountry adoption from Central and South America increased (Davis, 2011). Political strife, violence, and unstable economies created conditions for an intercountry adoption industry rife with abuse (Davis, 2011). Guatemala was the main sending country from Latin America starting in 1999, with almost 30,000 children adopted into the United States (U.S. Department of State—Bureau of Consular Affairs, 2017), until intercountry adoption from Guatemala was closed in 2008 as a consequence of high rates of baby trafficking (Davis, 2011). Additionally, between 1971 and 2009, more than 15,000 children were adopted from Colombia (Davis, 2011). Other top sending countries to the United States, listed in descending order, include Mexico, Brazil, Chile, El Salvador, Peru, Paraguay, and Honduras.

## African Intercountry Adoptees

In recent years, there has been a growing trend for White parents to adopt Black children from Africa or the Caribbean, rather than domestically (Davis, 2011). This is partially explained by the perception of "less social distance" between White Americans and foreign-born Black individuals (Raleigh, 2016, p. 89) than between White Americans and native-born Blacks. From 2000 to 2009, Ethiopia was the main sending country from Africa to the United States, with more than

7,000 children adopted (Davis, 2011). However, in the last decade, adoption rates from Ethiopia to the United States declined (U.S. Department of State—Bureau of Consular Affairs, 2017), and the Ethiopian government banned intercountry adoption in 2018, due to continued irregularities and abuse in the adoption process.

## TRANSRACIAL SOCIALIZATION FOR ADOPTEES

While sometimes used interchangeably, the terms racial, ethnic, and cultural socialization are distinct and nuanced constructs. Harrison, Wilson, Pine, Chan, and Buriel (1990) described cultural socialization as a lifelong developmental process in which one learns about the meaning of race and ethnicity in one's life through direct observation of family behavior and practice of customs, traditions, values, and languages, which over time are internalized and become part of one's identity. For the purpose of this chapter, we use the following definitions: "Racial" refers to physical characteristics and internalized societal racial perception; "ethnic" refers to shared beliefs and history based on national or regional origins; and "cultural" refers to sense of belonging based on personal experience and behaviors (Baden & Steward, 2007; Robinson, 2012). The three categories typically intersect within any individual. The following sections discuss racial, ethnic, and transracial socialization patterns.

### Racial Socialization

Transracial adoptees are subject to both racial (Sue et al., 2007) and adoption-related (Baden, 2016) microaggressions, yet unlike their non-adopted peers of color, they may feel ill equipped to cope with racial discrimination because of limited racial socialization by their parents, most of whom are White (Langrehr, 2014). Racial socialization is the degree to which parents foster racial pride and prepare their children to cope with discrimination (Montgomery & Jordan, 2018). This process is positively correlated with transracial adoptees' psychological well-being (e.g., comfort with adoptive status and high self-esteem) (Mohanty, 2013). However, being socialized in a White environment while being treated as a person of color ("transracial adoption paradox"; Lee, 2003), makes racial socialization particularly challenging. Adoptees must learn to cope with a mismatch between self-identification and others' perceptions.

In transracial adoptive families, racial socialization is affected by the extent to which White parents acknowledge the racial differences between themselves and their adopted children (Barn, 2013). While adoptive parents play a crucial role in adoptees' racial identity development (Bergquist, Campbell, & Unrau, 2003), White adoptive parents' effectiveness in racial socialization remains controversial (Dolan, 2015). Three-quarters of White adoptive parents never or rarely talk about race with their children (Brown, Tanner-Smith, Lesane-Brown, & Ezell, 2007), perhaps because racial dialogues may elicit feelings of guilt and shame for these parents (Langrehr, 2014). White adoptive parents must examine their own racial bias and privilege in order to model open and honest communication for their children. Their avoidance of or ambivalence about discussing race, racism, and White privilege increases adoptees' own discomfort in these areas (Chang, Feldman, & Easley, 2017). As a result of perceived White fragility, adoptees may choose not to share experiences of discrimination with their parents for fear of burdening them (Chang et al., 2017).

Three main approaches to racial socialization in transracial adoptive families have been identified: avoidant, ambivalent, and engaged (Chang et al., 2017). Parents choosing avoidance, also known as humanitarianism (Barn, 2013), de-emphasize the role of race in the adoptee's life. These parents raise their children from a colorblind or White savior perspective (Chang et al., 2017). Colorblindness denies the racial difference between parents and their child (Kim et al., 2013) and does not acknowledge the discrimination to which the child may be subjected (Morgan & Langrehr, 2018). Dolan (2015) found that one-third of White parents denied that their adopted child experienced racism.

Adoptive parents who take an ambivalent approach express hesitation about acknowledging the adoptee's racial background (Barn, 2013). Although these parents may recognize the existence of racism, they have difficulty effectively engaging in "race talk" with their child (Dolan, 2015). They may encourage the adoptee to connect with the birth culture without considering the adoptee's lack of interest or discomfort. Adoptees may develop a distorted perception that race and culture are "performed" only in certain spaces and with other people of color (Goss, Byrd, & Hughey, 2017), in place of a deeper sense of self.

While avoidant and ambivalent approaches are most common, engaged racial socialization or transculturalism (Barn, 2013) is associated with positive identity development of transracial adoptees (Chang et al., 2017). It is consistent with the shared fate theory (Kirk, 1984) in which White parents recognize and value the racial differences within the family, viewing their own as "multiracial" (Kim et al., 2013). These parents are likely to move to diverse communities to give their children support and role models (Barn, 2013). White parents' ability to talk about racial bias and to validate adoptees' feelings of anger provides a safe space for adoptees of color to explore the complex dynamics of their transracial adoptive background (Langrehr, Yoon, Hacker, & Caudill, 2015; Mohanty, 2013). Adoptive parents may not experience racism themselves, but adoptees of color learn that they are not alone in confronting racial bias.

## Ethnic Socialization

While transracial adoptees may have a strong desire to connect with individuals from similar racial and ethnic backgrounds (Goss et al., 2017), White adoptive parents often prefer to live in predominantly White neighborhoods, limiting the opportunities for interaction with people from diverse cultures (Mohanty, 2013). White parents frequently report not having a person of color in their lives to confide in and receive guidance from about race-related issues (Dolan, 2015). White parents having more frequent contact with people of color and endorsing less colorblind beliefs are more likely to expose their children to their birth culture (Hrapczynski & Leslie, 2018). However, mere exposure to diverse groups does not necessarily result in transracial adoptees developing meaningful connections with other people of color.

Steinberg and Hall (2000) defined ethnic socialization as consisting of three objectives: (a) developing an understanding of one's culture of origin, (b) learning and understanding how to function in majority society, and (c) acquiring ways to deal with racism and xenophobia. Mohanty and Newhill (2008) added that ethnic socialization is a process by which primary caregivers teach children about their race, ethnicity, and culture. Many adoptive parents may themselves be very interested in learning about their adopted child's ethnicity and culture. These definitions of ethnic socialization directly overlap with the definition of racial socialization.

## Transracial Socialization

According to Barn (2013), children of color are less likely to experience racial or ethnic socialization to their culture of origin without a minority parent. This is of particular concern for transracial adoptees raised in dominant White cultures and spaces. White adoptive parents raising adoptees of color have the added responsibility to prepare their children not only for the adoption-related challenges that await them but also for the highly racialized social situations that the children will inevitably be exposed to through everyday interactions at school and in the community. Without developmentally appropriate discussion and preparation for bias, racial/ethnic discrimination, and xenophobia, children will grow up lacking the tools and resources to navigate the murky waters of school, work, the community, and even social media.

Reynolds et al. (under review) interviewed eight transracial Chinese adoptees adopted by families in the northeastern United States about their experiences with racial, ethnic, and cultural socialization practices. Across the sample, adoptees reported that their White adoptive parents incorporated some level of cultural and ethnic socialization practices (i.e., enrolling the adoptee in Chinese language lessons, "return" trips to China, learning about and participating in Chinese holidays and cuisine, watching documentaries featuring Chinese history, and/or purposefully living in the Chinatown area of their city). Participants discussed the importance of finding a balance between being provided cultural learning opportunities and being forced to engage in cultural learning. Participants indicated that they would have preferred to be offered more options and to have more agency about participating in cultural and ethnicity-based practices growing up. Additionally, participants reported that their parents did not engage in "race talk" with them while growing up and, therefore, they were not prepared for racial bias and discrimination. In the rare instances that the adoptees did share experiences of racial discrimination with their adoptive parents, the parents were not well versed in how to respond in supportive ways, often minimizing, dismissing, or attempting to empathize with the child's experience of marginalization despite being White. Thus, adoptive parents may be actively engaged in ethnic socialization while ignoring the racial socialization of their child.

## CLINICAL IMPLICATIONS

There are many important factors to consider for parents, clinicians, teachers, and others working with transracial adoptive families. Given that a large proportion of domestic adoptions and the overwhelming majority of international adoptions are transracial, it is imperative that individuals working with adoptees and their families learn about racial identity development as well as the history of racism and institutional discrimination. In addition, it is important to keep in mind that there is no one-size-fits-all manual for how to work with transracially adopted individuals. While one's adoptive status should be recognized as an important aspect of identity, affecting the adoptee in many conscious and unconscious ways, it must not be overemphasized. Instead, the various intersections of identity (e.g., race, ethnicity, gender, sexual orientation, ability, socioeconomic status, religion, age, geographic location, documentation status) must be considered. These dimensions significantly impact an adoptee's lived experience (e.g., a Black, heterosexual, cisgender female adoptee adopted at age 5 by a White middle-class Baptist family in rural Oklahoma, versus a South Asian of Indian descent, gay, transgender male adoptee adopted at 5 months by an upper-middle-class Jewish White family in Washington, DC). Salient aspects of identity may fluctuate over the course of an individual's life.

Another important recommendation is that White adoptive parents who adopt children of color engage in self-exploration and continue to develop in their multicultural journey. Adopting a child of color requires considerable lifelong reflection and acknowledgment of institutional racism and discrimination, an experience White parents may never have had to deal with personally. Parents can prepare for this by reading about adoption and critical discourse, watching documentaries about adoption and the history of race relations in the United States, and maintaining diverse friendships. Developing a critical consciousness about the world will undoubtedly help in understanding some of the challenges an adoptee of color may be experiencing in predominantly White families, communities, and school spaces. Being in touch with school counselors and psychologists may also be important, as these trained professionals may help ease the transition for the adopted child and, more broadly, raise awareness of adoption experiences for teachers and other professionals in the school community.

Preliminary research has also explored the importance of the naming process for adoptees. The majority of individuals adopted earlier in life experience name changes at the time of adoption; most commonly, they are given an Anglicized name chosen by the adoptive parents. This change often represents a loss of connection to race, ethnicity, and culture, and may lead to questions regarding one's name and even increase the likelihood that the adoptee experiences microaggressions related to their name not "matching" their ascribed racial and ethnic background (Reynolds et al., 2017). Thus, it is recommended that adoptive parents seriously consider the long-term impact that changing the adoptee's name may have on the adoptee.

It is recommended that adoptive parents provide adopted children with opportunities to learn about their culture of origin and country of birth (if born outside the United States) in as many ways as possible (e.g., culture camps, language lessons, cultural celebrations, movies/documentaries, books, foods) while avoiding cultural exoticization and appropriation. Research has suggested that an overemphasis on birth culture as well as racial and ethnic identity differences early in life may negatively impact adoptee psychological well-being (Mohanty, 2015). Therefore, finding some balance or middle ground is recommended, as well as being patient and supportive of the adopted individual's decision to engage or not. In addition, ensuring that transracial adoptees have access to other transracial adoptees and individuals who look like them (e.g., diverse peers and mentors from their community) and seeking therapists who are experts on transracial adoption may help facilitate the adoptee's development.

## CASE VIGNETTE

Jenn Hall is a 33-year-old, heterosexual, cisgender female who was born in Seoul, South Korea. Her biological mother became pregnant with Jenn out of wedlock, and due to cultural stigma and lack of government support for single mothers in Korea in the 1980s, her biological mother decided that at birth she would place her child with Holt Adoption Agency. Jenn (originally named Minjee Kim) was born full term and healthy and was placed in foster care for 3 months while she awaited placement. Minjee Kim was adopted by a loving Christian family in a small town outside of Potsdam, New York in 1985. They changed her name to Jenn Hall. She was raised in a family of four, with one older brother (John), the biological child of Jenn's adoptive parents. Jenn's parents (Tom and Kelly) had always been interested in the idea of adoption. After having significant difficulties becoming pregnant and a series of birth-related complications with John, they decided to move forward with international adoption.

Jenn was generally a happy child. She was a well-rounded student, excelling in her academic and extracurricular activities, which included music, sports, and school clubs. In addition, Jenn was actively involved in her church community. Despite these positive supports and her forward trajectory in life, Jenn experienced many challenges growing up in Potsdam. In addition to being one of the only people of color in her school and community, she also recognized from very early on that she was one of the only Korean and Asian individuals in her school. On top of that, it was rare that she saw any type of media representation of people who looked like her, with the exception of stereotypes about Asians (e.g., Asians performing martial arts, "model minority" representations of Asians, Asians being good at math, exotic docile Asian women married to White men). While she was somewhat curious about Asian and Korean cultures, she did not feel a strong connection to them, nor did she have any access to learning about her birth culture. The only other people in her town who were of Asian descent were a Chinese family that owned a Chinese restaurant and a South Asian family with two children in the neighboring town who had emigrated from India. Thus, Jenn's upbringing in a White, middle-class, Christian home without any exposure to Asian or Korean cultures led to her internalizing a White consciousness and perception of the world. Jenn's parents were very supportive of her, and were relatively open with Jenn about her adoption story, given the limited information they received from her adoption paperwork. However, her parents largely practiced a colorblind approach ("I don't see race") in raising both Jenn and John.

While it is common for children of color adopted by White parents to integrate into mainstream White American culture, Jenn, like many others in her situation, also experienced dissonance related to her racial and ethnic identity. Jenn felt White inside, although she recognized that she was different on the outside and was quite self-conscious about her Asian physical traits. In addition, she lacked Asian role models or mentoring within her family, school, or community, as well as any positive reinforcement of her physical attributes through the media. Over time, this led to a core belief that she was less physically attractive than her White counterparts, as well as a dislike of herself, particularly the Asian parts of herself (i.e., internalized racism). It also manifested in a distancing from all activities and behaviors that made her "Asianness" stand out from others, including interactions with other Asian people. Throughout high school, Jenn had multiple long-term romantic relationships with White males.

Jenn attended college at a state university in New York a few hours from her hometown. The college was relatively small, and, while there were other Asian students at her school, the majority of them were either international students or from families that had recently immigrated to the United States. Jenn felt little to no connection with them given her lack of cultural and linguistic literacy, as well as her limited racial and ethnic socialization. In college, she majored in Secondary Education and English, and pledged at a sorority, in which she was the only woman of Asian descent. During her junior year, she met Peter, a White male, and the two became romantically involved. After graduating, Jenn accepted a teaching position in Albany. When Peter and Jenn relocated to Albany, Peter found employment in business.

Four years after graduation at the age of 26, the two were happily married. Jenn kept her maiden name. The two worked for several years and attended graduate school part time, Jenn receiving a Master's of Education in Teaching and Peter a Master's of Business Administration. Although Jenn was relatively open about her adoptive status, she became increasingly frustrated when she had to explain her lack of Korean linguistic abilities and lack of connection to Korean culture, particularly when meeting new people in graduate school and work environments. In addition, she grew tired of explaining her Anglicized American name, as it did not "match" her racial appearance. Around the age of 30, Jenn and Peter decided they wanted to start a family. Both pregnancies were healthy and full term. Jenn and John welcomed two children, David and Mary, into the world 2 years apart.

Following her second pregnancy with Mary, Jenn experienced some postpartum depression. It was recommended that Jenn see a counselor. In her first experience in treatment at the age of 33, she began to explore some challenges she had had in life, including those related to adoption and navigating the experience of having biracial children. Throughout this significant, albeit short-term 10-session experience, she began to become interested in exploring Korean culture and her adoption background. Through online group forums, she connected with other Korean adoptees and local adoptees in the Albany area. This was profound, as she began to learn about the long and complicated history of adoption between Korea and the United States and other Western nations. She slowly began to gain a critical consciousness about the world, becoming interested in combating institutionalized racism and fighting for social justice. In addition, she began considering a return trip to Korea and a birth family search, as other adoptees spoke of their own searches and, in some cases, reunification with their birth families. While Jenn was excited to reconnect with her roots and join a community by she felt fully understood, she recognized the increasing distance this placed between her and Peter, as well as between her and her adoptive parents and many of her friends. They were a bit hurt and could not fully understand why Jenn was interested in reconnecting to her roots at this phase in her life. Some were in disbelief that Jenn had experienced racism throughout her life. Thus, Jenn decided to seek out a long-term therapist to help her further reflect on and process some of her experiences.

## Discussion Questions

- As a counselor/therapist, what are some of the most important factors to consider?
- What could you do to take a strengths-based adoption-competent approach when working with Jenn?
- How do you support Jenn in her desire to reconnect with her Korean/Asian heritage?
- How might you help Jenn explore her racial, ethnic, and cultural identity development as a 33-year-old married woman with two biracial children and a White partner?
- How might you assist Jenn in exploring her connection to her names, specifically the name her adoptive parents gave her that frequently resulted in questions and assumptions, as well as her Korean birth name and the meaning that Jenn ascribes to this name?

## REFERENCES

Arnold, T., Braje, S. E., Kawahara, D., & Shuman, T. (2016). Ethnic socialization, perceived discrimination, and psychological adjustment among transracially adopted and non-adopted ethnic minority adults. *American Journal of Orthopsychiatry, 86*(5), 540–551. https://doi.org/10.1037/ort0000172

Baden, A. (2016). "Do you know your real parents?" and other adoption microaggressions. *Adoption Quarterly, 19*(1), 1–25. doi:10.1080/10926755.2015.1026012

Baden, A. L., & Steward, R. J. (2007). The cultural-racial identity model: A theoretical framework for studying transracial adoptees. In R. A. Javier, A. L. Baden, F. A. Biafora, & A. Camacho-Gingerich (Eds.), *Handbook of adoption: Implications for researchers, practitioners, and families* (pp. 90–112). Thousand Oaks, CA: Sage Publications, Inc.

Barn, R. (2013). "Doing the right thing": Transracial adoption in the U.S.A. *Ethnic and Racial Studies, 36*(8), 1273–1291. doi:10.1080/01419870.2013.770543

Barnes, A. R., Constantine Brown, J. L., & McCarty-Caplan, D. (2019). The unintended consequences of the Indian Child Welfare Act: American Indian trust in public child welfare. *Children and Youth Services Review, 98*, 221–227. doi:10.1016/j.childyouth.2019.01.012

Bergquist, K. J. S., Campbell, M. E., & Unrau, Y. A. (2003). Caucasian parents and Korean adoptees: A survey of parents' perceptions. *Adoption Quarterly, 6*(4), 41–58. doi:10.1300/J145v06n04_03

Brown, T. N., Tanner-Smith, E., Lesane-Brown, C. L., & Ezell, M. E. (2007). Child, parent, and situational correlates of familial ethnic/race socialization. *Journal of Marriage and Family, 69*(1), 14–25. doi:10.1111/j.1741-3737.2006.00340.x

Chang, D. F., Feldman, K., & Easley, H. (2017). "I'm learning not to tell you": Korean transracial adoptees' appraisals of parental racial socialization strategies and perceived effects. *Asian American Journal of Psychology, 8*(4), 308–322. doi:10.1037/aap0000091

Davis, M. A. (2011). Intercountry adoption flows from Africa to the U.S.: A fifth wave of intercountry adoptions? *International Migration Review, 45*(4), 784-811. doi:10.1111/j.1747-7379.2011.00868.x

Dolan, J. H. (2015). How White adoptive parents of Asian-born youth talk about racism within the family. *Journal of Social Distress and the Homeless, 24*(2), 81–92. doi:10.1179/1053078915Z.00000000025

Donaldson Adoption Institute. (2009). *Beyond culture camp: Promoting healthy identity formation in adoption.* Retrieved from https://affcny.org/wp-content/uploads/2009_11_BeyondCultureCamp.pdf

Donaldson Adoption Institute. (2011). *Adoption Institute e-newsletter.* Retrieved from http://www.adoptioninstitute.org/old/newsletter/2011_04.html

Dowling, M., & Brown, G. (2009). Globalization and international adoption from China. *Child & Family Social Work, 14*(3), 352–361. doi:10.1111/j.1365-2206.2008.00607.x

Engel, M. H., Phillips, N. K., & DellaCava, F. A. (2012). Indigenous children's rights: A sociological perspective on boarding schools and transracial adoption. *International Journal of Children's Rights, 20*, 279–299. doi:10.1163/157181811X612873

Garber, K. J., & Grotevant, H. D. (2015). "YOU Were Adopted?!": Microaggressions toward adolescent adopted individuals in same-race families. *The Counseling Psychologist, 43*(3), 435–462. doi:10.1177/0011000014566471

Goss, D. R., Byrd, W. C., & Hughey, M. W. (2017). Racial authenticity and familial acceptance among transracial adoptees: A bothersome bargain of belonging. *Symbolic Interaction, 40*(2), 147–168. doi:10.1002/symb.282

Harrison, A. O., Wilson, M., Pine, C. J., Chan, S., & Buriel, R. (1990). Family ecologies of ethnic minority children. *Children Development, 61*, 347–367. doi:10.1111/j.1467-8624.1990.tb02782.x

Hesketh, T., Lu, L., & Xing, Z. W. (2005). The effect of China's one-child family policy after 25 years. *New England Journal of Medicine, 353*(11), 1171–1176. doi:10.1056/NEJMhpr051833

Hrapczynski, K. M., & Leslie, L. A. (2018). Engagement in racial socialization among transracial adoptive families with White parents. *Family Relations, 67*(3), 354–367. doi:10.1111/fare.12316

Jacobs, M. D. (2013). Remembering the "forgotten child": The American Indian child welfare crisis of the 1960s and 1970s. *American Indian Quarterly, 37*(1–2), 137–159. doi:10.5250/amerindiquar.37.1-2.0136

Kim, E. J. (2010). *Adopted territory: Transnational Korean adoptees and the politics of belonging.* Durham, NC: Duke University Press.

Kim, O. M., Reichwald, R., & Lee, R. (2013). Cultural socialization in families with adopted Korean adolescents: A mixed-method, multi-informant study. *Journal of Adolescent Research, 28*(1), 69–95. doi:10.1177/0743558411432636

Kirk, H. D. (1984). *Shared fate.* Port Angeles, WA: Ben-Simon.

Kreider, R. M., & Lofquist, D. A. (2014). Adopted children and stepchildren: 2010. *United States Census Bureau.* Retrieved from https://www.census.gov/content/dam/Census/library/publications/2014/demo/p20-572.pdf

Langrehr, K. J. (2014). Transracially adoptive parents' color-blind attitudes and views toward socialization: Cross-racial friendships as a moderator. *Cultural Diversity and Ethnic Minority Psychology, 20*(4), 601–610. doi:10.1037/a0036528

Langrehr, K. J., Yoon, E., Hacker, J., & Caudill, K. (2015). Implications of transnational adoption status for adult Korean adoptees. *Journal of Multicultural Counseling and Development, 43*(1), 6–24. doi:10.1002/j.2161-1912.2015.00061.x

Lee, R. M. (2003). The transracial adoption paradox: History, research, and counseling implications of cultural socialization. *Counseling Psychology, 31*(6), 711–744. doi:10.1177/0011000003258087

Lee, B. J. (2007). Adoption in Korea: Current status and future prospects. *International Journal of Social Welfare, 16*(1), 75–83. doi:10.1111/j.1468-2397.2006.00421.x

Ma, K. (2017). Korean intercountry adoption history: Culture, practice, and implications. *Families in Society: The Journal of Contemporary Social Services, 98*(3), 243–251. doi:10.1606/1044-3894.2017.98.25

McRoy, R., & Griffin, A. (2012). Transracial adoption policies and practices: The U.S. experience. *Adoption & Fostering, 36*(3–4), 38–49. doi:10.1177/030857591203600305

Mohanty, J. (2013). Ethnic and racial socialization and self-esteem of Asian adoptees: The mediating role of multiple identities. *Journal of Adolescence, 36*(1), 161–170. doi:10.1016/j.adolescence.201210.003

Mohanty, J. (2015). Ethnic identity and psychological well-being of international transracial adoptees: A curvilinear relationship. In E. E. Pinderhughes & R. Rosnati (Eds.), *Adoptees' ethnic identity within family and social contexts. New Directions for Child and Adolescent Development, 150*, 33–45. doi:10.1002/cad.20117

Mohanty, J., & Newhill, C. (2008). A theoretical framework for understanding ethnic socialization among international adoptees. *Families in Society: The Journal of Contemporary Social Services, 89*(4), 543–550. doi:10.1606/1044-3894.3817

Montgomery, J. E., & Jordan, N. A. (2018). Racia–ethnic socialization and transracial adoptee outcomes: A systematic research synthesis. *Child and Adolescent Social Work Journal, 35*(5), 439–458. doi:10.1007/s10560-018-0514-9

Morgan, S. K., & Langrehr, K. J. (2018). Transracially adoptive parents' colorblindness and discrimination recognition: Adoption stigma as moderator. *Cultural Diversity and Ethnic Minority Psychology, 25*(2), 242–252. doi:10.1037/cdp0000219

National Association of Black Social Workers. (2013). *Position statement on trans-racial adoptions*. Retrieved from https://cdn.ymaws.com/www.nabsw.org/resource/collection/E1582D77-E4CD-4104-996A-D42D08F9CA7D/NABSW_Trans-Racial_Adoption_1972_Position_(b).pdf

Oh, A. H. (2012). From war waif to ideal immigrant: The Cold War transformation of the Korean orphan. *Journal of American Ethnic History, 31*(4), 34–55. doi:10.5406/jamerethnhist.31.4.0034

Raleigh, E. (2016). The color line exception: The transracial adoption of foreign-born and biracial Black children. *Women, Gender, and Families of Color, 4*(1), 86–107. https://doi.org/10.5406/womgenfamcol.4.1.0086

Reynolds, J. D., Elimelech, N. T., Miller, S. P., Anton, B. M., Bhattacharjee, C., & Ingraham, M. E. (under review). A qualitative exploration of names, identity, and transracial socialization for Chinese American adoptees.

Reynolds, J. D., Kim, O. M., & Ponterotto, J. G. (2019). Authenticity among adult transracial Korean adoptees: The influences of identity, thoughts about birth family, and multicultural personality dispositions. *Journal of Asia Pacific Counseling, 19*(1), 21–37. doi:10.18401/2019.9.1.2

Reynolds, J. D., Ponterotto, J. G., & Lecker, C. (2016). Displacement, identity, and belonging for Ibyangin: The personal journey of transracial Korean-born adoptees. *The Qualitative Report, 21*(2), 228–251. Retrieved from https://nsuworks.nova.edu/tqr/vol21/iss2/5

Reynolds, J. D., Ponterotto, J. G., Park-Taylor, J., & Takooshian, H. (2017, November 27). Transracial identities: The meaning of names and the process of name reclamation for Korean American adoptees. *Qualitative Psychology*. Advance online publication. doi:10.1037/qup0000115

Robinson, L. (2012). Identity development and transracial/ethnic adoption: Some challenges for practice. *Asia Pacific Journal of Social Work and Development, 22*(1–2), 116–126. doi:10.1080/02185385.2012.681150

Roemer, N. R. (2019). Finding harmony or swimming in the void: The unavoidable conflict between the interstate compact on the placement of children and the Indian Child Welfare Act. *North Dakota Law Review, 94*, 149–180.

Selman, P. (2002). Intercountry adoption in the new millennium; the "quiet migration" revisited. *Population Research and Policy Review, 21*(3), 205–225. doi:10.1023/A:1019583625626

Selman, P. (2009). The rise and fall of intercountry adoption in the 21st century. *International Social Work, 52*(5), 575–594. doi:10.1177/0020872809337681

Selman, P. (2015). Intercountry adoption of children from Asia in the twenty-first century. *Children's Geographies, 13*(3), 312–327. doi:10.1080/14733285.2015.972657

Spence, M. T. (2013). "Whose stereotypes and racial myths? The National Urban League and the 1950s Roots of color-blind adoption policy." *Women, Gender, and Families of Color, 1,* 143–179. https://doi.org/10.5406/womgenfamcol.1.2.0143

Steinberg, G., & Hall, B. (2000). *Inside transracial adoption.* Indianapolis, IN: Perspective Press.

Sue, D. W., Capodilupo, C. M., Torino, G. C., Bucceri, J. M., Holder, A. M. B., Nadal, K. L., & Esquilin, M. (2007). Racial microaggressions in everyday life: Implications for clinical practice. *American Psychologist, 62*(4), 271–286. doi:10.1037/0003-066X.62.4.271

Sweeney, K. A., & Pollack, R. L. (2017). Colorblind individualism, color consciousness, and the Indian Child Welfare Act: Representations of adoptee best interest in newspaper coverage of the baby Veronica case. *The Sociological Quarterly, 58*(4), 701–720. doi:10.1080/00380253.2017.1331717

U.S. Department of Health and Human Services. (2015). Adoption and foster care analysis and reporting system (AFCARS) report number 22 FY 2014. *Children's Bureau.* Retrieved from http://www.acf.hhs.gov

U.S. Department of State—Bureau of Consular Affairs. (2017). [Graph illustration and chart of adoption statistics 1999-2016]. *Adoption statistics.* Retrieved from https://travel.state.gov/content/travel/en/Intercountry-Adoption/adopt_ref/adoption-statistics.html

Vandivere, S., Malm, K., & Radel, L (2009). *Adoption USA: A chartbook based on the 2007 National Survey of Adoptive Parents.* Washington, DC: U.S. Department of Health and Human Services, Office of the Assistant Secretary for Planning and Evaluation. Retrieved from https://aspe.hhs.gov/pdf-report/adoption-usa-chartbook-based-2007-national-survey-adoptive-parents

# 4

# The DSM-5 From a Multicultural Perspective

*Betty Garcia and Zsuzsanna Monika Feher*

## INTRODUCTION

Effective diagnostic practice requires knowledge of the *Diagnostic and Statistical Manual of Mental Disorders, Fifth Edition* (*DSM-5*), as well as strong engagement skills in implementing a process that thoughtfully explores disorder criteria in relation to the unique factors, psychological and contextual, related to the client's experience. In the best of all worlds, effective practice is characterized by a quality of client participation that supports joint decision-making by the client and the clinician on diagnostic considerations. Clarity on the client's clinical issues are particularly challenging in situations where there are differences between the clinician and client; for example, in relation to ethnicity, social identity, socioeconomic status, privilege, and target status. The U.S. Census Bureau projects that by "2044, more than half of all Americans are projected to belong to a minority group" (Colby & Ortman, 2015, p. 1), "and by 2060, 29% of the United States is projected to be Hispanic—more than one quarter of the population" (Colby & Ortman, 2015, p. 9).

Current data show the Latinx[1] population represented 58.6 million out of the 325,344 million U.S. population in 2017, making it the second largest ethnic population in the United States (Krogstad, 2017). These data and projections heighten the necessity of clinicians to be prepared to practice with Latinx and diverse others as clients. For one, the heterogeneity within the Latinx population highlights a wide range of generational, socioeconomic, and psychosocial factors. The differences within the Latinx population result in diversity in social identity (e.g., traditional and/or dominant culture identifications) based on length of time the family has been in the United States and other identifications arising from

---

[1] Latinx refers to Latino and Latina individuals; here it is used interchangeably with Hispanic and Latinx, and refers to individuals of Spanish language heritage from the Americas and the Caribbean.

lived experience; for example, related to gender identity, social media, and popular culture. The idea of forming and testing hypotheses (Sue, Zane, Nagayama Hall, & Berger, 2009) in clinical assessment is particularly useful for clinicians as they form impressions based on cultural knowledge that are then systematically applied and altered to their perception of the client as the client's complexity becomes clear. The Latinx population in the United States is highly diverse based on multiple factors related to immigrant status, generation in the United States, and acculturation, to name a few variables.

Attention to the client's language preference, social identity, and acculturation level are critical in making what might have been invisible, visible. Assumptions about a first-generation client's (i.e., immigrant) sole identification with their traditional culture could lead to stereotyping the client and miss what potentially could be a source of stress.

This chapter focuses on clinical practice with Latinx women, with particular attention to immigrant status. We highlight diversity and contextual factors such as globalization and intersectionality that are helpful to grasp and explore in clinical practice. The Diversity/Resilience Formulation (DRF) (Petrovich & Garcia, 2016) is presented as a format for systematically exploring a client's strengths. Its application to a case study is discussed. First, in line with presenting clinical issues within a contextual framework, we will review Latinx and immigration demographics and then proceed to discuss globalization, intersectionality, and acculturation. The interrelationship of these factors is discussed for the purpose of proposing clinical considerations.

## LATINX POPULATION DEMOGRAPHICS

According to the Pew Research Center analysis of 2014 U.S. Census Bureau data, in the United States, Hispanics were the youngest major ethnic group, with 17.9 million, a third, under the age of 18, and 14.6 million, a quarter of all Hispanics, Millennials, meaning between the ages of 18 and 33 (Patten, 2016). Pew Research Center research highlights key Latinx population facts, such as young Latinxs are largely U.S. born; Latinxs account for a quarter of the nation's 54 million K-12 students in 2016; 14% of Americans aged 18–35 with Hispanic ancestry do not identify as Hispanic; and English use is on the rise among young Hispanics, even though approximately 60% of the youth say they use Spanish (Lopez, Krogstad, & Flores, 2018).

In 2017, according to Pew Research Center estimates, 11.6 million, a quarter of all U.S. immigrants, came from Mexico, there are less than 5 million non-documented immigrants from Mexico, which is a 2 million drop since 2007, and they comprise less than half of all U.S. unauthorized immigrants (Gonzalez-Barrera & Krogstad, 2019). Based on the data by the U.S. Department of Homeland Security, in 2017, out of the 1,127,167 people obtaining lawful permanent resident status, 424,743 people's country of birth was Asia, and respectively, 413,650, North America; 118,824, Africa; 84,335, Europe; 79,076, South America; and 5,071, Oceania. Moreover, in 2017, 1,127,167 of these individuals who received new permanent residency, 170,581 people were born in Mexico, 71,565 in China, 65,028 in Cuba, 60,394 in India, 58,520 in the Dominican Republic, and 49,147 in the Philippines (U.S. Department of Homeland Security, 2019). In 2017, a total of

53,691 refugees arrived in the United States; of these, 26,648 came from Asia, 20,248 from Africa, 5,026 from Europe, 1,455 from North America, and 233 from South America (U.S. Department of Homeland Security, 2019). These data highlight the reduction in immigration from Mexico, the demographics of legal immigration and refugee status, and assist in placing perspective on where Mexican and Central American immigrants fit into the larger immigration picture.

## GLOBALIZATION

The reality of immigration as a large scale, global phenomenon suggests that some understanding of globalization and its role in influencing immigration is necessary. Globalization was originally viewed in relation to the first and second globalization, respectively of finance and trade between 1870 and 1914, and in the 1970s (Piketty, 2014). Mullaly's (2007, p. 189) review of Giddens (1998) discussion points out that the second globalization "include[d] the development of the knowledge economy, telecommunications technology, and the decline in traditional social identities." That viewpoint would most likely include social media and other engaging technologies such as Facebook, Twitter, and Instagram.

The recent view of globalization is more diverse and diffuse and includes dynamic and multidirectional relationships. Sen (2009, pp. 172–173) observed that globalization leads us to find ourselves in "a new neighborhood" and that this status links us all, internationally, through "trade, commerce, literature, language, music, arts, entertainment, religion, medicine, healthcare, politics, news reports, media communications and other ties." The specific relevance of globalization for human service providers, including clinicians, is articulated in three publications on The Global Agenda for Social Work and Social Development, which focuses on the need to "provide equitable standards of decent well-being for the whole of the world's population" (International Association of Schools of Social Work, International Council on Social Welfare, and International Federation of Social Workers, 2014, p. 3). These publications focus on promoting social and economic equalities, promoting the dignity and worth of peoples, and promoting community and environmental sustainability. A subsequent publication, referred to as the fourth pillar, is intended to focus on the importance of human relationships (International Association of Schools of Social Work, International Council on Social Welfare, and International Federation of Social Workers, 2014).

## IMMIGRATION IN A GLOBAL PERSPECTIVE

Understanding immigration to the United States as part of a larger global phenomenon can assist clinicians in putting perspective on comprehending the subjective experience of their clients. According to the United Nation's International Migration Report (United Nations, Department of Economic and Social Affairs, Population Division [UN DESA], 2017), there was an estimated 258 million international migrants worldwide in 2017, 105 million more than in 1990, which is a 69% increase. In 2017, international migrants accounted for 3.4% of the world's population, compared to 2.9% in 1990. In 2017, the largest number of international migrants was living in Asia (80 million), 89% of whom were born in other Asian countries. Europe hosted 78 million, the second largest number of international migrants in 2017. North America hosted the third largest number of international migrants in 2017 (58 million), followed by Africa (25 million), Latin America and the Caribbean (10 million), and Oceania (8 million) (UN DESA, 2017). Clearly, immigration has been on the rise and continues to grow on a global level.

In Europe and North America, international migrants' countries of origins showed diversified patterns. In North America, 16 million out of the 30 million international migrants from 1990 to 2017 were born in Latin America and the Caribbean, 11 million from Asia, and over 2 million from Africa (UN DESA, 2017).

More than half (51%) of all international migrants were living in 10 countries. The largest number of migrants (49.8 million), nearly a fifth of the world total, resided in the United States. The second and third largest number of migrants were hosted by Saudi Arabia and Germany (12.2 million each), a fourth by Federation of the United Kingdom of Great Britain and Northern Ireland (nearly 8.8 million), and the United Arab Emirates (8.3 million), followed by France, Canada, Australia, and Spain (UN DESA, 2017).

The scale of immigration on a global level highlights the importance of clinicians exploring the motivation for the immigration as well as recognizing their feelings, perceptions, and countertransference that are evoked in their work with immigrants. It is recognized that the majority of immigration is motivated by war, poverty, drought, drug cartel activity, violence, and other factors that put the individual and their family at risk if they were to remain in their country of origin.

## INTERSECTIONALITY

Intersectionality highlights the unique constellation of various group membership identities that combine into an individual's social identity and recognition of the discrimination, marginalization, privilege, and target status experienced by individuals based on their social identity (Crenshaw, 1991). O'Neal and Beckman (2017) discussed the intersections of race, ethnicity, and gender, emphasizing the cultural, socioeconomic, and legal barriers to social services that Latinx female victims of intimate partner violence (IPV) face. They emphasized the importance of race, ethnicity, and the gender intersectional framework in IPV research, and emphasized the National Intimate Partner and Sexual Violence Survey (NISVS) result, that 37% have experienced IPV in their lifetime (Black et al., 2011). O'Neal and Beckman (2017) described cultural barriers that Latinx female IPV victims experience in connection to social services experiences, such as language, social isolation, and gender norms, via gender, race, and ethnicity. For example, language barriers may stop Latinx women from reporting IPV, while social and gender norms may isolate IPV victims; some victims are physically isolated as well. Additionally, there are socioeconomic barriers, such as educational attainment, unemployment, poverty, and distribution of resources in conjunction with gender, race, and ethnicity (O'Neal & Beckman, 2017).

The 2018 U.S. Census Bureau Educational Attainment data of the adult population on Latinx indicate the low proportion of Latinx individuals with degrees in higher education. Out of the 51,406,000 baccalaureate degree holders 18 years of age or older, there were 40,818,000 White individuals, 4,765,000 Hispanics, 4,731,000 Blacks and 4,673,000 Asians. Out of 21,280,000 master's degree holders in the same population, there were 16,560,000 Whites, 2,464,000 Asians, 1,910,000 Blacks, and 1,397,000 Hispanics. Out of 4,487,000 doctoral degrees, 3,403,000 were White, 686,000 Asians, 326,000 Blacks, and 196,000 Hispanics, retrospectively (U.S. Census Bureau, 2019).

A number of contextual factors such as poverty, legal and financial barriers to citizenship, and fear of deportation can undermine access to options. Other factors that create potentially insurmountable hurdles are law enforcement, anti-immigration beliefs and laws, and racial and ethnic discrimination (O'Neal & Beckman, 2017). Clinical practice that incorporates an intersectionality approach promotes exploring the presence of these combined factors, and supporting the client informs individuals as understanding the effects of and their choices in relation to IPV, victimization, and justice processes. It is essential for IPV victims to have support and affirmation in receiving services as the bureaucratic processes can potentially make them vulnerable to abuse as the proof of victimization is established (O'Neal & Beckman, 2017).

O'Neal and Beckman (2017) stated that IPV services need to follow the complex needs of Latinx populations and recommended greater numbers of social service providers and increased future research as well as culturally competent law enforcement, IPV shelters and programs, establishing support networks, and finally, Collaborative Community Response (CCR) and Community-Based Participatory Research (CBPR).

Intersectionality and globalization contribute perspectives that enhance understanding the complexity of Latinx by illuminating the multitude of contextual factors that comprise their lived experience. These two concepts highlight the importance of clinicians avoiding assumptions about the Latinx population based on documented, undocumented, or generational status, from the point of view of *DSM-5* diagnosis considerations and in identifying strengths.

## ACCULTURATION

The heterogeneity and social identities of Latinxs are influenced by numerous factors such as those discussed earlier (e.g., generation in the United States, level of education, economic and social status), as well as geographic region, gender identity, and disability status. Clinical understanding of a client's acculturation level may highlight that a Latinx social identity perhaps reflects traditional values; however, it could also be comprised of a wide variety of identifications that challenge making assumptions about someone who is Spanish language dominant. Acculturation refers to various distinctions and thus has different definitions. Sam and Berry (2010) described acculturation as a process of cultural and psychological changes that are the results of the meeting between cultures. Ferguson (2013, p. 249) defines acculturation as "what happens when groups or individuals of different cultures come into contact (continuous or intermittent, firsthand or indirect) with subsequent changes in the original culture patterns of one or more parties."

Ozer and Schwartz (2016) reviewed the history of acculturation models and found that the early initial *unidimensional models* referred to acculturation on a single continuum with two heritage cultures and receiving cultures on its extreme ends. Researchers then developed the *bi-dimensional model*, where acculturation processes were characterized along two dimensions, where individuals valued their relationship to their host culture and whether they valued their original identity (i.e., culture). Along these two dimensions they proposed four different acculturation possibilities: assimilation, integration, marginalization, and separation (Sam & Berry, 2010). Ryder, Alden, and Paulhus (2000) empirically demonstrated that the bi-dimensional model constitutes a broader more functional approach in comparison to the unidirectional model. Ozer and Schwartz's study (2016) created and validated a *tri-dimensional acculturation measure* to capture globalization-induced multicultural orientations in India. They studied acculturation processes, for example, that a student from a rural Indian area experienced in an urban setting. Results showed that the tri-dimensional acculturation scale significantly better fit this globalization-based acculturation data than the bi-directional acculturation scale due to capturing more of its complexity (Ozer & Schwartz, 2016).

Arnett (2002) referred to *globalization's* psychological consequences, stating that most people in the world now develop a bicultural identity, which involves their local identity and their identity tied to the global culture. Identity perplexity associated with globalization may escalate specifically among non-Western youth (Arnett, 2002). In their acculturation studies, Sam and Berry (2010) emphasized the general issue of treating individual-level and society-level acculturation characteristics separately. Ozer and Schwartz (2016) suggest that while the majority of acculturation studies focus on international migrants, such as immigrants, refugees, asylum seekers (Sam & Berry, 2010), it is important to distinguish between globalization and acculturation. Based on their review on acculturation studies, they agree with Arnett (2002) that globalization can generate acculturative change. Ozer and Schwartz (2016) pointed out Fergusson and Bornstein's (2017) view on different forms of cultural change, stating that globalization-based and remote acculturation differ from the classically studied immigration-based acculturation.

## Globalization, Acculturation, and Diversity

Ozer and Schwartz (2016) described globalization-based acculturation as global cultural streams without international migration, which refers to immigration-based acculturation. In their recent study, they added a third dimension, namely internal, within the same country, migration under the globalization-based type of acculturation. Kashima (2007) mentioned that the process of globalization often refers to a greater amount of and bigger volume interactions between those people who otherwise would only have limited knowledge of each other. Giddens (1991) described globalization as the "intensification of worldwide social relations which link distant localities in such a way that local events are shaped by events occurring many miles away and vice versa" (p. 64). Some scientists emphasized the risks of globalization, for example, growing uniformity and standardization, and inflaming cultural divisions and conflict (Kashima, 2007). Other researchers called teachers to be culturally self-aware, to teach globalization in schools (Buskist, Zuckerman, & Busler, 2012), to support the use of online technology in the classroom, to facilitate classroom interaction between the locals and students from overseas, and to encourage students' critical thinking about foreign and different perspectives (Velayo, 2012).

Some findings suggest that multicultural experiences make people more flexible, capable to analyze, and to solve problems from different cultural approaches (Chao, Kung, & Yao, 2015). Other studies found that these diverse experiences make people more close-minded and more likely to show hostility toward foreign cultures, which may be due to their perceived incompatibility and the "epistemic threat to individuals and the collectives that they belong to"; additionally, cultural conflicts may cause identity problems (Chao et al., 2015).

Globalization may be seen as a unifying force, while diversity highlights the differences between people. Based on conditioning theories within psychology, when people are taught to emphasize how they and their culture differ from others (ingroup/outgroup), they may get conditioned to these types of divergent viewpoints. Sociologists have initiated the integration of consensus theory, which focuses on social stability and shared values and norms (Kretchmar, 2014, p. 51). Dahrendorf described conflict theory, referring to unequal distribution of authority in all organizations, dividing those who are ruled and those who have authority and are dominant (Kretchmar, 2014, p. 50). Shared values may refer to globalization, while conflict theory emphasizes the diversity of power. The United Nations has emphasized the importance of balancing the benefits of integrating into a globalized world and protecting the uniqueness of local culture by facilitating "local resources, knowledge, skills and materials, creativity and sustainable progress" (United Nations, Educational Scientific and Cultural Organization [UNESCO], 2017). UNESCO (2017) also emphasized that respecting the diversity of cultures also "creates the conditions for mutual understanding, dialogue and peace."

Globalization affects our lives in extremely diffuse ways; not only is our material world affected by it but also our science, psychology, perception, emotions, cognitions, and behavior, as well as many aspects of our cultures and everyday lives. Ghosh (2011) summarized globalization-initiated cultural challenges in India and described its impact on consumer culture, mass media, knowledge, society, and popular culture, as well as the influence of technology such as mobile phones, the Internet, social networking, and increasing coverage of film and music, food diversity, cosmopolitan food, fashion, body appearance, and dress, mobility, risk, and rising disparity, referring to intensified processes, for example, the feminization of the workforce.

The study of modern globalization is in an early phase, which could lead people to question its existence. However, the question is not whether globalization exists, but how people need to approach it and deal with its impacts on their lives. For example, when a social worker or clinician has a client from an unfamiliar culture, acknowledging their own perception, feelings, and being aware of and accepting them may be the best first steps in order to establish a fruitful relationship with the client.

## CONTEXT OF CULTURALLY RELEVANT CLINICAL PRACTICE AND DIAGNOSTICS

A multicultural approach to a *DSM-5* diagnosis with a Latinx assumes an approach that is culturally relevant, recognizes the implications of intersectionality, globalization, and acculturation in the life of the client. This approach includes interpersonal engagement skills that reflect cultural competence and is characterized by a process that implements inquiry into multilevels of their experience on personal and intergenerational levels, and access to the other, that is, the clinician (Fowers & Davidov, 2006).

Culturally competent practice emphasizes development of effective skills, the significance of macro level, contextual factors such as the cultural proficiency of the organization within which clinicians work (Cross, Bazron, Dennis, & Issacs, 1989) and that it is not a status than can be achieved, but rather engages individuals in a life-long process about self and diversity. Conceptually, cultural humility (Mosher et al., 2017) furthers several perspectives in the cultural competence literature by highlighting cultural competency as a learning process, awareness of recognition of one's limitations, and awareness of the limits of their knowledge so as to recognize when to seek additional information (Tervalon & Murray-Garcia, 1998). Client perceptions of a clinician's cultural humility have been found to promote a therapeutic relationship and positive outcomes (Hook, Davis, Owen, Worthington, & Utsey, 2013). Tormala, Patel, Soukup, and Clarke (2018) found that pedagogy intended to improve cultural considerations in preparation of cultural formulations led to change that included greater perspective taking, awareness of intersectionality, and cultural self-awareness.

## DIAGNOSIS AND CULTURE

The significant role of culture as a core contextual factor in mental wellness and mental disorders requires that diagnostic assessments systematically explore the individual's subjective experience in relation to cultural influences, such as "values, orientations, knowledge and practices that individuals derive from membership in diverse social groups" (Lewis-Fernandez & Aggarwal, 2017, p. 2460). Lack of appreciation for an individual's various identifications and subjective experiences in relation to those identifications results in disembedding that person from their experience and thus making invisible to the clinician potentially significant information such as sources of resilience. Moreover, culture impacts an individual's openness to type and length of treatment (Lewis-Fernandez & Aggarwal, 2013). The purpose of the *DSM-5* Cultural Formulation Interview (CFI) is to provide a protocol that will assist clinicians in avoiding the pitfall of stereotyping clients, attending to contextual factors that affect how the symptomatic behavior is experienced and described, and making the individual's perspective on their symptoms a significant part of the diagnostic process.

Several crucial assumptions underlie a culturally relevant approach that include the use of interpreters in instances where clients are not English dominant and the clinician is not sufficiently conversant in the client's language. Also, in working with traditional culture families, it is essential to determine the significance of family involvement for that individual and their family. With practice with individuals from traditional cultures, it is essential to explore language preference and family involvement. Acculturation theory and globalization also highlight that the complexities of individuals remind us to inquire rather than make assumptions based on an individual's sociocultural profile.

Finally, a culturally relevant approach based on intersectionality emphasizes the importance of exploring the individual's cultural context that includes various dimensions such as gender identity, disability, ethnicity, race, nationality, religion, and socioeconomic class. For example, in relation to LGBTQ immigrant clients, intersectionality suggests exploring the combined effects of homophobia, xenophobia as well as threats of violence or violence in their current situation and in their country of origin, prior to immigration. Findings that LGBTQ youth are at greater risk for homelessness, mental health issues, and suicidality (Rhoades, Rusow, Bond, Lanteigne, Fulginiti, & Goldbach, 2018), and the significance for ethnic LGBTQ youth to have family support (Swendener & Woodell, 2017), highlight the importance of exploration of the LGBTQ individual's context. Also, Musicaro et al. (2019) recommend trauma-informed care for LGBTQ clients who may be polyvictims because of the threat of future revictimization.

## Diversity/Resilience Formulation

Petrovich and Garcia (2016) propose a DRF as a format to systematically develop a strength-based *DSM-5* diagnosis. The DRF proposes that where there are stressors, there are also corollary strengths, talents, and resources. The DRF complements the *DSM-5's* diagnostic dimension-driven format in the following domains:

A. *Intrapersonal:* Strengths, capabilities, interests, and talents, educational/occupational attainment, past successes and effective coping experiences, physical and emotional wellness practices such as exercise, healthy diet, and altruistic behaviors.
B. *Interpersonal:* Availability of support from family members, friendships, social life, and community network.
C. *Community*: Affiliation with and/or access to supportive, prosocial informal and formal networks and organizations.
D. *Spiritual*: Identification with spiritual beliefs/practices and/or formal religious organizations, spiritual leaders, and/or spiritual practices; perception of and ability to utilize support from these sources. The meaning-making aspect of spirituality is associated with beliefs, faith, and practices that provide a basis for ever significant hope. What hope is present and where does the person draw from for hope or a sense of wellness? What does the person hope for?
E. *Diversity:* Positive sources of self-definition and meaning as well as emotional and social support via diverse identifications (i.e., beliefs, values, and practices) and memberships. Depending on the cultural identification, there may be cultural leaders and healers as resources. All cultures have culture-specific definitions of strength and well-being and a framework for understanding symptoms and their expression. Occupational and other identity cultures (e.g., membership in the deaf community, participation in social action or community service networks or causes) can provide rich sources of personal and social empowerment to the individual.

## CASE VIGNETTE[2]

Maria is a recent immigrant to the United States. She arrived a month ago from a Central American country with her two daughters, age 7 and 11. At the Texas border, she was detained by Homeland Security Immigration and Customs Enforcement (ICE) for a month and her children were placed in a New York detention center. Upon release, she immediately went to the detention center in New York where her children were housed; however, the authorities would not release the children to her. Detention center staff informed her that the fingerprints her husband and her sister, who were in New York, had sent had not arrived. She was also asked for her own fingerprints. She felt exasperated, overwhelmed, and needing to get her children released quickly. She told staff "I need my children to be with me. My family has spent a month fighting to get my children released, and so far, it hasn't been possible. My family hasn't been able to do anything. My husband and my sister have come here several times, but they keep being told that the fingerprints haven't arrived yet. I am so worried about how my children are doing and I want to be with them. This separation is very difficult for my children and my suffering as a mother feels unbearable."

She was aware of the advocacy by many local and national groups on behalf of families like hers and asked for help from one of these groups, hoping to move the process along faster so that she and her children could be reunited quickly. She felt gratitude and wished she could personally say thank you to all who had a role in assisting her. She felt hope that they will continue their support for families like hers, so separated families can reunite quickly.

While going through the process of reconnecting with her children, Maria was referred by an advocacy agency to mental health services, because she had difficulty sleeping and was having crying spells. She was also preoccupied with memories of the violence that led to immigration as well as the threats she experienced and violence she observed on the journey to the United States. The pain of separation from her children at the border, not knowing where the children were or how they were doing, and the realization of the loss of hopefulness for a new life oftentimes felt unbearable.

In therapy, Maria reflected on her hope that support for families like hers will continue and could help move her process along. She also talked about how difficult the struggle is to get her children back and the disbelief she feels after coming to this country to seek protection, only to see how she and others have ended up. She tells the [clinician]:

> They've taken our children from us. This is so difficult, as a mother, I've been so hurt by what they've [U.S. officials] done to me, all because I left my country, fleeing from the gangs, after seeing family and friends killed. I sold my house to protect my children. I can't sleep, and have a hard time concentrating. And now, here, they've separated me from them. It's so hard living through this. . . . All I've asked for is compassion, and to the president, to give me my children back as soon as possible. That is what I need the most.

---

[2] The case vignette is derived and modified from a Democracy Now! 2019 story (Feltz, 2019).

As a refugee, Maria worried about many possible future hurdles such as not reuniting with relatives, expenses for DNA testing, concerns about fingerprints and their acceptance. In instances when parents reunite with their children, several challenges can arise regarding feelings of abandonment or attachment dynamics. And, developmental factors can play a role in children not remembering their parents or relatives. Worse yet, parents may have to decide whether they are going to return to their country of origin with their children or leave their children behind to face a separate asylum case in the United States.

## APPLICATION OF THE DRF TO *DSM-5* DIAGNOSIS

Consider how the DRF contributes to exploring and integrating relevant factors and dynamics that support acknowledging Maria's context and seeing her as a whole person. By integrating greater breadth and depth in these areas, the diagnostic process can address her uniqueness and value the diversity that she brings in relation to the dominate society as well as within the cultural groups that her social identity reflects. The following are some relevant clinical considerations that could come to form the DRF:

*Intrapersonal:* Hopeful, feels gratitude for assistance, commitment to her children, capacity for coping, and perseverance in the face of diversity, planning and follow through; also potential areas of interest (e.g., music, reading) or special skills (e.g., computer). It's not clear how much education she has or what employment she has had.

> *Interpersonal*: Close relationships with children, strong identity as a mother.
>
> *Community*: Close ties in her neighborhood and former neighbors.
>
> *Spiritual:* Catholic, strong sense of hopefulness and focusing on today what is possible in the present.
>
> *Diversity:* Strong identification with her nationality and with the United States as her new home. Places high value on traditional cultural healing processes for coping with and managing emotional pain such as that she has experienced via the numerous losses that she has experienced and could experience.

Other factors discussed in this chapter contribute additional perspectives that further illuminate Maria's complexity. *Intersectionality* highlights the necessity of exploring the various array of identifications Maria holds, their meaning for her, and her experience related to each of these regarding where she has felt target status (i.e., discrimination) and privilege (e.g., support by advocacy groups by virtue of connecting with them). *Acculturation* considerations direct us to explore the various combination of identifications that include her national and American culture. Her motivation to immigrate to the United States in part could be motivated by sharing values that she sees are embedded in the United States, as well as the necessity of escaping from violence. The Cultural Formulation Interview (CFI) emphasizes the necessity to see the client in their complexity and uniqueness, particularly in relation to contextual factors for the purpose of avoiding stereotyping the person. The CRF and CFI both promote utilizing an approach that affirms and includes the client's perspective on how they perceive and understand their symptoms. For instance, how do they talk to their friends about their symptoms?

## REFERENCES

Arnett, J. J. (2002). The psychology of globalization. *American Psychologist, 57*(10), 774–783. doi:10.1037/0003-066X.57.10.774

Black, M. C., Basile, K. C., Breiding, M. J., Smith, S. G., Walters, M. L., Merrick, M. T., . . . Stevens, M. R. (2011). *The National Intimate Partner and Sexual Violence Survey (NISVS): 2010 summary report.* Atlanta, GA: National Center for Injury Prevention and Control, Centers for Disease Control and Prevention.

Buskist, W., Zuckerman, C., & Busler, J. (2012). Globalization and the teaching of psychology: A call to action. *Psychology Learning & Teaching, 11*(3), 306–315. doi:10.2304/plat.2012.11.3.306

Chao, M. M., Kung, F. Y., & Yao, D. J. (2015). Understanding the divergent effects of multicultural exposure. *International Journal of Intercultural Relations, 47*, 78–88. doi:10.1016/j.ijintrel.2015.03.032

Colby, S. L., & Ortman, J. M. (2015). *Projections of the size and composition of the U.S. population: 2014 to 2060: Population estimates and projections.* Current population reports. U.S. Census Bureau. Retrieved from https://census.gov/content/dam/Census/library/publications/2015/demo/p25-1143.pdf

Crenshaw, K. (1991). Mapping the margins: Intersectionality, identity politics, and violence against women of color. *Stanford Law Review, 43*(6), 1241–1299. doi:10.2307/1229039

Cross, T., Bazron, B., Dennis, K., & Issacs, M. (1989). *Towards a culturally competent system of care* (Vol. 1). Washington, DC: Child and Adolescent Service System Program (CASSP) Technical Assistance Center, Georgetown University Child Development Center.

Feltz, R. (2018). Will parents separated from their children at the border be forced to separate again to win asylum? *Democracy Now!* Retrieved from https://www.democracynow.org/2018/7/13/will_parents_separated_from_their_children

Ferguson, G. M. (2013). The big difference a small island can make: How Jamaican adolescents are advancing acculturation science. *Child Development Perspectives, 7*(4), 248–254. doi:10.1111/cdep.12051

Fowers, B. J., & Davidov, B. J. (2006). The virtue of multiculturalism: Personal transformation, character, and openness to the other. *American Psychologist, 61*, 581–594. doi:10.1037/0003-066X.61.6.581

Giddens, A. (1991). *The consequences of modernity* (p. 64). Cambridge, UK: Polity Press.

Gonzalez-Barrera, A., & Krogstad, J. M. (2019). *What we know about illegal immigration from Mexico.* Pew Research Center: Fact Tank. Retrieved from https://www.pewresearch.org/fact-tank/2019/06/28/what-we-know-about-illegal-immigration-from-mexico

Ghosh, B. (2011). Cultural changes and challenges in the era of globalization: The case of India. *Journal of Developing Societies, 27*(2), 153–175. doi:10.1177/0169796X1102700203

Hook, J., Davis, D., Owen, J., Worthington, E., & Utsey, S. (2013). Cultural humility: Measuring openness to culturally diverse clients. *Journal of Counseling Psychology, 60*(3), 353–366. doi:10.1037/a0032595

International Association of Schools of Social Work, International Council on Social Welfare, and International Federation of Social Workers. (2014). Global agenda for social work and social development: First report – Promoting social and economic equalities. *International Social Work, 57*(S4), 3–16. doi:10.1177/0020872814534139

Kashima, Y. (2007). Globalization, diversity and universal Darwinism. *Culture & Psychology*, *13*(1), 129–139. doi:10.1177/1354067X07073666

Kretchmar, J. (2014). Conflict theory. In Editors of Salem Press (Eds.), *Sociology reference guide: Deviant behavior and the violation of social norms* (pp. 50–51). Ipswich, MA: Salem Press.

Krogstad, J. M. (2017). *U.S. Hispanic population growth has leveled off*. Philadelphia, PA: Pew Charitable Trusts.

Lewis-Fernandez, R., & Aggarwal, N. (2017). Cultural assessments in psychiatry. In H. S. Akiskal, D. V. Jeste, J. H. Krystal, L. Lewis-Fernandez, K. R. Merikangas, K. R. Nemeroff, C., . . . Tamminga, C. A. (Eds.), *Kaplan & Sadock's comprehensive textbook of psychiatry* (10th ed., Vol. 1, pp. 2460–2471). Philadelphia, PA: Wolters Kluwer.

Lopez, M. H., Krogstad, J. M., & Flores, A. (2018). Key facts about young Latinos, one of the nation's fastest-growing populations. *Pew Research Center: Fact Tank*. Retrieved from https://www.pewresearch.org/fact-tank/2018/09/13/key-facts-about-young-latinos

Mosher, D. K., Hook, J. N., Farrell, J. E., Watkins, C. E., & Davis, D. E. (2017). Cultural humility. In E. L. Worthington, D. E. Davis, & N. Hook (Eds.), *Handbook of humility: Theory, research and applications* (pp. 91–104). New York, NY: Routledge.

Mullaly, B. (2007). *The new structural social work* (3rd ed.). New York, NY: Oxford University Press.

Musicaro, R. M., Spinazzola, J., Arvidson, J., Swaroop, S. R., Goldblatt Grace, L., Yarrow, A., & Ford, J. D. (2019). The complexity of adaptation to childhood polyvictimization in youth and young adults: Recommendations for multidisciplinary responders. *Trauma, Violence, & Abuse*, *20*(1), 81–98. doi:10.1177/1524838017692365

O'Neal, E. N., & Beckman, L. O. (2017). Intersections of race, ethnicity, and gender: Reframing knowledge surrounding barriers to social services among Latina intimate partner violence victims. *Violence Against Women*, *23*(5), 643–665. doi:10.1177/1077801216646223

Ozer, S., & Schwartz, S. J. (2016). Measuring globalization-based acculturation in Ladakh: Investigating possible advantages of a tridimensional acculturation scale. *International Journal of Intercultural Relations*, *53*, 1–15. doi:10.1016/j.ijintrel.2016.05.002

Patten, E. (2016). The nation's Latino population is defined by its youth: Nearly half of U.S.-born Latinos are younger than 18. *Pew Research Center: Hispanic Trends*. Retrieved from https://www.pewresearch.org/hispanic/2016/04/20/the-nations-latino-population-is-defined-by-its-youth

Petrovich, A., & Garcia, B. (2016). *Strengthening the DSM: Incorporating resilience and cultural competence* (2nd ed.). New York, NY: Springer Publishing Company.

Piketty, T. (2014). *Capital in the twenty-first century*. Cambridge, MA: The Belknap Press of Harvard University Press.

Rhoades, H., Rusow, J. A., Bond, D., Lanteigne, A., Fulginiti, A., & Goldbach, J. T. (2018). Homelessness, mental health and suicidality among LGBTQ youth accessing crisis services. *Child Psychiatry & Human Development*, *49*(4), 643–651. doi:10.1007/s10578-018-0780-1

Ryder, A. G., Alden, L. E., & Paulhus, D. L. (2000). Is acculturation unidimensional or bidimensional? A head-to-head comparison in the prediction of personality, self-identity, and adjustment. *Journal of Personality and Social Psychology*, *79*(1), 49. doi:10.1037/0022-3514.79.1.49

Sam, D. L., & Berry, J. W. (2010). Acculturation: When individuals and groups of different cultural backgrounds meet. *Perspectives on Psychological Science*, *5*(4), 472–481. doi:10.1177/1745691610373075

Sen, A. (2009). *The idea of justice*. Cambridge, MA: The Belknap Press of Harvard University Press.

Sue, S., Zane, N., Nagayama Hall, G., & Berger, L. (2009). The case of cultural competency in psychotherapeutic interventions. *Annual Review of Psychology*, *60*, 525–548. doi:10.1146/annurev.psych.60.110707.163651

Swendener, A., & Woodell, B. (2017). Predictors of family support and well-being among Black and Latina/o sexual minorities. *Journal of GLBT Family Studies, 13*(4), 357–379. doi: 10.1080/1550428X.2016.1257400

Tervalon, M., & Murray-Garcia, J. (1998). Cultural humility versus cultural competence: A critical distinction in defining physician training outcomes in multicultural education. *Journal of Health Care for the Poor and Underserved, 9*, 117–125. doi:10.1353/hpu.2010.0233

Tormala, T., Patel, S., Soukup, E., & Clarke, A. (2018). Developing measurable cultural competence and cultural humility: An application of the cultural formulation. *Training and Education in Professional Psychology, 12*(1), 54–61. doi:10.1037/tep0000183

United Nations, Department of Economic and Social Affairs, Population Division. (2017). *International Migration Report 2017* (ST/ESA/SER.A/403). Retrieved from https://www.un.org/en/development/desa/population/migration/publications/migrationreport/docs/MigrationReport2017.pdf

United Nations, Educational Scientific and Cultural Organization. (2017). Culture for sustainable development. In *The future we want: The role of culture: UNESCO, Globalization and culture.* Retrieved from http://www.unesco.org/new/en/culture/themes/culture-and-development/the-future-we-want-the-role-of-culture/globalization-and-culture

U.S. Census Bureau. (2019). Educational attainment of the population 18 years and over, by age, sex, race, and Hispanic origin: 2018: Educational attainment in the United States: 2018. [Table 1.]. *Demo.* Retrieved from https://www.census.gov/data/tables/2018/demo/education-attainment/cps-detailed-tables.html

U.S. Department of Homeland Security. (2019). 2017 yearbook of immigration statistics. [PDF file]. *Office of Immigration Statistics.* Retrieved from https://www.dhs.gov/sites/default/files/publications/yearbook_immigration_statistics_2017_0.pdf

Velayo, R. S. (2012). Internationalizing the curriculum. In J. E. Groccia, M. A. T. Alsudairy, & W. Buskist (Eds.), *Handbook of college and university teaching: A global perspective* (pp. 268–278). Thousand Oaks, CA: Sage.

# 5

# Evidence-Based Practice With Ethnically Diverse Clients

*Manny John González*

## INTRODUCTION

Treatment outcome studies in the discipline of social work, psychology, and psychiatry have demonstrated the efficacy and effectiveness of differential psychotherapy approaches in addressing the psychological needs of individuals across the life span (Beutler & Crago, 1991; Hibbs & Jensen, 1996). Throughout the last four decades, scholar-practitioners have engaged in a professional quest to find evidence to support the efficacy of psychotherapy in ameliorating an array of clinical symptoms and levels of distress in identified patient or client populations. La Roche and Christopher (2009) contend that this quest began largely as a response to Eysenck's (1952) review of the treatment outcome literature, from which he concluded that the success rate of psychotherapeutic models of treatment was not greater than spontaneous remission. Eysenck's (1952) review set the stage for systematic therapy outcome studies aimed at demonstrating the efficacy and effectiveness of clinical interventions and selected psychotherapy approaches. Evidence-based practice and the current state of empirically supported psychosocial therapies are a by-product of this quest.

While it is evident that treatment outcome studies and the development of evidence-based psychosocial therapies have contributed to significant improvement in the delivery of clinical and mental health services (see Whaley & Davis, 2007), clinical researchers (e.g., Bernal, Jimenez-Chafey, & Domenech Rodriguez, 2009; Hwang, 2009; Rossello & Bernal, 1999) have raised concerns about the applicability of evidence-based practices to the psychosocial treatment of culturally diverse patient populations. At the root of the concern is the issue of whether evidence-based treatments developed within a particular cultural and linguistic context are appropriate for ethnocultural patient populations that do not share the same cultural values, mores, and language of the patient or client cohort for whom the treatment was developed. Because culture and specific socioethnographic variables influence the effective delivery of clinical services and the diagnostic and treatment process (see González & González-Ramos, 2005), the noted concern must always be in the forefront of competent psychosocial practice. In addition to this concern, some mental health scholars (Atkinson, Bui, & Mori, 2001; Miranda, Bernal, Lau, Kohn, Hwang, & LaFromboise, 2005) have documented the absence of ethnic and racial minority sample groups in studies of evidence-based treatments. The recruitment and retention of ethnically, racially, and linguistically diverse sample populations in psychotherapy research studies are of vital importance for the cultural adaptation of evidence-based practices.

This chapter presents an overview of evidence-based practice with ethnically diverse clients. Predicated on an integrative understanding of evidence-based practice and cultural competency in mental health and clinical care settings and the importance of intersectionality as the guiding theoretical perspective for effective delivery of patient-centered services, selected conceptual frameworks for the cultural adaptation of evidence-based treatments will be presented. Culturally adapted cognitive-behavioral therapy (CBT) will also be highlighted as an exemplar of evidence-based treatment for ethnic and racially diverse patient populations.

## EVIDENCE-BASED PRACTICE AND CULTURAL COMPETENCE IN MENTAL HEALTHCARE

Evidence-based practice—to a significant extent—is guided by Paul's (1967) seminal practice-informed research questions: "*What* treatment, by *whom*, is most effective for *this* individual, with *that* specific problem, and under *which* set of circumstances?" (p. 111). Consistent with the evidence-based movement in medicine (see Sackett, Straus, Richardson, Rosenberg, & Haynes, 2000), evidence-based practice in the professional disciplines of social work and psychology has as its major aim the improvement of patient outcomes—across specific psychological and social domains—through the integration of clinical practice with relevant research and patient values. Directed by this aim, the American Psychological Association (APA) Presidential Task Force on Evidence-Based Practice has defined this type of practice as "the integration of the best available research with clinical expertise in the context of patient characteristics, culture and preferences" (APA Presidential Task Force on Evidence-Based Practice, 2006, p. 273). This definition—with its emphasis on the clinical expertise of the practitioner in the context of client characteristics, culture, and preferences—resonates well with the value base of the helping professions. Evidence-based practice is a collaborative process for making treatment decisions (see Drisko & Grady, 2012, 2018) and its purpose, according to the Task Force, "is to promote effective psychological practice and enhance public health by applying empirically supported principles of psychological assessment, case formulation, therapeutic relationship and intervention" (p. 284). If this purpose is to be implemented by clinical practitioners and systems of care, the individual and cultural characteristics, preferences, and values of ethnically and racially diverse populations must converge with the overall intent of evidence-based practice: improved patient outcomes and effective delivery of psychosocial treatment. The convergence will be facilitated by understanding the need for cultural competence in the provision of mental health and clinical services.

The need for cultural competence in the provision of psychosocial services is justified by two important factors: (a) the increasing cultural diversity and multicultural population within the United States and (b) the well documented ethnic, racial, and linguistic disparities in the utilization of mental health services (Bernal & Scharron-del-Rio, 2001). From a clinical and organizational perspective, Sue and Torino (2005) define cultural competence in the following manner:

> Cultural competence is the ability to engage in action or create conditions that maximize the optimal development of the client and client systems. Multicultural counseling competence is achieved by the counselor's acquisitions of awareness, knowledge, and skills needed to function effectively in a pluralistic democratic society (ability to communicate, interact, negotiate, and intervene on behalf of clients from diverse backgrounds) and on an organizational/societal level, advocating effectively to develop new theories, practices, policies, and organizational structures that are more responsive to all people. (p. 8)

Culture, the major variable in culturally competent practice, is a complex and multidimensional construct that directly influences the process of psychotherapy and the understanding of the human condition. It has not always received, however, adequate attention as a construct that is of paramount importance in the development of culturally sensitive psychotherapy and culturally competent mental health services (Guarnaccia & Rodriguez, 1996; La Roche & Christopher, 2009). Evidence-based practice with ethnic minorities or ethnically and racially diverse clients must be guided by the recognition that culture is a phenomenon that impacts the bio-psychosocial functioning of the human organism across time and space. In acknowledgment of the role that culture plays in the development and implementation of evidence-informed psychosocial interventions, the APA Presidential Task Force on Evidence-Based Practice (2006) has articulated the following definition of this construct:

> Culture . . . is understood to encompass a broad array of phenomena (e.g., shared values, history, knowledge, rituals, and customs) that often results in a shared sense of identity. Racial and ethnic groups may have shared a culture, but those personal characteristics are not the only characteristics that define cultural groups (e.g., deaf culture, inner-city culture). Culture is a multifaceted construct, and cultural factors cannot be understood in isolation from social class, and personal characteristics that make each patient unique. (p. 278)

The integration of evidence-based practice and cultural competence can lead to the implementation of culturally sensitive psychotherapy in clinical settings. Drawing on the work of Hall (2001) on psychotherapy research with ethnic minorities, La Roche and Christopher (2009) note that: "Cultural sensitive psychotherapy is the tailoring of psychotherapy to specific cultural groups, so that persons from one group may benefit more from a specific type of intervention than from interventions designed for another cultural group" (p. 398). Culturally sensitive psychotherapy is composed of three interrelated domains. The first domain is composed of carefully defined ethnic, racial, and cultural factors that are unique to a specific patient population. The second domain encompasses the constellations of characteristics that are unique or more prominent in certain cultural groups relative to others. The last domain includes culturally sensitive clinical interventions that are targeted to address the needs of an identified culturally diverse patient group. Evidence-based practices that are adapted or created to meet the mental health or psychosocial needs of the ethnically diverse should include these noted domains.

## INTERSECTIONALITY, EVIDENCE-BASED PRACTICE AND CULTURALLY COMPETENT CLINICAL CARE

Recent research (see Araújo, Oliveira, & Araújo, 2018; Turan et al., 2019) on health and mental health disparities underscores the importance of individual social identities—such as race, ethnicity, gender, socioeconomic status—on treatment outcomes. The examination of these social identities in combined form—within the context of a socio-political-economic environmental context—is vital for understanding the social determinants of health and the negative treatment outcomes that often impact marginalized and oppressed populations. Intersectionality, as a theoretical perspective, provides the conceptual underpinnings required for such an examination. It is useful for understanding how different forms of privilege and oppression exist simultaneously in shaping an individual's experiences in the social world and as a recipient of health or mental health services. Importantly, it also helps practitioners and clinical scholars to see that perceived and disparate socio-cultural-economic forces (e.g., race, gender, class) are mutually dependent and co-constitutive (see Bowleg, 2012; Jackson, Williams, & Vander Weele, 2016). Developed by legal scholar Kimberlé Crenshaw, intersectionality draws attention to the "multidimensionality of marginalized subjects' lived experiences" (Crenshaw, 1989, p. 139), and Dill and Zambrana (2009) have identified it as a "systematic approach to understanding human life and behavior that is rooted in the experiences and struggles of marginalized people" (p.4).

In implementing evidence-based models of mental health treatment with diverse patient populations, it is important to consider how the combined effects of racism, discrimination, poverty and gender differences produce treatment inequalities and access to timely and critical care. Viruell-Fuentes et al. (2012), for example, have noted how racism yields social and economic inequities that, in turn, become a fundamental cause of physical and emotional disease. Emerging research appears to suggest that there is a correlation between perceived discrimination and lower levels of physical and emotional well-being and detrimental health behaviors among immigrant groups—such as Hispanics, Black immigrants and Asians (see Perez, Fortuna, & Alegría, 2008; Ryan, Gee, & Laflamme, 2006). Incorporating, therefore, the conceptual principles of intersectionality in the provision of both culturally competent and evidence-based mental health care may serve to reduce the health-related stigma that is often experienced by patient populations who experience perceived discrimination. Weiss and Ramakrishna (2006) have defined health-related stigma as "a social process or related personal experience characterized by exclusion, rejection, blame, or devaluation that results from experience or reasonable anticipation of an adverse social judgment about a person or group identified with a particular health problem" (p. 536). Models of evidence-based practice, therefore, must be informed by both the tenets of cultural competence and the transactional relationship that exists between health and mental health treatment outcomes and stigma. Operationalizing this noted interrelationship in practice will ensure that the principles of intersectionality inform the delivery of humane and effective care.

## CONCEPTUAL FRAMEWORKS FOR THE CULTURAL ADAPTATION OF EVIDENCE-BASED TREATMENTS

Integrating culturally competent practice with evidence-informed psychosocial therapies is a complex task. The integration, however, is not impossible—and it may serve to provide a systematic approach to treatment that takes into account the sociocultural and socioeconomic context of ethnically diverse patients. Bernal et al. (2009) argue that the integration can be achieved through the use of cultural adaptation procedures. They define cultural adaptation as "the systematic modification of an evidence-based treatment . . . or intervention protocol to consider language, culture, and context in such a way that it is compatible with the client's cultural patterns, meanings, and values" (p. 362). Cultural adaptation serves as a unifying bridge between scientis-practitioners who state that the psychosocial problems of ethnically diverse patients should primarily be treated with new treatment approaches (see Comas-Díaz, 2006) and those scholars (see Elliot & Mihalic, 2004) who believe that existing psychosocial treatments should be tested, unchanged, with culturally diverse populations before embarking on any type of adaptation task.

A number of conceptual frameworks (e.g., Bernal, Bonilla, & Bellido, 1995; Hwang, 2006, 2009) have been developed with the intent of facilitating the integration of cultural competence and evidence-based treatments, thereby making psychotherapy or psychosocial treatment culturally malleable for patient populations of diverse ethnic, racial, and linguistic backgrounds. Rogler, Malgady, and Rodriguez's (1989) framework for culturally competent mental health research provides the seminal domains on which current cultural adaptation psychotherapy frameworks rest. Rogler et al. (1989) recommended improving cultural understanding in mental health research, practice, and treatment innovation along five domains: (a) cultural factors in the emergence of a clinical/mental health presenting problem, (b) help seeking and service utilization, (c) factors that may affect an accurate diagnosis, (d) therapeutic and treatment issues, and (e) posttreatment adjustment of the patient. Hwang (2006) notes that this seminal framework is important in providing effective treatment to ethnic minorities because "it underscores the temporal sequence of problem development in relation to service delivery and highlights areas where culture is likely to play a role" (p. 703).

### Ecological Validity and Culturally Sensitive Framework

Developed by Bernal et al. (1995), the Ecological Validity and Culturally Sensitivity framework is predicated on the proposition that in the provision of culturally competent and evidence-based treatment, it is necessary to increase the congruence between the experience of the client's ethnocultural world and the properties of a particular psychotherapy as assumed by the therapist. The framework focuses on eight culturally sensitive elements: language (whether it is appropriate and culturally syntonic), person (role of ethnic similarities and differences between client and therapist in shaping therapy relationships), metaphors (symbols and concepts), content (cultural knowledge of the therapist), concepts (treatment concepts consistent with culture and context), goals (support of positive and adaptive cultural values), methods (cultural enhancement of treatment methods), and context (consideration of the economic and social contexts that might increase the risk of acculturative stress problems, disconnection for social support systems and reduction of social mobility for specific ethnocultural diverse client populations). Rossello and Bernal (1999) were able to successfully use this framework to culturally adapt cognitive-behavioral and interpersonal treatments for depressed Puerto Rican adolescents, and these adapted treatments have been shown to be efficacious in clinical trials. Similarly, the framework has been used to culturally adapt cognitive-behavioral group treatment for Haitian American adolescents (see Nicolas, Arntz, Hirsch, & Schmiedigen, 2009).

## Psychotherapy Adaptation and Modification Framework

Hwang (2006) created the Psychotherapy Adaptation and Modification Framework (PAMF) to help guide therapeutic adaptations of empirically supported treatments. A major conceptual underpinning of PAMF is that culture affects different mental health domains including: (a) the prevalence of mental illness, (b) etiology of disease, (c) phenomenology of distress, (d) diagnostic and assessment issues, (e) coping styles and help-seeking pathways, and (f) treatment and intervention. The framework incorporates six therapeutic domains and 25 therapeutic principles (see Hwang [2006] for a complete review of the therapeutic principles). The six therapeutic domains of the framework are: (a) dynamic issues and cultural complexities; (b) orientating clients to psychotherapy and increasing mental health awareness; (c) understanding cultural beliefs about mental illness, its causes, and what constitutes appropriate treatment; (d) improving the client–therapist relationship; (e) understanding cultural differences in the expression and communication of distress; and (f) addressing cultural issues specific to the patient population. Examples of the 25 therapeutic principles include: orienting clients to a bio-psychosocial or holistic model of disease development, focusing on psychoeducational aspects of treatment, finding ways to integrate extant cultural strengths and healing practices into the client's treatment, and aligning with traditional and indigenous forms of healing. While PAMF was created to meet the mental health needs of recently arrived Asian American immigrants, it may be used to adapt evidence-based practices for many diverse ethnocultural groups. In fact, in one treatment outcome study, PAMF has been use to adapt CBT for Mexican American students who suffer from anxiety disorders (Wood, Chiu, Hwang, Jacobs, & Ifekwunigwe, 2008). The framework may also be used to improve the clinical training of practitioners across the helping professional disciplines.

## Formative Method for Adapting Psychotherapy

As a by-product of the PAMF, Hwang (2009) also developed the Formative Method for Adapting Psychotherapy Framework (FMAPF). FMAPF is a community-based bottom-up approach for culturally adapting psychotherapy. According to Hwang (2009), FMAP

> was developed to be used in conjunction with the top-down PAMF ... to generate ideas for therapy adaptation, provide additional support for theoretically identified modifications, and help flesh out and provide more specific and refined recommendations for increasing therapeutic responsiveness. (p. 370)

Consistent with the principles of practice-based evidence (see Fox, 2003), the FMAPF approach consists of five phases: (a) generating knowledge and collaborating with stakeholders, (b) integrating generated information with theory and empirical and clinical knowledge, (c) reviewing the initial culturally adapted clinical intervention, (d) testing the culturally adapted intervention, and (e) finalizing the culturally adapted intervention. This framework has been used to create a manualized treatment for depressed Chinese Americans.

## CULTURALLY ADAPTED CBT

CBT is based on the premise that thoughts, actions, and feelings are closely related (see Beck, Rush, Shaw, & Emery, 1979). CBT is an evidence-based, short-term therapy approach for the treatment of depression, anxiety, and other related mental health and psychosocial disorders. To treat depressive feelings, this treatment approach attempts to identify those thoughts and actions that influence these feelings. In the treatment of depression, the primary aims of CBT are: to diminish depressive feelings, shorten the time the identified client feels depressed, teach alternative ways of preventing depression, and increase the person's sense of self-control over their life. Treatment is directed at assisting the identified client to understand how thoughts influence mood, how daily activities influence mood, and how interactions with other people influence mood as well.

Recent reviews of the literature (see Miranda et al., 2005; Voss Horrell, 2008) on the impact of evidence-based mental healthcare on ethnic minorities provide support for the effectiveness of CBT for African American, Hispanic, and Asian American patients suffering from anxiety and depressive disorders. Culturally adapted CBT approaches are also effective in reducing symptoms of distress among ethnocultural patient populations. Wood et al. (2008), for example, documented via a detailed case study how cultural modification of CBT can lead to positive outcomes for Mexican American students who suffer from anxiety disorders. In their study, Wood et al. (2008), integrated the following cultural competence principles in their adaptation of CBT: (a) spend time learning about the client's cultural practices, acculturative status, migration history, language proficiencies and preferences, and other relevant background history; (b) respect the client's and the family's conceptualization of mental illness and its treatment to increase acceptance of CBT techniques; (c) establish CBT goals that are valued by the client and family to improve the working relationship; (d) actively collaborate with school staff to alleviate parental apprehension; (e) provide an orienting session early on to increase family understanding and participation; (f) learn about the cultural context of parenting to facilitate engagement in CBT; (g) engage the extended family in the child's CBT treatment; (h) align CBT techniques with family cultural beliefs and traditions to enhance commitment to treatment; (i) consider whether culturally based conversational norms are masking poor adherence to treatment; and (j) remain attuned to the role of acculturation gaps in children's adjustment problems, but consult with cultural experts before addressing this topic with families. The integration of these principles with an evidence-based model of treatment increased the probability of a positive treatment outcome for an ethnically diverse client group that underutilizes mental health services and is more likely to drop out of treatment prematurely.

In a pilot study of a 12-session, culturally adapted CBT for Hispanics with major depression, Interian, Allen, Gara, and Escobar (2008) reported a 57% mean reduction of depressive symptoms at posttreatment among patients who completed the intervention. Cultural adaptations that were made in the treatment protocol included: (a) the use of an ethnocultural assessment, which involved inquiring about the patients' number of years in the United States, their adaptation to the migration, whereabouts of family members and changes in social support; (b) providing the treatment in Spanish including the phraseology commonly used by Hispanics to describe therapeutic phenomena; and (c) allowance for the centrality of the family in treatment. Based on the findings of the study, Interian et al. (2008) note that cultural adaptations to existing treatments may be clinically beneficial, and they recommend that clinicians complement CBT with an ethnocultural assessment.

Similar to the study by Interian et al. (2008), Kohn, Oden, Munoz, Robinson, and Leavitt (2002) adapted a manualized, 16-week cognitive-behavioral group therapy intervention for depressed, low-income, African American women. Adaptation of the CBT group intervention took place along two domains: structural and didactic. Adaptations at the structural level included: (a) limiting the group to African American women, (b) keeping the group closed to facilitate cohesion, (c) adding experiential meditative exercises during treatment and a termination ritual at the end of the 16-week intervention, and (d) changes in some of the language used to describe CBT techniques. For instance, rather than using the term "homework," the group participants preferred the term "therapeutic exercises." At the didactic level four culturally specific sections of content were added to the therapy modules: (a) creating healthy relationships, (b) spirituality, (c) African American family issues, and (d) African American female identity. At termination of the intervention, women in the group exhibited a significant decrease in their depressive symptoms as measured by the Beck Depression Inventory (BDI).

The cited studies provide a level of evidence for the effectiveness of culturally adapted CBT in reducing symptoms of depression and anxiety in some ethnocultural patient populations. While the noted studies are primarily applicable to Hispanic and African American patients, some published case studies would seem to suggest that culturally adapted CBT may be the treatment of choice for other ethnically diverse populations such as Japanese clients (see Toyokawa &

Nedate, 1996) and Orthodox Jews (see Paradis, Friedman, Hatch, & Ackerman, 1996). As a treatment model, culturally adapted CBT is illustrative of a treatment approach that is informed by both research evidence and cultural competence. The model also demonstrates the type of integrative and complementary relationship that can exist between empirically supported therapies and the reality of culture.

## CONCLUSION

The integration of science with the phenomenon of culture and social context are equally important in the development, testing, and implementation of evidence-based practices. If this integration is overlooked in clinical research and in the delivery of clinical services, clients from diverse ethnic, racial, and linguistic backgrounds may be placed at risk for receiving psychosocial care that is not adequate or appropriate. Cultural adaptation frameworks—in conjunction with the conceptual underpinnings of intersectionality—must be employed to evaluate the appropriateness of evidence-based models of psychosocial treatment. The psychotherapy adaptation frameworks highlighted in this chapter—together with intersectionality as a theoretical perspective—serve to bridge the gap between evidence-based therapies and cultural competence. As demonstrated by the cited studies on the effectiveness of culturally adapted CBT, the literature on evidence-based treatment with ethnocultural patients is increasing and points to positive treatment outcomes. The positive treatment outcomes with culturally adapted evidence-based therapies are welcome in an era where there is growing recognition that mental health services must mirror the diverse and changing demographic profile of the nation. Cultural competence and evidence-based practice are two critical issues that will continue to shape clinical services in the near future. This chapter has addressed both issues and the need for their integration.

## DISCUSSION QUESTIONS

1. What is the relationship between evidence-based practice and cultural competence in the mental health field?
2. How does intersectionality inform the integration of evidence-based practice and cultural competence?
3. Why should the mental health/psychotherapy field adapt its models of treatment to diverse cultural populations?

## REFERENCES

American Psychological Association Presidential Task Force on Evidence-Based Practice. (2006). Evidence-based practice in psychology. *American Psychologist, 61*(4), 271–285. doi:10.1037/0003-066X.61.4.271

Araújo, E. M., Oliveira, N. F., & Araújo, T. M. (2018). Intersectionality of race, gender and common mental disorders in northeastern Brazil. *Ethnicity & Disease, 28*(3), 207–214. doi:10.18865/ed.28.3.207

Atkinson, D. R., Bui, U., & Mori, S. (2001). Multicultural sensitive empirically supported treatments: An oxymoron? In J. G. Ponterotto, J. M. Casas, L. A. Suzuki & C. M. Alexander (Eds.), *Handbook of multicultural counseling* (2nd ed., pp. 542–574). Thousand Oaks, CA: Sage.

Beck, A. T., Rush, A. J., Shaw, B. F., & Emery, G. (1979). *Cognitive therapy of depression.* New York, NY: Guilford Press.

Bernal, G., Bonilla, J., & Bellido, C. (1995). Ecological validity and cultural sensitivity for outcome research: Issues for the cultural adaptation and development of psychosocial treatments with Hispanics. *Journal of Abnormal Child Psychology, 23*(1), 67–87. doi:10.1007/BF01447045

Bernal, G., & Scharron-del-Rio, M. R. (2001). Are empirically supported treatments valid for ethnic minorities? Toward an alternative approach for treatment research. *Cultural Diversity and Ethnic Minority Psychology, 7*(4), 328–342. doi:10.1037/1099-9809.7.4.328

Bernal, G., Jimenez-Chafey, M. I., & Domenech Rodriguez, M. (2009). Cultural adaptation of treatments: A resource for considering culture in evidence-based practice. *Professional psychology: Research and practice, 40*(4), 361–368. doi:10.1037/a0016401

Beutler, L. E., & Crago, M. (Eds.). (1991). *Psychotherapy research: An international review of programmatic studies.* Washington, DC: American Psychological Association.

Bowleg, L. (2012). The problem with the phrase *women and minorities*: Intersectionality—an important theoretical framework for public health. *American Journal of Public Health, 102*(7), 1267–1273. doi:10.2105/AJPH.2012.300750

Comas-Díaz, L. (2006). Latino healing: The integration of ethnic psychology into psychotherapy. *Psychotherapy: Theory, Research, Practice, Training, 43*(4), 436–453. doi:10.1037/0033-3204.43.4.436

Crenshaw, K. (1989). Demarginalizing the intersection of race and sex: A Black feminist critique of antidiscrimination doctrine, feminist theory and antiracist politics. *University of Chicago Legal Forum, 1,* 139–167.

Dill, B. T., & Zambrana, R. E. (2009). Critical thinking about inequality: An emerging lens. In B. T. Dill & R. E. Zambrana (Eds.), *Emerging intersections: Race, class, and gender in theory, policy, and practice* (pp. 1–21). Piscataway, NJ: Rutgers University Press.

Drisko, J., & Grady, M. D. (2012). *Evidence-based practice.* New York, NY: Springer Publishing Company.

Drisko, J., & Grady, M. D. (2018). Teaching evidence-based practice using cases in social work education. *Families in Society: The Journal of Contemporary Social Services, 99,* 269–282. doi:10.1177/1044389418785331

Elliot, D. S., & Mihalic, S. (2004). Issues in disseminating and replicating effective prevention programs. *Prevention Science, 5*(1), 47–53. doi:10.1023/B:PREV.0000013981.28071.52

Eysenck, H. J. (1952). The effects of psychotherapy: An evaluation. *Journal of Consulting Psychology, 16*(3), 319–324. doi:10.1037/h0063633

Fox, N. J. (2003). Practice-based evidence: Towards collaborative and transgressive research. *Sociology, 37*(1), 81–102. doi:10.1177/0038038503037001388

González, M. J., & González-Ramos, G. (Eds.). (2005). *Mental health care of new Hispanic immigrants: Innovations in clinical practice.* New York, NY: Haworth.

Guarnaccia, P. J., & Rodriguez, O. (1996). Concepts of culture and their role in the development of culturally competent mental health services. *Hispanic Journal of Behavioral Sciences, 18*(4), 419–443. doi:10.1177/07399863960184001

Hall, G. C. (2001). Psychotherapy research with ethnic minorities: Empirical, ethical and conceptual issues. *Journal of Consulting and Clinical Psychology, 69*(4), 502–510. doi:10.1037/0022-006X.69.3.502

Hibbs, E. D., & Jensen, P. (Eds.) (1996). *Psychosocial treatments for child and adolescents disorders.* Washington, DC: American Psychological Association.

Hwang, W. C. (2006). The psychotherapy adaptation and modification framework: Application to Asian Americans. *American Psychologist, 61*(7), 702–715. doi:10.1037/0003-066X.61.7.702

Hwang, W. C. (2009). The formative method for adapting psychotherapy (FMAP): A community-based developmental approach to culturally adapting therapy. *Professional Psychology: Research and Practice, 40*(4), 369–377. doi:10.1037/a0016240

Interian, A., Allen, L. A., Gara, M. A., & Escobar, J. I. (2008). A pilot study of culturally adapted cognitive behavior therapy for Hispanics with major depression. *Cognitive and Behavior Practice, 15*(1), 67–75. doi:10.1016/j.cbpra.2006.12.002

Jackson, J. W., Williams, D. R., & Vander Weele, T. J. (2016). Disparities at the intersection of marginalized groups. *Social Psychiatry and Psychiatric Epidemiology, 51*(10), 1349–1359. doi:10.1007/s00127-016-1276-6

Kohn, L. P., Oden, T., Munoz, R. F., Robinson, A., & Leavitt, D. (2002). Adapted cognitive behavioral group therapy for depressed low-income African American women. *Community Mental Health Journal, 38*(6), 497–504. doi:10.1023/A:1020884202677

La Roche, M. J., & Christopher, M. S. (2009). Changing paradigms from empirically supported treatment to evidence-based practice: A cultural perspective. *Professional Psychology: Research and Practice, 40*(4), 396–402. doi:10.1037/a0015240

Miranda, J., Bernal, G., Lau, A., Kohn, L., Hwang, W. C., & LaFromboise, T. (2005). State of science on psychosocial interventions for ethnic minorities. *Annual Review of Clinical Psychology, 1*(2), 113–142. doi:10.1146/annurev.clinpsy.1.102803.143822

Nicolas, G., Arntz, D. L., Hirsch, B., & Schmiedigen, A. (2009). Cultural adaptation of a group treatment for Haitian American adolescents. *Professional Psychology: Research and Practice, 40*(4), 378–384. doi:10.1037/a0016307

Paradis, C. M., Friedman, S., Hatch, M. L., & Ackerman, R. (1996). Cognitive behavioral treatment of anxiety disorders in Orthodox Jews. *Cognitive and Behavioral Practice, 3*(4), 271–288. doi:10.1016/S1077-7229(96)80018-6

Paul, G. (1967). Strategy of outcome research in psychotherapy. *Journal of Consulting Psychology, 31*(2), 109–118. doi:10.1037/h0024436

Perez, D. J., Fortuna, L., & Alegría, M. (2008). Prevalence and correlates of everyday discrimination among U.S. Latinos. *Journal of Community Psychology, 36*(4), 421–433. doi:10.1002/jcop.20221

Rogler, L. H., Malgady, R. G., & Rodriguez, O. (1989). *Hispanics and mental health: A framework for research.* Malabar, FL: Krieger.

Rossello, J., & Bernal, G. (1999). The efficacy of cognitive-behavioral and interpersonal treatments for depression in Puerto Rican adolescents. *Journal of Consulting and Clinical Psychology, 67*(5), 734–745. doi:10.1037/0022-006X.67.5.734

Ryan, A. M., Gee, G. C., & Laflamme, D. F. (2006). The association between self-reported discrimination, physical health and blood pressure: Findings from African Americans, Black immigrants, and Latino immigrants in New Hampshire. *Journal of Health Care for the Poor and Underserved, 17*(2), 116–132. doi:10.1353/hpu.2006.0079

Sackett, D. L., Straus, S. E., Richardson, W. S., Rosenberg, W. M., & Haynes, R. B. (2000). *Evidence-based medicine: How to practice and teach EBM* (2nd ed.). London: Churchill Livingstone.

Sue, D. W., & Torino, G. C. (2005). Racial-cultural competence: Awareness, knowledge, and skills. In R. T. Carter (Ed.), *Handbook of racial-cultural psychology and counseling: Training and practice* (Vol. 2, pp. 3–18). Hoboken, NJ: Wiley.

Toyokawa, T., & Nedate, K. (1996). Application of cognitive behavior therapy to interpersonal problems: A case study of a Japanese female client. *Cognitive and Behavioral Practice, 3*(4), 289–302. doi:10.1016/S1077-7229(96)80019-8

Turan, J. M., Elafros, M. A., Logie, C. H., Banik, S., Turan, B., Crockett, K.B., Pescosolido, B., & Murray, S.M. (2019). Challenges and opportunities in examining and addressing intersectional stigma and health. *BMC Medicine, 17*(7), 1–15. doi:10.1186/s12916-018-1246-9

Viruell-Fuentes E. A., Miranda P. Y., & Abdulrahim, S. (2012). More than culture: Structural racism, intersectionality theory, and immigrant health. *Social Science & Medicine, 75*(12), 2099–2106.

Voss Horrell, S. C. (2008). Effectiveness of cognitive-behavioral therapy with adult ethnic minority clients: A review. *Professional Psychology: Research and Practice, 39*(2), 160–168. doi:10.1037/0735-7028.39.2.160

Weiss, M. G., & Ramakrishna, J. (2006). Stigma interventions and research for international health. *Lancet, 367*(9509), 536–538. doi:10.1016/S0140-6736(06)68189-0

Whaley, A. L., & Davis, K. E. (2007).Cultural competence and evidence-based practice in mental health services: A complementary perspective. *American Psychologist, 62*(6), 563–574. doi:10.1037/0003-066X.62.6.563

Wood, J. J., Chiu, A. W., Hwang, W. C., Jacobs, J., & Ifekwunigwe, M. (2008). Adapting cognitive behavioral therapy for Mexican American students with anxiety disorders: Recommendations for school psychologists. *School Psychology Quarterly, 23*(4), 515–532. doi:10.1037/1045-3830.23.4.515

# Part II

## Administrative and Legal Perspectives

# 6

# Managing Agencies for Multicultural Services

MANOJ PARDASANI AND LAURI GOLDKIND

## THE CHANGING DEMOGRAPHICS OF THE NATION AND THE SOCIAL WORK PRACTICE FIELD

The nation's human services agencies mirror the cultural diversity of the U.S. population today. Multicultural workforces and clients are no longer atypical. Currently the non-Hispanic Caucasian population comprises 60.4% of the total population (U.S. Census Bureau, 2018). However, by the mid-21st century, about 50% of Americans will be racial and ethnic minorities (Poston & Saenz, 2019). Hispanic/Latinx are the largest minority ethnic group, while Asian Americans have the highest rate of growth among racial/ethnic groups (U.S. Census Bureau, 2018). In 2017, the Hispanic/Latinx cohort comprised 18.3% of the population while the Black/African American cohort comprised 13.4% of the population (U.S. Census Bureau, 2018). Asian Americans comprise 5.9% of the population, while a fast growing cohort is one that comprises individuals who identify with two or more races (2.4%) (U.S. Census Bureau, 2018). Immigrants and refugees are also changing the demographic composition of America as individuals and families from a wide variety of cultures, ethnicities, and nationalities relocate throughout the states in search of better opportunities and conditions. Currently, the U.S. Census Bureau estimates that there are nearly 43.7 million documented immigrants living in the United States and projects that another 70 million foreign-born individuals will immigrate to the country by 2050 (U.S. Department of Labor, 2017). What was once regarded as an urban phenomenon can now be seen across the country in towns and rural communities. Moreover, this trend toward a more diverse population, and thereby a diverse workforce, is expected to continue.

Social service agencies continue to face two challenges in this multicultural environment: (a) managing workplaces in which workforces have become increasingly heterogeneous in terms of gender, race, age, religion, sexual orientation, ethnicity, and national origin and (b) meeting the service needs of client populations who may represent a wide range of very different cultures, languages, values, religions, and preimmigration or refugee experiences. While there is wide agreement with regard to changing U.S. demographics, less is understood about how to successfully create organizational cultures that embrace diversity and serve multicultural populations well.

## THE CHANGING U.S. WORKFORCE

The U.S. workforce (aged 25 to 64 years) is in the midst of a sweeping demographic transformation. From 2014 to 2024, the non-Hispanic Caucasian working-age population is projected to increase by 2.3%. During the same period, the minority proportion of the workforce is projected to increase by 10.1% for the African American/Black cohort, by 23.2% for the Asian American cohort, and by 28% for the Hispanic/Latinx cohort (Bureau of Labor Statistics, 2015). The Bureau of Labor Statistics also reports that four out of 10 (40.5%) individuals working in social work, social service, or community practice are non-Caucasian (2018). A national survey of professional master's level social workers conducted by the Council of Social Work Education (CSWE) found that the profession was disproportionately female (85%) and Caucasian (72.6%) (2017). They reported that Asian American, Hispanic/Latinx, and Black/African American social workers comprised less than 30% of the professional workforce; however, they predicted that this cohort would increase significantly in the next few decades (CSWE, 2017). There is inadequate information on the proportion of LGBT individuals and religious backgrounds within social work at this time. Nonetheless, it is easy to see why diversity and multiculturalism in the workplace is a critical issue.

## WHO ARE THE LEADERS IN HUMAN SERVICES?

While all indicators overwhelmingly point to growing multicultural and multiracial population trends, human services organizational leadership at the senior executive and board levels remain overwhelmingly Caucasian and male. Many nonprofit boards are cut off from the public they serve by an ethnically homogeneous membership and a failure to engage in externally oriented activities. Eighteen percent of nonprofits whose clientele is more than 50% Black/African American have no Black/African American trustees, while 32% of their Hispanic/Latinx counterparts have no Hispanic/Latinx board members. On average 86% of board members are Caucasian, 7% are Black/African American, 3.5% are Hispanic/Latinx, and the balance are from other ethnic groups (Ostrowerer, 2007).

Little is known about the demographic characteristics of social work agency leadership. Best practice models of multicultural management suggest that leadership mirror the racial/ethnic distribution of social work staff, and that staff represent some reflection of a similar demographic as clients. Yet the leadership of social work and social service agencies continues to be overwhelmingly Caucasian at 78.4% of all social and community service managers (Bureau of Labor Statistics, 2018). Male leaders of such agencies are in higher proportion than their overall proportion of the professional social work workforce (Bureau of Labor Statistics, 2018). A survey of nearly 200 social service agencies in the tri-state area (New York, New Jersey, and southern Connecticut) conducted by the authors found that nearly 78% of the leaders identified as Caucasian, while only 2.4% identified as Hispanic/Latinx and 7.1% as Black/African American, which is not reflective of the racial/ethnic compositions of these communities. One-third of the leaders surveyed (34%) identified as male (Goldkind & Pardasani, 2010).

But social work agencies are not limited to just social work professionals. Most human service organizations now function in an interdisciplinary format, whereby individuals from different professional backgrounds are required to work in teams. Thus, organizations and agencies are even more challenged today to accommodate a varied workforce while simultaneously tending to the needs of a diverse clientele.

## DEFINING CULTURAL COMPETENCE AND MULTICULTURALISM

Multiculturalism is defined as

> a general rejection of the straight-line assimilation norm, the promotion of equality for racial and ethnic groups, respect for, tolerance of, and celebration of cultural diversity, the facilitation of cultural difference, and an assertion of rights and protections for particular racial and ethnic groups. (Bass, 2008)

But the social work profession does not just celebrate diversity and difference. The profession strives to engage cultural norms and beliefs into the conceptualization of human suffering and utilize them to inform individual and societal transformation. In fact, the National Association of Social Workers (NASW) *Code of Ethics* directs social workers to obtain education and seek to understand the nature of social diversity, as well as uphold social justice standards and actively fight against oppressive forces.

Culture is an essential component in the helping process because it is embedded in how problems are defined and manifested, how individuals seek help, and how providers conceive of and offer treatment options (Pinderhughes, 1989). Cultural competence involves both ethical and legal social work practice as it is a set of behaviors, attitudes, and policies that enable social work agencies and professionals to effectively serve individuals by incorporating the values and belief systems of those being served. Cultural competence is a process whereby individuals are challenged to recognize their internal biases and how they distort their own worldview. Some researchers question the very concept of cultural competence because they believe it does not take into account contextual and structural inequities (Fisher-Borne, Cain, & Martin, 2015). They prefer the concept of cultural humility "which takes into account the fluidity of culture and challenges both individuals and institutions to address inequalities" (Fisher-Borne, Cain, & Martin, 2015). Cultural competence should be built into our agencies' organizational cultures to create welcoming climates and work environments for employees as well as clients. While Saunders, Haskins, and Vasquez (2015) refer to cultural competence in organizations as an elusive goal, they believe that, rather than a static end-goal, it is a constantly shifting benchmark that requires continuous learning in organizations.

Individuals and organizations may be at various levels of awareness, knowledge, and skills along the cultural competence continuum, and this may impact their effectiveness (Cross, Bazron, Dennis, & Isaacs, 1989). A culturally competent practitioner or agency develops a deep respect for other cultures, is willing to learn about other cultures, is ready to engage people's different world views, is willing to use appropriate engagement skills, and is willing to tailor and adapt interventions for culturally diverse individuals and groups (Cross et al., 1989).

In recent years, the discussion of cultural competence has moved away from the concept of multiculturalism and diversity to an implicit understanding of intersectionality (Bubar, Caspedes, & Bundy-Fazioli, 2016). Intersectionality compels us to engage in a complex analysis of diversity and difference. Intersectionality hones in on the connection between privilege and oppression, and the complex ways those intersections influence and are influenced by social identities (Bubar, Caspedes, & Bundy-Fazioli, 2016). Rather than focus on one aspect of social identity, such as race, gender, or religion, intersectionality examines the complex interplay between various identities (some privileged and some oppressed) existing within an individual and between individuals. In other words, cultural competence is not about gaining knowledge of one social identity or another individually but examining the cumulative impact of various social identities and experiences of marginalization in those identities. To underscore this paradigm shift in our field, in 2008, CSWE's Standards on Engaging Diversity and Difference in Practice added intersectionality to promote the learning of power, privilege, and oppression by social work students as a critical foundation of responsive and ethical practice.

## MULTICULTURAL CHALLENGES IN THE WORKPLACE

There are two main challenges faced by leaders and managers in social work agencies discussed here.

### Culturally Competent Service Delivery

The need for culturally competent service delivery has been recognized by several researchers and service providers (Furman et al., 2009; Ramos-Sanchez, 2009; Switzer, Scholle, Johnson, & Kelleher, 1998; Taylor, Garcia, & Kingson, 2001). Zeitlin, Altschul, and Samuels (2016) posit that with a greater emphasis on evidence-based practices in social work services, administrators need to ensure that the adopted interventions are culturally competent for the populations they serve. Studies have found that Black/African American and Hispanic/Latinx clients are most likely to not have access to, and limited knowledge of, available resources (Furman et al., 2009; Martin & Bonder, 2003; Ramos-Sanchez, 2009). The most common barriers reported by minority clients to receiving services are provider insensitivity, minority consumer distrust of providers who may be from different socioeconomic and ethnic backgrounds, reluctance of providers to incorporate a consumer's spiritual and religious beliefs into care, lack of outreach by providers, and communication barriers (Hodge & Bushfield, 2006; Martin & Bonder, 2003; Williams, 2006; Yan & Wong, 2005). Bandyopadhyay and Pardasani (2011) found that clients of interdisciplinary community health centers highlighted cultural sensitivity on the part of staff, an understanding of the unique needs of different genders, recognition of the importance of religion and spirituality in treatment plans, and culturally appropriate communication (translators, bilingual reading materials, etc.) were critical tools to serving diverse clients effectively. Barney (2017) argues that a critical underpinning of a culturally competent organization is its mission (and practice) to encourage participatory decision-making. He argues that this not only helps address the power differential between provider and consumer but also addresses the structural inequities that impact cultural competence in service delivery (Barney, 2017). Commitment to such practices also incorporates the concept of intersectionality and power within the workplace, both with clients and providers. Dominelli and Ioakimidis (2015) believe that addressing the marginalization experienced by our clients is the most effective method to enhance cultural competence in social work.

In addition to issues of race/ethnicity, greater attention is being paid to sexual identity and sexual orientation in social work practice. Davies (1996) highlighted culturally competent practice as one that "affirms a lesbian, gay, or bisexual identity as an equally positive human experience and expression to heterosexual identity" (p. 25). Affirmative practitioners celebrate, advocate, and validate the identities of LGBT individuals (Crisp & McCave, 2007; Moone et al., 2014; Tozer & McClanahan, 1999). Frequently though, the issues of gender identity are lost in the maze of discussion about gay and lesbian clients. Markman (2011) and Vanderburgh (2009) have highlighted the critical need to prepare social workers to conduct outreach, comprehensively assess needs, and develop interventions specifically tailored for transgendered clients.

There is a growing emphasis on assessing and incorporating the spirituality or religious beliefs into practice with clients (Gilligan & Furness, 2006; Husain, 2017). They posit that incorporating the religious and spiritual beliefs and practices of clients into the service delivery model is necessary for culturally competent practice. Hodge (2006) coined the term "spiritual interventions," which called for the incorporation of a religious/spiritual component as a central dimension of treatment if it was important to the clients. Gilligan and Furness (2006) posit that social workers need to respond appropriately to the needs of service users for whom religious and spiritual beliefs are crucial. They argue that culturally competent practice depends on an understanding of the impact of faith and belief on an individual's decisions in life (Gilligan & Furness, 2006).

Finally, in a country historically built on immigration, the needs and concerns of immigrants and refugees within the purview of social service are also of paramount concern. Understanding the complex process of migration is necessary as it has been shown to impact individual experiences and challenges (Foster, 2001; Furman et al., 2009; Shier, Engstron, & Graham, 2011). The nature of migration with respect to choice (voluntary vs. involuntary), past trauma, separation from family, pressure of assimilation, and adaptation to an alien culture, legal status of residency, and exploitation influence help-seeking decisions made by refugee and immigrant clients.

## Culturally Competent Leadership and Human Resources Management

As mentioned earlier, social work managers are increasingly challenged with creating an inclusive organizational culture by welcoming and promoting diversity in their organizations (Cox, 2001; Findler, Wind, & Mor Barak, 2007; Miller & Katz, 2002). Social work agencies are increasingly multidisciplinary, and leaders need to manage a diverse workforce with respect to gender, race/ethnicity, age, national origin, sexual orientation and sexual identity, religious affiliation, and social class, as well as educational backgrounds. And rather than dealing with each of these factors as separate, they need to understand the complex interplay of these various identities and their impact on the work environment.

Reviews of existing diversity research suggest that demographic differences can have both positive and negative effects on how organizational members interact and perform (O'Leary & Weathington, 2006). A diverse workforce (in terms of race/ethnicity, education, and work experience) has been found to be positively associated with creative problem solving (McLeod & Lobel, 1992; Watson, Kumar, & Michaelsen, 1993), innovative practice techniques (Bantel & Jackson, 1989), cooperation between staff (Cox, Lobel, & McLeod, 1991), and a readiness to consider diverse perspectives and values (O'Reilly, Williams, & Barsade, 1997). Acquavita, Pitman, Gibbons, and Castellanos-Brown (2009) conducted a national survey of social workers and found that organizational diversity actually increased social workers' job satisfaction.

However, simply having a diverse workforce in itself does not guarantee greater productivity or job satisfaction. In fact, diverse workplaces have also been linked to greater interpersonal conflict, lack of team cohesion, poor communication, and lowered job satisfaction (O'Leary & Weathington, 2006). In order to utilize the diversity inherent in the workforce to create a healthy environment and effectively serve clients, social work managers and leaders need to pay attention to their own role in cultivating a culturally competent workplace. In other words, organizational culture needs to embrace and commit to promoting cultural competence. Findler, Wind, and Mor Barak (2007) reported "organizational-culture variables such as fairness, inclusion, and social support to employee outcomes of well-being, job satisfaction, and organizational commitment" (p. 64). Mamman (1996) also identified situational factors (attitudes toward others from different backgrounds, exposure to diverse groups, organizational culture, and management attitudes toward diversity), and interaction strategies employed by staff in dealing with differences (avoidance vs. action) as mediating the experiences of an individual working in a diverse workplace. Mamman (1996) posited that while an individual's cultural background cannot be changed, factors identified as mediating variables could be addressed by the management of an organization to enhance worker motivation and teamwork while serving diverse clients more competently. Acquavita et al. (2009) also reported that supervisory support of employees and perception of inclusion/exclusion in the workplace played a significant role in workers' satisfaction on the job and their motivation to do good work.

Blitz and Kohl Jr. (2012) suggested racial affinity group meetings that could act as effective tools against racism within the workplace and help initiate organizational cultural shifts toward cultural responsiveness. Other researchers posit that making sure organizations incorporate practices that empower clients, build their self-reliance and actively address social problems encountered by them would make them responsive to diverse settings (Robaeys, Raeymaeckers, & van Ewijk, 2018).

## Strategies for Developing Cultural Competence

Edewor and Aluko (2007) identified several steps to creating a multicultural workplace—managing by example, explicit policies regarding diversity, training programs, awareness and acknowledgment of differences, actively seeking input from minority groups, rewarding culturally competent behavior, increasing opportunities for socialization among staff, flexible work environment, and consistent monitoring of staff interactions and performance. In this section, we identify strategies to develop and/or enhance cultural competence within organizations on two levels:

1. Service delivery
2. Leadership within organizations and human resources management

In order to create a culturally competent and inclusive organization, leaders (board members and managers) need to engage in some soul-searching with regard to their motives for transforming the workplace. This introspection is important as it will determine the plan of action undertaken by the leadership. Ely and Thomas (2001) identified three perspectives that inform the actions of organizational leaders: discrimination-and-fairness, integration-and-learning, and access-and-legitimacy. The discrimination-and-fairness perspective suggests that cultural diversity is essentially a moral imperative that should be implemented because of its inherent virtue, and not be tied to financial outcomes. The integration-and-learning perspective proposes that the diversity of ideas arising from diverse backgrounds and experiences can benefit the organization in a variety of ways. Finally, the access-and-legitimacy perspective espouses the benefits of "matching the organization's cultural diversity to that of its surrounding area or customer base" (as cited in O'Leary & Weathington, 2006, p. 6). The authors of this chapter believe all three perspectives need to be incorporated into any process of change, as they underscore the basic professional values and mission of social work.

Once the organizational motives have been clearly espoused, leaders need to conduct a comprehensive assessment of services, personnel, board of directors, and the consumer base. This involves several steps: (a) collecting demographic information about managers, board members, staff, and clients; (b) developing a profile of the community in which the organization is located; (c) assessing whether the current service model meets the needs of diverse clients and other members of the community; (d) evaluating staff morale and cohesiveness; (e) assessing the level of awareness, knowledge, and skills of staff with respect to working with diverse groups; (f) reviewing organizational mission and policies regarding diversity in the workplace; and (g) collecting a historical perspective on how the organization has dealt with diversity. Once this assessment has been completed and reviewed by the management, board of directors, and staff members, the organization can begin the process of transformation and growth.

1. Ensuring culturally competent service delivery:
    In order to ensure that the services and programs offered by an organization are meeting the needs of diverse clients, the following steps are critical:

    a. *Hiring staff that reflects the demographic profile of clients and/or community.* The staff profile needs to reflect the diversity of their consumer base to the greatest extent possible. Clients from minority groups, especially those who belong to disenfranchised, oppressed, or discriminated groups, may be wary of staff members who have difficulty in "connecting" with them. Trust is an essential component of building worker–client therapeutic rapport, and this can be enhanced by recruiting personnel from the clients' respective groups. We are not advocating for matching every client with staff that has the same demographic characteristics. Similarly, concurrent with our discussion of intersectionality, it is not as simple as matching staff–client characteristics by ethnicity, gender, sexual orientation, or religious affiliation. We believe that the presence of competent staff from diverse backgrounds could enhance outreach and relationships between the agency and clients. The diversity of experiences with marginalization, oppression, and privilege are necessary to have a nuanced understanding of our target populations. It is also important to ensure that staff members speak the languages most prevalent in the community in which the agency operates. If bilingual staff is not available, efforts should be made to offer translation services through interns, community peers, or volunteers. Agency forms could also be translated into a format that encourages accurate and comprehensive information sharing. Informational materials such as flyers and brochures need to be linguistically appropriate, but more importantly, the pictures needs to reflect the clients who are being served.

b. *Training for staff and managers.* Becoming a culturally competent professional requires developing self-awareness and enhancing one's practice knowledge and skills. In this regard, training for staff is critical. Training would challenge staff and managers to confront their own biases, prejudices, long-held stereotypes, and values. Being able to verbalize and understand one's own beliefs about others is necessary in order to unlearn what is not helpful and integrate new information and ideas. The second goal of training would be to enhance one's awareness and knowledge of diverse client populations and develop critical skills for effective practice. This requires dialogue between staff members themselves, dialogue between staff and current clients, and dialogue with community leaders and representatives of the groups being served. Agencies can invite community leaders, professional trainers, and experts who can inform and educate the staff. One issue to keep in mind is that training needs to be consistent. Very often, agencies will offer training in response to a crisis or serious complaint, and then there is no follow-up. Since developing cultural competence is a long-term, continuous learning process, training needs to be offered strategically and consistently. In other words, training must become part of the organizational culture and be a crucial component of the job responsibilities of staff, managers, and even board members. Furthermore, the concepts of power, privilege, marginalization, and intersectionality have to be grappled with by staff and administrators. Openness to address these issues can be challenging but is critical to any effective impact in the workplace.

c. *Including evidence-based interventions.* There is an increasing awareness and incorporation of evidence-based interventions in social work agencies. There is also a significant body of research on effective interventions with diverse groups. It would behoove agencies to investigate these documented practices and service models, and adapt them to suit the specific needs of their consumer base. These models can provide ideas for effective recruitment, engagement, assessment, and practice with members of historically underserved, oppressed, or stigmatized populations.

d. *Setting up a consumer advisory group.* Client empowerment is a critical goal of social work, and allowing clients to collaborate in their treatment is an important strategy to realize that mission. A consumer advisory group that is reflective of client diversity would be an effective tool to building trust among management, staff, and clients. An advisory group could also serve as a vehicle to test out new program ideas, assess current perceptions of staff competence, identify unmet needs, and evaluate consumer satisfaction with services. This group could provide ideas and guidance to the agency to enhance their services and provide maximum benefit to the community. Management would have to be cognizant of the fact that group members may feel vulnerable to backlash or be treated in a patronizing manner. All efforts must be made to protect the advisory group members from staff persecution, and any ideas generated by the group must be given full and serious consideration. Otherwise, the advisory group will be viewed as "spokespersons" for management and will lack the support of their fellow clients.

e. *Cultivating community leaders and peer mentors.* Developing partnerships and linkages within a community is important if an agency wishes to thrive. Partnerships with other community organizations need to be strategic and coordinated in order to increase access to new clients, enhance services for current clients (through referrals to partners), and building goodwill in the community. Similarly, cultivating leaders of minority groups or peers from underserved groups would assist the agency in reaching out to a wider cross-section of clients. These members of the community can act as gatekeepers for referrals, help reduce community suspicions and/or opposition, and provide valuable guidance for effective service.

f. *Recruitment and outreach of underserved, marginalized, and vulnerable groups.* As discussed earlier, some members of a community may be resistant to seek help from agencies due to a lack of trust or knowledge of an agency's services. Additionally, societal stigmatization of their identity, status, or problems may lead to avoidance of assistance. Developing specialized outreach efforts that speak to members of underserved groups would be essential. The agency can use their staff, community partners, and peer mentors to build inroads into the community. Incorporation of evidence-based engagement techniques with diverse populations could be helpful and effective. Recruitment materials (posters, advertisements, presentations at various sites, etc.) should be designed to keep the linguistic abilities, demographic characteristics (race/ethnicity, sexual orientation, sexual identity, religious affiliation, health status, etc.), and needs of the people being reached. Additionally, if practices within an organization reflect shared or participatory decision-making, that ensures respect for the inherent strengths/resilience of the target populations and enhances their motivation to engage with the organization.

2. Ensuring culturally competent leadership and human resources management: In order to develop and maintain a workforce that is culturally competent, the following steps are critical:

a. *Recruitment of a diverse board of directors.* The board of a nonprofit organization like a social work agency should be comprised of volunteers from diverse backgrounds. However, board members do not always reflect the diversity of the clients served. This directly impacts the motivation and ability of an organization to engage in the exhaustive process of developing cultural competence. Board members from diverse backgrounds could provide guidance on, and raise awareness of, cultural differences. They could assist the management in making inroads into underserved communities and help build agency credibility. Awareness of the intersectionality of social identities and the implicit privilege enjoyed by potential members of the board (due to their professional and social status) must be a part of the selection process.
b. *Ensuring concise and specific written policies.* All organizations have a policy and procedures manual. Usually, organizations have clearly spelled out policies regarding promotion of diversity in human resources and prevention of discrimination in the workforce. These written policies are strongly influenced by the various human resource laws that exist and with which social work agencies need to be in compliance. Clearly written policies can be effective in preventing all forms of harassment from taking root and creating hostile work environments. The reputation and public image of agencies can easily be tarnished, while worker morale is damaged, because of racially motivated remarks, ethnic slurs, and subtle forms of intimidation that fall within the definition of sexual harassment. Agencies need to develop policies (and monitor compliance) that acknowledge the dignity of each worker and the right to work in an environment free of personal harassment, stress, and interpersonal friction. These policies should specifically forbid all forms of harassment and discriminatory behavior, and spell out the penalties, including dismissal or personal legal and financial liability. A policy manual should also provide guidance to employees to report incidents of abuse or harassment and assure them of protection for doing so.
c. *Providing training for staff, managers, and board members.* This type of training is different from the one proposed earlier to enhance the cultural competence of service delivery. This training would specifically center around providing information on what constitutes a culturally competent organization, existing laws, and agency policies regarding discrimination and harassment and options available to employees for reporting such incidents. The trainings would also engage managers and staff in confronting their own biases and stereotypes about each other in a safe environment while learning effective means of legal and ethical communication. It would also be helpful if staff and managers can learn techniques of conflict resolution and team building in order to increase group cohesion.
d. *Providing mentoring for staff members.* Frequently, staff members belonging to minority groups feel estranged from their colleagues or excluded from strategic alliances. It is very difficult for a new staff member from any background to break into or join an existing group. However, it is exceptionally hard for members of minority groups to feel accepted. This may be due to disinterest, wariness, or the reluctance of other staff members to engage a person they deem "different." This reluctance could stem from existing biases about the group the new staff member belongs to, or a fear of offending the person by saying the wrong thing. At other times, the new staff

member may be peppered with questions about their beliefs and practices, making them feel like they need to be spokespersons for their community. Dialogue and exchange of information is a positive means of building a cohesive team and enhancing cultural competence, but this process needs to be supervised. Managers could offer mentoring to all staff members to facilitate the process of inclusion. Care must be taken to not just mentor staff members from minority groups as this may lead to conflict or envy. But a general mentoring process would allow all staff members to feel valued and respected.

e. *Creating opportunities for socialization.* Opportunities for socialization outside of daily work responsibilities makes staff feel valued for their contributions and allows staff to get to know each other personally. A typical workday can be quite hectic or frenzied, allowing little time for staff members to engage with one another in a meaningful manner. Socializing away from the workplace, staff members are more relaxed and are able to communicate freely. This allows for a free and open exchange of ideas, increases awareness and empathy, and helps develop rapport. If staff members are left to socialize on their own, they may only invite individuals they like or are comfortable with. But events organized by management would ensure that all employees are invited and have the opportunity to engage with one another. Such events would increase staff morale and help build team spirit. These events also help staff members and administrators understand each other as complex, nuanced human beings who are not simply a representative of one social identity but an amalgamation of experiences and values. This enhances cross-cultural understanding and rapport.

f. *Consistently monitoring policy compliance and organizational morale.* It is the ethical and moral responsibility of the board and management to ensure that an agency is constantly working on enhancing its cultural competence. Provisions need to be made to consistently and systematically monitor compliance with agency policies regarding staff recruitment, development and training, prevention of harassment or discrimination, and optimum service delivery. Furthermore, the leadership needs to engage in a process of routinely assessing the morale of both staff and clients, evaluating complaints and grievances, and ensuring the promotion of participatory decision-making at all levels.

## Building a Multicultural Perspective Into the Organizational Culture

As we have discussed, creating an agency culture that optimizes heterogeneity is considered to be one of the major challenges facing human service administrators and leaders today (Brody, 1993; Hasenfeld, 1996; Menefee, 1997). Hyde (2004) uses the phrase "diversity climate" to begin to explain the diversity and multicultural dimensions of an organization's culture and as a framing conceptualization to explore the organizational characteristics that contribute or detract from building a functional and flourishing climate of diversity. They define diversity climate as a construct designed to capture the breadth and depth of organizational diversity measured by both the literal degree of staff diversity and also the efforts to promote and further an environment that maximizes the benefits of such diversity.

An organization's diversity climate reflects the degree to which a primary goal of most diversity intention models is achieved: the creation of a culturally pluralistic setting in which all workers perform at their optimal levels. (Hyde & Hopkins, 2008, p. 27)

Organizations with more robust diversity climates engage in efforts that reflect a long-term orientation and commitment to infusing the organization's culture with a multicultural perspective. This includes reflecting diversity in outreach efforts (both staff and clients), staff accountability, resource allocation, and planning (Cox, 2001; Hyde, 2003, 2004; Iglehart, 2000; Norton & Fox, 1997). While long-range orientations toward building a diversity climate tend to yield the most robust and lasting results, more frequently organizations engage in sporadic training (including occasional training on cultural sensitivity and communication), and developing nondiscriminatory policies that tend to result in only weak to moderate changes in organizational culture. Similar to other organizational change or development strategies, diversity initiatives seem to be most sensitive to sabotage by a lack of leadership, high workload demands, staff resistance, and a failure to engage the community (Hayles & Russell, 1997; Hyde, 2003, 2004; Iglehart, 2000).

## Barriers to Cultural Competency

We have outlined several strategies for increasing cultural competency both internally by creating climates respectful of difference and externally in terms of thinking about how we are employing culturally competent treatment modalities. However, we must also have a realistic understanding of the barriers to creating organizational climates and cultures that respect difference and where a diverse range of staff can succeed as human services professionals. Two well-documented barriers or challenges to effective multicultural climates are microaggressions and aversive racism. These two forms of subtle racism and oppression may be perpetrated on the staff to staff level as well as on the staff to client level. As human services managers we must be aware of how these unconscious oppressive mechanisms operate and begin to develop strategies for creating respectful and welcoming climates for all staff and clients.

Racial microaggressions are brief and commonplace daily verbal, behavioral, or environmental indignities, whether intentional or unintentional, that communicate hostile, derogatory, or negative racial slights and insults toward people of color and people with different religious affiliations. Perpetrators of microaggressions are often unaware that they engage in such communications when they interact with racial/ethnic minorities (Sue et al., 2007). Microaggressions are unconsciously delivered as subtle snubs, dismissive looks, gestures, and tones. These exchanges are so pervasive and automatic in daily conversations and interactions that they are often dismissed and glossed over as being innocent and innocuous. Yet, as indicated previously, microaggressions are detrimental because they impair performance in a multitude of settings by sapping the psychic and spiritual energy of recipients and by creating inequities (Franklin, 2004; Sue, 2004).

Sue et al. identify three main types of microaggressions: microassault, microinsult, and microinvalidation. A microassault is an explicit racially motivated attack, characterized primarily by a verbal or nonverbal assault meant to hurt the intended victim through name-calling, avoidant behavior, or purposeful discriminatory actions. Microassaults are most similar to what has been called "old fashioned" racism conducted on a micro or individual level. They are most often conscious and deliberate, although they are generally expressed in limited "private" situations (micro) that allow the perpetrator some degree of anonymity. A microinsult is characterized by communications that convey rudeness and insensitivity and demean a person's racial heritage or identity. Microinsults represent subtle snubs, frequently unknown to the perpetrator, but clearly convey a hidden insulting message to the recipient of color. Microinvalidations are characterized by communications that exclude, negate, or nullify the psychological thoughts, feelings, or experiential reality of a person of color (Sue et al., 2008).

It is clear that any plan for creating a culturally competent management practice must help managers to overcome their fears and their resistance to talking about race or other social identities by fostering safe and productive learning environments (Sanchez-Hucles & Jones, 2005). It is important that any training or development program be structured and facilitated in a manner that promotes inquiry and allows managers to experience discomfort and vulnerability (Young & Davis-Russell, 2002). The prerequisite for cultural competence has always been racial self-awareness. This is equally true for understanding microaggressions. This level of self-awareness brings to the surface possible prejudices and biases that inform racial microaggressions. Education and training must aid managers in achieving the following: (a) increase their ability to identify racial microaggressions in general and in themselves in particular; (b) understand how racial microaggressions, including their own, detrimentally impact clients of color; and (c) accept responsibility for taking corrective actions to overcome racial biases (Sue et al., 2008).

### Future Directions for Culturally Competent Management

Social work agencies are charged with creating and sustaining culturally competent, multicultural organizations. "An organization which simply contains many different cultural groups is just a plural organization, but it is considered multicultural only if the organization values this diversity" (Edewor & Aluko, 2007, p. 190). A culturally competent organization is one that integrates diverse staff at all levels within an organization, promotes the human rights of staff and clients, prevents discrimination and harassment, addresses the concept of intersectionality, builds bridges with the community in which they exist, offers programs and services that meet the needs of their constituents, and advocates for a just and equitable society. It is important that agencies not just accommodate diversity but also value and incorporate that diversity.

### REFERENCES

Acquavita, S. P., Pittman, J., Gibbons, M., & Castellanos-Brown, K. (2009). Personal and organizational diversity factors' impact on social workers job satisfaction: Results from a national Internet based survey. *Administration in Social Work, 33,* 151–166. doi:10.1080/03643100902768824

Bandyopadhyay, S., & Pardasani, M. (2011). Do quality perceptions of health and social services vary for different ethnic groups? An empirical investigation. *International Journal of Non-Profit and Voluntary Sector Marketing, 16*(1), 99–114. doi:10.1002/nvsm.404

Bantel, K., & Jackson, S. (1989). Top management and innovations in banking: Does composition of the team make a difference? *Strategic Management Journal, 10*, 107–124. doi:10.1002/smj.4250100709

Barney, R. (2017). South African HIV/AIDS service providers' perceptions of participatory decision-making and empowerment: Exploring the role of power distance. *International Social Work, 60*(4), 914–926. doi:10.1177/0020872815594219

Bass, S. (2008). Multiculturalism, American style: The politics of multiculturalism in the United States. *Journal of International Diversity in Organizations, Communities and Nations, 7*(6), 133–141. doi:10.18848/1447-9532/CGP/v07i06/39498

Blitz, L., & Kohl, Jr. B. (2012). Addressing racism in the organization: The role of Caucasian affinity groups in creating change. *Administration in Social Work, 36*, 479–498. doi: 10.1080/03643107.2011.624261

Brody, R. (1993). *Effectively managing human service organizations.* Newbury Park, CA: Sage.

Bubar, R., Cespedes, K., & Bundy-Fazioli, K. (2016). Intersectionality and social work: Omissions of race, class and sexuality in graduate school education. *Journal of Social Work Education, 52*(3), 283–296. doi:10.1080/10437797.2016.1174636

Bureau of Labor Statistics. (2015). *Labor force projections to 2024: The labor force is growing, but slowly.* Retrieved from https://www.bls.gov/opub/mlr/2015/article/labor-force-projections-to-2024.htm

Bureau of Labor Statistics. (2018). *Labor Force Statistics From the Current Population Survey.* Retrieved from https://www.bls.gov/cps/cpsaat11.htm

Council of Social Work Education. (2017). *Profile of the Social Work Workforce.* Washington, DC: Author

Cox, T. H. (2001). *Creating the multicultural organization: A strategy for capturing the power of diversity.* San Francisco, CA: Jossey-Bass.

Cox, T. H., Lobel, S. A., & McLeod, P. L. (1991). Effects of ethnic group cultural differences on cooperative, and competitive behavior on a group task. *Academy of Management Journal, 34*, 827–847. doi:10.5465/256391

Crisp, C., & McCave, E. L. (2007). Gay affirmative practice: A model for working with gay, lesbian and bisexual youth. *Child and Adolescent Social Work Journal, 24*, 403–421. doi:10.1007/s10560-007-0091-z

Cross, T., Bazron, B., Dennis, K., & Isaacs, M. (1989). *Towards a culturally competent system of care: A monograph of effective services for minority children who are severely emotionally disturbed.* Washington, DC: Georgetown University Child Development Center.

Davies, D. (1996). Towards a model of gay affirmative therapy. In D. Davies & C. Neal (Eds.), *Pink therapy: A guide for counselors and therapists working with lesbian, gay and bisexual clients.* Buckingham, UK: Open University Press.

Dominelli, L., & Iaokimidis, V. (2015). Social work on the frontline in addressing disasters, social problems and marginalization. *International Social Work, 58*(1), 3–6. doi:10.1177/0020872814561402

Edewor, P. A., & Aluko, Y. A. (2007). Diversity management: Opportunities and challenges in multicultural organizations. *International Journal of Diversity, 6*(6), 189–195. doi:10.18848/1447-9532/CGP/v06i06/39285

Ely, R., & Thomas, D. (2001). Cultural diversity at work: The effects of diversity perspectives on work group processes and outcomes. *Administrative Science Quarterly, 46*(2), 229–273. doi:10.2307/2667087

Findler, L., Wind, L. H., & Mor Barak, M. E. (2007). The challenge of workforce management in a global society: Modeling the relationship between diversity, inclusion, organizational culture, and employee well-being, job satisfaction and organizational commitment. *Administration in Social Work, 31*(3), 63–94. doi:10.1300/J147v31n03_05

Fisher-Borne, M., Cain, J., & Martin, S. (2015). From mastery to accountability: Cultural humility as an alternative to cultural competence. *Social Work Education, 34*(2), 165–181. doi:10.1080/02615479.2014.977244

Foster, R. P. (2001). When immigration is trauma: Guidelines for the individual and family clinician. *American Journal of Orthopsychiatry, 71*(2), 153–170. doi:10.1037/0002-9432.71.2.153

Franklin, A. J. (2004). *From brotherhood to manhood: How Black men rescue their relationships and dreams from the invisibility syndrome.* Hoboken, NJ: Wiley.

Furman, R., Negi, N., Iwamoto, D., Rowan, D., Shukraft, A., & Gragg, J. (2009). Social work practice with Latinos: Key issues for social workers. *Social Work, 54*(2), 167–174. doi:10.1093/sw/54.2.167

Gilligan, P., & Furness, S. (2006). The role of religion and spirituality in social work practice: Views and experiences of social workers and students. *British Journal of Social Work, 36*(4), 617–637. doi:10.1093/bjsw/bch252

Goldkind, L., & Pardasani, M. (2010). *Assessing the core competencies of social service administrators and managers.* Paper presented at the Council on Social Work Education (CSWE) Annual Program Meeting, Portland, Oregon.

Hasenfeld, Y. (1996). The administration of human services. In P. Raffoul & C. McNeece (Eds.), *Future issues in social work practice* (pp. 191–202). Boston, MA: Allyn & Bacon.

Hayles, R., & Russell, A. (1997). *The diversity directive: Why some initiatives fail & what to do about it.* New York, NY: McGraw-Hill.

Hodge, D. R. (2006). Spiritually modified cognitive therapy: A review of the literature. *Social Work, 51,* 157–166. doi:10.1093/sw/51.2.157

Hodge, D., & Bushfield, S. (2006). Developing spiritual competence in practice. *Journal of Ethnic and Cultural Diversity in Social Work, 15*(3/4), 101–127. doi:10.1300/J051v15n03_05

Husain, A. (2017). Islam in the 21st century: Challenges and opportunities for social work with Muslims. *Journal of Religion & Spirituality in Social Work: Social Thought, 36*(1/2), 1–5. doi:10.1080/15426432.2017.1324699

Hyde, C. (2003). More harm than good? Multicultural initiatives in human service agencies. *Social Thought, 8,* 23–43. doi:10.1080/15426432.2003.9960324

Hyde, C. (2004). Multicultural development in human services: Challenges and solutions. *Social Work, 49,* 7–16. doi:10.1093/sw/49.1.7

Hyde, C. & Hopkins A. (2008). Diversity climates in human service agencies: An exploratory assessment. *Journal of Ethnic and Cultural Diversity in Social Work, 13*(2), 25–43.

Iglehart, A. (2000). Managing for diversity and empowerment in social services. In R. Patti (Ed.), *The handbook of social welfare administration* (pp. 425–444). Thousand Oaks, CA: Sage.

Mamman, A. (1996). A diverse employee in a changing workplace. *Organization Studies, 17*(3), 449–477. doi:10.1177/017084069601700305

Markman, E. R. (2011). Gender identity disorder, the gender binary and transgender oppression: Implications for ethical practice. *Smith College Studies in Social Work, 81*(4), 314–327. doi:10.1080/00377317.2011.616839

Martin, L., & Bonder, B. (2003). Achieving organizational change within the context of cultural competence. *Journal of Social Work in Long Term Care, 21*(1/2), 81–94. doi:10.1300/J181v02n01_06

McLeod, P. L., & Lobel, S. A. (1992). *The effects of ethnic diversity on idea generation in small groups.* Paper presented at the Annual Academy of Management Meeting, Las Vegas, Nevada.

Menefee, D. (1997). Strategic administration of nonprofit human service organizations: A model of executive success in turbulent times. *Administration in Social Work, 21,* 1–19. doi:10.5465/ambpp.1992.17515639

Miller, F. A., & Katz, J. H. (2002). *The inclusion breakthrough.* San Francisco, CA: Berret-Koehler.

Moone, R., Cagle, J., Coghan, C., & Smith, J. (2014). Working with LGBT older adults: An assessment of employee training practices, needs and preferences of senior service organizations in Minnesota. *Journal of Gerontological Social Work, 57*, 322–334. doi: 10.1080/01634372.2013.843630

Norton, J., & Fox, R. (1997). *The change equation: Capitalizing on diversity for effective organizational change*. Washington, DC: American Psychological Association.

O'Leary, B. J., & Weathington, B. L. (2006). Beyond the business case for diversity in organizations. *Employee Responsibilities and Rights Journal, 18*(4), 283–292. doi:10.1007/s10672-006-9024-9

O'Reilly, C., Williams, K., & Barsade, S. (1997). Group demography and innovation: Does diversity help? In E. Mannix & M. Neale (Eds.), *Research in the management of groups and teams*. Greenwich, CT: JAI Press.

Ostrowerer, F. (2007). *Non-profit governance in the United States: Findings on performance and accountability from the first national representative study*. Washington, DC: Center on Nonprofits and Philanthropy, The Urban Institute.

Pinderhughes, E. (1989). *Understanding race, ethnicity and power: The key to efficacy in clinical practice*. New York, NY: Free Press.

Poston, D., & Saenz, R. (2019). The U.S. Caucasian majority will soon disappear forever. *The Chicago Reporter*, May 16.

Ramos-Sanchez, L. (2009). Counselor bilingual ability, counselor ethnicity, acculturation, and Mexican Americans' perceived counselor credibility. *Journal of Counseling and Development, 87*(3), 311–318. doi:10.1002/j.1556-6678.2009.tb00112.x

Robaeys, B., Raeymaeckers, P., & van Ewijk, H. (2018). Contextual-transformational social work in super-diverse contexts: An evaluative perspective by clients and social workers. *Qualitative Social Work, 17*(5), 676–691. doi:10.1177/1473325016683793

Sanchez-Hucles, J., & Jones, N. (2005). Breaking the silence around race in training, practice, and research. *Counseling Psychologist, 33*, 547–558. doi:10.1177/0011000005276462

Saunders, J., Haskins, M., & Vasquez, M. (2015). Cultural competence: A journey to an elusive goal. *Journal of Social Work Education, 51*, 19–34. doi:10.1080/10437797.2015.977124

Shier, M. L., Engstrom, S., & Graham, J. R. (2011). International migration and social work—A review of the literature. *Journal of Immigrant and Refugee Studies, 9*, 38–56. doi:10.1080/15562948.2011.547825

Sue, D. W. (2004). Caucasianness and ethnocentric monoculturalism: Making the "invisible" visible. *American Psychologist, 59*, 759–769. doi:10.1037/0003-066X.59.8.761

Sue, D. W., Capodilupo, C. M., Nadal, K. L., & Torino, G. C. (2008). Racial microaggressions and the power to define reality. *American Psychologist, 63*(4), 277–279.

Sue, D. W., Capodilupo, C. M., Torino, G. C., Bucceri, J. M., Holder, A. M. B., Nadal, K., & Esquilin, M. (2007). Racial microaggressions in everyday life: Implications for clinical practice. *American Psychologist, 62*(4), 271–286. doi:10.1037/0003-066X.62.4.271

Switzer, G., Scholle, S., Johnson, B., & Kelleher, K. (1998). The Client Cultural Competence Inventory: An instrument for assessing cultural competence in behavioral managed-care organizations. *Journal of Child and Family Studies, 7*(4), 483–491. doi:10.1023/A:1022910111022

Taylor, B., Garcia, A., & Kingson, E. (2001). Cultural competence versus cultural chauvinism: Implications for social work. *Health and Social Work, 26*(3), 185–187. doi:10.1093/hsw/26.3.185

Tozer, E. E., & McClanahan, M. K. (1999). Treating the purple menace: Ethical considerations of conversion therapy and affirmative alternatives. *Counseling Psychologist, 27*, 722–742. doi:10.1177/0011000099275006

U.S. Census Bureau. (2018). *Ethnicity and race: Quick facts*. Washington, DC: U.S. Department of Commerce. Retrieved from https://www.census.gov/quickfacts/fact/table/US/PST045218

U.S. Department of Labor. (2017). *Selected characteristics of the native and foreign-born populations*. Washington, DC: U.S. Bureau of Labor Statistics. Retrieved from https://factfinder.census.gov/faces/tableservices/jsf/pages/productview.xhtml?src=bkmk

Vanderburgh, R. (2009). Appropriate therapeutic care for families with pre-pubescent transgender/gender-dissonant children. *Child and Adolescent Social Work Journal, 26*(2), 135–154. doi:10.1007/s10560-008-0158-5

Watson, W. E., Kumar, K., & Michaelsen, L. K. (1993). Cultural diversity's impact on interaction process and performance: Comparing homogeneous and diverse task groups. *Academy of Management Journal, 36*, 590–602. doi:10.2307/256593

Williams, C. (2006). The epistemology of cultural competence. *Families in Society, 87*(2), 209–220. doi:10.1606/1044-3894.3514

Yan, M., & Wong, Y. (2005). Re-thinking self-awareness in cultural competence: Toward a dialogic self in cross-cultural social work. *Families in Society, 86*(2), 181–188. doi:10.1606/1044-3894.2453

Young, G., & Davis-Russell, E. (2002). The vicissitudes of cultural competence: Dealing with difficult classroom dialogue. In E. Davis-Russell (Ed.), *The California School of Professional Psychology Handbook of multicultural education, research, intervention, and training* (pp. 37–53). San Francisco, CA: Jossey-Bass.

Zeitlin, W., Altschul, D., & Samuels, J. (2016). Assessing the utility of a toolkit for modifying evidence-based practice to increase cultural competence: A comparative case study. *Human Service Organizations: Management, Leadership and Governance, 40*(4), 369–381. doi:10.1080/23303131.2016.1153551

# 7

# Legal Issues in Practice With Immigrants and Refugees

*Fernando Chang-Muy*

## INTRODUCTION

Given the evolving demographics with the movement of people across borders, nonprofit organizations and their social service staff must adapt and ensure that programs and services respond to meet the needs of these clients. As a best practice, organizations that are effective regularly evaluate their boards of directors, management and line staff, programs, and operations to ensure that all of these areas take into account newcomer strengths and challenges and meet the needs of the populations served.

In order to be effective, providers should have a working knowledge of immigration issues that their clients face regardless of the providers' areas of expertise, be it health, mental health, employment, education, or housing, and regardless of populations served—women, youth, elderly, and homeless. Providers' lack of knowledge of clients' legal immigration challenges may result as a barrier to care, adding to mental and physical health stressors in the client, and impeding resolution of other core issues that the social service provider is trying to resolve.

This chapter hopes to raise service providers' knowledge by providing a framework of immigration policies, with a focus on three particular newcomer populations—women, youth, and refugees. Understanding newcomer clients' strengths as well as challenges, including legal immigration challenges, will allow providers to develop, in partnership with the client, a comprehensive action plan to move forward. To do so, this chapter first provides a brief overview of key legal classifications in U.S. immigration law, such as definitions for undocumented, immigrant, and citizen. Then the chapter focuses on women, youth, and refugees and their particular legal challenges as well as strengths. As refugees are a particularly vulnerable group, the chapter details the process for applying for refugee status and how service providers can support asylum seekers. The chapter concludes with overall suggestions on cultural competency in serving newcomer communities.

The ultimate desired outcome is to enable newcomers to have agency in their own life and contribute to their community. Given the tools to understand key aspects of immigration law, social service providers, in collaboration with legal services and other human service providers, can support newcomers so that they in turn can build on their strengths and resilience, and contribute to their own well-being, their families, and their new host communities.

## U.S. IMMIGRATION LEGAL CLASSIFICATIONS: NONIMMIGRANT AND UNDOCUMENTED

U.S. immigration law[1] sets out a variety of methods in which newcomers can enter the country legally. This section deals with *short-* and *long-term* methods of entry. Typically, foreigners (to be called "newcomers" in this chapter) can enter the United States for a short term or long term. The law sets out reasons for entering for a short term, such as (a) tourism, (b) education, (c) short-term employment, or (d) humanitarian reasons. This section focuses only on humanitarian reasons for entering, as these are the types of newcomers that a social service agency may usually encounter.

In order to enter the United States legally, that is, with documents, newcomers must have a passport and some may need a visa. Just as in order to enter a room, one needs a door and a key—a passport (issued by the country of origin) is analogous to a door, and a visa (issued by the U.S. embassy or consulate in the country of origin) is the "key" permitting newcomers to enter the room (in this context, the United States). The U.S. Visa Waiver Program (VWP)[2] allows citizens of specific countries to travel to the United States for up to 90 days *without* having to obtain a visa. In turn, and as a reciprocal agreement, U.S. citizens similarly do *not* have to apply for a visa to enter those countries. All countries participating in the VWP are regarded as developed countries (i.e., most European countries).

The Immigration Act classifies as "illegal" (to be called "undocumented" in this chapter) those individuals who enter without a passport or visa. There are situations, however, where persons do enter *with* the proper documents (passport and visa) but could later become *undocumented*[3] if the visa expires and/or the person does not return to their country of origin under the terms of the visa types described here. It is estimated that there may be 11 million undocumented individuals in the United States.[4]

In this decade, the predominant country of origin for undocumented newcomers is Mexico, where estimates indicate that Mexicans make up over half of undocumented immigrants—57% of the total, or about 5.3 million. Another 2.2 million (23%) are from other Latin American countries. About 10% are from Asia, 5% from Europe and Canada, and 5% from the rest of the world. Almost two-thirds of the undocumented population lives in just six states: California (26%), Texas (12%), Florida (10%), New York (8%), Illinois (4%), and New Jersey (4%). Estimates indicated that the undocumented populations of Arizona, Georgia, and North Carolina have grown so rapidly that they may already have surpassed New Jersey's undocumented population.[5]

As to entering with documents, a visa enables newcomers to approach the United States at a port of entry (airport or land border-crossing) and then be allowed to enter if the passport and visa are in order. Executing Congress' immigration laws falls under the jurisdiction of the U.S. Department of Homeland Security (DHS). The U.S. immigration officials working for the DHS, Immigration and Customs Enforcement (ICE) branch, have the authority to permit newcomers to enter the United States. Officers from ICE decide how long newcomers can stay for any particular visit depending on their visa types.

When meeting with newcomer clients, social service providers may want to ascertain first *how* the person first entered the country and *what* immigration status the person has now, as a way to later determine possible legal remedies. By gathering the relevant legal information, and with the client's consent sharing the information with a nonprofit legal services immigration agency, the collaboration between the client, social service provider, and legal service provider can be made smoother as all can then work toward resolution and stabilization of the immigration status.

Of special interest to social services providers is the nonimmigrant or short-term visas given to persons who may have entered legally and their visa expired or who entered without visas. They are now undocumented or "illegal," but for the reasons described in the following, the government gives them permission to remain.

### Humanitarian Short-Term Visas: Victims of Trafficking

Some persons, especially women, may be in the United States because they are or have been a victim of some forms of trafficking. If such a person is physically present in the United States, American Samoa, or the Commonwealth of the Northern Mariana Islands, or at a port of entry, on account of such trafficking, and has complied with any reasonable request for assistance in the federal, state, or local investigation or prosecution of these acts, the person is allowed to remain. When the government designates a person a victim of trafficking, he or she may be given a document, or their passport (if they have one) may be stamped with the letter "*T*," which is a designation that they have been classified as a victim of trafficking and allowed to remain in the United States legally.[6]

### Humanitarian Short-Term Visas: Victims of Crimes

In addition, there may be newcomers in the United States who, like victims of trafficking, have also suffered, not because of trafficking, but because they have endured substantial physical or mental abuse as a result of having been a victim of *criminal* activity. Examples of such activity include:

> Rape; torture; trafficking; incest; domestic violence; sexual assault; abusive sexual contact; prostitution; sexual exploitation; female genital mutilation; being held hostage; peonage; involuntary servitude; slave trade; kidnapping; abduction; unlawful criminal restraint; false imprisonment; blackmail; extortion; manslaughter; murder; felonious assault; witness tampering; obstruction of justice; perjury; or attempt, conspiracy, or solicitation to commit any of the above mentioned crimes.

If the newcomer cooperates with a federal, state, or local law enforcement official investigating or prosecuting a criminal, the government may allow the person to remain in the United States. When the government designates a person a victim of such crimes, the government may give the individual a document, or in their passport (if they have one) it may be stamped with the letter "U," which is a designation that they have been classified as a victim of crimes and allowed to remain in the United States legally.[7] As will be described, individuals who obtain short-term visas due to being victims of trafficking or crimes can later apply to stay in the United States permanently.

For both T and U visas, a provider's role can be to provide psychological and other case management support, such as helping the client gather the necessary documents to apply for lawful permanent residence later on.

## U.S. IMMIGRATION LEGAL CLASSIFICATIONS: IMMIGRANTS AND CITIZENS

In addition to being allowed to remain in the United States as a nonimmigrant for a short term in the humanitarian categories already briefly described (e.g., trafficked, victim of crime), individuals may enter the United States, or be allowed to remain, as immigrants. This status allows newcomers to live permanently in the United States. If they choose, they never have to return to their country of origin. Just like nonimmigrant visas are for individuals who want to enter temporarily, immigrant visas on the other hand are for the people who intend to live permanently in the United States. Terms such as obtaining a "green card" or a "lawful permanent residence" are all synonymous.

There are a number of methods by which newcomers can enter and remain in the United States legally and permanently. This section describes the main avenues for lawful permanent residence that are relevant to social work practice. The key methods to remain in the country permanently include the following:

*a.* Family sponsorship
*b.* Surviving domestic violence
*c.* Being adjudicated a minor who is dependent on the foster care system
*d.* Applying for refuge/asylum

### Family Sponsorship as a Path to Lawful Permanent Residency

Newcomers who wish to become lawful permanent residents may do so if they have a close relative who can sponsor them. As part of a comprehensive intake with newcomers, social services providers may want to assess if a client has an immediate family member, both for immigration reasons as well as for family support reasons (though the family member may be a factor in causing trauma and not a source of social support or immigration support).

U.S. immigration law recognizes only specific types of relationships for purposes of obtaining lawful permanent residence. In other words, only a U.S. citizen or permanent resident mother/father, brother/sister, husband/wife, or child over 21 can sponsor a foreigner.[8] Procedurally, the U.S. citizen or permanent resident needs to file the appropriate documentation and, depending on the nature of the relationship (e.g., husband sponsoring wife vs. parent sponsoring child), there may be a long waiting period for the family to be reunited.

The United States or lawful permanent resident relative in the United States will need to sponsor the newcomer, and prove that the petitioner has enough income or assets to support the person who wishes to immigrate. By ascertaining whether the client has immediate relatives as described previously, the social worker can make a more efficient referral to an immigration nonprofit provider or private attorney as a way to help the client remain in the United States. The relative sponsor and the intending immigrant must successfully complete certain steps in the immigration process in order to come to the United States. Some of the key steps that service providers can help with include the following:

- Completing the Immigration Form I-130 Petition for Alien Relative.[9]
- Gathering information to prove the relationship between the sponsor and the newcomer (e.g., marriage certificates, birth certificates).
- Assisting with proving that the petitioner has adequate income or assets to support the intending immigrant, by completing and signing a document called an Affidavit of Support Immigration Form I-134.10. For low-income families, this may prove an obstacle in helping newcomers obtain permanent residence through family sponsorship.

Even if income status is not an obstacle in obtaining permanent residence, there may still be a backlog in obtaining an immigrant visa (or green card). The U.S. government sets annual minimum family-sponsored visas in the following categories:

*Immediate Relatives of U.S. Citizens* (IR): The spouse, widow(er), and unmarried children under 21 of a U.S. citizen, and the parent of a U.S. citizen who is 21 or older.
*First preference:* Unmarried sons and daughters of citizens.
*Second preference:* Spouses and children, and unmarried sons and daughters of permanent citizens.
*Third preference:* Married sons and daughters of citizens.
*Fourth preference:* Brothers and sisters of adult citizens.

The U.S. Department of State publishes the Visa Bulletin, updated monthly, which lays out categories and backlogs describing waiting periods for family members to be reunited.[11] The service provider can share this resource with the petitioner and intending immigrant so that they can assess the waiting period, if any, for obtaining lawful permanent residence.

## Violence Against Women Act (VAWA) as a Path to Lawful Permanent Residency

Service providers are also important in supporting newcomer women who are survivors of violence. Before Congress amended the Immigration Act, U.S. and permanent resident husbands could exploit newcomer women by dangling the application for a lawful residence as a carrot, forcing the woman to endure physical, mental, and sexual abuse. Through the provisions of the Violence Against Women Act,[12] Congress amended the Immigration Act to stop this abuse. As a result, newcomer women, married to lawful permanent residents or U.S. citizens, can *self*-petition without the need of the abusive sponsor/husband to petition for them. The immigrant woman can now flee domestic violence, obtain permanent residence, and even prosecute their abusers.

In addition, the law now also extends immigration relief to immigrant victims of sexual assault, human trafficking, and other violent crimes who agree to cooperate in criminal investigations or prosecutions. A key goal of VAWA's immigration protections is to cut off the ability of abusers, traffickers, and perpetrators of sexual assault to coerce their victims with threats of deportation, and thereby avoid prosecution. VAWA allows immigrant survivors to obtain immigration relief without the need of their abusers' cooperation or knowledge.

Social service providers can assist individuals who have been victims to prove abuse by helping the client put together the evidence required to prove a case of abuse, which may ultimately result in lawful permanent residence. The survivor of domestic violence can now self-petition if married to a U.S. citizen or lawful permanent resident. Unmarried children under the age of 21, who have not filed their own self-petition, may be included in petitions as *derivative beneficiaries*. Social service providers can assist the applicant to prove abuse through affidavits and other documents by:

- Submitting affidavits that the marriage was ended within the past 2 years for reasons connected to domestic violence;
- Getting copies of the Protection from Abuse Order;
- Obtaining hospital records, if any, of medical treatment because of the abuse;
- Obtaining police records to show that the police had been called; and
- Submitting affidavits that the social worker is providing counseling as a result of the trauma suffered through abuse.

## Special Juvenile Immigrant Status (SJIS) Act as a Path to Lawful Permanent Residency

Newcomer children who are dependent on the state, because they are victims of abuse, neglect, or abandonment, are among the most vulnerable people in the United States. But in many cases, the children or their advocates can obtain a critical legal immigration benefit that will help the children gain control of their lives and successfully transition to adulthood.

Newcomer children who have experienced abuse suffer the same emotional and physical problems as abused U.S. citizen children—and often more. Added to the other insecurities facing them, youth without documentation will not be able to work legally or qualify for in-state tuition at college, and face the constant threat of deportation. In addition, the counties caring for the children will not qualify for federal foster care matching funds if the children remain undocumented.

To address these challenges, the immigration law now provides that newcomer children in permanent placement can apply for lawful permanent residency status as "special immigrant juveniles."[13]

The social service providers' role, especially those working with children and youth, is crucial in raising awareness of this benefit both to clients, as well as to government agencies and other nonprofit providers who work with children. If the children have legal counsel or county caseworkers, they too can help to complete and submit the necessary paperwork to help the child obtain lawful permanent residence.

As mentioned, abused immigrant children who are *not* county dependents may still be eligible for immigration benefits. An immigrant who was battered or abused by a U.S. citizen or permanent resident parent or spouse may be able to apply for permanent residence under the provisions of VAWA. In this case, the child (or spouse) does not have to have been taken in by the county or made a court dependent. However, the abuser must have been a permanent resident or U.S. citizen.

The service provider's role can be to assist in completing the application for this immigration status resulting in lawful permanent residence. Social service providers can assist in proving abuse through affidavits and other documents by ensuring that the child:

- Obtains an order from a dependency court confirming that the child is eligible for long-term foster care due to abuse, neglect, or abandonment;
- Completes USCIS forms[14] (although there is a fee for the application process, a fee waiver is available);
- Obtains a special medical exam; and
- Provides fingerprints, a photograph, and proof of age.

The federal government will grant the applicant employment authorization (if relevant to the youth) as soon as the application is filed, and schedule a date for the SIJS interview. Generally, the government will decide the case at the time of the SIJS interview. While the child is a juvenile court dependent, it is important to apply for SIJS because the process may take from 6 to 18 months after submitting the application to get an SIJS interview. If the child is released and is no longer an adjudicated dependent *before* the immigration interview takes place, the current government policy is to deny the case.

## Refugee Protection as a Path to Lawful Permanent Residency

The service provider's role in providing support to newcomers is perhaps most relevant in applications for asylum. More than 140 nations have signed a United Nations international treaty: the 1951 Convention and 1967 Protocol relating to the Status of Refugees.[15] By signing this refugee treaty, the signatory countries agree to provide refuge to persons who meet the definition of refugee. The United States signed the treaty in 1967 and incorporated the principles of the treaty into domestic law through Congress's enactment of the 1980 U.S. Refugee Act.[16] The international and U.S. definition of a "refugee" is a person who is outside of their country of origin and has a well-founded fear of persecution because of:

- Race,
- Religion,
  - Nationality,
  - Membership in a particular social group, or
  - Political opinion.

Depending on certain procedural issues, applicants for asylum can file for protection from persecution either before an asylum officer or an immigration judge. The social worker's role can be crucial in helping the client to obtain legal assistance in filing the case, and later, in helping both the client (and attorney) in drafting the affidavit[17] describing the past or future persecution to support the application for asylum. No matter the venue, whether in front of an asylum officer or an immigration judge, the service provider's experience in trauma-informed interviewing skills can help the applicant complete the needed affidavit.[18] The service provider's role can be especially helpful in proving the first criterion of the refugee test: that the applicant is indeed afraid and that the provider is providing therapy to alleviate the fear of past (and future) persecution if deported to the country of origin. In addition, the service provider may also be helpful in conducting research on information on human rights abuses to support the second prong of the definition: persecution as substantiated through reported human rights violations.[19]

Under the U.S. Refugee Act, in alignment with the internationally accepted definition, a refugee is a person who has fled his or her country of origin because of past persecution or a well-founded fear of future persecution based upon race, religion, nationality, political opinion, or a membership in a particular social group. If the person is not in the United States, he or she may apply overseas to *enter as an already recognized* refugee. If the person is *already within* the United States, for example, having entered as a visitor, or a student, or even entered without documents (passport and/or visa), he or she is applying for *asylum*.[20] The legal standard is the same: "well-founded fear of persecution" on any of the five grounds presented. The designation of which word to use—refugee or asylee—simply depends on where the applicant is physically at the time of the application.

In order to obtain refugee status (outside the United States so as to be resettled to the United States) or obtain protection as an asylee (inside the United States so as to be allowed to remain), applicants must prove each of the prongs of the international and U.S. definition of "refugee":

Well-founded fear of persecution, linked to the applicants' race, religion, nationality, social group, or political opinion.

For newcomers entering the United States who are already recognized as refugees, the service provider's role could ensure that the applicant has access to mental health (and if necessary physical health) and other types of counseling support and referrals. Many refugees have suffered triple trauma: in the country of origin suffering violations of human rights on themselves or their families; in flight (crossing mountains, sea, borders); and now in the host country due to factors such as language, customs, and alienation, resulting in depression. Hence, ensuring access to culturally competent services can be an important role for the provider. Refugees have many strengths—business acumen, language, and education. The service provider can play a role in helping to restore the refugee's assets and build on their strengths.

For those individuals who did not enter as refugees (e.g., entered as students, tourists, or even without documents), social service providers can also support newcomers in their goal of obtaining protection so as to be able to remain in the United States. An individual who enters the United States as a nonimmigrant (e.g., student, visitor, or even without documents) may apply for asylum through the "affirmative" asylum process as described in the following.

### Step One: Arrive in the United States

The service provider can assist newcomers wishing to apply for asylum by first ensuring that the application is filed within 1 year of the client's last arrival in the United States. Although the law states that applicants must apply within 1 year of arriving, an exception to the rule is if the applicant can prove "changed circumstances" materially affecting the applicant's eligibility for asylum or "extraordinary circumstances" related to the delay in filing.[21] If one year has passed and the applicant wishes to apply for protection, the social service provider can support the applicant by helping to gather information relating to changed or extraordinary circumstances explaining why the applicant is applying *after* the 1 year deadline.

### Step Two: Complete the Application for Asylum

The applicant must complete Form I-589, "Application for Asylum and for Withholding of Removal." This form requires the applicant to explain the fear of returning, the persecution suffered or to be suffered, and on what grounds. The social service provider can help the applicant relive the trauma, with care, so as to be able to draft an Affidavit in support of the Application for Asylum. In collaboration with legal counsel, the service provider can use this first draft as the foundation for a final affidavit to be submitted as part of the application.

In addition to assisting the applicant in drafting his or her own affidavit with the narrative of what happened, the service provider can also write an affidavit attesting to the provider's own clinical support being offered to the applicant. The affidavit can go into detail as to the assessment and diagnoses of physical scars or mental health trauma that the provider has observed. The provider's affidavit will be used by the government as one more bit of evidence to assist in the U.S. government's final determination: grant or deny asylum.

### Step Three: Asylum Interview

The government notifies applicants of an interview with an Asylum Officer typically at one of the eight Asylum Offices or at a USCIS field office,[22] depending on where the applicant lives and where the application is filed. Service providers can support applicants by accompanying the applicant and providing psychological support, serving as interpreters, and/or serving as a bridge between the applicant and the attorney. An asylum interview may last about an hour, although the time may vary depending on the case. Applicants may also bring witnesses to testify on the applicant's behalf. Service providers can testify as to the applicant's fear of being persecuted based on clinical, social, and psychological services rendered.

At the interview, the asylum officer will determine whether the applicant meets the definition of a refugee as listed previously, and also assesses whether the applicant is barred from being granted asylum for reasons such as the applicant can return to another safe third country or is filing long than 1 year after the date of the alien's arrival in the United States. (If, however, the applicant demonstrates the existence of changed circumstances or extraordinary circumstances relating to the delay in filing the application, the applicant may still be able to file for asylum.[23]) If, for example, the applicant did not file before the 1 year deadline due to posttraumatic stress disorder, a provider's affidavit can be useful in proving "extraordinary circumstances," which caused the filing delay.

### Step Four: Applicant Receives Decision

In most cases, the government advises the applicant within 1 or 2 months of the interview to return to the asylum office to pick up the decision. The decision may also be to deny or to refer to the Immigration Judge.[24]

In addition to applying for asylum before an Asylum Officer in an "affirmative" setting, depending on the situation, individuals may have to apply for asylum in a "defensive" setting before an Immigration Judge. The provider's role is similar to that described previously in helping the applicant draft an affidavit, as well as the provider drafting his or her own affidavit in support of the application.[25]

## U.S. Citizenship

The final portions of the Immigration Law of relevance to social service providers deal with how immigrants can become citizens. The United States, unlike other countries, grants citizenship under three circumstances:

1. Citizenship by parentage
2. Citizenship by birth on U.S. soil
3. Citizenship by application

Many countries provide for passing on citizenship through parentage or blood; for example, if the parents are German, then the child is German at birth. Similarly, U.S. immigration laws follow the principle of *jus sanguine*: Citizenship is conferred even if the child is born *outside* of the United States (e.g., if a child is born in China to U.S. missionaries, the child is considered a U.S. citizen).

Other countries provide for citizenship if the individual is born on their soil. Similarly, U.S. immigration laws, pursuant to the U.S. Constitution, follow the principle of *jus solis*.[26] Thus, a child born in the United States, regardless of whether the parent is with or without documents, is considered a U.S. citizen. Given the perception of the rise in undocumented newcomers, a segment of the native-born population has been calling for an end to "birthright citizenship" and is advocating for an amendment to the Fourteenth Amendment of the U.S. Constitution.

Finally, unlike other countries, U.S. immigration laws provide a third path toward citizenship and also allows citizenship by *application*, even if the applicant had neither U.S. parents (*jus sangine*), or was not born on U.S. soil (*jus solis*). In this third possibility for gaining citizenship, a newcomer arrives in the United States as a student or refugee. The person then becomes a lawful permanent resident based on a sponsorship by a family member or employer or gaining asylum as described previously. In these cases, after a 3- to 5-year period of being a lawful permanent resident, the individual can *apply* for naturalization—hence a third route to citizenship is by *application*.

# 7. LEGAL ISSUES IN PRACTICE WITH IMMIGRANTS AND REFUGEES

Social service providers can assist applicants who wish to become citizens by helping to gather information required by law. The provider can assist to prove that the applicant

a. Is at least 18 years old;
b. Is a permanent resident of the United States;
c. Has had lawful permanent residency for 3 to 5 years;
d. During the last 5 years has been inside the United States for 30 months or more;
e. Has the ability to read, write, and speak basic English;
f. Has the ability to pass the civics test; and
g. Is a person of good moral character.

For clients who are English-language learners, passing the test of reading, writing, and speaking basic English may be a problem. This is especially true for elderly newcomers, who may have been residents for a long period of time but are not able to speak English for a number of reasons. However, for elderly persons who are already residents and are older than 65 years and have resided in the United States as permanent residents for at least 20 years, they have different requirements for history and government knowledge: They may also be tested in the language of their choice because they are exempt from the English literacy requirements.

Social service providers may want to urge their lawful permanent clients to seriously consider applying for U.S. citizenship since benefits include:

- The right to vote;
- Faster family sponsorship;
- Public benefits/entitlements;
- Educational grants and scholarships;
- U.S. travel document passport; and
- Nondeportation if convicted of a crime.

## RECOMMENDATIONS ABOUT THE ROLE OF SOCIAL SERVICE PROVIDERS IN ASSISTING REFUGEES

Service providers can play specific roles to support newcomers, depending on the legal remedy available as to whether the applicant is a survivor of domestic violence, an unaccompanied minor, or an asylum seeker. Regardless of the specific group, some general principles that will assist the provider in becoming more culturally competent include the following:

Micro advocacy competencies to advocate for *the client:*

1. Listening skills so as to develop trusting relationships with the woman, child, or asylum seeker.[27]
2. Ability to refer clients to legal services providers to navigate the legal systems.
3. Crisis intervention skills and finding culturally appropriate partners to assist in areas such as housing, health, mental health, education, immigration, and legal services.
4. Ability to seek and access emotional and stress support for oneself.

Mezzo advocacy competencies to advocate *in-house* within the organization:

5. Securing organizational commitment to ensure newcomer access and participation (newcomer board members; bilingual bicultural staff; bilingual external communications tools [web; brochures; signage]).
6. Staff and board continuous learning and professional development as to diverse cultures and belief systems.
7. Staff and board knowledge of the difference between integration versus assimilation.
8. Multiagency partnerships built around the needs of refugees and asylum seekers, at both strategic and operational levels, which will facilitate access to and development of appropriate social care provision.

Macro advocacy competencies to advocate for *change in systems:*

9. Political understanding of the larger picture including the triple trauma of country-of-origin events the client faced in the country of origin which resulted in the client leaving; the trauma encountered in flight; and the trauma in the host country.[28]

In the end, providers can listen to and partner with newcomers to ensure their engaged participation in leading their own lives in the host community. When providers raise their awareness of immigration laws, then, in collaboration with legal service providers and other service providers, with newcomers leading the way, newcomers will be able to play to their strengths, and contribute to their own well-being, their families, and their host communities.

## NOTES

1. 8 U.S.C.
2. 8 U.S.C. §1103,1187), and 8 CFR 235.1, 264, and 1235.1.
3. 8 U.S.C. § 1325 Improper entry by alien.
4. For estimates of numbers of undocumented, see http://pewhispanic.org/files/reports/46.pdf; www.uscis.gov
5. http://www.urban.org/publications/1000587.html
6. In October 2000, Congress created the "T" nonimmigrant status by passing the Victims of Trafficking and Violence Protection Act (VTVPA). The legislation strengthens the ability of law enforcement agencies to investigate and prosecute human trafficking, and also offers protection to victims.
7. 8 U.S.C. § 101(a) (15) (U).
8. 8 U.S.C. § 201(b).
9. See www.uscis.gov to obtain copy of the form.
10. Ibid.
11. See https://travel.state.gov/content/travel/en/legal/visa-law0/visa-bulletin.html for monthly updates as to waiting periods/backlogs from time of filing to date government issues visa to relatives.
12. 42 *U.S.C.* § 13981.
13. 8 U.S.C. § 203(b)(4).
14. See www.uscis.gov to obtain copy of the form.

# 7. LEGAL ISSUES IN PRACTICE WITH IMMIGRANTS AND REFUGEES 113

15. UN General Assembly, *Convention Relating to the Status of Refugees*, 28 July 1951, United Nations, Treaty Series, vol. 189, p. 137.
16. Refugee Act of 1980 (Public Law 96-212).
17. 8 C.F.R. 208.1 et seq.
18. See www.uscis.gov/portal/site/uscis for forms, specifically Form I-589 Application for Asylum and Withholding of Removal.
19. For sample supporting affidavits, see www.immigrationequality.org/issues/law-library/lgbth-asylum-manual/sample-cover-letter/ for sample applications, and Corroborating Client-Specific Documents; see https://www.theadvocatesforhumanrights.org/uploads/pro_bono_asylum_representation_manual_2009.pdf
20. www.dhs.gov/xlibrary/assets/statistics/publications/ois_rfa_fr_2010.pdf
21. 8 U.S.C. § 208(a)(2)(D); 8 C.F.R. § 208.4(a).
22. For list of locations for asylum office see: https://egov.uscis.gov/crisgwi/go?action=offices.type&OfficeLocator.office_type=ZSY
23. INA Section 208(b)(2).
24. For more information on the "affirmative" asylum process see: www.uscis.gov/portal/site/uscis/menuitem.5af9bb95919f35e66f614176543f6d1a/?vgnextoid=888e18a1f8b73210VgnVCM100000082ca60aRCRD&vgnextchannel=f39d3e4d77d73210VgnVCM100000082ca60aRCRD
25. For more information on the "Defensive" asylum process see http://trac.syr.edu/immigration/reports/159
26. U.S. Constitution, Fourteenth Amendment: All persons born or naturalized in the United States, and subject to the jurisdiction thereof, are citizens of the United States and of the State wherein they reside . . .
27. Social worker role in "listening" https://books.google.com/books?id=e3uMDwAAQBAJ&pg=PA172&lpg=PA172&dq=Social+worker+role+in+%E2%80%9Clistening%22++blackwell&source=bl&ots=I10oIh41Wr&sig=ACfU3U2aArtGr785kqaPeAjQH6boLocjKQ&hl=en&sa=X&ved=2ahUKEwil55anqqnoAhVHmXIEHRLbATEQ6AEwAHoECA0QAQ#v=onepage&q=Social%20worker%20role%20in%20%E2%80%9Clistening%22%20%20blackwell&f=false
28. https://www.communitycare.co.uk/2010/07/02/social-care-for-refugees-and-asylum-seekers/

# Part III

## Life Cycle Perspectives

# 8

# The Multicultural Triangle of the Child, the Family, and the School: Culturally Competent Approaches

CARMEN ORTIZ HENDRICKS[‡] AND MANNY JOHN. GONZÁLEZ

## INTRODUCTION

Social work and psychology in urban public schools is one arena of multicultural practice in which knowledge of a client group's culture and status in society is central to service delivery. With rapidly increasing racial and ethnic diversity in cities throughout the United States, there is an urgent need to increase the numbers of bilingual, bicultural, and culturally competent school social workers and psychologists and to decrease the cultural dissonance often found between mainstream school systems and the communities they serve. From a mental health perspective, Shahidullah (2019) has observed that

> the school system is an important setting for child development—and school-based providers, such as school psychologists, are positioned to address behavioral health issues (i.e., mental health, behavioral and social/emotional development, behavioral factors associated with medical conditions) within the school setting. (p. 279)

This chapter looks at the complex interplay of cultures present when families and children from diverse cultural backgrounds interact with public school professionals—each representing different values, beliefs, and historical experiences—a factor frequently overlooked in the process of assessing and helping children with their learning needs. Freire (1998) considers teachers to be

---
[‡] Deceased.

"cultural workers" and exhorts them to think "about the learners' cultural identity and about the respect that we owe it in our educational practices" (p. 71). The same can be said of school social workers and psychologists who are required to be culturally competent practitioners and "cultural mediators" (de Anda, 1984), since they are the primary school professionals who work with children while simultaneously mediating the environmental dynamics of the family and the school (Bronstein & Abramson, 2003; Hughes, Minke, & Sansosti, 2017). Culturally competent school social workers and psychologists, for instance, know their personal and professional identities and values, and are in the best position to function as interpreters of the language, experiences, and beliefs of diverse families, children, and the schools they attend (American Psychological Association, 2003; Constable & Montgomery, 1985; Franklin, 2000; Garrett, 2006; Lopez & Rogers, 2007; Staudt, 1991).

The school setting has a major impact on the lives of children and families. Public schools have traditionally been held responsible for transmitting the dominant, mainstream U.S. cultural values and beliefs, and promoting acculturation and assimilation to that culture—and they are often the best sites for providing clinical services to children (see Hughes et al., 2017). Schools have the power to strongly influence children, especially when the child's cultural background is different from the mainstream culture of the society or the school. These differences may be the result of recent immigration to the United States or bicultural/bilingual life experiences. Schools also exert enormous power over families that have limited understanding of the school system as a whole, or families that have to deal with underfunded, overcrowded inner-city schools. These families may already feel powerless and alienated within their communities. Take, for example, an immigrant family whose children are removed and placed into foster care because of a myriad of family issues and concerns (Jackson & McParlin, 2006; Johnson-Reid et al., 2007; Trout, Hagaman, Casey, Reid, & Epstein, 2008). Given the current anti-immigrant mood of the country, how are these families and their children's needs attended to by the school system and school social worker or psychologist? Freire's renowned *Pedagogy of the Oppressed* (1993) urges educators and schools to be a liberating and enlightening force in the lives of children, families, and communities rather than perpetuating the oppressive broader environmental conditions. As potential liberating agents, educators and schools must balance the importance of educating children with the recognition that there is a transactional relationship between emotional and psychological well-being and academic success. From an intersectionality approach, this noted transactional relationship is both sustained and challenged by the internal and external worlds of school-aged children, youth, and their families. Intersectionality is a sociological approach that draws attention to the multiple threats of discrimination when an individual's sense of self overlaps with a number of variables—such as race, gender, age, ethnicity, health, and other sociocultural and contextual characteristics (Crenshaw, 1991; Viruell-Fuentes, Miranda, & Abdulrahim, 2012). The approach also draws attention to both intragroup and intergroup differences, while underscoring the reverberating effects of oppression and its impact on optimal human development and psychosocial functioning—and the manifestation of individual and family maladaptive coping and psychopathology. As an approach to both clinical practice and service delivery, intersectionality is a useful conceptual guide in understanding the ways in which the multiple aspects of

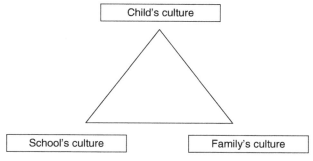

Figure 8.1 *The child/family/school triangle.*

a child's emerging identity intersects, influences, and creates unique lived experiences that can only be assessed via a transactional lens that takes into account the inner and outer world of the human organism.

## THE MULTICULTURAL TRIANGLE

A multicultural triangle (see Figure 8.1) invariably forms when the child, the family, and the school conflict over measures of a child's ability, intelligence, or educability (Compher, 1982; Constable & Walberg, 1988; Douglas, 2011). Each feels the tensions of differing cultural values and objectives, and each encompasses a culture that needs to be understood and negotiated in order to promote positive learning experiences for children (Aponte, 1976; Woolley, Kol, & Bowen, 2009). To begin with, there may exist radically different cultural assumptions and expectations by the family and the school regarding the following questions:

- How does a particular cultural group view children?
- What is it like to be a child of a particular cultural group?
- How does it feel to not belong to the "dominant" mainstream cultural group?
- What is it like to grow up feeling different or "less than"?
- What is the particular culture of the school?
- What value is placed on the parents' role in educating children?
- How do different cultural groups measure intelligence?
- What value do different cultural groups place on education?
- How do professionals define "normalcy" or a normal range of development?
- How are different behavioral norms understood and applied?
- In what context are learning needs and problems defined?
- How culture-bound are the labels and definitions of educability?

These questions also point to the interrelationship between a child's school performance, the family's identity, and the school's policies and practices (Figure 8.2). Many immigrant families value education for their children. The children's educational performance is considered to be a family matter, and it is given prominence and recognition in their community (Appleby, Colon, & Hamilton, 2001; Ryan & Smith, 1989).

From a systemic point of view, what affects one part of the system has a reverberating impact on other parts of the system. Therefore, assessment of a child's

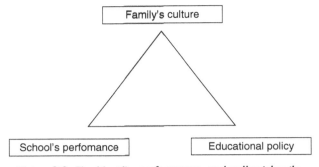

Figure 8.2 *The identity, performance, and policy triangle.*

school performance cannot be separated from assessment of a family's self-identity or evaluation of a school's educational policies and practices (Douglas, 2011; Dowling & Osborne, 1985). The problems or positions of one by necessity affect the other. This triangle, like most triangles in family systems theory, provides many convenient issues to focus upon while avoiding the fundamental cross-cultural conflicts at hand. For example, school programs like Head Start and other early childhood intervention programs frequently expect or mandate parental participation in a child's educational plan, but these expectations are not enough to ensure parental participation. School professionals tend to focus attention on a child's educational needs while ignoring the important aspects of the parent/school relationship (Correa, 1989; Hill & Torres, 2010). Parent/professional interactions are sometimes so structured as to render parents effectively powerless as partners in their children's educational careers. Culturally competent approaches can build shared understanding and shared responsibilities between parents and school professionals. When parents are genuinely invited and their participation is properly utilized, they are an invaluable resource and highly effective collaborators in the educational process (Aponte, 1976; Chavkin & Garza-Lubeck, 1990; Correa, 1989). Parents are in the best position to assist educators and social workers in decision-making while protecting and advocating for their children.

Overburdened parents may be limited in the time available to attend school conferences, or their lack of understanding may be misinterpreted as resistance or lack of interest (Delgado & Rivera, 1997; Delgado-Gaitan, 1987). Limited English proficiency combined with the lack of bilingual, bicultural, and culturally competent school personnel also limits parental participation. Language usage and professional jargon further alienate parents from participating in their child's educational plans. There are many different interpretations for such terms as *bilingual education, special education, learning disability, speech or developmental delays, attention deficit disorder, hyperactivity,* and *special needs children.* These technical terms have been socially constructed in the United States and have different meanings and interpretations. They also do not always translate accurately for parents (Bennett, 1988). School professionals freely use these diagnostic categories or labels that are based on mainstream, middle-class, Western standards of measurement for evaluating intelligence. In the United States, these terms are used uniformly across a range of cultural and social class groups with little appreciation for the different life experiences that contribute to or could assist with educational difficulties.

A perfect example is the use of the term *disability*, which inevitably suggests a deficit in the individual. "The moral and medical models define disability as a pathological individual characteristic. In contrast, the social model defines disability as a diverse attribute in society" (Mackelprang, 2008, p. 39). Social workers and psychologists deal with neurocognitive, physical, and psychiatric disabilities. Most parents will resist such categorizations of their child, and will seek to protect the child's identity from labels that appear to stigmatize the child completely rather than describe a particular difficulty in some aspect of the child's learning capacity. In *The Learning Differences Sourcebook* (1998), Boyles and Contadino list a range of learning difficulties including speech and language disorders, attention deficit/hyperactivity disorders, obsessive compulsive disorders, Tourette syndrome, oppositional defiant or conduct disorders, autism, mental retardation and developmental delays, visual or hearing impairments, and environmentally induced impairments such as those resulting from lead poisoning or fetal alcohol syndrome. When a parent denies a diagnosis or categorization, it should not be automatically assumed that the educational assessment is correct and the parent is misguided or resistant to recognizing that the child is suffering from a mild to serious learning problem (Dowling & Osborne, 1985; Golden & Cupuzzi, 1986; Hill & Torres, 2010). Rather, parents should be asked to provide their own explanation for their child's learning difficulties. School personnel may learn some valuable information to assist them and the parents in addressing the child's needs (Bennett, 1988; Harry, 1992b; Kalyanpur & Rao, 1991). The parent's point of view may be a more accurate representation of the child's needs as well as the parent's experience of the world. For example, parents of color can see with their own eyes the disproportionate placement of children of color in special education classes. This supports the parental perception of the arbitrary nature of such designations as learning disabled and promotes the view that special education programs are discriminatory or oppressive (Dao, 1991; Delgado-Gaitan, 1987; Gandara & Contreras, 2009; Kalyanpur & Rao, 1991).

Culturally competent school social workers and psychologists are aware that placement in special education programs may be a more accurate reflection of the school's culture or social values than objective reality, especially when it relates to the underachievement of children of color from inner-city neighborhoods (Kurtz & Barth, 1989; Woolley et al., 2009). Often underachieving children of color experience academic difficulties as a by-product of toxic stress. Toxic stress in children is caused by strong, frequent, and/or prolonged adversity without adult support—and it has been found to disrupt the development of brain anatomy and function, while increasing the risk for poor health, limited social-emotional skills, and cognitive impairment (National Scientific Council on the Developing Child, 2012; Rojas-Flores, Clements, Koo, & London, 2017). Problems in school performance have a range of meanings to parents, children, and teachers alike—and are a by-product of complex, interacting sources. A few example case vignettes can help underscore these issues:

## CASE VIGNETTES

> Eight-year-old Maria came home sobbing that her teacher did not like her anymore and was sending her to another classroom. The

mother, with her 15-year-old son as interpreter, went to the school to explain to the teacher that Maria was a good girl, she worked hard at her homework, and she could read and speak both English and Spanish quite well. The teacher tried to explain the learning disability that had been diagnosed in Maria, but to this Dominican mother, a disability was some kind of severe incapacity like being blind or paralyzed. Her daughter was not incapacitated like that, so she continued to resist the change to a special classroom.

Elementary school teachers were frustrated with an Asian mother whose child was severely delayed in speech and language development, but she steadfastly refused all efforts to move her child to a remedial educational placement outside the immediate neighborhood. The school social worker learned that this mother had lost four children in a devastating flood that destroyed her village in Bangladesh a few years earlier. Losing a child, even to a nearby school, was too stressful for this mother, and other arrangements had to be made to meet the child's needs.

A mother, raised and educated in Jamaica, was finally able to bring her 8-year-old son to live with her in the United States. Before leaving Jamaica, she consulted the village wise man who told her that her son would experience many difficulties during his first year in the United States. She was convinced that when the year ended, her son's health problems and learning difficulties would cease as well.

These examples demonstrate the kinds of multicultural misunderstandings that can arise when there are different definitions of the problem at hand (Lynch & Stein, 1987). Parents may be interpreting or naming the child's difficulties in their own way, and are trying to help their child by reframing the issues in words that are more compatible with their cultural values and beliefs and less harmful to the child's self-image (Greene, Jensen, & Jones, 1996; Harry, 1992a; McAdoo & McAdoo, 1985). These redefinitions and clarifications need to be respected no matter how strange they may seem to school officials. Parents use any number of phrases or personal narratives to explain to school professionals how they view a child's learning difficulties:

- "He's just the way my brother was at this age."
- "She'll grow out of it, the way I did."
- "His father was just like him."
- "She is much smarter than she lets on to the teachers."
- "My child knows to not boast about his abilities."
- "She just needs time to catch on."

These perceptions should be utilized in the child's individual educational assessment and plan and included when discussing such things as genetic predisposition, developmental or maturational factors, different historical evolutions, medical and psychological progress, and individual or family strengths. The focus is on the strengths of parents' perceptions rather than on the pathology or deficits perspectives of school professionals (Hill & Torres, 2010; Tower, 2000). This focus is aimed at engaging parents in the educational and clinical process that will yield academic and emotional well-being in the identified child. The strength-based focus does not negate the fact that children and adolescents in the United States face significant challenges related to academic achievement and mental health (Williams Splett, Fowler, Weist, McDaniel, & Dvorsky, 2013). In fact, in the Congressional mandated annual report—*The condition of education*—which summarizes important developments and trends in education, McFarland et al. (2017) found that one out of every 17 students will not complete high school and about 6.6. million youth enrolled in school require special education services for one or more learning disabilities. Learning disabilities or challenges clearly impact mental health and academic outcomes.

Bicultural and bilingual children who hear conflicting comments about their cognitive–behavioral abilities from their parents and teachers are frequently torn between the demands of two cultures—the culture of home and the culture of school (Freeman & Pennekamp, 1988). As bicultural/bilingual children, they struggle daily to live up to teacher expectations, to learn new ways of solving problems and relating to others (Bennett, 1988; Lynch & Stein, 1987), to deal with peer demands for mainstream behavioral responses, and to remain true to family admonitions to put their culture of origin first regardless of what they experience around them. These children need "culture brokers" (Ortiz Hendricks, Haffey, & Asamoah, 1988)—persons who can teach them how to negotiate conflicts and facilitate resolution of multicultural dilemmas and opportunities. When the child is biracial, they are forced to deal with the additional task of choosing one racial identity over another, an enormously stressful and difficult experience for children and youth faced with multiple developmental tasks.

When school professionals and parents use different culturally based and culturally biased criteria for describing a child's behavior, it is the child who gets caught between their respective interpretations (Ryan & Smith, 1989). "For the most part, school curricula are designed to have each student achieve certain academic milestones along a predetermined timetable . . . The problem? Not every child is on this developmental schedule" (Boyles & Contadino, 1998, p. 1). The same authors describe a number of biases in instruments that are used to assess intelligence such as "value bias," which involves designing tests so that answers reflect the responses acceptable to the dominant culture, and "linguistic bias," which means assessment of a child's knowledge of a particular language like English rather than assessment of their general language development. Before resorting to biased criteria to evaluate a child's difficulties in school, school professionals would do well to pay careful attention to the parents' criteria for normalcy and intellectual ability, which holds special meaning for the families they serve. There are different cultural meanings to what school professionals may believe are uniform and universally accepted definitions of intelligence, competence, and disability (Dao, 1991; Kalyanpur & Rao, 1991). Many parents are incredulous when they are first told that their child is learning disabled or suffers from a more severe neurological impairment (Bennett, 1988). They see a healthy body, a child who can use common sense, a child who has achieved elementary academic skills in two languages, and a child who has already exceeded a parent's educational attainments (Ryan & Smith, 1989). These accomplishments clearly deny a diagnosis that is designed for someone whose competence is impaired or who is mentally deficient. Parents cannot view their child as anything but intellectually superior when a 7-year-old's homework is harder than anything the parents have experienced in their own education (Spener, 1988). From a strengths perspective, by working with the definitions offered by parents, school professionals can reinforce the fact that the child is not severely incapacitated. This positions the school to motivate children and parents to address learning needs in a more empowering manner.

When examining a child's difficulties in school, educational experts point to several important themes that emerge as children and parents struggle to understand why a child is having trouble. Family identity, school performance, and educational policies are culturally bound and culturally interwoven aspects of school-based clinical services (Harry, 1992a, 1992b; Hughes et al., 2017; Williams Splett et al., 2013). Together, these factors contribute to narrow definitions of a child's difficulties and rigid triangulations of communication among all parties concerned.

## FAMILY IDENTITY

Family identity is very important when interpreting a child's developmental patterns or learning needs. The Coleman Report of 1966, a national study, reported that family background influenced an individual's school achievement more than any other factor (Andersen & Collins, 1998). Wherever there is a strong cultural value placed on the family as a whole, there is an equally strong value placed on the family's identity as a group rather than as a collection of individuals. Problems are viewed as family problems rather than as issues solely of the individual. The family feels a collective shame when school professionals inadvertently or intentionally give the impression that the child's learning difficulties result from some deficit in the home or other family problem. Parents may associate the child's difficulties as tied to some family trait or characteristic or even to some past wrongdoing by a relative. On the other hand, a strong family identity diffuses the stigma on a child who is having school problems. While a strong family identity engenders vulnerability in the whole family, it also serves to protect the child's identity. The child is not different because he or she is just like everyone else in the family. Lynch and Stein (1987) found that Latino and African American children were described in terms of family traits and were often not considered to be outside the family's normal range of behavior. Culturally competent practitioners recognize that family group identity has to be taken into consideration when addressing a child's learning needs. For example, a child who is withdrawn or hyperactive may be demonstrating behavior that is viewed as culturally syntonic to the family. The family may see the quiet or overactive child as exhibiting some inherited aspect of family behavior, or a part of the family's preferred mode of behavior. In other words, the child has always been this way, and it is an inherited characteristic from the grandfather or aunt. The family has always accommodated the child, and will continue to help the child deal with this behavior. They do not view the behavior as a problem or symptomatic of any other condition. Culturally competent practitioners need to build on the strength of family identity while securing remedial services for the child (Douglas, 2011).

## SCHOOL PERFORMANCE

When looking at the school performance of diverse children, especially immigrant and refugee children, an appreciation of the advantages and disadvantages of second language acquisition in a child's education is essential. Children can experience problems simply from the confusion associated with changing from one language at home to another language in school (Cummins, 1984; Spener, 1988). It is the school that generally assesses whether a child enters into regular English-speaking classes with a bilingual aide or whether they need English as a second language (ESL) classes, or a comprehensive bilingual education program. The point of immigration in the child's life cycle has a great deal to do with how a child adjusts to English and American schools. Parents may feel that their children were doing well academically in schools in their country of origin, and see their children's problems now as emerging from the high demands or tough expectations of teachers. They may even feel like their children are being singled out because of their limited English proficiency (LEP) and no other learning difficulties. Some parents are so proud of their children's ability to speak and read English that they see American teachers as overly critical of accents or mispronunciations, or expecting their children to speak English perfectly (Correa, 1989).

Parents are further confused by such terms as ESL, LEP, and IEP (individualized educational plan), and special programs like bilingual education, special education, and resource rooms; they have many misconceptions about these terms or programs. The battles fought over bilingual education had parents believing that these programs held children back rather than helping them learn better. In truth, bilingual education is ill-defined in practice and inconsistently implemented.

> Critics complain that it [bilingual education] produces low-scoring students with poor English language skills. Supporters counter that . . . ultimately language minority children who learn to read and write in their native tongue will be more cognitively developed than language minority children who learn to read and write in English. (Ravitch & Viteritti, 2000, p. 187)

There is limited research to support either point of view. Historically, bilingual education has focused on Hispanic children, whereas Asian students have been allowed to learn primarily in English. These distinctions need to be thoroughly researched in a culturally sensitive way in order to determine what is in the best interest of bilingual/bicultural students. Many immigrant parents are adamant that their children learn English even if the parents themselves are resistant to learning the new language (Dao, 1991; Spener, 1988). These same parents are concerned that their children maintain their language of origin and not forget it. To lose the ability to speak the language of origin or native tongue frequently means losing the ability to speak to relatives and friends back home. These factors put enormous pressure on children to be bilingual at all costs. At the same time, the broader social environment in the United States today, with growing support for English-only laws and anti-immigrant sentiment, communicates a less than welcome environment for immigrants, migrants, and refugees. Young children often have to struggle alone with the demands of their parents and families, the school, and the broader society. Cultural sensitivity is necessary to help children succeed in their school performance and to navigate their bilingual and bicultural identities.

## EDUCATIONAL POLICIES AND PRACTICES

The school's culture extends to things like how curricula are delivered, how reading and math are taught, and how children are evaluated. Parents frequently complain about how unstimulating curricula can be, how inflexible teaching methods can be, and how frequently a child's classrooms, programs, teachers, and even schools are changed due to some new evaluation of a child's learning needs (Gandara & Contreras, 2009; Sarason, 1982). Mainstream as well as immigrant parents are not always able to assert their parental authority, and they are reluctant to refuse to go along with educational practices recommended by school professionals. Parents and children get confused and frustrated when educational changes occur without their approval or understanding or without any credence given to their position or interpretation. Some parents fight back, but they are not always successful. A perfect example of this was discussed in a *New York Times* article entitled, "City Retools Special Education, But Pupils Are Slipping Through Cracks":

> Under special education law, when children do not get services, parents can request a hearing . . . Siow Wei Chu and her husband, Harry Sze, Chinese immigrants, asked that their daughter Jane be given a bilingual aide in her second-grade class at P.S. 203 in Queens, along with daily academic support. The City agreed that Jane should have a bilingual aide, but wanted to move her to another school: one that used a teaching model with a mix of 25 special ed and general ed students, and two teachers . . . At one point, the parents' lawyer asked a teacher if the family's request to keep Jane in P.S. 203, where she had been since kindergarten, was a better plan than the city proposal to move her. "Of course," said the teacher . . . Immediately before the [second] hearing, the city agreed to give the parents exactly what they had requested. Their victory was bittersweet. Instead of getting the bilingual aide at the I.E.P. meeting on October 7, 2003, Jane would get one in September—one school year later. (Winerip, 2004, p. 26)

This example demonstrates that even when parents are able to advocate for their children, inefficient and ineffective school policies and overburdened and underfunded schools are barriers to achieving educational goals. Some parents who have struggled with public schooling in the United States are determined that the only way to secure adequate education for their children is to avoid school policies that hinder and obstruct this objective. They try to outsmart the educational system by falsifying or losing their child's records from the country of origin in their eagerness to have their child seen as possessing normal intelligence and placed in regular, age-appropriate grades. When parents and schools are caught up in family identity issues and school policies, the child's school performance suffers.

## CULTURALLY COMPETENT SCHOOL SOCIAL WORKERS AND PSYCHOLOGISTS

Achieving cultural competence is an ongoing, lifelong process for all mental health professionals, as no one is born culturally competent. "Cultural competence does not come naturally to any social worker [or psychologist] and requires a high level of professionalism and sophistication, yet how culturally competent practitioners are trained is not clear in professional education or practice" (Ortiz Hendricks, 2003, p. 75). More bilingual, bicultural, and culturally competent professionals are needed to meet the needs of fast-growing, diverse client populations, and to help ensure unbiased and culturally sensitive assessments for educational, familial, and social services. Cultural competence is a fundamental necessity for school-based mental health practitioners, including school social workers, who must mediate between the client's culture and the agency's culture while increasing their sensitivity and knowledge of the values, practices, customs, and beliefs of each culture and simultaneously appreciating their own personal and professional values and beliefs (Figure 8.3).

Culturally competent school clinicians need to be culturally aware, culturally sensitive, and culturally knowledgeable practitioners who are open to new ways of defining and evaluating children and their learning needs. They do this over time and in several ways. First, they can begin by recognizing that there are many important ways in which the meanings of terms such as *learning* and *learning disabled* differ among cultural groups, and they need to examine these meanings and their significance to the parents and the communities they serve. Second, they should examine the parameters of what is *normal* in child development and integrate much broader explanations of normalcy than those utilized by educational institutions. Third, they can best help parents by listening carefully to their theories about their children's difficulties, and from a constructivist approach work with parents to bridge the fine distinctions between learning difficulties and measurements of emotional and mental stability. Lastly, culturally competent school-based clinicians have a role in advocating alternative school policies and practices that welcome parents' participation in the educational plans for their children, and that are culturally sensitive and friendly to diverse populations. Cummins (1984) supports this holistic approach that incorporates the cultural, linguistic, and community needs of populations served and calls for a collaborative versus an exclusionary approach to working with parents. "Children's seeming unpreparedness

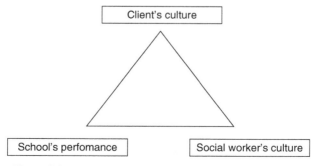

Figure 8.3 *The cultural triangle of client/school/clinician.*

for mainstream schooling is only a measure of the rigidity and ignorance of our school system which creates handicap out of social and cultural difference" (p. 70).

A major contribution by school social workers involves sharing their assessment of the social and cultural needs of children and families with other school professionals. These assessments include comprehensive data and evaluation about

1. Family structures and functions;
2. Generations and length of stay in the United States;
3. Trauma experienced in the country of origin and in the process of immigration itself;
4. Socioeconomic conditions of the family in the country of origin and in the United States;
5. Educational history of all family members;
6. Racial identity; and
7. Language proficiency among all family members.

In addition, school social workers (and school psychologists) should pay attention to parents' attitudes toward education. Initially, they may be filled with great hope and faith in the educational system in the United States, but gradually they become disillusioned and develop a negative attitude toward education in general. Understanding these patterns can help school professionals intervene to prevent or explain the frustration parents encounter in meeting the educational needs of their children.

Lynch and Hanson (1992) propose a specific methodology for competent cross-cultural practice that includes appreciating the impact of cultural assumptions on the intervention process, enhancing cultural self-awareness, understanding the factors that contribute to cultural identification and acculturation, gathering information on other cultures, and establishing guidelines for using interpreters or translators. It is equally important to understand how a particular culture views the helping relationship, how cultural traditions affect problem solving, and "what specific intervention skills and ways of thinking work more effectively with particular groups than those based primarily on the Euro-American frame of reference" (Dungee-Anderson & Beckett, 1995, p. 460).

Furthermore, social workers and psychologists need to engage in an ongoing self-evaluation of their own cultural backgrounds and values (Aponte, 1991; American Psychological Association, 2003; Lum, 1999; Lopez & Rogers, 2007; National Association of Social Workers [NASW], 2007; Pinderhughes, 1989). This ensures their ability to listen to and hear different cultural perspectives and not just the prerogatives of their own cultural heritage or of the school clinician's profession that is in and of itself a cultural point of view. A broad definition of cultural self-awareness includes an appreciation of the following factors:

- Personal values, beliefs, attitudes, biases, prejudices, knowledge paradigms, and how these may differ from other worldviews or values orientations.
- Differences within broad categories of diversity and differences between these groups; for example, Hispanic/Latino encompasses 19 or more different nationalities, social classes, histories, immigration experiences, and geographic locations.

- Definitions of diversity that include race, skin color, ethnicity, gender, gender expression, sexual orientation, religious and spiritual beliefs, social class and status, age, abilities, language, national origin, political beliefs, and geographic and regional locations that interact and combine in complex and significant ways. The challenge for social workers is to be cognizant of individual features of diversity while understanding the multifaceted and intersecting nature of these factors.
- Power, privilege, and oppression and how these affect people, and define who they are, especially as members of oppressed or dominant groups.
- The impact of trauma, colonialism, dominance, and exploitation on human development and mental health.
- Identity development issues, including stages of racial identity formation, and stages of "coming out" and the formation of sexual orientation identity and gender expression.
- Multiple status integration and intersecting identity issues (e.g., a biracial adolescent struggling to solidify their identity).
- Cultural competence in all aspects of practice including work with individuals, families, groups, and communities; clinical work, research, administration, program development, policy analysis and advocacy, and community organizing.
- Culture as a part of personality development and mental health and not just an economic, social, or political variable.
- The impact of bias and discrimination, especially racism, ethnocentrism, sexism, ableism, and heterosexism, on the beneficiaries and survivors of these unequal power relationships.

The development of culturally competent knowledge, skills, and values is critical for social workers and psychologists particularly given certain social, political, economic, and professional realities operating today. Among these realities are changing population demographics and data on the continuing underutilization of mental health services by clients of color. The social work profession, for example, has also advanced cultural competence through its recent accreditation and ethical standards on diversity (NASW, 1999). NASW has developed *Standards for Cultural Competence in Social Work Practice* (2000) that was endorsed by the Council on Social Work Education in 2003. In 2007, NASW developed *Indicators for the Achievement of Cultural Competence in Social Work Practice*. The indicators now give social workers the ability to evaluate their individual strengths and weaknesses in the arena of cultural competence. There are also indicators for what constitutes a culturally competent organization. Similarly, the American Psychological Association (2003) has established guidelines aimed at advancing multicultural education, training, research, practice and organizational change for psychologists. Hirman (2010) aptly notes if school psychologists are to be culturally competent, they must first recognize the limits of their expertise and competencies with ethnically and racially diverse populations.

Diversity is creating many new tensions in North American societies where it is often experienced as a threat rather than as an opportunity to open up dialogue on intergroup conflicts, and enhance intergroup relationships. Greene (1994) speaks of *cross-cultural* and *culturally diverse* as "umbrella terms for the diversity of human experience that is rooted in ethnic, national, or religious identity, race, gender, and social class membership" (p. xii). Along similar lines, this author proposes the following definition of culturally competent social work practice (CCSWP) for consideration:

> CCSWP encompasses a range of professional knowledge, skills, and values that address the complex cultures emerging in a society from the interplay of power, privilege, and oppression associated with race and ethnicity, gender and sexual orientation, religious and spiritual beliefs, social class and status, and age and abilities. (Greene, 1994, p. 8)

This definition recognizes that all people have a cultural group identity, and that many types and forms of group membership in society take on varying significance depending on the societal context. A societal context in which difference is not merely "different from" but is associated with "better or less than," is a society in which differences are not viewed as the norm for human behavior but rather differences are viewed as deviant or deficit. Power and privilege are then used to minimize these differences or oppress characteristics that are simply a part of human diversity. Whoever has power or is in a dominant position contributes to the oppression of those not considered within the mainstream of society (e.g., immigrant women), or those that are part of the mainstream society (e.g., White women), or those who are relegated to an inferior status (e.g., undocumented immigrants).

CCSWP involves a dynamic, interactive assessment of a client's particular lifestyle, which moves from universal categories of cultures (Latino, African American, Asian, Jewish American, Irish Catholic, etc.) to more specific, individualized, and complex categories of cultures within cultures (Fong & Frito, 2001; Lum, 1999). Gould (1995) proposes that a multicultural framework refutes the basic assumption that cultural identity has to be unidimensional or that becoming more of something automatically means becoming less of the original. "A multicultural framework goes beyond encouraging intercultural learning and multicultural competency to building a multicultural identity for all groups" (Gould, 1995, pp. 202–203). A specific situation can help to clarify exactly what is entailed in such a multicultural framework:

> A Cuban school psychologist is assigned to work with a family from the Dominican Republic. Each can be viewed from very broad class, racial, ethnic, or gender categorizations, but these distinctions do not do justice to the multifaceted cultures each uniquely encompasses. The psychologist is a 42-year-old Latina clinician who was born in Cuba and raised in New York City. She considers herself a White, middle class, Hispanic American professional. The Velasquez family is composed of a 27-year-old woman who is a laboratory technician and a 28-year-old man who works in his cousin's food market. They are married and have two children aged 7 and 5. The family has recently re-migrated for the third time to New York City from the Dominican Republic for a variety of family reasons. A referral is made because of suspected incidents of family violence, excessive

school absences, and a recently diagnosed learning disability for the 7-year-old child. The case is automatically referred to the only Latina psychologist in the school because of ethnic and linguistic commonalities.

A multicultural framework can help this social psychologist appreciate the similarities and differences between her and the Velasquez family. As Hispanics, they share experiences of oppression both within and outside their countries of origin. Yet each has distinct experiences—as Dominicans and Cubans in the United States, including different historical and social evolutions, English and Spanish language proficiencies, skin colors, immigration patterns, and citizenship status. The psychologist can best help this Dominican family and others like them by recognizing the oppression experienced by immigrant Latinos who deal with the stress of immigration, resettlement, and family reorganization in addition to economic hardships and discrimination in the United States (Organista, 2009). Together, the psychologist and clients will engage in a multicultural encounter in which understanding each other's unique experiences will be integral to the work they do in confronting an inner-city public school system (Falicov, 1995).

## CONCLUSION

As cultural diversity increases in the United States, school social workers and psychologists are on the front lines of empowering children and families to deal effectively with a public school system that has the power to influence the lives of children and families in positive and negative ways. The development of bilingual, bicultural, and culturally competent social workers is critical for a positive interaction and healthy relationship among the child, the family, and the school systems, especially when a child demonstrates some form of learning difficulty. Culturally competent school clinicians play a central role in appreciating and dealing with the power, powerlessness, and unequal power relationships that are inherent in these systems. All school professionals need to recognize that enhancing the parents' power to understand and attend to their children's educational needs is in the best interests of the children served. "True empowerment benefits both the client system and the practitioner in that client and [clinician] experience a sense of each other's freedom and individuality which includes a real appreciation of each other's differences and similarities" (Pinderhughes, 1989, p. 240). Empowering diverse families will result in vast numbers of children experiencing more satisfying and productive relationships with the educational system, and will help them reconcile the various cultural challenges presented by the home, the community, and the school.

> As we look into the future of school social work [and school psychology], concerns about the quality and cost of education, student learning outcomes, accountability, increased demand to serve more diverse student populations, and increased social problems among children and families, will challenge the profession to think creatively and differently about their services and how to organize them for greater effectiveness and efficiency. (Allen-Meares, 2008, p. 6)

This is difficult but extremely rewarding work as school professionals, children, and families help each other to live in a multiculturally diverse society.

## DISCUSSION QUESTIONS

1. Describe the importance of the multicultural triangle (child, family, and school) in providing culturally competent care to children and families within urban public schools.
2. What role do educational policies and practice play in supporting or hindering the academic outcomes of children?
3. How can school psychologists and school social workers achieve cultural competence in their practice with children and families?
4. Define cultural self-awareness and state why it is an important component of culturally competence practice within school settings.

## REFERENCES

Allen-Meares, P. (2008). School social work. In T. Mizrahi & L. E. Davis (Eds.-in-chief), *Encyclopedia of Social Work* (20th ed., Vol. 4, pp. 3–7). Washington, DC: NASW Press and Oxford University Press.

Andersen, M. L., & Collins, P. H. (Eds.). (1998). *Race, class, and gender: An anthology.* Boston, MA: Wadsworth.

Aponte, H. J. (1976). The family-school interview: An ecostructural approach. *Family Process, 15*(3), 303–312. doi:10.1111/j.1545-5300.1976.00303.x

Aponte, H. J. (1991). Training on the person of the therapist for work with the poor and minorities. *Journal of Independent Social Work, 5*(3/4), 23–39. doi:10.1300/J283v05n03_04

Appleby, G. A., Colon, E., & Hamilton, J. (2001). *Diversity, oppression, and social functioning: Person-in-environment assessment and intervention.* Boston, MA: Allyn & Bacon.

American Psychological Association. (2003). Guidelines on multicultural education, training, research, practice and organizational change for psychologists. *American Psychologist, 58*(5), 377–402. doi:10.1037/0003-066X.58.5.377

Bennett, A. T. (1988). Gateways to powerlessness: Incorporating Hispanic deaf children and families into formal schooling. *Disability, Handicap and Society, 3*(2), 119–151. doi:10.1080/02674648866780131

Boyles, N. S., & Contadino, D. (1998). *The learning differences sourcebook.* Los Angeles, CA: Lowell House.

Bronstein, L. R., & Abramson, J. S. (2003). Understanding socialization of teachers and social workers: Groundwork for collaboration in the schools. *Families in Society, 84*(3), 323–332. doi:10.1606/1044-3894.110

Chavkin, N. F., & Garza-Lubeck, M. (1990). Multicultural approaches to parent involvement: Research and practice. *Social Work in Education, 13*(1), 22–23. doi:10.1093/cs/13.1.22

Compher, J. V. (1982). Parent-school-child systems: Triadic assessment and intervention. *Social Casework, 63*(7), 415–433. doi:10.1177/104438948206300705

Constable, R., & Montgomery, E. (1985). Perceptions of the school social worker's role. *Social Work in Education, 7*(4), 244–257. doi:10.1093/cs/7.4.244

Constable, R., & Walberg, H. (1988). School social work: Facilitating home, school, and community partnerships. *Urban Education, 22*(4), 429–443. doi:10.1177/004208598802200404

Correa, V. I. (1989). Involving culturally different families in the education process. In S. H. Fradd & M. J. Weismantel (Eds.), *Meeting the needs of culturally and linguistically different students* (pp. 130–144). Boston, MA: College-Hill.

Crenshaw, K. W. (1991). Mapping the margins: Intersectionality, identity politics, and violence against women of color. *Stanford Law Review, 43*, 1241–1299. doi:10.2307/1229039

Cummins, J. (1984). *Bilingualism and special education: Issues in assessment and pedagogy.* San Diego, CA: College-Hill.

Dao, M. (1991). Designing assessment procedures for educationally at-risk Southeast Asian-American students. *Journal of Learning Disabilities, 24*(10), 594–601. doi:10.1177/002221949102401002

de Anda, D. (1984). Bicultural socialization: Factors affecting the minority experience. *Social Work, 29*(2), 101–107. doi:10.1093/sw/29.2.101

Delgado, M., & Rivera, H. (1997). Puerto Rican natural support systems: Impact on families, communities, and schools. *Urban Education, 3*(1), 81–97. doi:10.1177/0042085997032001005

Delgado-Gaitan, C. (1987). Parent perceptions of schools: Supportive environments for children. In H. T. Trueba (Ed.), *Success or failure? Learning and the language minority student* (pp. 131–155). New York, NY: Newbury House.

Douglas, S. T. (2011). *The relationship between parenting styles, dimensions of parenting and academic achievement of African American and Latino students.* Dissertation, New York University, PhD Program, New York.

Dowling, E., & Osborne, E. (1985). *The family and the school: A joint systems approach to problems with children.* London: Routledge & Kegan Paul.

Dungee-Anderson, D., & Beckett, J. (1995). A process model for multicultural social work practice. *Families in Society: The Journal of Contemporary Human Services, 76*, 459–466. doi:10.1177/104438949507600802

Falicov, C. J. (1995). Training to think culturally: A multidimensional comparative framework. *Family Process, 34*, 373–388. doi:10.1111/j.1545-5300.1995.00373.x

Fong, R., & Furuto, S. (Eds.). (2001). *Culturally competent practice: Skills, interventions, and evaluations.* Boston, MA: Allyn & Bacon.

Franklin, C. (2000). Predicting the future of school social work practice in the new millennium. *Social Work in Education, 22*(1), 3–8. doi:10.1093/cs/22.1.3

Freeman, E. M., & Pennekamp, M. (1988). *Social work practice: Toward a child, family, school, community perspective.* Springfield, IL: Charles Thomas.

Freire, P. (1993). *Pedagogy of the oppressed.* New York, NY: Seabury Press.

Freire, P. (1998). *Teachers as cultural workers: Letters to those who dare to teach.* New York, NY: Westview Press.

Gandara, P. C., & Contreras, F. (2009). *The Latino education crisis: The consequences of failed social policies.* Cambridge, MA: Harvard University Press.

Garrett, K. (2006). Making the case for school social work. *Children & Schools, 28*(2), 115–122. doi:10.1093/cs/28.2.115

Golden, L., & Cupuzzi, D. (1986). *Helping families help children: Family interventions with school related problems.* Springfield, IL: Charles Thomas.

Gould, K. H. (1995). The misconstruing of multiculturalism: The Stanford debate and social work. *Social Work, 40*(2), 198–205.

Greene, R. R. (1994). *Human behavior theory: A diversity framework.* New York, NY: Aldine de Gruyter.

Greene, G. J., Jensen, C., & Jones, D. H. (1996). A constructivist perspective on clinical social work practice with ethnically diverse clients. *Social Work, 41*(2), 172–180. doi:10.1093/sw/41.2.172

Harry, B. (1992a). *Culturally diverse families and the special education system.* New York, NY: Teachers College Press.

Harry, B. (1992b). Making sense of disability: Low-income, Puerto Rican parents' theories of the problem. *Exceptional Children, 59*(1), 27–40. doi:10.1177/001440299205900104

Hill, N. E., & Torres, K. (2010). Negotiating the American dream: The paradox of aspirations and achievement among Latino students and engagement between their families and schools. *Journal of Social Issues, 66*(1), 95–112. doi:10.1111/j.1540-4560.2009.01635.x

Hirman, J. (2010). *The role of school psychologists in mental health services with underserved students.* Unpublished Master's Thesis, The Graduate School, University of Wisconsin-Stout, Menomonie, WI.

Hughes, T. L., Minke, K. M., & Sansosti, F. J. (2017). Expanding school psychology service delivery within the context of national health and mental health reform. *Journal of Applied School Psychology, 33*(3), 171–178. doi:10.1080/15377903.2017.1317139

Jackson, S., & McParlin, P. (2006). The education of children in care. *Psychologist, 19*(2), 90–94.

Johnson-Reid, M., Jiyoung, K., Barolak, M., Citerman, B., Laudel, C., Essma, A., & Thomas, C. (2007). Maltreated children in schools: The interface of school social work and child welfare. *Children & Schools, 29*(3), 182–191. doi:10.1093/cs/29.3.182

Kalyanpur, M., & Rao, S. S. (1991). Empowering low-income black families of handicapped children. *American Journal of Orthopsychiatry, 61*(4), 523–532. doi:10.1037/h0079292

Kurtz, P. D., & Barth, R. P. (1989). Parent involvement: Cornerstone of school social work practice. *Social Work, 39*, 407–413.

Lum, D. (1999). *Culturally competent practice: A framework for growth and action.* Pacific Grove, CA: Brooks/Cole.

Lopez, E., & Rogers, M. R. (2007). Multicultural competencies and training in school psychology: Issues, approaches, and future directions. In G. E. Esquivel, E. Lopez, & S. G. Nahari (Eds.), *Multicultural handbook of school psychology* (pp. 47–66). Mahwah, NJ: Lawrence Erlbaum Associates.

Lynch, E. W., & Hanson, M. J. (Eds.). (1992). *Developing cross-cultural competence: A guide for working with young children and their families.* Baltimore, MD: Paul H. Brookes.

Lynch, E. W., & Stein, R. C. (1987). Parent participation by ethnicity: A comparison of Hispanic, Black and Anglo families. *Exceptional Children, 54*, 105–111. doi:10.1177/001440298705400202

Mackelprang, R. W. (2008). Disability overview. In Mizrahi T. & L. E. Davis (Eds.-in-chief), *Encyclopedia of Social Work* (20th ed., Vol. 2, pp. 36–43). Washington, DC: NASW Press and Oxford University Press.

McAdoo, H., & McAdoo, J. L. (1985). *Black children: Social educational and parental environments.* Beverly Hills, CA: Sage.

McFarland, J., Hussar, B., de Brey, C., Snyder, T., Wang, X., Wilkinson-Flicker, S., . . . Hinz, S. (2017). *The condition of education.* Washington DC: Department of Education, National Center for Education Statistics.

National Association of Social Workers. (1999). *Code of ethics.* Washington, DC: NASW Press.

National Association of Social Workers. (2000). *Standards for cultural competence in social work practice.* Washington, DC: NASW Press.

National Association of Social Workers. (2007). *Indicators for the achievement of cultural competence in social work practice.* Washington, DC: NASW Press.

National Scientific Council on the Developing Child. (2012). *Establishing a level of foundation for life: Mental health begins in early childhood: Working paper 6.* Cambridge, MA: Harvard University Press.

Organista, K. C. (2009). New practice model for Latinos in need of social work services. *Social Work, 54*(4), 297–305. doi:10.1093/sw/54.4.297

Ortiz Hendricks, C. (2003). Learning and teaching culturally competent social work practice. *Journal of Teaching in Social Work, 23*(1/2), 73–86. doi:10.1300/J067v23n01_06

Ortiz Hendricks, C., Haffey, M., & Asamoah, Y. (1988). *The roles of culture bearer and culture broker in social work practice with culturally diverse families.* Paper presented at the Annual Program Meeting of the Council on Social Work Education, Atlanta, GA.

Pinderhughes, E. B. (1989). *Understanding race, ethnicity, and power: The key to efficacy in clinical practice.* New York, NY: Free Press.

Ravitch, D., & Viteritti, J. P. (Eds.). (2000). *Lessons from New York: City schools*. Baltimore, MD: The Johns Hopkins University Press.

Rojas-Flores, L., Clements, M. L., Koo, H., & London, J. (2017). Trauma and psychological distress in Latino citizen children following parental detention and deportation. *Psychological Trauma: Theory, Research, Practice, and Policy, 9*(3), 352–361. doi:10.1037/tra0000177

Ryan, A. S., & Smith, M. J. (1989). Parental reactions to developmental disabilities in Chinese American families. *Child and Adolescent Social Work Journal, 6*(4), 283–299. doi:10.1007/BF00755222

Sarason, S. B. (1982). *The culture of the school and the problem of change*. Boston, MA: Allyn & Bacon.

Shahidullah, J. D. (2019). Behavioral health care coordination across child-serving systems: A burgeoning role for school psychologists. *School Community Journal, 29*(1), 279–296.

Spener, D. (1988). Transitional bilingual education and the socialization of immigrants. *Harvard Educational Review, 58*, 133–152. doi:10.17763/haer.58.2.x7543241r7w14446

Staudt, M. (1991). A role perception study of school social work practice. *Social Work, 36*(6), 496–498.

Tower, K. (2000). A study of attitudes about school social workers. *Social Work in Education, 22*(2), 83–95. doi:10.1093/cs/22.2.83

Trout, A., Hagaman, J., Casey, K., Reid, R., & Epstein, M. (2008). The academic status of children and youth in out-of-home care: A review of the literature. *Children and Youth Services Review, 30*, 979–974. doi:10.1016/j.childyouth.2007.11.019

Viruell-Fuentes, E. A., Miranda, P. Y., & Abdulrahim, S. (2012). More than culture: Structural racism, intersectionality theory, and immigrant health. *Social Science & Medicine, 75*, 2099–2106. doi:10.1016/j.socscimed.2011.12.037

Williams Splett, J., Fowler, J., Weist, M. D., McDaniel, H., & Dvorsky, M. (2013). The critical role of school psychology in the school mental health movement. *Psychology in the Schools, 50*(3), 245–258. doi:10.1002/pits.21677

Winerip, M. (2004, July 4). City retools special education, but pupils are slipping through cracks. *The New York Times*, pp. 1, 26.

Woolley, M. E., Kol, K. L., & Bowen, G. L. (2009). The social context of school success for Latino middle school students—Direct and indirect influences of teachers, family, and friends. *The Journal of Early Adolescence, 29*(1), 43–70. doi:10.1177/0272431608324478

# 9

# Cross-Cultural Perspectives on Working With Adolescents

DANIEL KAPLIN AND UWE P. GIELEN

## INTRODUCTION

During recent decades, ethnic and racial variability has increased greatly in classic immigration countries such as Australia, Aotearoa-New Zealand, Canada, and the United States. In Western Europe as well, immigration from North Africa, Asia, and neighboring European countries has accompanied the economic rise and decrease in birthrates characterizing that part of the world. In all these countries, minority and immigrant groups may include a disproportionate percentage of young people who need to find a place in society while developing complex and evolving forms of identity. This chapter introduces a variety of culturally informed models of identity development that may be useful to social workers, clinical and counseling psychologists, and educators. They may be in a position to support adolescents from a broad range of ethnic, religious, and bicultural groups as well as youth differing in their sexual orientation and gender identity.

In Erikson's (1968) psychosocial stage theory, he proposes eight periods of development. Within each of these stages, a person has a life task (or crisis) that needs to be resolved to promote successful development across the lifespan. In adolescence, the primary challenge is to develop an understanding of one's sense of self. This is often referred to as the *identity versus role confusion* conflict.

In modern post-industrial societies, the developing adolescent begins to leave childhood behind around 12 to 13 years of age and transitions into emerging adulthood when he or she reaches the age of 18 to 19 years. However, in traditional societies with limited or no schooling, many girls were—and in countries such as Niger and Bangladesh still are—married off in their middle teenage years (Gielen & Kim, 2019). Consequently, they are expected to perform many adult tasks at an earlier age than is typical for economically developed societies with their elaborate educational systems and late marriage ages. In these societies and mediated by a broad range of information and communication technologies, many adolescents are exposed to a broad range of both local and global cultural influences. This, in turn, can lead to complex, multicultural, and at times contradictory forms of identity. The struggles of adolescents and "emerging adults" (18–25 years old; cf. Arnett & Tanner, 2006) to achieve a coherent identity were initially discussed by psychologists such as Erikson (1968) and Marcia (1966), but in more recent decades, social scientists have increasingly emphasized the cultural, ethnic–racial, and gender related dimensions of identity development.

Influenced by Erikson's theory, Marcia (1966, 1980) notes that adolescents and young adults go about their search for the self in different ways. He examined adolescents' level of exploration and commitment as a way to determine their identity status. Marcia (1966) noted that adolescents could be categorized in one of four ways. *Foreclosure* is characterized by low exploration and high commitment. *Moratorium* is characterized by high exploration, low commitment, and a sense of crisis. *Diffusion* is marked by low exploration and low commitment. Lastly, *achievement* often follows a period of exploration that culminates in high commitment.

## INDIVIDUALISTIC VERSUS COLLECTIVISTIC CULTURES

Both Erikson and Marcia fail to fully capture the impact of culture on one's understanding of identity/self-concept. Hofstede (2001) notes that cultures can be evaluated on their relative power inequalities, degree of interdependence, drive to be the best, ability to tolerate the uncertainty of the future, interest in remaining connected to their past, and desire to regulate people's impulses. Individualistic societies tend to favor individual freedoms over the group. Collectivistic societies, on the other hand, are giving a group priority over each individual in it. Western countries tend to be more individualistic than Eastern communities (Riemer, Shavitt, Koo, & Markus, 2014).

Triandis (2001) and Triandis and Suh (2002) propose that members of individualistic and collectivistic communities will differ in personality. More specifically, culture will impact a person's definition of self, adoption of social norms, self-esteem, personal versus situational attributions, ethnocentrism, dominance, expression of emotions, view of morality, and Big Five personality traits (i.e., openness, conscientiousness, extraversion, agreeableness, and neuroticism). Thus, the cultural context one is raised in usually impacts one's sense of self (Markus & Kitayama, 1994; Triandis, 2001).

## TIGHT AND LOOSE CULTURES

Gelfand (2018) discusses the contrast between tight and loose cultures and societies. Tight societies such as Malaysia and Pakistan encourage obedience to strict social norms in a variety of domains while sanctioning those members who do not live up to them. While not as tight as Pakistani society, traditional Chinese society is regarded as tighter (and more collectivistic) than present-day American society in domains such as family organization, child rearing practices, dating practices, and permissible behavior in educational institutions. Tight societies encourage self-control for children, adolescents, and adults that may, for instance, be intertwined with firm sexual norms especially for unmarried females. In contrast, loose cultures accept a considerable range of behaviors as admissible. One can observe this, for instance, in New York City's highly diverse local cultures where individual behaviors and dress codes can be quite variable. In a related fashion, some of the City's subcultures encourage public displays of various sexual orientations and identities that may be less acceptable in the southern and central areas of the United States. Moreover, loose societies tend to encourage openness as a personality trait, whereas tight societies tend to reinforce traits such as conscientiousness and firm self-control. The contrast between tight and loose societies is especially pertinent for minority group members and bicultural individuals. They frequently have to struggle with a variety of potentially contradictory identities, which majority group members may not always judge to be preferable or even acceptable. Minorities, women, adolescents attending strict schools, and those living at the bottom of the economic order tend to live in more tightly regulated worlds especially when compared to those occupying elite positions within the majority culture.

## ETHNIC/RACIAL IDENTITY MODELS

Another consideration is that Erikson's (1968) and Marcia's (1966, 1980) views on identity development underestimate the impact racism, ethnic prejudice, sexism, classism, and other "isms" have on one's sense of self. Several racial identity models have been developed to remedy this shortcoming. For example, Cross (1971) proposed the *Black Racial Identity Model* to address how African Americans develop an appreciation for their ethnic identity. In its most recent form, this model includes pre-encounter (low racial identity salience), encounter (exposure to a race-related incident), immersion/emersion (begins to develop a Black identity), and internalization (high racial identity salience) stages (Cross & Vandiver, 2001; Jackson, 2012). Several limitations have emerged in regards to Cross's model (Constantine, Richardson, Benjamin, & Wilson, 1998). Barnes, Williams, and Barnes (2014) emphasize the importance of exploring racial identity with African Americans.

In Helms's (1990, 1995) *White Racial Identity Development Model*, individuals attempt to reconcile their White identity with the racist backdrop of being White in America. The end product is that White individuals become allies in the process to dismantle some of the structural racism ethnic minorities experience. Accordingly, this model explains how to appreciate the impact one's "Whiteness" has on others and the process of moving toward an anti-racist identity. Helms's model includes *contact* (obliviousness of racism), *disintegration* (ambivalence), *reintegration* (starts to denigrate the out-group), *pseudo-independence* (recognition of unfairness on an intellectual level), *immersion/emersion* (recognition of White privilege and reshaping continues), and *autonomy* (moves toward a non-racist and flexible understanding of race). Several researchers have expressed concern about the suggested stage-like progression of White identity development (Miller & Fellows, 2007; Rowe, Bennett, & Atkinson, 1994). Nevertheless, incorporating this model into training could help White students to process their resistance around multicultural topics (Suthakaran, 2012).

Ruiz (1990) proposed a *Latin American Identity Development Model* that includes five stages. In the *casual* stage, the individual receives messages that result in the denigration of their ethnic identity, which results in the failure to identify as Latinx. In the *cognitive* stage, individuals develop distorted thinking that being Latinx will result in poverty/prejudice and assimilation into the larger White society is the only way to successfully avoid this poverty. During the *consequence* stage, members of the Latinx community start to develop a sense of shame and embarrassment toward their ethnic identity and culture. In the *working through* stage, due to the cognitive dissonance of identifying with an alien ethnic identity, individuals start to begin to reclaim and reintegrate their Latinx identity. Finally, in the *successful resolution* stage, individuals develop more positive views of their Latinx identity. This results in increased self-esteem.

Kim's (1981) *Asian American Identity Development Model* includes five stages. In the *ethnic awareness* stage, the child has positive or neutral attitudes toward their Asian identity. During the *White identification* stage, children start to become aware of their ethnic differences and attempt to identify with White society. In the *awakening* stage, Asians start to recognize various forms of oppression and stop identifying with White identity. In the *redirection* stage, they reconnect with their Asian American heritage and culture. Finally, in the *incorporation* stage, Asian Americans grow comfortable with their Asian identity. Other researchers (Kodama, McEwen, Liang, & Lee, 2002) focusing on Asian Americans proposed a domain-based psychosocial developmental model. At its core, identity and having a sense of purpose are intertwined. In this model, they reflect on how family/cultural (e.g., deferring to authority, guilt, humility, language, educational value, gender roles, and generational status) and societal factors (e.g., perpetual minority, model minority, homogenization, gender stereotypes, and invisibility) impact identity. These authors note that Asian Americans' identity is also driven by maintaining a sense of interdependence, harmonious relationships, and integrity.

Poston's (1990) *Biracial Identity Development Model* divides the development of biracial identity into five successive stages. In the personal identity stage, individuals do not attach their sense of self to their race. When a person moves to the *choice of group* stage, they start to feel compelled to select one racial identity. The *enmeshment/denial* stage includes guilt feelings around not being able to fully embrace one's racial identity. The *appreciation* stage results in increased awareness of multiple identities. Lastly, in the *integration* stage, the individual accepts his or her multiple racial identities.

## BICULTURAL IDENTITY

Berry's (1980, 1997) acculturation model is often used to address identity for those who immigrate from another country and are trying to adapt to their new environment. Four outcomes emerge as a function of a person's acceptance or rejection of their native and host country's culture (Berry, 1997; Berry, Kim, Minde, & Mok, 1987). More specifically, *integration* occurs when a person is able to maintain a connection with their native country's culture, while being able to also adopt aspects of their host culture. *Assimilation* occurs when the person adopts the culture of their host country and rejects their native culture. *Separation* takes place when a person maintains their native culture, but rejects their host culture. Finally, *marginalization* occurs when the person rejects or withdraws from both their native and host cultures. Marginalization often leads to a sense of disorientation and unhappiness, whereas integration tends to work well for individuals residing in multicultural immigration societies such as Canada.

## GENDER AND SEXUAL IDENTITY MODELS

Downing and Roush (1985) proposed the Feminist Identity Development Model. At first, *passive acceptance* involves accepting the structural oppression of women. During the *revelation* stage, a crisis occurs which results in a sense that men are bad and women are good. Afterwards, during the *embeddedness and emanation* stage, women start to develop a connection with other women. During the *synthesis* stage, women develop a positive feminist identity. Lastly, during the *active commitment* stage, there develops a stronger focus on societal change. This includes commitment to a non-sexist world. Some researchers have hesitated to support the stage-like nature of this theory (Erchull et al., 2009; Hyde, 2002).

There exist several sexual identity development models (Cass, 1979; Coleman, 1982; Troiden, 1979). Cass's Identity Model (1979, 1984) postulates six stages, which include *identity confusion* (recognition of gay or lesbian thoughts), *comparison* (examination of the implications of being gay or lesbian), *tolerance* (seeking out relationships with other gay or lesbian individuals), *acceptance* (beginning to embrace one's gay or lesbian identity), pride (minimizing one's contact with heterosexuals), and *synthesis* (integration of sexual identity with other identities).

Troiden's Gay Identity Acquisition Model (1979) includes four stages of development. In the *sensitization* stage, a person starts to feel different. During the *self-recognition* stage, the individual realizes they are attracted to people of the same sex. During the *identity assumption* stage, the person starts to become more certain of their sexual orientation. Lastly, during the *commitment* phase, the person begins to adopt a homosexual way of life. Coleman's (1982) Developmental Stages of Coming Out has five successive stages: *pre-coming out, coming out, exploration, first relationships,* and *integration*.

Pollock and Eyre (2012) proposed a model for transgender identity development. In the first stage, a person develops a *sense of gender*. In this stage, a person has a sense that their gender identity does not match their sexual characteristics. In the second stage, the person develops *recognition* of their transgender identity. The person begins to explore transgender possibilities. In the third stage, the person begins a *social adjustment* process. This involves coming out, physical transition, and integrating their trans-identity with other aspects of their sense of self.

## CASE VIGNETTE

Suzie[1] is a 16-year-old, single, Chinese American female, who lives in Manhattan with her mother and older brother, was referred for services by her teacher

---

[1] For the sake of maintaining confidentiality, the name "Suzie" was given as a pseudonym. Several other aspects of her history have been modified.

because she wrote a note in music class stating that "she wanted to die." Suzie reported feeling this way because she felt that she was being teased because she was making mistakes on the drums. She reported that this was triggered because a fellow student persistently bullied her. Suzie reports that she wrote that note in October, but the thoughts persisted for several weeks afterward. However, she denied the presence of intent or plan. Suzie also denied the history of suicidal or self-harm behaviors (e.g., cutting, self-mutilation). Suzie denied receiving psychological services or psychiatric hospitalizations.

Suzie's parents were born in Fuzhou, which is the capital of the Fujian Province of China. However, they immigrated to New York City prior to the birth of Suzie and her older brother. Suzie's parents are both U.S. citizens. Suzie's mother reports that they immigrated to the United States for greater financial opportunities. Suzie's parents predominantly speak Chinese, but her mother has mastery of conversational English. Suzie noted that she feels more Americanized relative to her mother.

Suzie's mother and father are divorced and she has limited contact with her father. Suzie's mother reported that the reason for the divorce was that Suzie's father engaged in domestic violence and drank heavily. Suzie's mother works as a patient care technician in a nursing home. Suzie's father worked in a local restaurant as a dishwasher, but has not provided much financial or emotional support for the family since their divorce. Suzie's mother reports that they struggle financially, but can pay their current bills.

Suzie's older brother is a senior in high school. Record review indicated that her brother was in treatment for depression several years prior. Suzie notes that her mother shows a bias in favor of her older brother. Suzie says that when she misbehaves, her mother yells at her. She reports that there have been several occasions where she experienced corporal punishment, but denied the presence of child abuse, neglect, and maltreatment. Overall, Suzie says that she is close to her mother and older brother.

Suzie's mother reported that her developmental history is unremarkable. Suzie is in the 10th grade in a regular education classroom. Suzie noted, "her mother puts considerable pressure on her to maintain her grades so that she can get into a good college" and "make the family proud." She reports having perfect attendance and being a B student on average. However, Suzie struggles with math, which is a source of distress. She denies ever having been suspended or the presence of conduct problems.

Suzie is a post-pubertal adolescent female. She reported normal adjustment to her physiological changes. She denies having any romantic relationships saying, "she would rather focus on her studies." However, she noted that she identifies as heterosexual. Suzie denied the use of alcohol, tobacco, and other drugs. She also denied the presence of compulsive gambling or video game/Internet use. She also denies having any legal problems.

Suzie reports that she has very few friends in school. However, she noted that this doesn't bother her. The friends she has are similar in age, mostly female, and come predominantly from the Asian community. Suzie notes that her parents were not religious in China, but adopted Christian principles when coming to the United States. She finds prayer to be helpful in times of distress, but does not consider herself overly religious. Suzie reported that one of her strengths is that she likes to draw.

## ASSESSING SALIENT FACTORS FROM SUZIE'S IDENTITY

In the following, we first introduce several salient treatment concerns in the context of Congress's (2008) culturagram. In doing so, we can gain further appreciation for sociocultural and/or environmental factors that could become relevant in treatment. In addition, we also assess Suzie's identity using Hays's (2016) ADDRESSING framework to identify potential areas of threats to Suzie's multidimensional identity.

### Assessing Suzie Using the Congress (2008) Culturagram

According to Congress (2008), one should assess 10 domains when evaluating a client on the basis of her culturagram. They are (a) the client and/or family's reason for relocation, (b) legal status, (c) time in the community, (d) language spoken at home and in the community, (e) health beliefs, (f) trauma and crisis events, (g) cultural and religious affiliation, (h) oppression, (i) values of education/work, and (j) the family structure. In the paragraphs that follow, we use this assessment mechanism to evaluate the impact Suzie's cultural experience has on her and her family.

As noted, Suzie's parents left China for greater financial opportunity. Consistent with Berry's (1980, 1997) bicultural identity model, Suzie's mother appears to be struggling to reconcile her Chinese and American identities. While Suzie views herself as American, her mother maintains fondness for China. In some sessions, Suzie's mom discussed how things might be easier if she were still in China because of the family and cultural ties. The cultural gaps between Suzie and her mother result in acculturative stress as they balance Suzie's mother's nostalgia of China and the adjustments to the United States (Ho & Gielen, 2016; Lui, 2015). Of notable interest is because Suzie and her brother are U.S. born, and they tend to be more assimilated than their mother. This created some tension within the family.

Suzie's mother and father used traditional routes of immigration and obtained U.S. citizenship before they had children. Because of this difference, Suzie's family is less likely to experience fears and isolation that have been linked to undocumented families (Tummala-Narra, 2020). Moreover, because their move to the United States was not due to war, trauma, or oppression, Suzie's family was not subjected to emotional distress and traumatic experiences many other immigrants and refugees experience (Kim-Prieto et al., 2018; Nosè et al., 2017; Rousseau & Drapeau, 2004).

Another source of distress for Suzie's mom is that her lack of English language proficiency makes her stand out. Although she has developed command of conversational English, Suzie's mother still feels uncomfortable due to her making grammatical errors, pragmatic language problems, and the feeling that her accent makes her stand out. This is a common concern for immigrants and refugees (Stewart et al., 2008). To reduce the discomfort, Suzie feels compelled to speak Chinese in the home. However, she prefers to speak English, which she reports is her more developed language. A second manifestation is that Suzie, like many children of immigrants, sometimes serves as a language broker for her mother's doctor's appointments (Hua & Costigan, 2012; Shen, Kim, & Benner, 2019; Tse, 1996). Recruitment of bilingual practitioners should be considered to ensure one provides culturally and linguistically appropriate services (Lin, Chiang, Lux, & Lin, 2018).

Coming from a traditional East Asian family, mental health stigma is common (Mellor, Carne, Shen, Mccabe, & Wang, 2013). Suzie and her family are no different. Suzie was apprehensive about entering therapy but felt obligated by the school. As such, there was some resistance around assessment and treatment. However, after processing the stigma around mental health treatment, Suzie became more comfortable and forthcoming in treatment.

Suzie's family structure is consistent with that of many East Asian families (Kodama et al., 2002). While divorced, her mother often emphasizes the importance of family cohesion (Kodama et al., 2002; Raymo, Park, Xie, & Yeung, 2015). Suzie reported in one session that sometimes she has to forego part of her individuality to conform to these expectations. This sense of interdependence is also common in Asian communities (Hofstede, 2001; Riemer et al., 2014; Triandis, 2001). Suzie also internalized pressure to excel in the classroom from her mother. Lastly, consistent with many traditional cultures, Suzie expressed that her brother receives preferential treatment within the family (Chung, 2017; Kodama et al., 2002). These factors could be further explored in therapy.

While Suzie has few friends, she reported meaningful relationships with them. She also uses religion and prayer practices as a source of strength. Suzie identifies as more Americanized, but participates in several Chinese holiday customs (e.g., Lunar New Year). These are protective factors for Suzie. Suzie appears to be in the redirection stage of Kim's (1981) Asian Identity Development model. The most salient factors for consideration are related to acculturation, language, mental health stigma, academic pressures, and the pressures that come from the family structure. In Figure 9.1, a complete analysis of Suzie's culturagram is presented.

## Assessing Suzie Using Hays's (2016) ADDRESSING Framework

Congress's (2008) culturagram places emphasis on sociocultural factors that impact a client's experience. Pamela Hays's (1996, 2016) ADDRESSING framework is designed to reflect overlapping domains that reflect cultural identity. Consideration of age, developmental disabilities, acquired disabilities, religion, ethnicity, sexual orientation, socioeconomic status, indigenous group membership, nationality, and gender contributes to a complete understanding of cultural identity (Hays; as cited in Kaplin, 2017, p. 16). According to Hays (2016), each aspect of cultural identity can result in privilege or marginalization. In the following, we isolate several prominent cultural identity factors that could impact the treatment process.

Suzie's areas of privilege are reflected in her lack of disability, religious majority status, sexual orientation, not being part of an indigenous group, and her national status. Nevertheless, she is also subject to marginalization. For example, in the East Asian tradition, there is an emphasis on honoring older adults for their wisdom (Löckenhoff et al., 2009). Yet, as an adolescent, Suzie could be subjected to a form of ageism called *adultism*, where children and adolescents' are exposed to prejudice and discrimination (Campos-Holland, 2017; John, 2013; Westman, 1991). This could result in rhetoric like, "What does she know, she is just a kid?" In doing so, Suzie's might feel like her perspectives are invalidated.

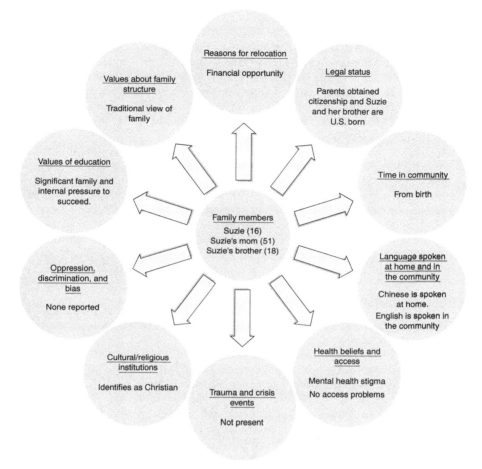

Figure 9.1 *A summary of Suzie's culturagram is presented.*

A second concern is that Suzie could be experiencing racism based on her ethnic identity and situation (Kim, 1981; Yoon et al., 2017). Interestingly, she noted that many of her friends come from within the Asian American community. This could be reflective of ethnic socialization messages from her family and community (Kodama et al., 2002; Yoon et al., 2017). One form of racism that Suzie could experience is the model minority stereotype (Grossman & Liang, 2008). This stereotype, coupled with the family pressure, might partially explain Suzie's pressure to excel in the classroom. Moreover, Suzie could be subjected to racial microaggressions, which could adversely impact her health (Atkin, Yoo, Jager, & Yeh, 2018; Ong, Burrow, Fuller-Rowell, Ja, & Sue, 2013).

A third potential concern for Suzie is classism. Suzie's mother expressed that they struggle financially to make ends meet. Poverty has a profound impact on one's psychological well-being. As such, clinicians should increase their awareness of the impact class has on one's client, use treatment modalities that address poverty, discuss their physical needs, and serve as an ally as they work toward self-determination (Appio, Chambers, & Mao, 2013).

A fourth concern issue is related to sexism. As noted, in East Asian communities, preferential treatment and greater freedom are rather frequently granted to males (Chung, 2017; Kim & Fong, 2014). As a female, Suzie expressed frustration that her brother is afforded special privileges based on his gender. Suzie appears to be in the revelation stage of Downing and Roush's (1985) Feminist Identity Development Model. Feminist therapy could help her to reconcile some of these injustices (Tummala-Narra & Yang, 2019).

As such, a person could be part of a majority group in one domain, but be a minority in another domain, or have multiple minority statuses (Crenshaw, 2019; Kaplin, 2017). In Suzie's case, it is important for clinicians to consider how her multiply stigmatized minority identities of being an adolescent, Chinese American, female who is part of a lower income community impacts her sense of self (Crenshaw, 2019; Hays, 2016). Yet, the scientific evaluation of how class intersects with gender and race is fairly limited (Block & Corona, 2014; Reimers & Stabb, 2015). In one study, researchers found these factors to have a direct impact on health outcomes (Brown, Richardson, Hargrove, & Thomas, 2016).

## Discussion Questions

1. Which of Marcia's developmental stages are most relevant to understanding Suzie's socioemotional development?
2. How is the concept of identity impacted by individualism and collectivism? How might this influence Suzie's concept of the self?
3. Which identity development models are most relevant for Suzie and her family?
4. What would your treatment priorities be when working with Suzie?
5. Keeping Congress's (2008) culturagram and Hayss' (2016) framework in mind, what sociocultural factors are most salient?
6. How might Suzie's multiple minority status and the concept of intersectionality impact your clinical case conceptualization and treatment plan?

## KEY TERMS

**Acculturative Stress**—psychological stress linked to adaptation to a new culture.

**ADDRESSING**—overlapping, multicultural identity domains of Age, Developmental disabilities, acquired Disabilities, Religion, Ethnicity, Sexual orientation, Socioeconomic status, Indigenous populations, Nationality, and Gender.

**Adultism**—prejudice and accompanying systematic discrimination against young people.

**Ageism**—prejudice or discrimination on the grounds of a person's age.

**Classism**—prejudice against or in favor of people belonging to a particular social class.

**Collectivism**—the practice or principle of giving a group priority over each individual in it.

**Culturagram**—a multidimensional approach to assessing a person and their family's cultural experience.

**Cultural Gap**—any systematic difference between two cultures that hinders mutual understanding or relations.

**Genderism**—a form of prejudice against gender minorities based on the premise that gender is binary.

**Indigenous Population**—originating from or native to a particular place.

**Individualism**—a sociocultural theory favoring freedom of action for individuals over the group.

**Language Broker**—used to describe children of immigrant families "who interpret and translate between culturally and linguistically different people and mediate interactions in a variety of situations" (Tse, 1996).

**Microaggression**—brief, everyday exchanges that send denigrating messages to certain individuals because of their group membership.

**Model Minority Stereotype**—a model minority is a demographic group (often applied to Asian Americans) whose members are perceived to achieve a higher degree of socioeconomic success than the population average.

**Privilege**—a special right, advantage, or immunity granted or available only to a particular person or group.

**Racial/Ethnic Identity Development Models**—a series of theoretical frameworks that were proposed to explain how individuals develop a sense of racial/ethnic identity.

**Racism**—prejudice, discrimination, or antagonism directed against someone of a given group based on their racial or ethnic identity.

**Sexism**—prejudice, stereotyping, or discrimination, often against women, on the basis of sex.

**Undocumented**—lacking documents required for legal immigration.

## REFERENCES

Appio, L., Chambers, D.-A., & Mao, S. (2012). Listening to the voices of the poor and disrupting the silence about class issues in psychotherapy. *Journal of Clinical Psychology*, 69(2), 152–161. doi:10.1002/jclp.21954

Arnett, J. J., & Tanner, J. L. (Eds.). (2006). *Emerging adults in America: Coming of age in the 21st century*. Washington, DC: American Psychological Association.

Atkin, A. L., Yoo, H. C., Jager, J., & Yeh, C. J. (2018). Internalization of the model minority myth, school racial composition, and psychological distress among Asian American adolescents. *Asian American Journal of Psychology*, 9(2), 108–116. doi:10.1037/aap0000096

Barnes, E. F., Williams, J. M., & Barnes, F. R. (2014). Assessing and exploring racial identity development in therapy: Strategies to use with Black consumers. *Journal of Applied Rehabilitation Counseling*, 45(4), 11–17. doi:10.1891/0047-2220.45.1.11

Berry, J. W. (1980). Acculturation as varieties of adaptation. In A. M. Padilla (Ed.), *Acculturation: Theory, models, and some new findings* (pp. 9–25). Boulder, CO: Westview.

Berry, J. W. (1997). Immigration, acculturation, and adaptation. *Applied Psychology: An International Review, 46*(1), 5–34. doi:10.1111/j.1464-0597.1997.tb01087.x

Berry, J. W., Kim, U., Minde, T., & Mok, D. (1987). Comparative studies of acculturative stress. *International Migration Review, 21*(3), 491–511. doi:10.2307/2546607

Block, D., & Corona, V. (2014). Exploring class-based intersectionality. *Language, Culture and Curriculum, 27*(1), 27–42. doi:10.1080/07908318.2014.894053

Brown, T. H., Richardson, L. J., Hargrove, T. W., & Thomas, C. S. (2016). Using multiple-hierarchy stratification and life course approaches to understand health inequalities: The intersecting consequences of race, gender, SES, and age. *Journal of Health & Social Behavior, 57*(2), 200–222. doi:10.1177/0022146516645165

Campos-Holland, A. (2017). Sharpening theory and methodology to explore racialized youth peer cultures. *Sociological Studies of Children & Youth, 22,* 223–247. doi:10.1108/S1537-466120180000022011

Cass, V. C. (1979). Homosexual identity formation: A theoretical model. *Journal of Homosexuality, 4*(3), 219–235. doi:10.1300/j082v04n03_01

Cass, V. C. (1984). Homosexual identity formation: Testing a theoretical model. *Journal of Sex Research, 20*(2), 143–167. doi:10.1080/00224498409551214

Chung, A. Y. (2017). Behind the myth of the matriarch and the flagbearer: How Korean and Chinese American sons and daughters negotiate gender, family, and emotions. *Sociological Forum, 32*(1), 28–49. doi:10.1111/socf.12316

Coleman, E. (1982). Developmental stages of the coming-out process. In W. Paul, J. D. Weinrich, J. C. Gonsiorek, & M. E. Hotvedt (Eds.), *Homosexuality: Social, psychological, and biological issues* (pp. 149–158). Beverly Hills, CA: Sage.

Congress, E. (2008). Using the culturagram with culturally diverse families. In A. Roberts & G. Greene (Eds.), *Social work desk reference* (2nd ed., pp. 57–61). New York, NY: Oxford University Press.

Constantine, M. G., Richardson, T. Q., Benjamin, E. M., & Wilson, J. W. (1998). An overview of Black racial identity theories: Limitations and considerations for future theoretical conceptualizations. *Applied & Preventive Psychology, 7*(2), 95–99. doi:10.1016/S0962-1849(05)80006-X

Crenshaw, K. (2019). *On intersectionality: Essential writings.* New York, NY: The New Press.

Cross, W. E., Jr. (1971). *Shades of Black: Diversity in African-American identity.* Philadelphia, PA: Temple University Press.

Cross, W. E., Jr., & Vandiver, B. J. (2001). Nigrescence theory and measurement: Introducing the Cross Racial Identity Scale (CRIS). In J. G. Ponerotto, J. M. Casas, L. M. Suzuki, & C. M. Alexander (Eds.), *Handbook of multicultural counseling* (2nd ed., pp. 371–393). Thousand Oaks, CA: Sage.

Downing, N. E., & Roush, K. L. (1985). From passive acceptance to active commitment. *The Counseling Psychologist, 13*(4), 695–709. doi:10.1177/0011000085134013

Erchull, M. J., Liss, M., Wilson, K. A., Bateman, L., Peterson, A., & Sanchez, C. E. (2009). The feminist identity development model: Relevant for young women today? *Sex Roles, 60,* 832–842. doi:10.1007/s11199-009-9588-6

Erikson, E. H. (1968). *Identity: Youth and crisis.* New York, NY: Norton.

Gelfand, M. (2018). *Rule makers, rule breakers: Tight and loose cultures and the secret signals that direct our lives.* New York, NY: Scribner.

Gielen, U. P., & Kim, S. (2019). *Global changes in children's lives.* Cambridge, UK: Cambridge University Press.

Grossman, J., & Liang, B. (2008). Discrimination distress among Chinese American adolescents. *Journal of Youth & Adolescence, 37*(1), 1–11. doi:10.1007/s10964-007-9215-1

Hays, P. A. (1996). Addressing the complexities of culture and gender in counseling. *Journal of Counseling & Development, 74*(4), 332–338. doi:10.1002/j.1556-6676.1996.tb01876.x

Hays, P. A. (2016). *Addressing cultural complexities in practice: Assessment, diagnosis, and therapy* (3rd ed.). Washington, DC: American Psychological Association.

Helms, J. E. (1990). *Black and White racial identity: Theory, research, and practice.* New York, NY: Greenwood Press.

Helms, J. E. (1995). An update of Helms' White and People of Color racial identity models. In J. G. Ponterotto, J. M. Casas, L. A. Suzuki, & C. M. Alexander (Eds.), *Handbook of multicultural counseling* (pp. 181–191). Thousand Oaks, CA: Sage.

Ho, J., & Gielen, U. P. (2016). Chinese American adolescents and emerging adults in New York City: Striving for a place in the sun. In U. P. Gielen & J. L. Roopnarine (Eds.), *Childhood and adolescence: Cross-cultural perspectives and applications,* (2nd ed., pp. 347–376). Santa Barbara, CA: Praeger/ABC-CLIO.

Hofstede, G. (2001). *Culture's consequences: Comparing values, behaviors, institutions, and organizations across nations* (2nd ed.). Thousand Oaks, CA: Sage.

Hua, J., & Costigan, C. (2012). The familial context of adolescent language brokering within immigrant Chinese families in Canada. *Journal of Youth & Adolescence, 41*(7), 894–906. doi:10.1007/s10964-011-9682-2

Hyde, J. S. (2002). Feminist identity development. *The Counseling Psychologist, 30*(1), 105–110. doi:10.1177/0011000002301007

Jackson, III., B. W. (2012). Black identity development: Influences of culture and social oppression. In C. L. Wijeyesinghe & B. W. Jackson (Eds.), *New perspectives on racial identity development: Integrating emerging frameworks* (pp. 33–50). New York, NY: New York University Press.

John, B. (2013). Patterns of ageism in different age groups. *Journal of European Psychology Students, 4*(1), 16–36. doi:10.5334/jeps.aw

Kaplin, D. (2017). Microaggressions and macroaggressions in religiously diverse communities. *NYS Psychologist, 29*(3), 16–24.

Kim, J. (1981). Processes of Asian American identity development: A study of Japanese American women's perceptions of their struggle to achieve positive identities as Americans of Asian ancestry. *Dissertation Abstracts International Section A: Humanities and Social Sciences, 42*(4-A), 1551.

Kim, S. W., & Fong, V. L. (2014). A longitudinal study of son and daughter preference among Chinese only-children from adolescence to adulthood. *China Journal, 71,* 1–24. doi:10.1086/674551

Kim-Prieto, C., Kim, G. S., Crane, L. S., Lowe, S. M., Phi Loan Le, & Dinh, K. T. (2018). Legacies of war: Asian American women and war trauma. *Women & Therapy, 41*(3/4), 203–218. doi:10.1080/02703149.2018.1425023

Kodama, C. M., McEwen, M. K., Liang, C. T. H., & Lee, S. (2002). An Asian American perspective on psychosocial development theory. *New Directions for Student Services, 97,* 45–59. doi:10.1002/ss.38

Lin, C.-H., Chiang, P. P., Lux, E. A., & Lin, H.-F. (2018). Immigrant social worker practice: An ecological perspective on strengths and challenges. *Children and Youth Services Review, 87,* 103–113. doi:10.1016/j.childyouth.2018.02.020

Löckenhoff, C. E., De Fruyt, F., Terracciano, A., McCrae, R. R., De Bolle, M., Costa, P. T., . . . Yik, M. (2009). Perceptions of aging across 26 cultures and their culture-level associates. *Psychology and Aging, 24*(4), 941–954. doi:10.1037/a0016901

Lui, P. P. (2015). Intergenerational cultural conflict, mental health, and educational outcomes among Asian and Latino/a Americans: Qualitative and meta-analytic review. *Psychological Bulletin, 141*(2), 404–446. doi:10.1037/a0038449

Marcia, J. E. (1966). Development and validation of ego-identity status. *Journal of Personality and Social Psychology, 3*(5), 551–558. doi:10.1037/h0023281

Marcia, J. E (1980). Identity in adolescence. In J. Adelson (Ed.), *Handbook of adolescent psychology* (pp. 159–187). New York, NY: Wiley.

Markus, H. R., & Kitayama, S. (1994). The cultural construction of self and emotion: Implications for social behavior. In S. Kitayama & H. R. Markus (Eds.), *Emotion and culture: Empirical studies of mutual influence* (pp. 89–130). Washington, DC: American Psychological Association.

Mellor, D., Carne, L., Shen, Y.-C., Mccabe, M., & Wang, L. (2013). Stigma toward mental illness: A cross-cultural comparison of Taiwanese, Chinese immigrants to Australia and Anglo-Australians. *Journal of Cross-Cultural Psychology, 44*(3), 352–364. doi:10.1177/0022022112451052

Miller, A. N., & Fellows, K. L. (2007). Negotiating White racial identity in multicultural courses: A model. In L. M. Cooks & J. S. Simpson (Eds.), *Whiteness, pedagogy, performance: Dis/placing race.* (pp. 49–66). Lanham, MD: Lexington Books/Rowman & Littlefield.

Nosè, M., Ballette, F., Bighelli, I., Turrini, G., Purgato, M., Tol, W., . . . Barbui, C. (2017). Psychosocial interventions for post-traumatic stress disorder in refugees and asylum seekers resettled in high-income countries: Systematic review and meta-analysis. *PLoS ONE, 12*(2), 1–16. doi:10.1371/journal.pone.0171030

Ong, A. D., Burrow, A. L., Fuller-Rowell, T. E., Ja, N. M., & Sue, D. W. (2013). Racial microaggressions and daily well-being among Asian Americans. *Journal of Counseling Psychology, 60*(2), 188–199. doi:10.1037/a0031736.supp

Pollock, L., & Eyre, S. (2012). Growth into manhood: Identity development among female-to-male transgender youth. *Culture, Health & Sexuality, 14*(2), 209–222. doi:10.1080/13691058.2011.636072

Poston, W. S. C. (1990). The Biracial Identity Development Model: A needed addition. *Journal of Counseling & Development, 69*(2), 152–155. doi:10.1002/j.1556-6676.1990.tb01477.x

Raymo, J. M., Park, H., Xie, Y., & Yeung, W. J. (2015). Marriage and family in East Asia: Continuity and change. *Annual Review of Sociology, 41*(1), 471–492. doi:10.1146/annurev-soc-073014-112428

Reimers, F. A., & Stabb, S. D. (2015). Class at the intersection of race and gender: A 15-year content analysis. *The Counseling Psychologist, 43*(6), 794–821. doi:10.1177/0011000015586267

Riemer, H., Shavitt, S., Koo, M., & Markus, H. R. (2014). Preferences don't have to be personal: Expanding attitude theorizing with a cross-cultural perspective. *Psychological Review, 121*(4), 619–648. doi:10.1037/a0037666

Rousseau, C., & Drapeau, A. (2004). Premigration exposure to political violence among independent immigrants and its association with emotional distress. *Journal of Nervous and Mental Disease, 192*(12), 852–856. doi:10.1097/01.nmd.0000146740.66351.23

Rowe, W., Bennett, S., & Atkinson, D. R. (1994). White racial identity models: A critique and alternative proposal. *The Counseling Psychologist, 22*(1), 120–146. doi:10.1177/0011000094221009

Ruiz, A. S. (1990). Ethnic identity: Crisis and resolution. *Journal of Multicultural Counseling & Development, 18*(1), 29–40. doi:10.1002/j.2161-1912.1990.tb00434.x

Shen, Y., Kim, S. Y., & Benner, A. D. (2019). Burdened or efficacious? Subgroups of Chinese American language brokers, predictors, and long-term outcomes. *Journal of Youth & Adolescence, 48*(1), 154–169. doi:10.1007/s10964-018-0916-4

Stewart, M., Anderson, J., Beiser, M., Mwakarimba, E., Neufeld, A., Simich, L., & Spitzer, D. (2008). Multicultural meanings of social support among immigrants and refugees. *International Migration, 46*(3), 123–159. doi:10.1111/j.1468-2435.2008.00464.x

Suthakaran, V. (2012). Integrating Helms's White Racial Identity Development Model with Cognitive-Experiential Self-Theory: Implications for multicultural education. *Multicultural Learning and Teaching, 7*(2). doi:10.1515/2161-2412.1095

Triandis, H. C. (2001). Individualism-collectivism and personality. *Journal of Personality, 69*(6), 907–924. doi:10.1111/1467-6494.696169

Triandis, H. C., & Suh, E. M. (2002). Cultural influences on personality. *Annual Review of Psychology, 53*(1), 133–160. doi:10.1146/annurev.psych.53.100901.135200

Troiden, R. R. (1979). Becoming homosexual: A model of gay identity acquisition. *Psychiatry: Journal for the Study of Interpersonal Processes, 42*(4), 362–373. doi:10.1080/00332747.1979.11024039

Tse, L. (1996). Language brokering in linguistic minority communities: The case of Chinese- and Vietnamese-American students. *Bilingual Research Journal, 20*(3–4), 485–498. doi:10.1080/15235882.1996.10668640

Tummala-Narra, P. (2020). The fear of immigrants. *Psychoanalytic Psychology, 37*(1), 50–61. doi:10.1037/pap0000245

Tummala-Narra, P., & Yang, E. J. (2019). Asian American adolescent girls: Navigating stress across multiple contexts. In T. Bryant-Davis (Ed.), *Multicultural feminist therapy: Helping adolescent girls of color to thrive* (pp. 113–153). Washington, DC: American Psychological Association. doi:10.1037/0000140-005

Westman, J. C. (1991). Juvenile ageism: Unrecognized prejudice and discrimination against the young. *Child Psychiatry and Human Development, 21*(4), 237–256. doi:10.1007/BF00705929

Yoon, E., Adams, K., Clawson, A., Chang, H., Surya, S., & Jérémie-Brink, G. (2017). East Asian adolescents' ethnic identity development and cultural integration: A qualitative investigation. *Journal of Counseling Psychology, 64*(1), 65–79. doi:10.1037/cou0000181

# 10

# Working With Culturally Diverse Older Adults

*Janna Heyman and Linda White-Ryan*

## INTRODUCTION

The growth of the older adult population in the United States has received increasing attention over recent years. With the anticipated increase in the aging population, the United State Census Bureau has described the 2030s as a "transformative decade" (U.S. Census Bureau, 2018). These changes are due to an anticipated decrease in the number of births, while the population will continue to age and become more racially and ethnically diverse. Roberts, Ogunwole, Blakeslee, and Rabe (2018) indicated that by 2030, "about 1 billion (12% of the projected total world population) and by 2050, 1.6 billion (17%) of the total population of 9.4 billion will be 65 and older" (p. 1). As the population changes, there needs to be a focus on the growing diversity of older adults. In 2019, the U.S. Census Bureau estimated that the 65 and older population represented 15.6% of the population. Roberts et al. (2018) provide the most recent data by age and race based on the U.S. Census Bureau definition. They reported that for older adults, 65 and over, 8% were Hispanic or Latino and 92% were Not Hispanic or Latino, with the following breakdown: White (77.3%), Blacks/African American (8.9%); Asian (4.2%), American Indian and Alaska Native (0.5%), Native Hawaiian and other Pacific Islander (0.1%), other races (0.1%), and 0.9% representing two or more races (Roberts et al., 2018).

While life expectancy in the United States is estimated at 78.6 years at birth (Xu, Murphy, Kochanek, Bastian, & Arias, 2018), it can also differ by race and ethnic group (Arias, 2016), educational attainment (Laditka & Laditka, 2015), income (Chetty et al., 2016), and other factors. The age-adjusted death rate was 724.6 per 100,000 (National Vital Statistics, 2016); however, racial and ethnic disparities need to be recognized (National Center for Health Statistics, 2016). For example, the age-adjusted death rate was 1.2 times greater for the non-Hispanic Black population than for the non-Hispanic White population (National Vital

Statistics, 2016). In addition to racial and ethnic disparities, health disparities may also be related to education, gender, place of residence, and sexual orientation (Adler et al., 2016).

It is critical to understand that it is not race or other factors that describe an individual but the lived experiences and multidimensional factors and dynamics that may shape peoples' lives (Crenshaw, 1991). This chapter highlights the importance of understanding different multicultural experiences and the challenges in addressing the needs and concerns of a diverse older population. The experiences of all people vary. Immigrants and refugees from around the world bring rich and vastly different cultural heritages. Differences within diverse populations should also be recognized. For example, while Hispanic older adults may share a common language, they come from many countries of origin and represent a diverse population. Furthermore, it is important to remember that race, ethnicity, language, and other cultural differences do not define an individual. The need to understand and respect different cultures and experiences of the older adults and their families should be in the forefront.

## INTERSECTIONALITY

Kimberlé Williams Crenshaw's work (1991) addressed the importance of intersectionality in this groundbreaking work which underscores that human lives and experiences cannot be described by categories (e.g., gender, race), but that individuals lives are multidimensional and shaped by different factors and dynamics. McCall (2005) suggested that "intersectionality is the most important theoretical contribution that women's studies, in conjunction with related fields, has made thus far" (p. 1771). Intersectionality has been tied to the principles of social work (Murphy, Hunt, Zajicek, & Hamilton, 2009) using the person-in-environment framework. The authors state that the "intersectional perspective acknowledges the breadth of human experiences, instead of conceptualizing social relations and identities separately in terms of either race *or* class *or* gender *or* age *or* sexual orientation" (Murphy et al., 2009, p. 5). It provides a lens that captures the complexity of different interrelated systems. Intersectionality can also help address social and health and other inequality and promote social justice (Hankivsky, 2014; Simien, 2007). For work with older adults and their families, this perspective is pivotal for shaping future direction in practice, policy, and research.

## SOCIAL DETERMINANTS OF HEALTH

Also, understanding social determinants of health can provide further insights into working with older adults and their families using multicultural practice. Social determinants of health are

> the circumstances in which people are born, grow up, live, work and age, and the systems put in place to deal with illness. These circumstances are in turn shaped by a wider set of forces: economics, social policies, and politics. (World Health Organization, 2017, p. 1)

Social determinants of health include health and healthcare, economics, education, social and community contexts, and neighborhood and environment (Office of Disease Prevention and Health Promotion, 2017). According to Heyman, Kelly, Reback, and Blumenstock (2018), it is important to understand social determinants of health when addressing diversity and differences among population groups.

## Health and Healthcare

Health and healthcare are two of the most common issues linked to aging, and this may vary for different groups and cultures. For many individuals, access to healthcare presents a challenge. The enactment of the 2010 Patient Protection and Affordable Care Act (ACA), is "the most important health care legislation enacted in the United States since the creation of Medicaid and Medicare in 1965" (Obama, 2016, p. 525). The ACA has helped many individuals access healthcare who previously had to wait until they became Medicare eligible. It may be years until we can fully understand how the enactment of the ACA may impact overall health, but it may have helped in preventing and addressing the outcomes for the future older population.

For older adults, chronic illness and disabilities are significant. The proportion of the older population with some disability increases with age. For example, for older adults 85 and older, 48% have serious difficulty walking or climbing stairs, and the percentage of people with a disability related to independent living has also increased (Roberts et al., 2018). Older persons have also reported significant difficulties with hearing, with 9.2% of 65- to 74-year olds, 17.4% of 75- to 84-year olds, and 34.6% of 85 and older persons indicating hearing as a problem (Roberts et al., 2018). A study by Pratt et al. (2009) found that that self-reported hearing loss differed by race, gender, and age. Being White and being male were related to higher loss.

These losses may be significant. For example, if older adults have hearing loss, they may feel unable to engage with family or friends in conversations. In addition, older adults with chronic health issues may have more difficulties socializing with family and friends. It can impair their ability to participate in social activities, possibly leading to a sense of isolation. If an older adult finds that they are no longer able to drive a car, this can cause some older adults to feel more dependent. Interestingly, Schryer, Boerner, Horowitz, Reinhardt, and Mock (2017) found that "driving cessation was associated with a decline in life satisfaction among social partners but not for the drivers" (p. 975).

Loss of memory can be significant for some older adults. It is estimated that 5 million Americans have Alzheimer's disease, an irreversible, progressive brain disorder that affects memory and thinking skills. Alzheimer's is also the most common cause of dementia among older adults (National Institute on Aging, 2019). Data from the Alzheimer's Association indicate that African Americans are about two times more likely to have Alzheimer's disease, and Hispanics are about one and a half times more likely to have the disease than non-Hispanic Whites (Alzheimer's Association, 2016). Stigma associated with the disease and its progression often deters individuals and their families from openly discussing the disease. Older adults and their families may be ashamed to discuss it with professionals and their support system, so seeking treatment is often delayed (Heyman, White-Ryan, & Kelly, 2018).

Depression and other mental health issues can also be stigmatizing for older adults and their families (U.S. Surgeon General, 2019). Depression is not a normal part of aging, but it is treatable when people are accurately assessed and diagnosed. Kok and Reynolds (2017) found that "older adults with depression more commonly have several concurrent medical disorders and cognitive impairment" (p. 2114). Also, individuals with depressive symptoms have greater disability and are often high users of healthcare resources (Federal Interagency Forum on Aging-Related Statistics, 2010) and experience other difficulties such as loneliness (Adams & Moon, 2009). Research on the link between race and depression among older adults is mixed. Hooker et al. (2018) found that while 10.2% of older adults age 65 or older screened at risk for depression, they found that depression was higher for persons who identified as Mexican, Puerto Rican, Cuban, or another Hispanic/Latino, when compared with non-Hispanic Whites. Also Hooker et al. (2018) found that Blacks/African Americans, Asians, Filipinos, Native Hawaiians/Pacific Islanders, or those of two or more races were also higher than non-Hispanic Whites, and state, "These disparities should inform distribution of health care resources; efforts to educate and ameliorate depression should be culturally targeted" (p. 1).

Substance abuse is also important when addressing health and healthcare for older adults and their families. Between 1988 and 2010, "the median number of prescription medications used among adults aged 65 and older doubled from 2 to 4, and the proportion taking ≥5 medications tripled from 12.8%" (Charlesworth, Smit, Lee, Alramedham, & Odeden, 2015, p. 989). White-Ryan (2018) highlights that sometimes older adults also may not realize the risks associated with alcohol and medication use, and this may increase risks of falls and other serious health issues. "The older adult cohort presents unique challenges for health care professionals regarding the stigma of substance abuse and such a nonjudgmental and nonconfrontational approach can be effective" (p.132).

Understanding the different individual experiences and cultural context can significantly impact practice with older adults and their families. Future healthcare policies need to be shaped by using an intersectionality perspective.

## Economics

Due to the numerous changes in our nation's economy, many older adults are not traditional retirees, choosing phased retirement or returning to work (Raymo, Warren, Sweeney, Hauser, & Ho, 2010). According to Roberts et al. (2018),

> for the total population aged 16 and over, 68% of males and 58% of females participated in the labor force. Comparatively, for the population 65 and older, 22% of men and 14% of women were in the labor force. (p. 16)

There are many older adults who work because of their financial need, personal desire, or other reasons.

Approximately 9.2% of older adults live in poverty, and more than 15 million older adults had incomes below 200% of poverty, representing 30.1% (Cubanski,

Koma, Damico, & Neuman, 2018). These data are based on the official measure in 2017, which was $11,756 for an individual age 65 or older. The Social Security Administration (2016) reported that 61% of older adult beneficiaries receive at least half their income from Social Security and that the 2.1 million older adults on Supplemental Security Income (SSI) receive, on average, just $435 each month (Social Security Administration, 2016). These data underscore the importance of financial challenges and the difficult struggle many older adults have to maintain their housing, healthcare, food, and access to transportation (National Council on Aging, 2019).

The challenge of economic need may vary for the different groups. In a recent study by the Kaiser Foundation, the poverty rate is significantly higher for Black and Hispanic adults over the age of 65. For example, more than 60% of older Black and Hispanic women have incomes below 200% of the poverty level compared to 41.4% of older White women (Cubanski et al., 2018, p. 6). Another study by Dumez and Derbrew (2011) similarly found 45% of older persons age 65+ fall into an economic insecurity gap. This gap varies by race/ethnic group, with 76% of Latinos, 69% of African Americans, and 67% of Asian Americans disadvantaged economically (Dumez & Derbrew, 2011). According to Dumez and Derbrew (2011), many older persons do not have enough money to meet basic needs but may not qualify for many public programs because of eligibility criteria.

For older adults, one of the primary barriers to accessing healthcare is financial. Although Medicare is the primary source of coverage for older persons, a significant amount of healthcare is not covered under Medicare. Older adults often pay out of pocket for these costs. The burden of out-of-pocket healthcare expense is high for older adults (Desmond, Rice, Cubanski, & Newman, 2007; Richard, Walker, & Alexandre, 2018).

## Education

McGill (2016) states, "Education is not just about what is learned in the classroom; it is also about the doors it unlocks to future well-being" (p. 1). The educational level of the older adult is increasing. According to McGill,

> the percentage who had completed high school varied considerably by race and ethnic origin in 2016: 90% of Whites (not Hispanic), 80% of Asians (not Hispanic), 77% of African Americans (not Hispanic), 71% of American Indians/Alaska Natives (not Hispanic), and 54% of Hispanics. The increase in educational levels is also evident within these groups. (p. 11)

Education can also help to inform health and health choices as an older adult ages. Education can be pivotal to helping older adults understand important health and healthcare information. For many diverse older adults, material that is sensitive to language and cultures can enrich their lives and experiences. Often having material available in different languages can help improve older adults' understanding about different healthcare issues and provide important information so they can make informed decisions. Sometimes jargon and terminology are used by professionals. Being sensitive about the way information is provided to older adults and their families is critical. Older adults who do not speak English may rely on a family member or friend to translate the information. This may put the family member/friend in a difficult position. Berkman, Stein, and Glajchen (2018) explain that it is important to check "the patient's understanding of what has been communicated, is especially critical when there is a cultural or language difference" (p. 155).

## Social Connections, Families, and Neighborhoods

Social connections matter. For older adults, families and friends are critical to their lives. Neighborhoods can provide an important sense of community and support for many older adults, a community and culture that have been part of their lives. Yet, as mentioned earlier, many older adults may experience losses of family and friends due to death, moves, or other factors. They may have to leave the homes, communities, and neighborhoods in which they have lived for years. These changes can represent another layer of loss. There may be a sense of loss due to changes in role status. At one point, the grandparent may be the caregiver for their grandchildren and families; however, due to illness, an older adult's role may change. For all cultures, families need to be supported. The Family and Medical Leave Act (FMLA) of 1993 enables workers to take up to 12 weeks of unpaid leave to care for a seriously ill family member, for one's own serious health condition, orthe care of a new child (U.S. Department of Labor, n.d.). The National Family Caregiver Support Program, which is under Title III-E of the Older Americans Act, is a federal program that provides services to families who care for frail older relatives, as well as grandparents and other relatives age 55 and over who are raising children. However, more needs to be done to assist family members who provide care for older adults.

Connections to families, friends, and neighborhoods are paramount. The National Institute on Aging (2019) highlights the value of Dr. Cacippo's research, noting, "Social isolation is the objective physical separation from other people (living alone), while loneliness is the subjective distressed feeling of being alone or separated" (p. 1). The Institute summarizes how important social isolation and loneliness are to health risks. Some protective factors, such as fostering connections through programs, services, and other outreach initiatives, have been recognized. Intergenerational programs can be effective (Canedo-Garcia, Garcia-Sánchez, & Pancheco-Sanz, 2017) and build connections and community. Heyman, Gutheil, and White-Ryan (2011) found that intergenerational programming can positively impact perceptions of older adults by young children, which may help to shape the future attitudes toward aging. As policies develop toward creating livable communities for all generations, it is important to take into consideration how connections impact society, cultures, and communities in which we live.

## MULTICULTURAL PRACTICE

Multicultural practice emphasizes the importance of working with diverse populations and addressing the concerns specific to their individual needs and concerns. For example, for social workers, the Council on Social Work

Education Educational Policy and Accreditation Standards (EPAS) competencies highlight the importance of engaging on diversity and differences in practice. This includes understanding the importance around culture and cultural differences as a key aspect of the human experience. For all helping professionals, it is critical to understand that culture can affect assessment of clients presenting concerns, perception of strengths and weaknesses, and development of interventions. This includes developing awareness and knowledge of the cultural experiences of others and strengthening skills at developing working relationships with those of differing cultural backgrounds. Equally important, professionals must examine their own values, cultural backgrounds, and life experiences, and assess the impact of these factors on their own view. Professionals should consider their own experiences with persons from other cultures and be aware of how this impacts their work. It is beneficial for professionals to be aware of their own possible biases in order to confront and address them. Self-awareness is essential for the helping professionals to be effective in practice.

As each individual may have different cultural backgrounds and experiences, it is important to avoid making assumptions that all persons from a diverse group experience the world in the same way or hold the same values. Professionals need to understand the rights to self-determination and respect a person's choice. An important skill is being able to be an active listener and open to all lines of communication. The engagement skills of professionals contribute to developing a trusting relationship. It is critical that professionals have cultural humility and respect. Culture has been defined as

> the way of life of a society and life patterns related to conduct or ways of behavior, beliefs, traditions, values, art, skills, and social relationships. Culture perpetuates the sharing of ideas, attitudes, values, and beliefs among individuals of that culture. (Lum, 2007, p. 54)

Cultural competency is defined as the process that promotes effective interactions with individuals of all cultures based on curiosity and respect about differences related to language, class, ethnicity (race), and religion. This perspective affirms the dignity of individuals, families, and communities and informs practice with individuals, families, groups, communities, and organizations in roles that include direct service providers, administrators, and change agents. Cultural humility was a term used by Tervalon and Murray-Garcia (1998) to focus on lifelong learning and self-reflection. Hook, Davis, Owen, Worthington, and Utsey (2013) discuss the importance of cultural humility and the process of other-oriented self-awareness and openness when working with culturally diverse clients.

Respect is a critical component of a therapeutic relationship. It is important to demonstrate respect by listening and adapting to individual sensory or cognitive limitations. The way a professional engages and works with an older adult may strongly influence the development of the relationship with both the older person and their family. Respecting differences in treatment options, use of interpreters, and communication strategies are important when working with culturally diverse populations (Yeo & Yoshikawa, 2019).

## Screening and Assessment

For different cultures, fear of stigma and other issues can impact treatment (O'Connor et al., 2010; U.S. Surgeon General, 2019). Yet, screening and assessment are critical in providing information that can result in appropriate referrals for an older person. Engaging older adults and their families is important to start the dialogue about the importance of screening and assessment. A complete assessment should include an understanding of biological, psychological, social, cultural, and spiritual factors, as well as information regarding their family and support system. Special attention must be paid to environmental factors because, in the face of changing or declining abilities, older persons are often profoundly impacted by their physical environments. Social workers play a critical role in assessment.

As part of the assessment, it is important to understand the support from family and friends. Jeong, Shin, Park, and Park (2019) examined Korean family caregivers' roles in a family-oriented culture when older adults were being treated for cancer. They found that multiple family caregivers played significant roles. They also found that the "older the patients were, the heavier reliance was on the adult children, including sons, daughters and daughters-in-law" (Jeong et al., 2019, p. 141). While families are understood to be the primary source of care for older adults, it is important to recognize that caregiving and support are not one directional. Often, it is the older adult who is providing care for younger family members. The most striking example of this phenomenon is grandparents raising grandchildren. Caregiving differs across diverse population groups (Chen, Mair, Bao, & Yang, 2015).

Assessment of older adults and their family caregivers must always include an understanding of the strengths that can be drawn upon. Older adults, dealing with the numerous challenges and losses of later life, are continuing lifelong patterns of coping and adaptation. Assessment and diagnosis leading to effective interventions and treatment are critical to positive outcomes.

Cultural issues are critical but often overlooked in assessment. Clarke and Smith (2011) underscore the importance of the cultural context in fostering psychological resources, a key factor in well-being. Accurate assessment must take into account the client's cultural values. Cultural values may also determine how health concerns are understood and how symptoms are interpreted. Berkman, Maramaldi, Breon, and Howe (2002) as well as Hooyman, Kawamoto, and Kiyak (2017) note that culturally sensitive assessment protocols are needed.

## Treatment

Access to services is a primary issue for older persons (Min, 2005). Higher service needs do not translate into greater service use. Although there are mixed findings regarding utilization of services by older persons of color, there is general concern that the service needs of these individuals are not being adequately met.

Hooyman et al. (2017) enumerate a range of barriers to service utilization. They divide these barriers into: (a) cultural and economic barriers, and (b) structural barriers in the service system. Among the cultural barriers are language differences, perceived stigma associated with service use, fear or lack of trust in care providers, and lack of knowledge.

Berkman et al. (2018), in their work with palliative care, state

> Diversity of cultures throughout the United States and globally demands awareness of differences in perceptions and preferences related to serious illness and its treatment. While it is not possible to become culturally competent in all the cultural groups encountered, aiming to be culturally sensitive, open-minded, and respectful of other cultures will result in more appropriate care. (p. 154)

It is effective to offer services in ways that are consonant with the cultures of diverse older adults. Professionals need to have the knowledge and skills necessary to engage, empower, and connect older adults to services that address their needs. Pardasani and Allen (2018) state, "Skills include working to understand diversity and tradition and the unique ways individuals, families, groups, and communities experience lifelong patterns of being, shaped by such forces as oppression for some people and privilege for some others" (p. 216).

The choice of treatment approach is based on the needs, capacity, and values of the older person and his or her family. Understanding of and respect for the lived experiences and wishes of the older adult is critical. The broader cultural context of the individual and the family must be considered. The professional needs to have cultural humility and be aware of a range of resources in order to provide the service and care most appropriate to the older person's cultural background.

## CASE VIGNETTE

Ms. C is an 88-year-old widow who lost her husband 2 years ago. Prior to moving to the United States in 2000 she lived in the Dominican Republic. She relied on her husband to help with their single family house in which she lives. Her husband used to take care of the finances and household expenses. Ms. C's primary language is Spanish, and she often relies on a neighbor to help translate when she goes to her physicians' offices. She has a daughter who lives in another state, and it is often hard for her daughter to help because of her daughter's own caregiver responsibilities. Ms. C lives alone and has been struggling with her health. She has chronic obstructive pulmonary disease (COPD), has difficulty going up and down her stairs, and is hard of hearing. She discusses her faith and culture as being extremely important to her. Recently, Ms. C has reported feelings of being depressed and being alone. She talks about difficulties with sleeping and is worried about what will happen to her in the future.

This case involves physical, social, spiritual, and mental health issues. An accurate assessment needs to be completed and appropriate services discussed with Ms. C. In working with older adults, helping professionals need to understand that older adults from diverse culture may have difficulties seeking mental health services. For some older persons, seeking mental health services would stigmatize the family. There may be issues involved in accepting other kinds of services as well. In the case of Ms. C, there was no family nearby. Her daughter is hesitant to become involved because she has so many challenges in her own life. With respect to Ms. C's living environment, there may be difficult challenges and a need to reassess priorities.

As mentioned, screening and assessment are important. While the professional may quickly be able to identify the "best" treatment approach for Ms. C, she and her family may have very different ideas of what they are willing to accept. Being an active listener and open to hearing about Ms. C's concerns is important. Professionals must listen to direct and indirect communications. There is a need to recognize cultural differences. Flexibility and a range of options may be necessary. In order to develop a treatment plan that meets the needs of Ms. C, professionals should collaborate with Ms. C and her family to discuss a plan that she feels works best for her.

## CONCLUSION

As helping professionals, it is important to recognize the rights of the older person, respect self-determination, and understand the strengths of the individual. An intersectional perspective recognizes the extent and breadth of human experiences. It is critical for professionals to understand the ways older adults and their families experience and cope with age-related changes. Professionals should understand that older adults' lives are multidimensional and may be shaped differently. Cultures and a range of other factors may influence the ways help is defined, whether help is sought outside the family, and how offers of help will be received. Incorporating a multidimensional lens in practice with older adults may have a significant impact on the lives and well-being of older adults and their families.

### Discussion Questions

1. Using the intersectionality lens, what are the important considerations that professionals should incorporate when working with older adults?
2. How can culture be incorporated in screening and assessment in multicultural practice?
3. What are the critical skills that professionals should use when working with older adults and their families?

## REFERENCES

Adams, K. B., & Moon, H. (2009). Subthreshold depression: Characteristics and risk factors among vulnerable elders. *Aging & Mental Health, 13*(5), 682–692.

Adler, N., Cutler, D., Fielding, J., Galea, S., Glymour, M., Koh, H., & Satcher, D. (2016). *Addressing social determinants of health and health disparities.* Discussion Paper, Vital Directions for Health and Health Care Series. National Academy of Medicine, Washington, DC. Retrieved from https://nam.edu/wp-content/uploads/2016/09/Addressing-Social-Determinants-of-Health-and-Health-Disparities.pdf

Alzheimer's Association. (2016). *Race, Ethnicity, and Alzheimer's Disease.* Retrieved from https://www.alz.org/media/greatermissouri/2015_Race_and_Ethnicity_Fact_Sheet (1).pdf

Arias, E. (2016). *Changes in life expectancy by race and Hispanic origin in the United States, 2013–2014.* NCHS Data Brief 244. Hyattsville, MD: National Center for Health Statistics.

Berkman, B., Maramaldi, P., Breon, E. A., & Howe, J. L. (2002). Social work gerontological assessment revisited. *Journal of Gerontological Social Work, 40*(1/2), 1–14. doi:10.1300/J083v40n01_01

Berkman, C., Stein, G. L., & Glajchen, M. (2018). Palliative and end-of- life care: Social determinants of health. In J. C. Heyman & E. P. Congress (Eds.), *Health and Social Work: Practice, Policy, and Research* (pp. 145–168). New York, NY: Springer Publishing Company.

Canedo-Garcia, A., Garcia-Sánchez, J., & Pancheco-Sanz, D. (2017). A systematic review of the effectiveness of intergenerational programs. *Frontiers in Psychology, 8*, 1882. doi:10.3389/fpsyg.2017.01882

Charlesworth, C. J., Smit, E., Lee, D. S. H., Alramadhan, F., & Odden, M. C. (2015). Polypharmacy among adults aged 65 years and older in the United States. *Journal of Gerontology Series A: Biology Science and Medical Science, 70*(8), 989–995. doi:10.1093/gerona/glv013

Chen, F., Mair, C. A., Bao, L., & Yang, Y. C. (2015). Race/ethnic differentials in the health consequences of caring for grandchildren for grandparents. *Journal of Gerontological: Series B. Psychological Sciences and Social Sciences, 70*(5), 793–803. doi:10.1093/geronb/gbu160

Chetty, R., Stepner, M., Abraham, S., Lin, S., Scuderi, B., Turner, N., . . . Cutler, D. (2016). The association between income and life expectancy in the United States, 2001-2004. *Journal of the American Medical Association, 315*(16), 1750–1766. doi:10.1001/jama.2016.4226

Clarke, P., & Smith, J. (2011). Aging in a cultural context: Cross-national differences in disability and the moderating role of personal control among older adults in the United States and England. *The Journals of Gerontology Series B: Psychological Sciences and Social Sciences, 66B*(4), 457–467. doi:10.1093/geronb/gbr054

Crenshaw, K. (1991). Mapping the margins: Intersectionality, identity politics, and violence against women of color. In M. A. Finemane, & R. Mykitiuk (Eds.), *The public nature of private violence* (pp. 93–118). New York, NY: Routledge.

Cubanski, J., Koma, W., Damico, A., & Neuman, T. (2018). *How many seniors live in poverty?* San Francisco, CA: The Henry J. Kaiser Family Foundation. Retrieved from https://www.kff.org/medicare/issue-brief/how-many-seniors-live-in-poverty

Desmond, K. A., Rice, T., Cubanski, J., & Newman, P. (2007). *The burden of out-of-pocket health spending among older versus younger adults: Analysis from the Consumer Expenditure Survey, 1998-2003.* Menlo Park, CA: The Henry J. Kaiser Family Foundation.

Dumez, J., & Derbrew, H. (2011). *The economic crisis facing seniors of color: Background and policy recommendations.* Berkeley, CA: The Greenlining Institute.

Federal Interagency Forum on Aging-Related Statistics. (2010). *Older Americans 2010: Key indicators of well-being.* Retrieved from https://bookstore.gpo.gov/agency/federal-interagency-forum-aging-related-statistics

Hankivsky, O. (2014). *Intersectionality 101.* Retrieved from http://vawforum-cwr.ca/sites/default/files/attachments/intersectionallity_101.pdf

Heyman, J. C., Gutheil, I. A., & White-Ryan, L. (2011). Preschool children's attitudes toward older adults: Comparison of intergenerational and traditional day care. *Journal of Intergenerational Relationships, 9*, 435–444. doi:10.1080/15350770.2011.618381

Heyman, J. C., Kelly, P., Reback, G., & Blumenstock, K. (2018). Social determinants of health. In J. C. Heyman & E. P. Congress (Eds.), *Health and Social Work: Practice, Policy and Research* (pp. 37–50). New York, NY: Springer Publishing Company.

Heyman, J. C., White-Ryan, L., & Kelly, P. (2018). *Impact of Alzheimer's disease awareness initiative.* West Harrison, NY: Author.

Hook, J. N., Davis, D. E., Owen, J., Worthington, E. L., Jr., & Utsey, S. O. (2013). Cultural humility: Measuring openness to culturally diverse clients. *Journal of Counseling Psychology, 60*(3), 353–366. doi:10.1037/a0032595

Hooker, K., Phibbs, S., Irvin, V. L., Mendez-Luck, C. A., Doan, L. N., Li, T., . . . Choun, S. (2018). Depression among older adults in the United States by disaggregated race and ethnicity. *The Gerontologist, 59*(5), 886–891. doi:10.1093/geront/gny159

Hooyman, N. A., Kawamoto, K. Y., & Kiyak, H. A. (2017). *Social gerontology: A multidisciplinary perspective.* (10th ed.). Boston, MA: Allyn & Bacon.

Jeong, A., Shin, D., Park, J. H., & Park, K. (2019). What we talk about when we talk about caregiving: The distribution of roles in cancer patient caregiving in a family-oriented culture. *Cancer Research & Treatment, 51*(1), 141–149. doi:10.4143/crt.2017.557

Kok, R. M., & Reynolds, C. F. (2017). Management of depression in older adults: A review. *Journal of the American Medical Association, 317*(202), 2114–2122. doi:10.1001/jama.2017.5706

Laditka, J., & Laditka, S. (2015). Associations of educational attainment with disability and life expectancy by race and gender in the United States: A longitudinal analysis of the Panel Study of Income Dynamics. *Journal of Aging and Health, 28*(8), 1403–1425. doi:10.1177/0898264315620590

Lum, D. (2007). *Culturally competent practice: A framework for understanding diverse groups and justice issues.* Belmont, CA: Thomson Books/Cole.

McCall, L. (2005). The complexity of intersectionality. *Signs. 30*(3), 1771–1800. doi:10.1086/426800

McGill, N. (2016). Education attainment linked to health throughout lifespan: Exploring social determinants of health. *The Nation's Health, 46*(6), 1–19.

Min, J. W. (2005). Cultural competency: A key to effective social work with racially and ethnically diverse elders. *Families in Society, 86,* 347–358. doi:10.1606/1044-3894.3432

Murphy, Y., Hunt, V., Zajicek, A. M., & Hamilton, L. (2009). *Incorporating intersectionality in social work practice, research, policy, and education.* Washington, DC: NASW Press.

National Center for Health Statistics. (2016). *Health, United States, 2015: With special feature on racial and ethnic health disparities.* Hyattsville, MD.

National Council on Aging. (2019). *Economic security.* Retrieved from https://www.ncoa.org/news/resources-for-reporters/get-the-facts/economic-security-facts

National Institute on Aging. (2019). *Alzheimer's disease fact sheet.* Retrieved from https://www.nia.nih.gov/health/alzheimers-disease-fact-sheet

National Vital Statistics. (2016). *Death: Final data for 2014.* Retrieved from https://www.cdc.gov/nchs/nvss/deaths.htm

Obama, B. (2016). United States health care reform: Progress to date and next steps. *Journal of the American Medical Association, 316*(5), 525–532. doi:10.1001/jama.2016.9797

O'Connor, K., Copeland, V. C., Grote, N. K., Koeske, G., Rosen, D., Reynolds, C. F., & Brown, C. (2010). Mental health seeking treatment among older adults with depression: The impact of stigma and race. *American Journal of Geriatric Psychiatry, 18*(6), 531–543. doi:10.1097/JGP.0b013e3181cc0366

Office of Disease Prevention and Health Promotion. (2017). *Social determinants of health.* Retrieved from https://www.healthypeople.gov/2020/topics-objectives/topic/social-determinants-of-health

Pardasani, M. P., & Allen, L. (2018). Health care and work with older adults and their caregivers. In J. C. Heyman & E. P. Congress (Eds.), *Health and Social Work: Practice, Policy, and Research* (pp. 213–233). New York, NY: Springer Publishing Company.

Pratt, S. R., Kuller, L., Talbott, E., McHugh-Pemu, K., Buhare, A., & Xu, X. (2009). Prevalence of hearing loss in Black and White elders: Results of the Cardiovascular Health Study. *Journal of Speech, Language and Hearing Research, 52,* 973–989. doi:10.1044/1092-4388(2009/08-0026)

Raymo, J. M., Warren, J. R., Sweeney, M. M., Hauser, R. M., & Ho, J. H. (2010). Later-life employment preferences and outcomes: The role of mid-life work experiences. *Research on Aging, 32,* 419–466. doi:10.1177/0164027510361462

Richard, P., Walker, R., & Alexandre, P. (2018). The burden of out of pocket costs and medical debt faced by households with chronic health conditions in the United States. *PLoS One, 13*(6), e0199598. doi:10.1371/journal.pone.0199598

Roberts, A. W., Ogunwole, S. U., Blakeslee, L., & Rabe, M. A. (2018). *"The Population 65 Years and Older in the United States: 2016,"* American Community Survey Reports, ACS-38, U.S. Census Bureau. Washington, DC. Retrieved from https://www.census.gov/content/dam/Census/library/publications/2018/acs/ACS-38.pdf

Schryer, E., Boerner, K., Horowitz, A., Reinhardt, J. P., & Mock, S. E. (2017). The social context of driving cessation: Understanding the effects of cessation on the life satisfaction of older drivers and their social partners. *Journal of Applied Gerontology, 32*, 975–996.

Simien, E. (2007). Doing intersectionality research: From conceptual issues to practical Examples. *Politics & Gender, 3*(2), 36–43. doi:10.1017/S1743923X07000086

Social Security Administration. (2016). *Facts and figures.* Retrieved from https://www.ssa.gov/policy/docs/chartbooks/fast_facts/2016/fast_facts16.html

Tervalon, M., & Murray-García, J. (1998). Cultural humility versus cultural competence: A critical distinction in defining physician training outcomes in multicultural education. Journal of Health Care for the Poor and Underserved, 9(2), 117–125. doi:10.1353/hpu.2010.0233

U.S. Census Bureau. (2018). *Older people to outnumber children. (CB18-41).* Retrieved from https://www.census.gov/newsroom/press-releases/2018/cb18-41-population-projections.html

U.S. Census Bureau. (2019). *U.S. Census Bureau quick facts.* Retrieved from https://www.census.gov/quickfacts/fact/table/US/PST045218

U.S. Department of Labor. (n.d.). *Family and Medical Leave Act.* Retrieved from https://www.dol.gov/whd/fmla

U.S. Surgeon General. (2019). *Mental health.* Retrieved from https://www.hhs.gov/surgeongeneral/reports-and-publications/mental-health/index.html

White-Ryan, L. (2018). Substance misuse, abuse, and substance-related disorders. In J. C. Heyman & E. P. Congress (Eds.), *Health and Social Work: Practice, Policy, and Research* (pp. 125–143). New York, NY: Springer Publishing Company.

World Health Organization. (2017). *Social determinants of health.* Retrieved from http://www.who.int/social_determinants/thecommission/finalreport/key_concepts/en

Xu, J.Q., Murphy, S.L., Kochanek, K.D., Bastian, B., & Arias, E. (2018). Deaths: Final data for 2016. *National Vital Statistics Reports, 67*(5). Hyattsville, MD: National Center for Health Statistics.

Yeo, G., & Yoshikawa, T. (2019). The future of the ethnogeriatric research and publications. *Journal of American Geriatrics Society, 67*(6), 1120–1122. doi:10.1111/jgs.15875

# Part IV

Practice With Individuals and Families From Different Racial/Ethnic Backgrounds and Gender Orientation

# 11

# Practice With African American Families

SAMUEL R. AYMER

## INTRODUCTION

The chapter discusses elements of Afrocentricity—pointing out that Afrocentric scholars de-emphasize the marginalization of people of African ancestry and place them at the center of all discourses (Akbar, 2004; Asante, 1987). In promulgating matters of culture, spirituality, nature, and collectivity, its philosophical underpinnings are rooted in the precepts of both African American culture and traditional Africa (Akbar, 1985; Schiele, 1996). The chapter, stressing that Afrocentricity is a social science framework, also focuses on the need to contextualize a treatment framework that encompasses the confluence of a family's idiosyncratic processes and the *Nguza Saba*—the seven principles of Kwanzaa. (These principles are discussed later in the chapter.) Developed by Karenga (1989), Kwanzaa is a cultural celebration and its self-affirming purpose can be used in clinical work to help African American families address facets of self-identity that have been affected by the effects of historical and present-day oppression.

In addition, this chapter also explores how an Afrocentric perspective can be used in family treatment with African Americans, and focuses on how the construct of intersectionality can be used to contextualize the lives of this group. It is understood that this group is not homogeneous, yet it is also understood that intersecting issues of race, racism, and White supremacy continue to penetrate their daily lives. Furthermore, what is common among African Americans is that because their ancestors were enslaved, the stain of slavery has informed their narratives. Thus, the chapter begins with a brief overview of slavery, highlighting the multiple ways in which families have been affected. Slave trauma syndrome (STS) and posttraumatic slaves syndrome (PTSS) are two relatively new constructs that are receiving attention from social scientists who have argued that the horrendous acts of physical and psychological violence perpetrated under the institution of slavery have culminated in psychic trauma (Akbar, 2004; Latif & Latif, 1994; Leary, 2005; Poussaint & Alexander, 2000).

## HISTORICAL OVERVIEW

From an epistemological perspective, the Afrocentric paradigm includes the history, culture, values, mores, and spirituality of people of African ancestry (Akbar, 2004; Asante, 1987). Because of this, an Afrocentric view—in relation to family treatment with African Americans—must pay attention to the varied ways in which the legacy of slavery affected family dynamics. Having knowledge of slavery adds context to the treatment process and prevents clinicians from assuming a historical stance when working with this population. Boyd-Franklin (2003) notes that "slavery set the tone for people of African descent to be treated as inferior" (p. 9). An in-depth discussion concerning the pernicious effects of enslavement on family life is beyond the scope of this chapter; nevertheless, it is hoped that this brief overview will provide a backdrop for increasing awareness of how the intersecting issues of enslavement and contemporary facets of racism converge, thus influencing the functioning of African American families.

Enslavement meant "the repeated separation of mothers and children and the loss of language, culture and natural religion worked to depose the real African self" (Akbar, 2004, p. 102). The notion of the real African self, as posited by Akbar, meant that indigenous African people had a range of cultural expressions and religious beliefs, and strong familial bonds that fostered self-efficacy (Johnson, 1982; Kardiner & Ovesey, 1962; Staples, 1982). Slavery undermined the concept of the real African self in that women were abducted, raped, and expected to produce as workers for slaveholders. Women were forced to witness the emasculation of men: fathers, sons, and mates. Staples (1982) writes:

> Beginning with the fact slave men and women were equally subjugated to the capricious authority of the slaveholder, the African male saw his masculinity challenged by the rape of his woman, sale of his children, the rations issued in the name of the woman and children bearing her name—which his presence went unrecognized. (p. 2)

Men's physical and psychological welfare were dangerously unstable (Kardiner & Ovesey, 1962, p. 45). Lynching was an inescapable truth for Black men—this practice, in conjunction with being sold, impelled men to flee—and this ruptured family stability (Johnson, 1982). For that reason, "[t]he mother-child family with the father either unknown, absent, or, if present, incapable of wielding influence, was the only type of family that could survive in the new environment" (Kardiner & Ovesey, 1962, p. 45). This familial configuration was known as the *uterine family* (or *uterine society*) and was not consonant with traditional African culture (Kardiner & Ovesey, 1962). Kardiner and Ovesey posit that "under the conditions of enslavement, the uterine family was not institutionalized, but incidental to a host of conditions that held priority of claim" (p. 46). As a result, slave women employed adaptive and maladaptive reactions to the circumstances relating to the institution of slavery (Billingsley, 1968; Kardiner & Ovesey, 1962).

## SLAVE TRAUMA SYNDROME

STS, a term coined by Latif and Latif (1994), is an area of research that is beginning to offer insights into the traumatic effects of slavery on African Americans whose ancestors were slaves. Latif and Latif (1994) refer to STS as the "psychic trauma" of African Americans, proclaiming that "the psychological trauma from slavery has never been addressed, and the resulting emotional scars have been passed down, generation to generation" (p. 20). They raised the following questions to explore the consequences of STS on African Africans whose bloodline is affected by slavery:

> What happens to those citizens who are smuggled away, locked in chains, and shipped off to a foreign land, where they are murdered, tortured, raped, beaten, and forced to labor in the fields under the lash of whip and the constant threat of death? What happens to them when they are forced to have sex with each other for the purposes of producing babies, who are then snatched away and sold, like puppies, to strangers? (p. 18)

Moreover, this question also helps frame the STS discourse. Latif and Latif (1994) believe that the essence of these questions draws attention to the psychological damages connected to slavery, and the dehumanizing activities that treated slaves as chattel and stripped them of their humanity. The traumatic conditions of slavery can be viewed through the prism of what Herman (1992) refers to as "the damaged self," which reflected how slavery impeded the mental lives of its victims by undermining their sense of agency, ego strengths, and the capacity to feel psychologically safe, whole, and secure. This viewpoint is supported by Poussaint and Alexander (2000) who assert that PTSS has affected the "minds and bodies of Black people" (p. 15).

In addition to Latif and Latif's (1994) research, Leary (2005) also calls attention to enslavement and its impact on African Americans, using PTSS to define a condition that exists when a population has experienced multigenerational trauma resulting from centuries of slavery and continues to experience oppression and institutionalized oppression. Likewise, research by Fanon (1963) and others (Akbar, 2004; Altman, 1995; Kardiner & Ovesey, 1962; Karenga, 1982) shows that the consequences of slavery have influenced African Americans' perception of themselves in relation to White American standards, which, in turn, reinforces Leary's (2005) observation that deep-rooted feelings of inferiority pervade the psyche of victims of slavery. Framed as multigenerational trauma, Leary's view of PTSS is that the injurious effects of enslavement create maladaptive behaviors in its victims, and, in turn, such effects have been passed on to succeeding generations, a view also held by Latif and Latif (1994). Such a postulation implies that the nexus of multigenerational trauma and the ongoing reality of racial oppression inevitably hamper the stability of African American families. Thompson and Neville (1999) make the same argument:

> Racism has evolved over time as a changing yet enduring outgrowth of American political and social life. Therefore, it is inaccurate to conclude that racism was essentially nonexistent during certain historical periods (e.g., following the Civil Rights Movement) and prevalent during other periods (e.g., slavery in the segregated U.S. South). (p. 168)

Indeed, it has been difficult for African Americans to work through the internalized feelings emanating from being the descendants of slaves and victims of contemporary oppression. The psychological and behavioral dynamics from enslavement and contemporary oppression that have been passed on to descendants of slaves (as delineated by Leary [2005]) are vacant self-esteem, ever-present anger, and racist socialization.

*Vacant self-esteem* speaks to the self-development of African American people, who must live in oppressive contexts that devalue their personhood. Leary (2005) believes that it is onerous to feel psychologically fortified in a society that promotes stereotypic images of African Americans. Implied in this idea is the notion that internalizations (negative or positive) of one's group are critical to fostering self-worth. And, when negative internalizations are combined with knowing that one's history is connected to enslavement, this can induce feelings of anxiety, shame, and self-loathing behaviors in African Americans.

*Ever-present anger* refers to African Americans' tendency to externalize angry feelings that may not be proportional to the situation that triggered the reaction. From a contemporary perspective, Leary (2005) contends that blocked resources and opportunities, linked to structural racism and oppression, deny African Americans access to rights and privileges. The degree to which African American individuals are able to manage this reality depends on how they have come to understand their social reality within a hostile environment. Ever-present anger can be traced back to slavery, and Leary states that "slavery was an inherently angry, violent process" (p. 137). The violence and inhumane treatment perpetrated against slaves induced a range of emotions, including anger and rage (Grier & Cobbs, 1968). Leary indicates that anger was modeled by slave owners, whose oppressive behaviors served as a catalyst for cultivating generalized anger in slaves. An important aspect of Leary's thesis is that anger observed in many African Americans should be contextualized from a historical and contemporary vantage point, and it should be acknowledged that it can be a coping mechanism to manage oppression.

Racist socialization has its beginnings in slavery—enslaved Africans endured egregious treatment that led to self-hatred (Leary, 2005). Slave owners, for instance, manufactured a system of discrimination based upon skin color, favoring lighter-skinned slaves (who were the product of rape) over darker-skinned ones. Leary (2005) argues that skin-color dynamics among African Americans persist and correlates it to the legacy of slavery and the devaluation of Negroid attributes, including skin color and hair texture. Other scholars have made similar claims and argue that such issues operate in African American families (Grier & Cobbs, 1968). Factors regarding skin color are discussed in the latter part of this chapter.

## AFROCENTRICITY

The utility of Afrocentric concepts in social work and human behavior theories has received attention over the last 10 years (Schiele, 1996). In academia, for instance, one of the aims of Afrocentric scholarship is to disrupt traditional Eurocentric paradigms that promote a one-dimensional view (i.e., White middle class) of normative human growth and development. Afrocentrists believe that it is critical to raise questions about the primacy of Eurocentric constructs in terms of their relevance to the social and psychic reality of people of African ancestry (Akbar, 2004; Davis, Williams, & Akinyela, 2010). By doing so, people of African ancestry are located at the center of all discourses, thus creating conditions for portraying their experiences in ways that obviate marginalization. Afrocentric theoreticians emphasize the centrality of Africa and its relationship to the collective consciousness of African Americans (Akbar, 2004). Afrocentricity espouses that culture, spirituality, nature, and the collective (or tribe) is inextricably linked to the social and psychological circumstances of people of African ancestry (Asante, 2007). Black psychology, a domain of social science that interrogates Black psychosocial functioning through the lens of culture, race, oppression, spirituality, racial identity development, and the developing practice of Afrocentric social work, subscribes to Asante's view of Afrocentricity (Akbar, 2004; Schiele, 1996). Correspondingly, Davis et al. (2010) concluded that "[a] basic premise of an Afrocentric approach is that culture matters—in the past, in the present, and in the future" (p. 4).

In addition, Schiele (1996) indicates that "[t]he Afrocentric paradigm is a social science paradigm that is embedded in the philosophical concepts of contemporary African America and traditional Africa" (p. 285). It underscores the salience of traditional African ethos, stressing that philosophical African assumptions about human existence are predicated on respect for spirituality and connectedness to people, nature, community, and the ancestors (Mazama, 2002; Mendes, 1982). In the purview of spirituality, for instance, Mazama maintains that it has been of paramount importance to African Americans throughout the diaspora, and has served to assuage the daunting effects of racial oppression and colonization. Further elaboration of Mazama's argument is as follows:

> Afrocentricity, as an emancipatory movement, then inscribes itself with a tradition of African resistance to European oppression. One commonly noted feature of African resistance is its reliance on spirituality. Indeed, spirituality has always historically played an important role in our many struggles for liberation, from Nanny in Jamaica to the Haitian revolutionary war and Nat Turner. Why, after all, should Afrocentricity differ? (p. 219)

## INTERSECTIONALITY

The construct of intersectionality has gained considerable attention in academia over the last 20 years, and often it is used to ground classroom discourses relative to White supremacy, race, racism, ethnocentricity, culture, homophobia, immigration, social class, and other sociocultural variables that impact on the psychological functioning of people within the social environment. Accordingly, Knudsen (2006, p. 61) stated that "intersectionality may be defined as a theory to analyse how social and cultural categories intertwine." Still, African American feminist legal scholar Crenshaw (1995), who developed this construct, posited that people's (African American individuals) social location, race, gender, and culture cannot be divorced from the myriad ways in which they must navigate and make sense of the terrain of social injustice in

America. Crenshaw underscored this position in her seminal essay, "Mapping the margins: Intersectionality, identity politics and violence against Black women," arguing that services (i.e., social or legal) for Black women affected by intimate partner violence (IPV), for example, should consider how interlocking factors of structural racism and patriarchy have shaped the vicissitudes of their personal and familial circumstances. And thus, a practitioner, who may identify a Black woman's ambivalence about pursuing police intervention to deal with issues of IPV, might strengthen their evaluation of the woman's experience by recognizing the fraught relationship that exists between the African American community and the police. This is an intersectional reality for this group of women who may want the violence to stop, but who may also have anxiety about the adverse effects (police brutality/killing of their male partners) of police involvement in familial matters. From an intersectional point of view, having this type of cultural knowledge could facilitate therapeutic attunement, allowing practitioners to grasp the psychosocial angst associated with the narratives of abused African American women who often grapple with such a duality, which is known as double consciousness (Du Bois, 1953). An amplification of this point is captured via Crenshaw's observation:

> Women of color are often reluctant to call the police, a hesitancy likely due to a general unwillingness among people of color to subject their private lives to the scrutiny and control of a police force that is frequently hostile. (p. 362)

Locating the aforementioned ideas within the context of intersectionality and Afrocentricity provides historical and contemporary contexts for understanding White supremacy and its influences on the lives of African American people during and after enslavement. Likewise, both theories can be used to explicate how clinical work with African American families should incorporate a treatment mode that addresses and alleviates the intrapersonal problems that are rooted in structural oppression (Alexander, 2010; Aymer, 2016). With this in mind, the practitioner attends to the emotional needs of family members by honoring their subjective truths concerning how they have been impacted by race-based stress, a phenomenon that has been researched by Carter (2007) who has studied intersecting issues of race, racism, and the lived issues of African American families. As a result, Carter's findings suggest that "the symptoms manifestations of race-based stress include having reactions of intrusions (re-experiencing), avoiding (numbing) of stimuli associated with the trauma, and increased arousal or vigilance" (p. 84). In treating African American families, Carter's research reminds us that it is critically important for practitioners to pay attention to how racial animus can undermine their mental health and well-being.

## RELATIONAL AND NARRATIVE LENSES IN FAMILY THERAPY

Aspects of relational and narrative family therapy tenets can be useful in treating African American families. Honesty, authenticity, and openness are relational attributes that can serve to establish a working alliance. Race and class notwithstanding, it is important for practitioners to reflect on how their subjective reality has been marred by similar forms of oppression (e.g., internalized oppression, exposure to daily microaggressions), a process that would occur due to a two-person psychological model (Altman, 1995). Likewise, Boyd-Franklin (2003, p. 179) advances the idea that "the person-to-person connection" can be effective in work with African American families because it engenders trust in the working alliance between the practitioner and the family. This idea is supported by Hadley (2008), who reminds us that in the sphere of relational work, mutuality and dynamic and interactional processes are salient to the interplay that occurs between the clinician and the client; it is necessary for the practitioners to be attuned to these variables so that the clinician can gain insights into how transferential and countertransferential issues are affecting the work. Finally, Altman (1995) notes that "[f]rom the perspective of relational psychoanalysis, patient and analyst inevitably bring their own predispositions to the encounter" (p. 132).

African American families are not homogeneous, and, therefore, they present a range of idiosyncrasies in treatment. It must be acknowledged, however, that this population is exposed to the deleterious effects of racial oppression, which creates a sense of shared vulnerability. Shared vulnerability means that many African Americans have some level of psychological consciousness about the potential physical and psychic danger of living in a society that has a history of racial animus toward them. In spite of this, there is variability in how African Americans attempt to cope with exposure to environmentally based toxins, for example, microaggressions (i.e., racial slights and discrimination). Shared vulnerability becomes a pivotal part of this group's narrative, and it shapes aspects of their social identities. Cooper and Lesser's (2008) formulation of narrative therapy is apt in that they contend that "[n]arrative therapy is about knowledge and how the client has 'storied' her life to make sense of it" (p. 162). Clinicians start from a point of not knowing, minimizing their inclination to be the expert on the client's circumstances; employing this orientation with oppressed populations can lead to a clearer understanding of their subjective truths about experiencing social injustice. "Constructivism is rooted in post modern thinking—which assumes that there no universal truths and that there are many realties as there are perceivers of reality" (Cooper & Lesser, 2008, p. 177). Negative stereotypic messages from society and the family erode family members' self-worth (Leary, 2005). Utilizing a constructivist perspective in treatment can enable families to develop a positive view of themselves, thus providing them with an alternative construction of psychic reality.

What makes a relational and narrative approach to work with families useful is that research (Boyd-Franklin, 2003) reveals that African American individuals and families tend to be suspicious and distrustful of professionals, especially if they sense insensitivity to and lack of understanding of historical and here-and-now experiences with oppression. Boyd-Franklin (2003) uses the concept of *vibe*, articulating that families develop uneasiness with professionals who may not be sensitive to the social and cultural contexts of their experiences. The notion of *vibe* means that families are hypersensitive to whether they can connect with the therapist and whether the therapist can relate to them. This phenomenon is rooted in a basic "gut level" feeling, which can either support or hinder the development of a treatment relationship (Boyd-Franklin, 2003, p. 178).

## THE *NGUZO SABA* AS FOUNDATION FOR TREATMENT

As noted, an Afrocentric emphasis on treating African American families needs a framework that addresses internal (i.e., intrapersonal/idiosyncratic processes) and external (i.e., historical and current forms of oppression) variables. Majors and Mancini Billson (1992) state that Afrocentricity "is not anti-White, but it is an ideology that encourage[s] Black Americans to transcend their problems by reclaiming traditional African values" (p. 11). Majors and Mancini Billson's goal can be achieved by infusing the *Nguzo Saba* (the principles of Kwanzaa [Karenga, 1989]) in family treatment. Kwanzaa, an annual cultural holiday (celebrated in December and January), is associated with practices designed to inculcate in African Americans positive messages about Africa and African American experiences. The seven principles of Kwanzaa can counteract feelings of marginalization and self-hatred, which foster poor self-esteem (Aymer, 2010). The seven principles are the following:

*Unoja* (unity): To strive for and maintain unity in the family, community, nation, and race.

*Kujuchagulia* (self-determination): To define ourselves, name ourselves, create for ourselves, and speak for ourselves instead of being defined, named, created by others.

*Ujima* (collective work and responsibility): To build and maintain our community together and make our sister's and brother's problems our problems and to solve them together.

*Ujamma* (cooperative economics): To build and maintain our own stores, shops, and other businesses and profit from them together.

*Nia* (purpose): To make our collective vocation and building the development of our community in order to restore our people to their traditional greatness.

*Kuumba* (creativity): To do always as much as we can in the ways we can, in order to leave our community more beautiful and beneficial than we inherited it.

*Imani* (faith): To believe with all our hearts in God, our people, our parents, our teachers, our leaders, and the righteousness and victory of our struggle (Karenga, 1989, p. 45).

The value of infusing the principles of Kwanzaa in treatment affirms self-efficacy, an important ego function that may have been affected by historical and contemporary issues of oppression. This underlines the importance of using an intersectional lens in order to recognize the pernicious effects of marginalization on the functioning of African American families. That said, Karenga (1989) indicates that *Nguzu Saba* is an Afrocentric value system akin to the following goals: (a) "organize and enrich our relations with each other on the persons and the community level; (b) establish standards, commitments and priorities that would tend to enhance our human possibilities as persons and a people; (c) aid in the recovery and reconstruction of lost historical memory and cultural legacy in the development of an Afrocentric paradigm of life and achievement; (d) serve as a contribution to a core system of communitarian ethical values for the moral guidance and instruction of the community, especially for children; (e) contribute to an ongoing and expanding set of Afrocentric communitarian values which would aid in bringing into being a new man, woman, and child who self-consciously participate in the ethical project of starting a new history of African people and humankind" (p. 44).

## TREATMENT IMPLICATIONS

Treatment themes that African American families may present include—but are not limited to—the following: parent–child difficulties, grandparents as "other mothers," marital discord, immigration and migration, financial anxiety, internalized oppression relating to skin color and hair texture anxieties, and paternal issues. An important caveat is that these are examples of presenting difficulties that may surface in therapy and should not be viewed as definitive concerns unique to African Americans.

Combining *Nguzo Saba* with Hill's (1999) groundbreaking work on African American strengths (e.g., strong achievement orientation, strong work ethic, flexibility of family roles, strong kinship attachment, and strong religious values) enable clinicians to address coping and adaptive factors relative to family functioning. Hill's assertion is that these strengths are the foundation of African American family stability because social and political institutions work against their interests. The strong kinship attachment system must be assessed by examining who is living in and out of the household, as well as the types of familial bonds that exist among family members, excavating the viability of the family social network (e.g., godparents, close friends of the family, deacons of the church). *Umoja* (unity) can be used to understand the closeness and connections among and between family members. Akbar (2004) states that "[t]he often-described extended family among African people is relevant to this notion of oneness" (p. 125). Under the conditions of slavery, families maintained a strong sense of kinship, underlining why clinicians should have historical insights into the African American experience (Kardiner & Ovesey, 1962). In addition, Hill's use of strong religious values complements the principle of *Imani* (faith) because it will enable practitioners to assess how families use faith-based coping (e.g., praying, calling on the ancestors for guidance, engaging in religious practices) to alleviate psychosocial stress (Mazama, 2002). It should be noted that Mazama indicates that the use of spirituality is a protective factor that has served an emancipatory function for diasporic people.

Afrocentrists believe that African Americans' esteem is nurtured by their attachment to family and the African American community (Akbar, 1985, 2004; Karenga, 1989; Mbiti, 1969). Individuals obtain high regard from the group or tribe, supporting Hill's views about a strong achievement orientation, strong work ethic, and flexibility of family roles. Moreover, *Ujima* (collective work and responsibility) builds on this premise because it emphasizes collectivism over individualism—a functional factor in clients who may appear to be dependent on their families and community for support—as opposed to public systems of care. Underpinning a central precept of Afrocentricity is Mbiti's (1969) stance: "I am because we are; and because we are, therefore I am" (p. 108).

Internalized oppression, which can take the form of self-loathing reactions manifested in anxieties about skin color, hair texture, and facial features has the potential to surface in psychotherapeutic work with African American families. As noted previously, skin color is a troublesome concern shaping identity and interpersonal and intrapersonal processes within families. Research (Akbar, 2004; Boyd-Franklin, 2003; Leary, 2005; Russell, Wilson, & Hall, 1992) reveals that lighter skin tones (and hair texture) within the families are imbued with a sense of privilege and beauty, causing turbulence among siblings and other family members. Russell et al. (1992) delineated a myriad of ways in which skin color dynamics are played out in the African American communities and families:

> Identity is a multifaceted and in some ways nebulous concept. Being Black affects the way a person walks and talks, his or her values, culture, and history, how that person relates to others and how they relate to him or her. It is governed by one's early social experience; history and politics, conscious input and labeling, and the genetic accident that dictates appearance. Skin color appears to affect identify, but in complex and seemingly unpredictable ways. (p. 62)

Boyd-Franklin (2003) echoes a similar view: Lighter-skinned children are revered in families, whereas dark-skinned children are sometimes ostracized and devalued. This phenomenon often culminates in secret keeping and can produce unspoken turmoil, undercutting family members' self-esteem (Boyd-Franklin, 2003). Emblematic of Latif and Latif (1994) and Leary (2005) discourses, skin-color issues are significant outgrowths of STS that can be traced to the institution of slavery (specifically, the rape of slave women that produced mulatto children who were privileged and worked in the master's house as opposed to working in the field). Boyd-Franklin (2003) suggests that contemporary African American families continue to grapple with skin-color anxieties and may be reluctant to share their feelings with a professional due to shame. Utilizing the principles of *Nia* (purpose), *Kujuchagulia* (self-determination), and *Kuumba* (creativity) in treatment enables individuals to consider self-acceptance, an important factor that can counteract internalized negative stereotypical societal projections. Akbar (1985) argues that:

> Self-acceptance is the beginning for all positive social activity. Knowing who you are acquaints you with the best of your human potential and leads to productive acceptance of self. Accepting self means that you like yourself and have a commitment to self. Accepting self means that you want to be yourself and not anyone else's self, the self-accepting person does whatever he can to express himself. From physical features to cultural features the objective is to express self. The non-self-accepting person tries to change their features to look like another self. (p. 31)

The point is that the infusion of the principles of Kwanzaa in treatment serves to raise psychological and cultural consciousness for many families—mitigating cognitive dissonance—stemming from daily encounters with environmental deficits.

## CONCLUSION

Utilizing an Afrocentric approach in treating African American families is one important way for clinicians to help families cope with stressors related to their familial idiosyncratic dynamics and racial oppression. An Afrocentric viewpoint to practice contextualizes the social location of families and provides insights into how the intersection of race, oppression, and family life cohere in order to shape their psychological reality. A clinical embrace of intersectional factors in treatment with African American families is quite prudent given the setbacks they have endured from the legacy of enslavement—and the resulting consequences of contemporary social injustices. The *Nguza Saba,* therefore, can be used to instill cultural, spiritual, and social awareness in the treatment process. Furthermore, an Afrocentric approach to treatment can enable families to connect with thematic elements of the *Nguza Saba*: cultural pride, heritage, spirituality, faith, coping, and self-efficacy. The empowering effects of these themes in work with African American families affirm their resilience and determination to survive and thrive despite the ubiquitous circumstances of institutionalized cultural and racial oppression.

## REFERENCES

Akbar, N. (1985). *The community of self.* Tallahassee, FL: Mind Productions.

Akbar, N. (2004). *Akbar papers in African psychology.* Tallahassee, FL: Mind Productions.

Alexander, M. (2010). *The new Jim Crow: Mass incarceration in the age of colorblindness.* New York, NY: New Press.

Altman, N. (1995). *The analyst in the inner city: Race, class and culture through a psychoanalytic lens.* Hillside, NJ: The Analytic Press.

Asante, M. K. (1987). *The Afrocentric idea.* Philadelphia, PA: Temple University Press.

Asante, M. K. (2007). *The Afrocentric manifesto: Towards an African resistance.* Cambridge, MA: Polity Press.

Aymer, S. R. (2010). Clinical practice with African-American men: What to consider and what to do. *Smith College Studies in Social Work, 80*(1), 20–34. doi:10.1080/00377310903504908

Aymer, S. R. (2016). "I can't breathe": A case study—Helping Black men cope with race-related trauma stemming from police killing and brutality. *Journal of Human Behavior in the Social Environment, 29*(3–4), 367–376. doi:10.1080/10911359.2015.1132828

Billingsley, A. (1968). *Black families in White America.* Englewood Cliffs, NJ: Prentice Hall.

Boyd-Franklin, N. (2003). *Black families in therapy: Understanding the African American experience.* New York, NY: Guilford Press.

Carter, R. (2007). Racism and psychosocial and emotional injury. Recognizing and assessing race-based traumatic stress. *Counselling Psychologist, 35*(1), 333–339. doi:10.1177/0011000006292033

Cooper, M. G., & Lesser, J. G. (2008). *Clinical social work practice: An integrated approach* (3rd ed.). Boston, MA: Allyn & Bacon.

Crenshaw, K. (1995). Mapping the margins: Intersectionality, identity politics, and violence against women of color. In K. Crenshaw, N. Gotanda, G. Peller, & K. Thomas (Eds.), *Critical race theory: The key writings that framed the movement.* New York, NY: Press.

Davis, A. K., Williams, A. D., & Akinyela, M. (2010). An Afrocentric to building cultural relevance in social work research. *Journal of Black Studies, 41*(2), 338–350. doi:10.1177/0021934709343950

Du Bois, W. E. B. (1953). *The souls of Black folks.* Greenwich, CT: Fawcett Publications.

Fanon, F. (1963). *The wretched of the earth.* New York, NY: Grove Press.

Grier, W. H., & Cobbs, P. M. (1968). *Black rage.* New York, NY: Basic Books.

Hadley, M. (2008). Relational theory: Inside out, and outside in, in between, and all around. In J. Berzoff & L. M. Flanagan (Eds.), *Inside out and outside in: Psychodynamic clinical theory and psychopathology in contemporary.* New York, NY: Jason Aronson.

Herman, J. L. (1992). *Trauma and recovery: The aftermath of violence from domestic to political terror.* New York, NY: Basic Books.

Hill, R. B. (1999). *The strengths of African American families: Twenty-five years later.* New York, NY: University Press of America.

Johnson, J. E. (1982). The Afro-American family: A historical overview. In B. N. Bass, G. E. Wyatt, & G. P. Powell (Eds.), *The Afro-American family: Assessment, treatment, and research issues.* New York, NY: Harcourt Brace Jovanovich.

Kardiner, A., & Ovesey, L. (1962). *The mark of oppression.* Cleveland, OH: World Publishing.

Karenga, M. (1989). *The African American holiday of Kwanzaa: A celebration of family, community and culture.* Los Angeles, CA: University of Sankofa Press.

Knudsen, S. (2006). Intersectionality: A theoretical inspiration in the analysis of minority cultures and in identities in textbooks, In B. M. Horsely, S. V. Knudsen, & B. Aamotsbakken (Eds.), *Caught in the web of lost in the textbook* (pp. 61–76). Paris, France: IUFM dcCaen.

Latif, S., & Latif, N. (1994). *Slavery: The African American psychic trauma.* Chicago. IL: Latif Communications Group.

Leary, J. G. (2005). *Post Traumatic Slave Syndrome: America's legacy of enduring injury and healing.* Milwaukie, WI: Uptone Press.

Majors, R., & Mancini Billson, J. (1992). *Cool pose: The dilemmas of Black manhood in America.* New York, NY: Lexington Books.

Mazama, M. A. (2002). Afrocentricity and African spirituality. *Journal of Black Psychology, 3,* 218–234. doi:10.1177/002193402237226

Mbiti, J. (1969). *African religions and philosophy.* Oxford, UK: Heinemann Educational Books.

Mendes, H. A. (1982). The role of religion in psychotherapy with Afro-Americans. In B. N. Bass, G. E. Wyatt, & G. P. Wyatt (Eds.), *The Afro-American family: Assessment, treatment, and research issues.* New York, NY: Harcourt Brace Jovanovich.

Poussaint, A. E., & Alexander, A. (2000). *Lay my burden down.* Boston, MA: Beacon Press.

Russell, K., Wilson, M., & Hall, R. (1992). *The color complex: the politics of skin color among African Americans.* New York, NY: Harcourt Brace Javanovich.

Schiele, J. H. (1996). Afrocentricity: An emerging paradigm in social work practice. *Social Work, 41*(3), 284–285.

Staples, R. (1982). *Black masculinity: The Black male's role in American society.* San Francisco, CA: Black Scholar Press.

Thompson, C. E., & Neville, N. (1999). Racism, mental health, and mental health practice. *Counseling Psychologist, 27*(2), 155–223. doi:10.1177/0011000099272001

# 12

# Practice With Hispanic Individuals and Families

MANNY JOHN GONZÁLEZ AND GREGORY ACEVEDO

## INTRODUCTION

The term Hispanic was created by the United States Census Bureau in 1970. Latino[1] is a self-ascribed term that emerged from the everyday interpretative and linguistic practices of Hispanics in the United States. The term Latino appeared on the United States census form for the first time in 2000. However it may be categorized or defined, the Hispanic rubric remains "under construction" (Torres-Saillant, 2002). More recently, the term "Latinx" has come into vogue. It attempts to adopt a non-gendered, multicultural form of the term Latino, but its usage is controversial and has not yet achieved the same popularity as the terms Hispanic or Latino. The pan-ethnic, Hispanic population in the United States varies in terms of such important characteristics as immigration status (foreign-born Hispanics comprise a substantial proportion of both the Latino and the total foreign-born population in the United States), national origin, racial and ethnic identification, language use and proficiency, place of residence, and socioeconomic status. Common elements of the Hispanic rubric and Latino identity include the preponderance of Spanish-language use; similarity in sociohistorical and geopolitical influences; the psychosocial influence of family origins, socialization, and personal feelings; and the geospatial context of barrio life.

In 2017, the Hispanic population in the United States was approximately 58.9 million, comprising 18.1% of the total population (U.S. Census Bureau, 2018). The Latino population has increased nearly ninefold since 1960, growing from 6.3 million to 56.5 million by 2015 (Flores, 2017). In 2015, 33.4% of Hispanics were foreign born, a decrease from a previous high of 40.1% in 2000 (Flores, 2017). Mexicans continue to comprise the lion's share of the overall Hispanic population.

---

[1] The terms "Latino" and "Latina" are the masculine and the feminine forms of the term Latino in the Spanish language.

Table 12.1 *Largest Hispanic Subgroups in the United States*

| Country of Origin | Population |
|---|---|
| Mexican | 35,371,314 |
| Puerto Rican | 5,319,961 (not including Puerto Rico) |
| Salvadoran | 2,100,433 |
| Cuban | 2,045,970 |
| Dominican | 1,763,651 |
| Guatemalan | 1,324,694 |
| Colombian | 1,046,332 |
| Honduran | 812,731 |
| Spaniard | 753,538 |
| Ecuadoran | 659,166 |
| Peruvian | 614,151 |
| Nicaraguan | 414,136 |
| Venezuelan | 302,778 |
| Argentinean | 268,099 |
| Panamanian | 189,748 |
| Chilean | 149,113 |
| Costa Rican | 140,581 |
| Bolivian | 110,101 |
| Uruguayan | 67,226 |
| Paraguayan | 27,590 |

*Source:* Reproduced with permission from Stepler, R., & Brown, A. (2016). *2014, Hispanics in the United States Statistical Portrait.* Washington, DC: Pew Hispanic Center.

That said, the population of other national-origin groups has increased substantially as well (see Table 12.1 for a detailed disaggregation of the largest Hispanic subgroups in the United States).

An essential thread in the history of the Latino experience in the United States is social marginalization, poverty, and political disenfranchisement. Due to the stigmas associated with "illegal" or undocumented immigration (although over half of the Hispanic population in the United States is native-born) the focus of public perceptions, debates, and policies have centered on Latino immigrants, and has cast a shadow over all Latinos, whatever their legal status or origin. Hispanic immigrants in the United States and, by default, their native-born Latino counterparts are currently embroiled in a number of policy-related debates. The issues that are the subject of these debates are quintessential illustrations of the practice of policy deployed to regulate the lives of people of color, including immigration and border control, and also policies related to citizenship, bilingual education, welfare reform, and labor rights (Acevedo, 2010).

Hispanics are an essential part of the sociocultural, political, and economic life of the United States and are altering the demographic landscape of the United States. Among the critical issues facing Latinos today, one of the most troubling is economic vulnerability. The overall poverty rate in the United States in 2017 was 12.3%, but it was 18.3% among Hispanics, second only to non-Latino Blacks (21.2%) (Fontenot, Semega, & Kollar, 2018). Given the Hispanic population's overall youthfulness, fertility rate, and levels of immigration, their socioeconomic well-being has tremendous consequences for the entire U.S. population and the nation's economic future.

In light of the overall profile of Hispanics in the United States, the sociocultural, political, and economic dynamics that determine the Latino experience, and the differences between and within the various Hispanic national-origin groups, including linguistic diversity and immigration status, the task of mastering competent social work practice with this population takes on increased significance. The psychosocial issues associated with the emigration experience and complex personal and social environment transactions are reason enough to justify the relevance and need for culturally competent treatment models or approaches to clinical practice that are attuned to Hispanic individuals and families. Compounding the acute stressors of emigration—that many Hispanics must face on a continual basis—is the silhouette of an enduring shortfall in the economic, educational, and social arenas, creating the oppressive context of daily life that, if unaddressed, erodes the psychosocial well-being and coping strengths of this large and growing population. Informed by the tenets of the ecological perspective and the life model of social work practice (Gitterman & Germain, 2008), this chapter presents an overview of clinical practice with Hispanic families. The ecological perspective helps to promote clinicians' understanding of the psychosocial problems experienced by culturally diverse client populations as well as the socioenvironmental variables (e.g., racism, discrimination, poverty) that impede optimal physical, psychological, and social well-being. Because the process of individual or family treatment cannot separate personality structures and issues from the cultural factors that influence the emotional health of the individual, this chapter also underscores the key cultural characteristics of Hispanic individuals and families and their relevance for culturally competent clinical practice. Treatment recommendations and strategies for effective psychosocial intervention with Hispanic families is emphasized throughout the chapter.

## CULTURAL CHARACTERISTICS OF HISPANIC INDIVIDUALS AND FAMILIES

The clinical care for Hispanic clients must be predicated on an understanding of the way specific cultural values or characteristics directly affect how practitioners can provide effective psychotherapeutic and culturally congruent treatment. Sandoval and De la Roza (1986), as well as other Hispanic scholars

(Gil, 1980; González & González-Ramos, 2005; Santiago-Rivera, Arredondo, & Gallardo-Cooper, 2002), have identified and described the salient cultural values or characteristics that may inform the treatment strategies employed in the amelioration of psychological distress and social functioning among Hispanics. The values or characteristics are those of *simpatía, personalismo, familismo, respeto,* and *confianza.* There are also two gender-specific roles (Gil, 1980) that are part of the traditional Hispanic experience that may influence therapeutic approaches and outcomes: *marianismo* (female self-sacrifice) and *machismo* (male self-respect and responsibility). *Marianismo* and *machismo* may be terms that have acquired such common and pejorative usage that their actual centrality in the Hispanic maintenance of intrapersonal and interpersonal coherence is obscured.

Religion or a sense of spirituality also informs the traditional Hispanic experience and may serve to enhance, or at times challenge, the curative process of clinical social work practice. Clinical practitioners must be mindful of the fact that, irrespective of differences within or among Latino ethnic groups (e.g., Cubans, Mexicans, Puerto Ricans), Hispanics do share similarities based on these traditional characteristics. Hispanics' level of acculturation, socioeconomic class, and family and gender roles, however, will affect both their adherence to traditional cultural values or characteristics and their utilization of clinical services and the broader applications of psychosocial care. Examples of traditional Hispanic cultural values/characteristics and how they may impact the provision of clinical and mental healthcare are described in the following:

- **Simpatía.** *Simpatía* relates to what many call *buenagente* (the plural form of a nice person). Hispanics are drawn to individuals who are easygoing, friendly, and fun to be with. *Simpatía* is a value placed on politeness and pleasantness. Avoidance of hostile confrontation is a vital component of this specific ethnocultural value.
- **Personalismo.** *Personalismo* as a cultural trait or value is reflected in the tendency of Hispanic patients to relate to their service providers personally rather than in an institutional or impersonal manner. Hispanic clients expect to develop a warm personal relationship with their clinician characterized by interactions that are authentic.
- **Familismo.** *Familismo* is a collective loyalty to the nuclear and extended family that outranks the individual. The extended family within the Hispanic culture includes members who are biologically related to each other, as well as members who join the family system via *compadrazco* (godparentage). Biological parents select *compadres* (godparents) before the baptism or christening ceremony of a child. Historically, this practice is directly linked to Catholicism. Godparents assume a vital resource role in the Hispanic family particularly during times of crisis when instrumental and emotional support may be needed. It is important to note that this cultural value (*familismo*) remains strong even among highly acculturated families (Santiago-Rivera et al., 2002).
- **Respeto.** *Respeto* (respect) dictates appropriate deferential behavior toward others based on age, gender, social position, economic status, and authority. Within the Hispanic community, older adults expect respect from youngsters, women from men, men from women, adults from children, teachers from students, employers from employees, and so on. Clinicians must keep in mind,

however, that respect within the Hispanic culture implies a mutual and reciprocal deference. The clinician receiving respect as a professional is equally obligated to observe deferential courtesies to the client based on age, gender, and other sociocultural characteristics.

- *Confianza*. *Confianza* (trust) refers to the intimacy and familiarity in a relationship. The term in Spanish implies informality and ease of interpersonal comfort. Clinicians who are able to develop a bond of trust with Hispanic clients may eventually notice a level of improvement in the patient's psychological status, and a willingness of the client to comply with mental health or psychosocial care recommendations.

It is important to note, especially regarding *confianza* as a kind of culminating relational state based on the other named cultural values and expectations, that engagement and maintenance of a clinical working alliance could be similarly defined. The culturally sensitive practitioner is assisted in the development and maintenance of a productive clinical process by bearing in mind that these Hispanic-specific concepts offer practical guidance in work with all populations. Their conscious centrality to the clinician and client in work with Hispanic clients may call for a more overt demonstration of cultural protocols, particularly where there is divergence from the clinician's cultural orientation. However, the essential features of sympathy/empathy, respect, individuality, and trust apply across most, if not all interpersonal lines.

The essence of the most common traditional Hispanic values or characteristics may be summarized in the following points: (a) unity and interdependence among members of the nuclear and extended family; (b) expectation that the family (nuclear and extended) will care for the young and the elderly; (c) flexible sense of time—many Hispanic clients adhere to a present-time orientation; (d) physical closeness and touching in an appropriate context can be expected during conversation or an interpersonal exchange; and (e) respect for tradition and traditional family and social roles (Taylor, 1989).

## Gender-Specific Roles

Gender role expectations and values constitute an area where transference and countertransference may create the strongest potential for cultural misalignment and misunderstanding within the client–clinician treatment relationship. Demarcated gender roles are an important component of the Hispanic relational matrix. Traditional gender roles within the Hispanic family structure have intrinsically been linked to the concepts of *marianismo* and *machismo*. *Marianismo*, the term associated with Hispanic female socialization, implies that girls must grow up to be women and mothers who are pure, long-suffering, nurturing, pious, virtuous, and humble, yet spiritually stronger than men (Gil, 1980). The concept of *marianismo* is religiously associated with the Virgin Mary and, therefore, it is directly tied to the Roman Catholic faith. Although *marianismo* has contributed to a view of Hispanic women as docile, self-sacrificing, and submissive, it is clear that from a family systems' viewpoint women (particularly mothers) are the silent power in the family structure.

Clinicians need to be alert to the temptation to view the submissiveness of female Hispanic clients as a deficiency in self-esteem or self-assertiveness. Much clinical potential can be lost if the clinician, to whom it is also apt to demonstrate deference, focuses on gender roles per se rather than deconstructing the ways in which the client's posture toward others is or is not inherent to the problem brought to clinical attention. In his seminal paper, "Masochism, Submission, and Surrender—Masochism as a Perversion of Surrender," Ghent (1990) clearly distinguishes deference from powerlessness or self-devaluation. The culturally sensitive and clinically skilled practitioner, seeking empathic understanding of the client's meanings and methods without superficial evaluation of manifest behavior, is well advised to understand that surrender of dominance is a legitimate relational–interpersonal dynamic, especially if matched by protective factors and relational reciprocity as Hispanic values dictate. Surrender to the cultural and individual attributions of meaning and worth of the client is a cornerstone of the constructivist, non-positivist, practice required particularly with clients of differing worldviews (Jordan, 2010).

The gender role socialization of Hispanic males has centered on the construct of *machismo*. *Machismo* has been defined in the general social science literature as the cult of virility, arrogance, and sexual aggressiveness in male-to-female relationships (Santiago-Rivera et al., 2002). From a Hispanic perspective, however, Sandoval and De la Roza (1986) state that *machismo* refers to a man's responsibility to provide for, protect, and defend his family. Loyalty and a sense of responsibility to family, friends, and the community make a Hispanic male a good man. Hispanic males are expected to be honorable and responsible men. Within the Hispanic family structure, men (especially fathers and husbands) command and expect respect from others. If clinical treatment initiatives are to succeed, practitioners must be skilled at proffering this expected respect to Hispanic adult male clients. This applies to male and female clinicians alike. It is important to note that the process of acculturation may determine the degree to which both Hispanic males and females adhere to the concepts and cultural definitions of *machismo* and *marianismo*. Thus, adherence to these traditional roles may be more visible among recent Hispanic immigrants than among third and fourth generation Hispanics. Sandoval and De la Roza (1986, p. 174) have noted the impact that *machismo* may have on the delivery of mental health services:

> Machismo is one of the Hispanic cultural traits which greatly affect therapeutic intervention, especially family therapy. Machismo might be the reason why the Hispanic male seeks help at a more advanced stage of deterioration than is typically the case with females. Apparently the Hispanic male needs to be in greater pain in order to seek mental health assistance. Machismo [may] negatively influence the therapeutic process. There is resistance by the male to get involved in couples or family therapy, since males [may] generally perceive this involvement as having a deteriorating effect on their integrity and authority.

## Religion and Spirituality

The literature on cross-cultural mental health and psychotherapeutic care (Flores & Carey, 2000; González & González-Ramos, 2005; Santiago-Rivera et al., 2002; Sue & Sue, 1999) has identified Hispanics as an ethnic-minority group whose adherence to an array of religious or spiritual beliefs impacts the clinical social work process. From a mental health perspective, religion and spirituality may shape how individuals view and relate to their psychological world and social environment. Comas-Diaz (1989), for example, has observed that for Hispanics, religion not only affects their conception of mental illness and treatment, but it also influences their health-seeking behaviors. In some instances, when a religious (denominational) value is placed on suffering and martyrdom (self-denial), certain Hispanics may opt not to seek mental health treatment (Acosta, Yamamoto, & Evans, 1982). As noted regarding *marianismo* and *machismo*, culturally sensitive practice principles (Harper & Lantz, 1996) prescribe open and co-constructed exploration of how a psychosocial problem can be approached in ways that are congruent with the client's cultural outlook.

Historically, Hispanics have self-identified themselves as Roman Catholics. However, conversion to Protestant sects/denominations is not an uncommon phenomenon within the Latino community. Currently, many Hispanics identify themselves as Pentecostal, Seventh-Day Adventists, or Evangelical. In addition to adhering to institutionally organized religious belief systems, some Hispanic may profess faith in ancestral spiritual practices such as *santería* (combined Yoruban–Catholic religious practice), *espíritismo* (spiritism), or *curanderismo* (rural folk medicine). The interpenetration of religious beliefs and self-definition or problem accessibility is the clinician's obligation to discern.

Hispanics have used religion and spirituality as survival mechanisms within the context of an often hostile social environment. For example, for many immigrants, religion has served as a buffer against the toxic emotional effects of entrance into the United States as unwelcome interlopers. Urrabazo (2000) has noted the curative potential of faith and religion in therapeutically assisting undocumented Hispanic immigrants who have been robbed, raped, and beaten while crossing the border into the United States. Religion appears to emotionally sustain Hispanics who are subjected to the realities of racism, discrimination, and social injustice on a continuous basis. During times of psychological crisis or environmental distress, the religious belief systems of Hispanics may be used as a complementary adjunct to conventional clinical social work practice. Clinicians must be cognizant of the fact that for many Hispanics the church provides an opportunity for mutual aid and social support. Urrabazo (2000), for example, has observed that the growth of storefront churches in urban Hispanic communities provides evidence for understanding the desire of many Hispanics to belong to a "healing community" where self-validation, connection to others, guidance, and social support may be found.

Because of the importance of religion and spirituality among individuals of Latin American and Caribbean descent, it is important to note that Hispanics do not dichotomize physical and emotional health or illness. Thus, the Hispanic culture tends to view health and psychological well-being from a more integrated or synergistic point of view. This view is expressed within a continuum that includes the body, mind, and *espíritu* (spirit). Therefore, many Hispanic folk concepts of disease etiology appear to be related to the ill effects of experiencing intensely negative emotional states, such as fright, anger, or envy (The National Alliance for Hispanic Health, 2001). Treatments for these cultural maladies, therefore, are based on a variety of sociospiritual rituals including purification, social integration, and—at times—penance (Kaiser Permanente Foundation,

2000). Hispanics may often consult *curanderos* (Mexican folk healers), *espíritistas* (spiritualists who are primarily Puerto Rican folk healers), or *santeros* (Cuban and/or Puerto Rican folk healers) in an attempt to seek symptom relief for physical and/or emotional complaints.

### Nervios: An Example of a Culturally Bound Physical and Emotional Syndrome

*Nervios* (nerves) refers to restlessness, insomnia, loss of appetite, headache, and nonspecific aches and pains (Kaiser Permanente Foundation, 2000; The National Alliance for Hispanic Health, 2001). *Nervios* is often linked to experiencing chronic, negative life circumstances particularly in the domain of interpersonal relationships. Thus, this culturally bound syndrome may be often noticed in individuals who are experiencing maladaptive patterns of interpersonal relationships and communication as well as high levels of social stress. Closely linked to *nervios* is *ataque de nervios* (nerve attacks), which is a seizurelike conversion syndrome characterized by mutism, hyperventilation, hyperkinesis, and uncommunicativeness (Guarnaccia, De la Cancela, & Carrillo, 1989; Lewis-Fernandez & Kleinman, 1994). *Ataque de nervios* may resemble a panic attack, but providers of mental healthcare should not confuse one with the other.

Folk healers (e.g., *curanderos*, *santeros*, or *espíritistas*) who are sought after for the treatment of the described culturally bound condition will often perform special religious/spiritual rituals using a variety of methods such as massage with special ointments, prayers, candles, herbal teas, baths, and invocations to specific Catholic saints or spirits. Adherence to the practice of folk healing is predicated on the cultural understanding that many Hispanics accept the possibility that illness and disease are linked to the supernatural world; therefore, spirits and witchcraft may cause or significantly contribute to psychological and physical distress. Illness and disease may also be linked to external environmental or internal (individual) factors such as bad air, excess cold and heat, germs, dust, fear, envy, and shame. Clinical efforts that are aimed at improving the psychological status of Hispanics in the United States must be based on an understanding that many Hispanics will probably conform to both a medical–biological model of help-seeking behavior and a spiritual model of symptom relief.

## ECOLOGICALLY INFORMED TREATMENT: STRATEGIES AND RECOMMENDATIONS

The ecological perspective with its emphasis on niche, adaptation, transactions, reciprocity and mutuality, and the goodness of fit between people and their environments is well suited for analyzing the lived experience of Hispanics. The life model (Germain & Gitterman, 1995; Gitterman & Germain, 2008), with its keen attention to social ecology, lifecycle development, and vertical and horizontal stressors, offers a practice approach that is able to account for the clinical challenges experienced by Hispanic clients in its assessment and intervention strategies. This is clearly demonstrated when the ecological perspective and the life model are deployed to understand the mental health and psychosocial needs of Hispanic individuals and families.

Informed by the science of ecology and ego psychology, the life model of social work practice views the human being as constantly adapting in an interchange with differential aspects of the social environment. Both the human being and the social environment react to each other and change within a transactional matrix (Gitterman & Germain, 2008). The person and the environment can be understood only in terms of their relationship, in which each continually influences the other within a particular context.

Gitterman (2009) has noted that throughout the life course people attempt to maintain a harmonious fit with their surrounding environments. This harmonious fit is usually achieved through a sense of self-efficacy—or when the individual feels positive and hopeful about his or her capacity to survive and thrive within multiple social contexts—and the environment's responsiveness to human need via provision of life-sustaining resources. Conversely, this noted harmonious fit may be seriously compromised when the individual lacks adaptive coping capacities or when such capacities have been placed at risk by psychosocial stress and toxic environmental conditions. Within the life model (Germain & Gitterman, 1980), stress is conceptualized as a psychosocial state spawned by inconsistencies between the human being's needs and capacities and environmental qualities. As a psychosocial condition, stress is the by-product of complex personal and environmental transactions.

A central tenet of life-modeled practice is that individuals will encounter stress or experience life stressors over the life course. From an ecological perspective, life stressors breed by complex and precarious life issues that human beings perceive as being greater than their coping capacities and environmental resources (Germain & Gitterman, 1995). According to the life model, stress or life stressors will arise or be manifested in the following three interrelated areas of living: life transitions and traumatic life events, environmental pressures, and dysfunctional interpersonal processes. Gitterman (1996) has underscored the fact that while these three life stressors are interrelated, each takes on its own "force" and "magnitude" and provides direction for multi-method (e.g., individual, family, group, and community practice) and integrative interventions with diverse client systems.

Intervention or treatment within the life model is informed by the historic purpose of the social work profession: to enhance the problem-solving and coping capacities of people, and to promote the effective and humane operation of systems that provide people with needed resources and services (Germain & Gitterman, 1980). While not prescriptive in nature, life-modeled practice recognizes that clinical practitioners require a broad repertoire of skills and techniques in addressing the needs of individuals and families who are overwhelmed by significant life stressors. These skills and techniques must be aimed at increasing a client's self-esteem and problem-solving and coping capacities; facilitating group functioning; and engaging and influencing organizational structures, social networks, and social environmental forces (Gitterman & Germain, 2008). Payne (2005) has noted the type of therapeutic and socioenvironmental skills or techniques that practitioners may employ when implementing a life model approach with identified clients. Some of these skills and techniques include: strengthening the client's motivation toward change, validation, support, management of emotionally laden content, modeling behavior, mobilization of environmental supports, case advocacy, mediation, and teaching problem-solving skills.

## Ego-Supportive Intervention

Consistent with the treatment principles of the ecological perspective and the life model, Comas-Diaz (1989) has stressed that regardless of the treatment approach/modality used with Hispanic clients, clinicians need to address the complex set of treatment expectations Hispanics have, which involve a multiplicity of psychological, physical, and environmental dimensions. Within the set of treatment expectations, clinical practitioners must effectively incorporate a client's individual worldview and the ethnocultural variables of language and religion (González, 2002). Le Vine and Padilla (cited in Padilla & Salgado De Snyder, 1985), for instance, have proposed a pluralistic counseling approach for the psychosocial treatment of Hispanics that encompasses these important variables. In describing the treatment approach they note:

> Pluralistic counseling is defined as a therapeutic intervention that recognizes and understands a client's culturally based beliefs, values, and behaviors. This approach encompasses the client's personal and family history as well as social characteristics and cultural orientation in order to evaluate all the ways in which culture affects the individual. The goal of pluralistic counseling is to help clients clarify their personal and cultural standards and to orient their behavior according to these standards. (p. 160)

Within this counseling approach, culture (which includes an individual's worldview, use of language, and belief systems) and environmental conditions prevail as the principal source for comprehending the client's psychosocial problems.

Because the psychosocial problems and needs of Hispanic clients are often exacerbated by socioeconomic stressors, racism, and political oppression, an ego-supportive therapeutic approach may also be effective in meeting the psychosocial needs of this population. According to Goldstein (1995, p. 168):

> Ego-supportive intervention focuses on the client's current behavior and on his conscious thought processes and feelings, although some selected exploration of the past may occur.... A here-and-now and reality-oriented focus identifies current stresses on the client; restores, maintains, and enhances the client's conflict-free areas of functioning, adaptive defenses, coping strategies, and problem-solving capacities; and mobilizes environmental support and resources.

Ego-supportive treatment stresses the empowerment of clients, and intervention within the social environment is promoted. In addition, the following practice principles, relevant to the lived experience of Hispanics in the United States, are endorsed: appreciating the impact of the sociopolitical context on the functioning of clients; balancing a focus on ethnic/cultural group membership and individualization of the client; enhancing client strengths; building self-confidence, self-esteem, and personal power; educating clients about options to problem resolution and maximizing choice; linking clients to needed resources; connecting clients to mutual aid groups and peer supports; and encouraging collective and political action (Goldstein, 1995). Ego-supportive treatment is carried out through the use of selected psychological and ecological techniques or strategies. These techniques or strategies include: support, ventilation, instillation of hope, use of structure, exploration, clarification, confrontation, education and advice, and environmental modification (Woods & Hollis, 2000).

## Social/Environmental Change Agent Role Model

Given that many Hispanic clients (especially new immigrants) often lack instrumental support from their U.S.-based extended families, many attempt to negotiate complex environmental conditions (e.g., employment, housing, medical care, learning English as a second language) with minimal appropriate guidance. Predicated on this notion, Atkinson, Thompson, and Grant (1993) developed a three-dimensional psychosocial intervention approach (social/environmental change agent role model) for the mental health treatment of ethnic–racial minority clients that recognizes the impact of the social environment in promoting or handicapping psychological growth and development. Within this treatment model, clinicians who treat Hispanic clients can function as agents of change or as consultants or advisors with the therapeutic aim of strengthening the identified client's support systems. Because the successful psychosocial treatment of Hispanics may also require case advocacy and home visits, both environmental manipulation and home-based treatment services are quite consistent with the tenets of this therapeutic approach.

Atkinson et al. (1993) recommend that the following three factors should be diagnostically assessed when treating an ethnic minority patient: (a) the client's level of acculturation, (b) the perceived cause and development of the presenting problem (internally caused versus externally environmentally caused), and (c) the specific goals to be attained in the treatment process. In implementing this treatment approach with Hispanic clients, clinicians should be prepared to extend their professional role of psychotherapist to that of advocate, mediator, and broker or resource consultant. As an advocate, the clinician targets his or her intervention at problems-in-living that are exacerbated by the dynamics of oppression, discrimination, and unequal access to community resources. In the role of a mediator, the clinician attempts to reduce the tension and conflict that may emerge between a client and a human service institution when psychosocial services are sought, but the delivery or nature of the services are inadequate or ineffective in meeting the needs of the client (Woods & Hollis, 2000). When treatment entails referring clients to community resources, the clinician assumes the role of a broker or resource consultant. In implementing this role, and consistent with the cultural value base of Hispanics, clinicians, at times, may need to refer clients to both indigenous support systems and indigenous systems of healing.

## Ecological–Structural Family Treatment

Hispanic families often experience psychosocial distress because of intergenerational and acculturation conflict. Because the locus of the family dysfunction is not only internal but also external in nature, ecological–structural family treatment is well suited for the amelioration of maladaptive family patterns that are often observed in Hispanic families that are attempting to cope with complex psychological and social issues. Predicated on the theoretical and clinical work of Aponte (1976) and Minuchin (1974), this family treatment approach highlights the stress of acculturation and its disruptive impact on the adaptive functioning of the Hispanic family. The approach draws attention to how normal family processes may interact with acculturation processes to create intergenerational differences that may exacerbate intrafamilial conflict.

Altarriba and Bauer (1997) note that when applying ecological–structural family treatment to Hispanic families an assessment of the interaction between the identified client or patient and their environment should be conducted early in the initial phase of treatment. The diagnostic assessment process should include an appraisal of the boundaries between and among family members, the strength of the relationships between and among family members, an understanding of the hierarchical and authority structure of the family, and an examination of any inherent contradictions in the request for service. Szapocznik et al. (1997) have empirically studied the value of ecological–structural family treatment in assisting Cuban families to address their interactional problems from both a content and a process level. At the content level, the cultural and intergenerational conflicts can be the focus of clinical attention. At the process level, the treatment approach aims to modify the breakdown in communication processes resulting from intensified cultural and intergenerational conflicts. The content and process distinction is crucial in treating Hispanic families who are attempting to cope with life transitional issues, maladaptive interpersonal interactions, environmental problems and needs, and adaptation to a host culture.

## CONCLUSION

To achieve and maintain an optimal degree of emotional equilibrium and social well-being, basic human needs, including a sense of usefulness, a sense of control over one's life, and healthy connections to others must be satisfied. In order to achieve this goal, culturally informed clinical practice must address the psychological needs of the individual while understanding how the social and cultural milieu informs the development and unfolding of the self. Because Hispanics represent one of the largest ethnically diverse groups in the United States, clinicians should be familiar with selected culturally sensitive treatment approaches that are appropriate in ameliorating psychosocial distress within this population. Culturally competent or culturally sensitive psychosocial treatment requires clinical skill, empathy, and an awareness of how cultural values, gender roles, and religion or spirituality impact the effective delivery of psychosocial services. This chapter has presented an overview of clinical practice with Hispanic individuals and families. Informed by the conceptual underpinnings of the ecological perspective and the life model of social work practice, the chapter has highlighted selected treatment approaches and strategies that may be used to address the transactions of individuals and families of Hispanic origin within the context of the social environment. The locus of problem etiology, the client's level of acculturation, and the goal of clinical intervention should always guide the culturally sensitive or culturally competent psychological and social treatment of Hispanic clients.

## REFERENCES

Acevedo, G. (2010). Latinas in the "public square": Understanding Hispanics through the prism of United States immigration policy. In J. H. Schiele (Ed.), *Social welfare policy: Regulation and resistance among people of color* (pp. 215–236). Thousand Oaks, CA: Sage Publications.

Acosta, F. X., Yamamoto, J., & Evans, L. A. (1982). *Effective psychotherapy for low-income and minority patients.* New York, NY: Plenum Press.

Altarriba, J., & Bauer, L. M. (1997).Counseling Cuban Americans. In D. R. Atkinson, G. Morten & D. W. Sue (Eds.), *Counseling American minorities* (pp. 280–296). New York, NY: McGraw-Hill.

Aponte, H. J. (1976). The family-school interview: An ecostructural approach. *Family Process, 15*(2), 303–311. doi:10.1111/j.1545-5300.1976.00303.x

Atkinson, D. R., Thompson, C. E., & Grant, S. K. (1993). A three-dimensional model for counseling racial/ethnic minorities. *The Counseling Psychologist, 21*(2), 257–277. doi:10.1177/0011000093212010

Comas-Diaz, L. (1989).Culturally relevant issues and treatment implications for Hispanics. In D. R. Koslow & E. P. Salett (Eds.), *Crossing cultures in mental health* (pp. 31–48). Washington, DC: SIETAR International.

Flores, A. (2017). *Facts on U.S. Latinos, 2015: Statistical portrait of Hispanics in the United States.* Washington, DC: Pew Research Center.

Flores, M. T., & Carey, G. (Eds.). (2000). *Family therapy with Hispanics: Toward appreciating diversity.* Boston, MA: Allyn and Bacon.

Fontenot, K., Semega, J., & Kollar, M. (2018). *Income and poverty in the United States: 2017.* Washington, DC: U.S. Census Bureau Current Population Reports.

Germain, C. B., & Gitterman, A. (1980). *The life model of social work practice.* New York, NY: Columbia University Press.

Germain, C. B., & Gitterman, A. (1995). Ecological perspective. In R. L. Edwards (Ed.), *Encyclopedia of social work* (19th ed., pp. 816–824). Silver Spring, MD: NASW Press.

Ghent, E. (1990). Masochism, submission, surrender—Masochism as a perversion of surrender. *Contemporary Psychoanalysis, 26,* 108–136. doi:10.1080/00107530.1990.10746643

Gil, R. M. (1980). *Cultural attitudes toward mental illness among Puerto Rican migrant women and their relationship to the utilization of outpatient mental health services.* Unpublished doctoral dissertation, Adelphi University, New York.

Gitterman, A. (1996). Life model theory and social work treatment. In F. J. Turner (Ed.), *Social work treatment: Interlocking theoretical perspectives* (4th ed., pp. 389–408). New York, NY: Free Press.

Gitterman, A. (2009). The life model. In A. R. Roberts (Ed.), *Social workers' desk reference* (2nd ed., pp. 231–234). New York, NY: Oxford University Press.

Gitterman, A., & Germain, C. B. (2008). *The life model of social work practice: Advances in theory and practice* (3rd ed.). New York, NY: Columbia University Press.

Goldstein, E. (1995). *Ego psychology and social work practice* (2nd ed.). New York, NY: Free Press.

González, M. J. (2002). Mental health intervention with Hispanic immigrants: Understanding the influence of the client's worldview, language, and religion. *Journal of Immigrant and Refugee Services, 1*(1): 81–92. doi:10.1300/J191v01n01_07

González, M. J., & González-Ramos, G. (Eds.). (2005). *Mental health care for new Hispanic immigrants: Innovations in contemporary clinical practice.* New York, NY: Haworth Press.

Guarnaccia, P. J., De la Cancela, V., & Carrillo, E. (1989). The multiple meanings of ataque de nervios in the Latino community. *Medical Anthropology, 11,* 47–62. doi:10.1080/01459740.1989.9965981

Harper, K. V., & Lantz, J. (1996). *Cross-cultural practice: Social work with diverse populations.* Chicago, IL: Lyceum Books.

Jordan, J. V. (2010). *Relational-cultural therapy.* Washington, DC: American Psychological Association.
Kaiser Permanente Foundation. (2000). *A provider's handbook on culturally competent care: Latino population.* Oakland, CA: Author.
Lewis-Fernandez, R., & Kleinman, A. (1994). Culture, personality and psychopathology. *Journal of Abnormal Psychology, 103*(1), 67–71. doi:10.1037/0021-843X.103.1.67
Minuchin, S. (1974). *Families and family therapy.* Cambridge, MA: Harvard University Press.
Padilla, A., & Salgado De Snyder, N. (1985). Counseling Hispanics: Strategies for effective intervention. In P. Pederson (Ed.), *Handbook for cross-counseling and therapy.* Westort, CT: Greenwood Press.
Payne, M. (2005). *Modern social work theory* (3rd ed.). Chicago, IL: Lyceum.
Sandoval, M. C., & De la Roza, M. (1986). A cultural perspective for serving the Hispanic client. In H. P. Lefley & P. B. Pedersen (Eds.), *Cross-cultural training for mental health professionals* (pp. 151–181). Springfield, IL: Charles C. Thomas.
Santiago-Rivera, A. L., Arredondo, P., & Gallardo-Cooper, M. (2002). *Counseling Latinos and la familia: A practical guide.* Thousand Oaks, CA: Sage.
Stepler, R., & Brown, A. (2016). *2014, Hispanics in the United States Statistical Portrait.* Washington, DC: Pew Hispanic Center.
Sue, D. W., & Sue, D. (1999). *Counseling the culturally different: Theory and practice.* New York, NY: John Wiley.
Szapocznik, J., Kurtines, W., Santisteban, D. A., Pantin, H., Scopetta, M., Mancilla, Y., . . . Coatsworth, J. D. (1997). The evolution of structural ecosystemic theory for working with Latino families. In J. Garcia & M. C. Zea, (Eds.), *Psychological interventions and research with Latino populations* (pp. 166–190). Boston, MA: Allyn and Bacon.
Taylor, O. (1989). The effects of cultural assumptions on cross-cultural communication. In D. R. Koslow & E. P. Salett (Eds.), *Crossing cultures in mental health* (pp. 18–30). Washington, DC: SIETAR International.
The National Alliance for Hispanic Health. (2001). *A primer for cultural proficiency: Towards quality health services for Hispanics.* Washington, DC: Estrella Press.
Torres-Saillant, S. (2002). Problematic paradigms: Racial diversity and corporate identity in the Latino community. In M. M. Suárez-Orozco & M. M. Páez (Eds.), *Latinos remaking America* (pp. 435–455). Berkeley, CA: University of California Press.
Urrabazo, R. (2000). Therapeutic sensitivity to the Latino spiritual soul. In M. T. Flores & G. Carey (Eds.), *Family therapy with Hispanics: Toward appreciating diversity* (pp. 205–227). Boston, MA: Allyn and Bacon.
U.S. Census Bureau. (2018). *Hispanic heritage month 2018.* Washington, DC: Author.
Woods, M., & Hollis, F. (2000). *Casework: A psychosocial therapy* (5th ed.). New York, NY: McGraw-Hill.

# 13

# Practice With Asian Immigrant Families and Intergenerational Issues

GRACE S. KIM AND JULIE M. AHNALLEN

## ASIANS IN THE UNITED STATES: DIVERSITY AND HISTORY

The history of Asians in the United States goes back to 1763, with the first arrival of the sailors from the Philippines in New Orleans (Chan, 1991). Since then, there have been various waves of immigration from many Asian countries, starting with India (1790) and China (1830). Immigration from Asia has been affected by employment opportunities (e.g., sugar plantations in Hawaii and railroads in California) and U.S. policies, ranging from exclusionary policies such as the Chinese Exclusion Act (1882), quota systems, and the 1965 immigration reform that eliminated the quota system and focused on immigration of highly skilled workers. World events such as wars and political conflicts have also influenced the migration from Asia (Chan, 1991). Currently, Asians in the United States are one of the fastest growing populations, indicating 72% growth from 2000 to 2015, and it is estimated that eventually this group will be the "nation's largest immigrant group" (López, Ruiz, & Patten, 2017). According to 2016 data, the estimated number of Asian alone-or-in-any combination (i.e., monoracial Asian and multiracial Asian) populations in the United States was 21.4 million (U.S. Census Bureau, 2018). Ethnically, Chinese (Chinese alone-or-in-any combination) were the largest detailed group (4.9 million), followed by Asian Indian (4.1 million), Filipino (3.9 million), Vietnamese (2.1 million), Korean (1.8 million), and Japanese (1.5 million) (U.S. Census Bureau, 2018).

Asian immigrant experiences are vastly diverse and intersectional, depending on the specific family's immigration/migration history, pre-immigration experiences, social class, generational and acculturation status, post-migration experiences, racial and ethnic identities, religious and linguistic traditions, legal status, and social identities (e.g., gender, sexual orientation). In general, as an aggregated group, Asians in the United States tend to have a relatively high income level. However, a closer look at the data illustrates a bimodal distribution of socialeconomic status (SES) variables, with significant variations among different ethnic groups. The Asian immigrant populations with the longest history in the United States (e.g., East and South Asians) tend to fair well, whereas refugees continue to experience economic hardships and poverty (e.g., Southeast Asian populations; López et al., 2017). Because past historical trauma, social class, post-migration stress, and English language proficiency tend to intersect, particular ethnic groups may face continued and ongoing stress more than other ethnic groups. Further, legal statuses should also be taken into consideration in working with Asian immigrant families. In 2015, undocumented immigrants from Asian countries comprised about 13% of the 11 million undocumented immigrants in the United States (López et al., 2017).

## Common Cultural Values and Psychosocial Experiences Among Asian Immigrants

In this section, we discuss cultural aspects that are often shared by Asian immigrant families, while acknowledging that the degree to which such cultural values are shared may vary within the population. Hence, practitioners are encouraged to assess and explore the specific contexts of each family. We note that while we focus our discussions on Asian immigrants, we also use the terminology Asian Americans to refer to Asians in the United States broadly (i.e., immigrants from Asia or children of immigrants who reside in the United States; Liu, Murakami, Eap, & Nagayama, 2009). We chose to use both terminologies in order to capture the experiences of families that may include both immigrants and their family members (e.g., their children) who were born and raised in the United States.

### Collectivism and Interdependent Self-Construal

Cultural and religious influences, such as those of Confucianism and Buddhism, affect values of collectivism and interdependent sense of self in Asian American families (Park & Kim, 2008). Interdependent self-construal is highly contextual, and people are encouraged to be attentive to group interests over individual interests. This may mean conforming to the group norms, seeking harmony within the group, and being sensitive to others' needs (Markus & Kitayama, 1991). Interdependent self-construal is often in contrast with what is common among the White European American (WEA) view of self, characterized by individualism and independent self-construal. Independent self-construal focuses on being a distinct individual, in which sense of self is largely individually constructed with an emphasis on autonomy. While others may be important in one's sense of self, they are not integral in their identity as a unique person (Markus & Kitayama, 1991). Phrases such as "Think for yourself," "Be your own person," or "Don't follow the crowd" are characteristic of individualism and independent self-construal.

## Communication Styles

Interdependent self-construal impacts how Asian American families communicate with each other, and the language and communication styles, in turn, reinforce collectivism. In general, Asian American communication styles are highly context-dependent and relational, less direct, and highly nuanced. Asian American families tend to be multigenerational and have hierarchical structures (Cheung & Jahn, 2017), and language is utilized to foster harmony within this structure. Different linguistic codes are used to speak to elders (e.g., honorifics and polite forms), peers, or to children (e.g., plain forms; Park & Kim, 2008). Silence may be valued as a signifier of thoughtfulness and having better control of oneself (Kim, 2002). The high context communication styles relate to collectivism in that one attempts to provide what others may need by reading contextual cues, even when needs are not overtly spoken out loud. The ability to be sensitive to others indicates one's closeness to them. Actions are considered more important in verbally expressing care and affection, and hence, direct expression of feelings may not be seen often. This is in contrast to the low context communication, which tends to be more direct, straightforward, and, at times, lacking in nuances, found more in European American cultures. Stating what one really thinks/feels in a direct way is valued in the low-context communication styles (Park & Kim, 2008). In counseling Asian American families, it would be important to observe communication styles among family members, as they may relate to levels of acculturation or cultural self-construals. Different communication styles could cause or exacerbate intergenerational family conflicts. Also, clinicians should self-assess their own communication styles, and consider how they might be experienced by Asian American clients.

## ACCULTURATION AND INTERGENERATIONAL FAMILY CONFLICTS IN ASIAN IMMIGRANT FAMILIES

Acculturation, the process of change and adjustment when two or more cultures come in contact with each other (Berry, 1997), is a common experience that Asian American families experience upon migrating to the United States. Acculturative stress, the psychological and social stress that comes with needing to adjust to cultural norms and values that are incongruent with the person's home culture, could greatly impact family dynamics. Acculturative stress can be triggered by experiences of discrimination, language barriers, downward social mobility, feelings of inferiority, and general feelings of otherness (Berry, 1997), and psychological distress can result from acculturative stress (Crockett et al., 2007).

Research suggests intergenerational differences in levels of acculturation (Cheung & Jahn, 2017). This differential rate of acculturation can mean disruption of typical family dynamics. Immigrant parents who may have typically been in the role of authority figures may lack cultural knowledge and language proficiency in the new country. They may end up relying on children to be the cultural brokers, needing help with navigating unfamiliar systems, such as schools, healthcare, and governmental agencies. Both immigrant parents and children may experience this shift as a "loss," in that parents lose the parental role of being the knower and supportive figures who can provide guidance, while the children lose their sense of security that comes with trusting that parents can navigate the world around them.

## Challenges and Complexities of Parentification

The shift in roles between parents and children can lead to parentification, where children are asked to attend to tasks or perform duties beyond their developmentally appropriate responsibilities (Mechling, 2011). Parentified children tend to prioritize the needs of the family over their own needs. Some children may take on these responsibilities during the family's acculturation process as a way to develop close relationships with parents and avoid feelings of loss and anxiety (Barnett & Parker, 1998). Parentification in Asian American families can be perceived as dysfunctional or lacking in appropriate boundaries. Considering the distinction between instrumental and emotional parentification (Hooper, 2007), however, provides a framework for better understanding different types and their impact. Instrumental parentification refers to parentification of children through functional responsibilities where children take on the everyday tasks to run the household such as cooking, shopping, cleaning, and caretaking siblings. Instrumental parentification, when paired with parental support and acknowledgment, can provide opportunities for growth in sense of accomplishment and competence (Aldridge, 2006). In contrast, emotional parentification assigns children to meet the emotional and psychological needs of a parent, being the confidante and emotional support in moments of crisis, often at the neglect of their own developmental needs (Hooper, 2007). This kind of parentification is associated with negative mental health outcomes in adulthood, including symptoms of anxiety and depression (Earley & Cushway, 2002).

## Conflict Over Parenting Styles

Parenting styles could be a major area of intergenerational conflict. In discussing Asian American parenting styles, there are a few overarching aspects to keep in mind. First, because of acculturation, Asian American parenting styles may be in the process of changing from those of Asian families in Asia. Second, parenting styles may also be influenced by acculturative stress and other intersecting life stressors, such as undocumented legal status, poverty, language barriers, or access to cultural capital (e.g., existence or connection with Asian immigrant communities in the area).

In general, Asian American parenting styles focus more on providing instrumental love and affection to their children (e.g., doing things for their children) than giving verbal expressions of affection (e.g., saying "I love you"). Russell, Chu, Crockett, and Doan (2010) explored the meaning of parent–adolescent relationship quality among Chinese American and Filipino American adolescents in northern California through focus groups with adolescents. They noted that the meaning of "good parenting" differed in Asian American and WEA parents. While the WEA parents noted warmth, affection, responsiveness, involvement, and firmness as factors that make for "good parents," Asian American parents' notion of good parents were those who "provide, sacrifice for, nurture, and monitor adolescents' activities" (Russell et al., 2010). Much of the monitoring may be seen as the parents' role to provide life instructions to their children, with the hope that when successful, children would internalize what they learned from their parents and make wise decisions themselves.

Different ideas about parental monitoring and control can contribute to intergenerational family conflicts. Much of stereotypes about Asian American parents rely on the notion of "overly involved" or "highly demanding" parents who are relentless in controlling their children's activities and pushing them for academic excellence. The notion of "tiger parenting," which has been popularized in recent years, further adds to this stereotype. According to Chua (2011), tiger parents push their children toward success with intensity because, as parents, they believe they know what is best for their children and parents can override children's preferences (e.g., pushing children to not give up on tasks prematurely when the tasks become difficult).

Empirical studies, however, have debunked the notion that tiger parenting is common or effective. Kim, Wang, Orozco-Lapray, Shen, and Murtuza (2013) examined parenting styles and adolescents' developmental outcomes through a three-wave longitudinal investigation with 444 Chinese American families. They noted four distinctive parenting styles: supportive, tiger, easygoing, and harsh. They found that the most common was the supportive parenting style, which was correlated with positive adolescent adjustment and outcomes (i.e., higher GPA, education attainment, low academic pressure, low depression, and strong family obligation), in comparison to the other three parenting styles. Adolescent adjustment was the best for the supportive parenting style, followed by easygoing, tiger, and harsh parenting styles. Results illustrated that while the tiger parenting style does exist, it is not the most common form of parenting, and this parenting style is not correlated with positive psychological adjustment and high academic achievement in adolescents (Kim et al., 2013). In other studies, SES and having cultural capital from the ethnic communities were found to contribute to the achievement of Asian American children, rather than the tiger parenting style (Lee & Zhou, 2014). Furthermore, research suggests that parenting styles are not fixed. In their study with 50 Chinese immigrant mothers with young children in the United States, Chea, Leong, and Zhou (2013) noted that Chinese American parents negotiated between the parenting styles of both Chinese and mainstream U.S. cultures, as they acculturated in the United States. Most mothers were able to note the different parenting styles and discussed attempting to find more balanced parenting goals and practices of both Chinese and U.S. cultures (Chea et al., 2013).

## Conflict Over Issues of Separation and Individuation

Issues of separation and individuation are another salient aspect that may result in family conflict. Separation and individuation from parents is a developmental milestone that is highly valued and expected within the WEA cultures that emphasize independence. In contrast, this process is more complex for Asian Americans, given the value of familial interdependence even when there is physical separateness (Shon & Ja, 1982). Due to interdependent self-construal, many Asian parents see their children as extensions of themselves, rather than a separate entity outside the family. Individual accomplishments and failures are reflections of the family system, and there is a shared ownership and participation in each other's lives, which from a WEA view can seem intrusive and lacking boundaries. Asian American children may be expected to stay closely connected to their families, and may have responsibilities to fulfill for the family, such as aiding with monetary contribution, taking care of younger siblings, and serving as the family interpreters. Asian American adolescents and young adults may find themselves in conflict with their desire to be independent while attending to the needs of the family. The normalization of the dominant culture's notion of "you are an independent adult when you turn 18" may feel like a mismatch from the familial role and expectations of Asian American families. For example, many Asian and Asian American college students choose to attend college closer to home or travel home frequently to attend to family needs.

## CHALLENGES IN WORKING WITH ASIAN AMERICAN FAMILIES

There are unique complexities and challenges in working with Asian American families. They relate to the cultural attitudes about mental health and low rates of help seeking, and systemic issues such as limited access to mental healthcare, experiences of racism and discrimination faced by the population, and distrust in healthcare professionals.

### Low Rates of Help-Seeking for Mental Healthcare

The low rates of help-seeking for Asian American populations for mental health issues are particularly notable (Sue, Cheng, Saad, & Chu, 2012). Because therapy is often seen as the last-resort effort, by the time Asian American families seek therapy, they tend to report severe problems. Abe-Kim et al. (2002) reported generational differences for help-seeking, with the first-generation or second-generation Asian Americans seeking mental health support at lower rates (30.4% and 28.8%, respectively) than those of third- or higher generation Asian Americans (62.6%). Culturally, Asian Americans tend to view physical health and mental health as interconnected. Somatization of symptoms is common, and so is seeking medical professionals for conditions many in the United States would consider mental health issues, such as depression. In addition, there may be a cultural emphasis of pressing on even when one is not "happy," because life is understood to be challenging. This stance encourages people to persevere in the face of hardship (e.g., *Gaman*, the Japanese term for perseverance in hardship is a good example) (Herreria, 2019), and may result in overlooking mental health concerns. Further, the cultural perception about ideology of mental illnesses may be different from the mainstream U.S. cultures; for example, there may be belief that depressive symptoms of low motivation and isolation are caused by personality defect or personal weakness. If there is a recognition of psychological distress, it tends to be categorized as severe mental illness, and hence seeking therapy may carry stigma among Asian American populations (e.g., seen as being weak, "crazy," or severely ill).

## Systemic Issues: Access to Mental Healthcare and Experiences of Discrimination

Systemic issues related to mental healthcare access and disparity, and issues related to discrimination and distrust contribute to challenges in working with Asian American families. Recent Asian immigrants may not have a clear understanding of how to seek therapy, utilize medical insurance, and what the goals of therapy might be, other than to solve immediate problems. The Western notion of problem-solving through "talk therapy" may not be culturally congruent with many Asian American families, and doing so with a stranger may seem even more peculiar. Further, due to the limited number of Asian American mental health clinicians (e.g., only 5% of psychologists in the U.S. workforce in 2015 were Asian Americans, whereas 86% were White) (Lin, Stamm, & Christidis, 2018) and bilingual services, needs of many Asian American families are not met in the mental health system. These access issues are compounded for individuals who are poor, are not proficient in English, undocumented, or do not have many community resources. In addition, Asian Americans' experience of racism and discrimination often go unnoticed due to the model minority myth; yet, both overt racism and everyday racial microaggressions are common (Chou & Feagin, 2010). Some ethnic or religious group members (e.g., Muslim immigrants) may face further discrimination, and feelings of loss and fear could lead to depressive symptoms (Akram-Pall & Moodley, 2016). Similarly, Asian American families who have undocumented status are especially reluctant to seek support from schools, clinics, and governmental agencies, for fear of deportation or other legal ramifications (Ling, Okazaki, Tu, & Kim, 2014).

## CULTURALLY RESPONSIVE INTERVENTIONS

Empathic understanding for the clients and their family, strategic intervention planning, and thoughtful self-understanding of therapists are crucial for culturally responsive interventions. Clinicians should be attuned to Asian American clients' developmental and family history, and how their sociocultural contexts have shaped both their adaptive and maladaptive thoughts and behaviors. Therefore, culturally responsive clinicians need to pay attention to the family system and provide collaborative strategic plans that can empower the whole family. Clinicians may need to serve as a cultural broker without undermining the functional and culturally relevant system that is already in place. This requires clinicians to practice cultural humility and deep self-reflection of their own biases, assumptions, and counter-transference.

### Bringing Empathy: Holistic View of Asian American Values and Parenting Styles

Effective work with Asian American families requires building strong rapport with all members. Understanding Asian American parents in relation to their parenting styles may feel challenging due to cultural values that may not be shared with the clinicians. We suggest the clinicians to consider and explore their clients' contexts about the immigration/migration to the United States, and what this decision has meant for them. Often, immigrant experiences encompass various losses. They could include loss of community, connections to the country of origin, proficiency in one's ability to communicate freely, and downward social mobility, which requires an immigrant to reframe one's vocational identities and lower social status in the new context. Immigrants who settle in areas where their ethnic communities do not exist or they are the only Asians or racial minority may experience another layer of losses. Refugees or immigrants who have experienced trauma of war or political conflict may experience yet another layer of deep losses. Nuanced and complex understanding of these losses are significant, as they impact how Asian immigrant parents understand and make meaning about their parenting (e.g., that they are willing to be strong through the challenges or "make sacrifices" for a better future of their children). Furthermore, because many Asian immigrant parents have not attended schools in the United States, they are not aware of how U.S. school systems operate, what issues are pertinent among youths, and how Asian Americans are perceived racially and culturally. Often the connections with teachers and staff at the school systems rely on active parental involvement. For many Asian immigrant families, especially among working-class families, attending school functions may not only be impossible given their long work hours, and could be challenging if there are language barriers. With limited knowledge and access to resources, Asian immigrant parents obtain information from other immigrant parents, who have similar immigration histories or cultural values about parent–child relationships (Lee & Zhou, 2014).

When there are intergenerational conflicts, Asian immigrant parents may experience these as another layer of loss and sadness. The emphasis on education seen in many Asian American parents may relate to the belief that education may be the only way through which the immigrant parents could foresee an improved future for their children, without their experiencing acculturative stress or downward social mobility that the parents experienced. However, because these rationales are not communicated and/or are communicated in a way that is felt as pressure for children of immigrants, intergenerational conflict could arise. The difficult decisions immigrant parents have had to make and the challenges they overcame, in spite of the significant losses, could be seen as a strength. Empathizing with parents could enable them to have a better relationship with their children by becoming more flexible.

### Bringing Allyship: Strategic Interventions and Relationships

Working with Asian immigrant families provides clinicians crucial opportunities to serve as cultural brokers and allies for both Asian immigrant parents and their children. Cultural brokerage refers to "bridging, linking to mediating between groups or persons from different cultures" (Lo, 2010, p. 487). In order to help bridge the gap between the different cultural orientation between clinicians and clients, clinicians need to engage in cultural translation in order to integrate and operate from the client's perspective. This also means developing trust and rapport, establishing positive long-term relationships, and utilizing the already existing supportive networks of the Asian American families (Lo, 2010). The task of cultural brokerage requires cultural labor on the part of the clinician in terms of time and learning, in order to meet the specific needs of the families. Becoming familiar about the vast diversity within Asian American groups, ethnic group differences, political histories, and referent groups in determining whether a behavior is typical, in comparison to whom, is crucial. Without the cultural labor from the clinician in determining referent group and cultural norms, it would be impossible to fully assess and treat families without pathologizing.

Moreover, clinicians could become allies for their clients (Case, 2015). Allies are members of privileged groups in various areas who take action to "dismantle any form of oppression from which they might benefit" and they work to "create equality consistently and intentionally" (Ayvazian, 1995, p. 7). Clinicians who have knowledge of and access to the U.S. cultures, societal structures, English language proficiency, U.S. citizenship, for instance, could use their privileges to support Asian immigrant families through providing psychoeducation about different concepts of mental health, societal norms, and legal aspects in the United States without pathologizing clients' experiences or belief systems. Further, a number of clinical approaches might be helpful to consider in working collaboratively with Asian American families. Solution-Focused Brief Therapy (SFBT) aims to foster conversations that lead to feasible and observable solutions for all family members, through the use of questions (Cheung & Jahn, 2017). Cultural adaptation of various therapy methods, such as culturally sensitive cognitive behavioral therapy that are adapted to utilize a cultural framework or technique that works well with the Asian American context (e.g., focus on mindfulness or cultural values), may also be effective intervention strategies (Sue et al., 2012).

### Bringing Cultural Humility: Clinician Self-Reflection and Use of Self

Grounding on the concept of cultural humility, clinicians should center their interpersonal stance around aspects of cultural identities most important to the client. Tervalon and Murray-Garcia (1998) outlined three major aspects of cultural humility: (a) lifelong commitment to self-evaluation and self-critique; (b) desire to fix power imbalances; and (c) develop partnerships with others to advocate for positive change. The first aspect of cultural humility speaks to the unending journey of learning and self-evaluation that is crucial to engaging with clients from a humble stance of a learner rather than a teacher or expert. In working with Asian American families, this stance allows the clinician to work with ongoing curiosity and exploration, inviting the families to share their experiences from their own cultural viewpoint. It also provides the important collaboration between families and clinician to brainstorm possible interventions without prescribing a solution that may be incongruent to the family's value system. For many Asian American parents who have experiences of being undermined or evaluated by various systems, working collaboratively with clinicians who are willing to acknowledge what they do not know and are engaged in learning more about the family can be powerful. Clinicians should also self-reflect their awareness of stereotypes and assumptions about Asian Americans in the society in general, and potential unconscious biases in the clinician themselves, in particular.

The second aspect of cultural humility involves correcting the imbalance of power. This involves recognizing that clients too have something unique to bring to the table and contribute to their own healing process. It reminds clinicians that clients are the experts in their own lives and hold power in their personal narratives and experiences. In working with Asian American families, this frame allows for families to fully share their rich and complex histories of pain as well as resiliency without fearing judgment from an authority or evaluative figure. If the clinician holds more power and privilege than the Asian American client, the clinician's responsibility is to name the difference and strive to equalize power differentials through self-reflection and conversation with the client.

Lastly, making connections to organizations and communities focused on social justice and advocacy work is an important part of cultural humility. When working with Asian American families, clinicians are often helping clients navigate issues around immigration, language and cultural barriers, discriminatory policies, and lack of appropriate support for housing or jobs. Connecting with community organizations enables clinicians to not only advocate for their own clients but also engage in activities that can have larger systemic impact.

## CASE VIGNETTE

The following case vignette hopes to highlight the ways in which holistic understanding of Asian American families, allyship that is grounded in shared and collaborative understanding of the cultural context, and cultural humility of the therapist can have meaningful impact on the process of therapy. Details of the case are representative narratives from various Asian American clients at a college counseling center setting.

Hye Jin is a 20-year-old, female, heterosexual, cisgender, first-generation Korean American college student from a working class family in New York City. She reported growing up in a religious Protestant family. She presented at a university counseling center with symptoms of depression and anxiety in the context of ongoing family conflicts. During the intake, she shared her ambivalence about therapy, noting that her previous therapy experience a year ago was not helpful. As we gathered developmental and family history, it became clear that Hye Jin played a particular role within her family. The intersection of her identities as the oldest daughter of a working class immigrant family placed her in a parentified role as her parents struggled to run a small business while negotiating an unfamiliar culture and language. Hye Jin grew up taking care of her younger sister, doing household chores, being the identified family translator, and helping out at her parents' business on the weekends. She reported that her parents also had high expectations when it came to education, often reminding her that her academic success is a reflection of the whole family's success and sacrifice. She felt that while her parents were supportive of her, sometimes it was difficult to "feel [their support]" given their lack of verbal or physical affirmation and affection.

When leaving for college, Hye Jin felt excited, relieved, and guilty. Adjusting to college was more difficult than she had expected. She experienced "culture shock" when she saw the socioeconomic privilege of her peers and felt lost being a first-generation college student, who had no family support in navigating the college experience. She started to feel depressed and anxious, not knowing how and to whom to ask for help as she struggled academically and socially. When she called home, she pretended that everything was fine and focused her energy on being the caretaker of her family, a role that felt familiar to her.

Hye Jin finally decided to seek treatment, at the urging of a good friend, and met with a White female therapist who attributed her struggle to her "unhealthy connection" to her family. She explained that the goal of her last therapy was on separating from her parents and becoming an independent adult, but the more she tried to separate from her family, the more depressed she felt. It increased tension with her parents, who could not understand why Hye Jin was distancing from them. Hye Jin reported that she spent most of last year feeling angry and resentful, then feeling guilty for feeling that way, which led to a cycle of helplessness and hopefulness. She explained how adjustment to college made her feel alone, and the growing tension and separation from family took away the grounding she needed to survive in college.

I observed and noted that Hye Jin's previous treatment made the assumption that in order for Hye Jin to fully adjust to college and be healthy, she needed to separate and disconnect from "intrusive and unhealthy parents." We discussed how this felt like an impossible task for Hye Jin as connection to family and being an integral part of her family's functioning was an important part of her identity that she did not want to lose. We also brought more curiosity into what contributed to the idea of parents being seen as intrusive and unhealthy and found that Hye Jin actually had strong reactions to this notion. She reported that she often felt as though she had to defend her parents in her previous therapy as the therapist seemed horrified by some of Hye Jin's childhood accounts, despite it being culturally normative (e.g., parents having a strong say in what she wants to major in, and not trusting mental health clinicians but encouraging prayer as a method of healing psychological distress). Hye Jin acknowledged holding complex feelings toward her parents, but she found it difficult to discuss her true feelings in her previous therapy, due to the fear that the therapist would pathologize her parents and her experiences.

Our treatment centered on dismantling the idea of having to choose family or independence and moving toward integration, holding the multiple parts of herself that felt pulled in different ways. We identified and normalized Hye Jin's core conflict of wanting to be a "good" daughter to her parents and meeting their expectations, while at the same time recognizing her desire to be her own person with particular passions and needs. Hye Jin noted that the ongoing internal conflict left her feeling helpless and hopeless because she had a hard time imagining how she would be able to have both. The initial work involved creating a safe space for her to bring in both anger as well as gratitude toward her parents. Being aware of the importance of family loyalty, protectiveness that children feel toward immigrant parents, and cultural norm of deference and respect for parents in Asian American families, I modeled curiosity without blaming the parents, and joined Hye Jin in her feelings of gratitude and pain around her parents' immigration experience. This allowed Hye Jin to explore negative feelings without worrying about my judgment. It was important for Hye Jin to feel that her parents were being honored and respected, even when discussing negative feelings toward them. Conversations regarding her parents' experiences and Hye Jin's adult understanding of their struggles that she may not have been able to fully comprehend as a child allowed for greater empathy and compassion, not only toward her parents but also toward her younger self.

When discussing the tension around separation and individuation, it was extremely helpful to consider the WEA normative script on this process and how it did not fit her experience. We used Hye Jin's interest in sociology to contextualize her experiences and understand her conflicts through the lens of Western norms on parenting and expectations about separation and individuation, as well as stereotypes regarding Asian parents and immigrant families. This allowed us to broaden the conceptualization of her internal conflict to tensions between cultural expectations for someone who grew up bicultural. We discussed the unrealistic task of Hye Jin, an Asian American oldest daughter of immigrant parents, having a life fully independent from her family. We also explored ways to incorporate cultural practices familiar to her and her family as a way to work toward symptom reduction, such as mindfulness practices that centered on prayer, incorporating imagery congruent to her cultural experience via relaxation exercises. We practiced strategies for improving communication with parents that reflected high-context and indirect style of communication.

Our work focused on empowering Hye Jin to grapple with what an independent and connected self within her cultural context would look like. For her, this meant seeking out mentors, giving voice to her own experience, and having more direct communication with her parents about her needs, despite her concern about burdening them. We discussed how she had kept a huge part of herself hidden from others, including her parents, in her attempt to compartmentalize home and college. This added to her overall sense of not being seen or understood. Treatment aimed to build stronger relationships and healthy boundaries that allowed her to integrate and hold all parts of herself and her needs. By explicitly discussing our relationships and issues of representation, identification, expectation, and power, therapy served as a place of exploration, modeling, and practice for new behaviors. We also noted our own identities as two Asian American women, which required us to assess our assumptions and wishes for each other, and be clear about points of connection as well as differences.

## DISCUSSION QUESTIONS

1. In Hye Jin's first therapy experience, what assumptions were made about her separation and individuation process? What were some negative consequences for the client, family, and therapist?
2. How does intersectionality of Hye Jin's various identities impact her clinical presentation and intervention?
3. What are the ways in which clinicians can contribute to pathologizing Asian American families? Can you locate examples from the case?
4. What are the ways in which this case illustrates the therapist as a cultural broker and an ally to the client and her family?

## REFERENCES

Abe-Kim, J., Takeuchi, D., & Hwang, W. C. (2002). Predictors of help seeking for emotional distress among Chinese Americans: Family matters. *Journal of Consulting and Clinical Psychology, 70*, 1186–1190. doi:10.1037/0022-006X.70.5.1186

Akram-Pall, S., & Moodley, R. (2016). "Loss and fear": Acculturation stresses leading to depression in South Asian Muslim immigrants in Toronto. *Canadian Journal of Counselling and Psychotherapy, 50*, (3-S), S137–S155.

Aldridge, J. (2006). The experiences of children living with and caring for parents with mental illness. *Child Abuse Review, 15*, 79–88. doi:10.1002.car.904

Ayvazian, A. (1995). Interrupting the cycle of oppression: The role of allies as agents of change. *Fellowship, January/February*, 7–10.

Barnett, B., & Parker, G. (1998). The parentified child: Early competence or childhood deprivation? *Child Psychology and Psychiatry Review, 3*, 146–155. doi:10.1111/1475-3588.00234

Berry, J. W. (1997). Immigration, acculturation, and adaptation. *Applied Psychology, 46*, 5–34. doi:10.1111/j.1464-0597.1997.tb01087.x

Case, K. A. (2015). White practitioners in therapeutic ally-ance: An intersectional privilege awareness training model. *Women & Therapy, 38*, 3–4, 263–278. doi:10.1080/02703149.2015.1059209

Chan, S. (1991). *Asian Americans: An interpretive history*. Boston, MA: Twayne Publishers.

Chea, C. S. L., Leong, C. Y. Y., & Zhou, N. (2013). Understanding "tiger parenting" through the perceptions of Chinese immigrant mothers: Can Chinese and U.S. parenting coexist? *Asian American Journal of Psychology, 4*(1), 30–40. doi:10.1037/a0031217

Cheung, C. W., & Jahn, S. A. B. (2017). Closing the acculturation gap: A solution-focused approach with East Asian American families. *The Family Journal, 25*(2), 170–178. doi:10.1177/1066480717697686

Chou, R. S., & Feagin, J. R. (2010). *The myth of the model minority: Asian Americans facing racism*. Boulder, CO: Paradigm Publishers.

Chua, A. (January, 8, 2011). Why Chinese mothers are superior. *The Wall Street Journal*. Retrieved from https://www.wsj.com/articles/SB10001424052748704111504576059713528698754

Crockett, L. J., Iturbide, M. I., Torres Stone, R. A., McGinley, M., Raffaelli, M., & Carlo, G. (2007). Acculturative stress, social support, and coping: Relations to psychological adjustment among Mexican American college students. *Cultural Diversity and Ethnic Minority Psychology, 13*, 347–355. doi:10.1037/1099-9809.13.4.347

Earley, L., & Cushway, D. (2002). The parentified child. *Clinical Child Psychology and Psychiatry, 7*, 163–178. doi:10.1177/1359104502007002005

Herreria, C. (May 25, 2019). *Why Asian Americans struggle to seek therapy*. Retrieved from https://www.huffpost.com/entry/asian-american-seek-therapy_n_5ce7632ae4b05c15dea9cbe0?ncid=fcbklnkushpmg00000098&fbclid=IwAR1yuGCeE_LrrW5ruO72283Nx55umZ7ZzMXKtOmbBe0uj8-47OJ0tbfvbwQ

Hooper, L. M. (2007). The application of attachment theory and family systems theory to the phenomena of parentification. *The Family Journal: Counseling and Therapy for Couples and Families, 15*, 217–233. doi:10.1177/1066480707301290

Kim, H. J. (2002). We talk, therefore we think? A cultural analysis of the effect of talking on thinking. *Journal of Personality and Social Psychology, 83*(4), 828–842. doi:10.1037/0022-3514.83.4.828

Kim, S. Y., Wang, Y., Orozco-Lapray, D., Shen, Y., & Murtuza, M. (2013). Does "tiger parenting" exist? Parenting profiles of Chinese Americans and adolescent developmental outcomes. *Asian American Journal of Psychology, 4*(1), 7–18. doi:10.1037/a0030612

Lee, J., & Zhou, M. (2014). The success frame and achievement paradox: The costs and consequences for Asian Americans. *Race and Social Problems, 6*(1), 38–55. doi:10.1007/s12552-014-9112-7

Lin, L., Stamm, K., & Christidis, P. (2018). *How diverse is the psychology workforce?: News from APA's Center for Workforce Studies*. Retrieved from https://www.apa.org/monitor/2018/02/datapoint

Ling, A., Okazaki, S., Tu, M., & Kim, J. J. (2014). Challenges in meeting the mental health needs of urban Asian American adolescents: Service providers' perspectives. *Race & Social Problems, 5,* 24–37.

Liu, C. H., Murakami, J., Eap, S., & Nagayama, G. C. (2009). Who are Asian Americans?: An overview of history, immigration, and communities. In N. Tewari & A. N. Alvarez (Eds.), *Asian American psychology: Current perspectives* (pp. 1–29). New York, NY: Taylor & Francis.

Lo, M. (2010). Cultural brokerage: Creating linkages between voices of life world and medicine in cross-cultural clinical settings. *Health, 14,* 484–504. doi:10.1177/1363459309360795

López, S., Ruiz, N. G., & Patten, E. (2017). *Key facts about Asian Americans, a diverse and growing population.* Retrieved from https://www.pewresearch.org/fact-tank/2017/09/08/key-facts-about-asian-americans

Markus, H. R, & Kitayama, S. (1991). Culture and self: Implications for cognition, emotion and motivation. *Psychological Review, 98*(2), 224–253. doi:10.1037/0033-295X.98.2.224

Mechling, B. M. (2011). The experiences of youth serving as caregivers for mentally ill parents: A background review of the literature. *Journal of Psychosocial Nursing, 49*(3), 28–33. doi:10.3928/02793695-20110201-01

Park, Y. S., & Kim, B. S. K. (2008). Asian and European American cultural values and communication styles among Asian American and European American college students. *Cultural Diversity and Ethnic Minority Psychology, 14*(1), 47–56. doi:10.1037/1099-9809.14.1.47

Russell, S. T., Chu, J. Y., Crockett, L. J., & Doan, S. N. (2010). The meanings of parents-adolescent relationship quality among Chinese American and Filipino American adolescents. In S. T. Russell, L. J. Crockett, & R. K. Chao (Eds.), *Asian American parenting and parent-adolescent relationships: Advancing responsible adolescent development* (pp. 79–100). New York, NY: Springer Publishing Company.

Shon, S. P., & Ja, D. Y. (1982). Asian families. In M. McGoldrick, J. K. Pearce, & J. Giordano (Eds.), *Ethnicity and family therapy* (pp. 208–228). New York, NY: Guilford.

Sue, S., Cheng, J. K. Y., Saad, C. S., & Chu, J. P. (2012). Asian American mental health: A call to action. *American Psychologist, 67*(7), 532–544. doi:10.1037/a0028900

Tervalon, M., & Murray-Garcia, J. (1998). Cultural humility versus cultural competence: A critical distinction in defining physician training outcomes in multicultural education. *Journal of Health Care for the Poor and Underserved, 9,* 117–125. doi:10.1353/hpu.2010.0233

U.S. Census Bureau. (2018). *Asian-American and Pacific Islander Heritage Month: May 2018.* Retrieved from https://www.census.gov/newsroom/facts-for-features/2018/asian-american.html

# 14

# Practice With Native American Families

HILARY N. WEAVER

## INTRODUCTION

Native Americans are the descendants of the original inhabitants of North America. Over 570 distinct Native American nations are recognized today by the federal government as existing within the boundaries of the United States (Salazar, 2018). Some of these Native nations straddle the borders with Canada and Mexico. Other Native nations such as the Unkechaug of New York and Houma of Louisiana are recognized by the states that surround them but are not acknowledged by the federal government. Native nations (also known as tribes) are diverse in terms of languages, cultures, social systems, forms of government, and spiritual belief systems.

While these diverse groups are often referred to by general labels such as Native American or American Indian, many Indigenous people prefer to be referred to as a member of a specific tribal nation such as Comanche or Arapaho. Some Indigenous people find the use of labels that include the term American (i.e., Native American, American Indian) to be offensive since Indigenous people predate the founding of the United States and the labeling of this continent. The terms Indigenous and First Nations are preferred by some Native people. While there is no consensus on one acceptable term, usage of some terms is more common in certain geographical areas. Additionally, individuals often have strong preferences about terminology. It is noteworthy that in recent years the United Nations has recognized that Indigenous Peoples are collective entities or Peoples, not simply populations or groupings of individuals. Within this chapter, the term Indigenous people refers to multiple individuals (as in people who may be receiving services at an agency) while Indigenous Peoples refers to nations or tribes. The terms Native, Native American, and Indigenous are used interchangeably.

## DEMOGRAPHIC PROFILE

Native Americans are a young and growing population. In 2017, the U.S. Census estimated there were 6.8 million Native Americans (U.S. Census Bureau, 2019). The Native American population is growing faster than the U.S. population as a whole and is projected to reach 10 million, or 2.5% of the population, by 2060 (U.S. Census Bureau, 2019). The average age of Native Americans was 33.5 in 2017, compared to 38.1 for the population as a whole. Approximately 22.6% of the Indigenous population is under age 18 and 15.6% is age 65 or older (U.S. Census Bureau, 2019).

While Indigenous populations exist throughout the United States, California has the largest Native population (723,225) followed by Oklahoma (482,760) and Arizona (353,386) (Norris, Vines, & Hoeffel, 2012). Although more than 300 reservations serve as Indigenous homelands and seats of tribal governments, 78% of Native Americans live outside tribally controlled areas (Norris et al., 2012). Urbanization of Indigenous populations is a trend, yet, many Native families have lived in cities for generations as a result of a federal relocation program that began recruiting Native Americans to cities after World War II (Venables, 2004). The Indigenous population that remains on reservations tends to be younger, poorer, and less educated than their urban counterparts.

Native Americans are disproportionately affected by poverty. They have the highest poverty rate in the United States at 27% compared to 14.3% of the general population (Macartney, Bishaw, & Fontenot, 2013). It should be noted, however, that poverty varies significantly among Native Americans, with the reservation communities in South Dakota typically having the highest rates of unemployment and poverty. Likewise, Native Americans lag behind others in the United States in terms of educational attainment with 80.2% earning a high school degree by age 25 (compared to 88% of the overall population) and 14.7% earning a college degree compared to 32% of the overall population (U.S. Census Bureau, 2019).

## Sovereignty Versus Colonization: The Legal and Policy Context for Native Americans

As Indigenous Peoples, Native Americans have a status distinct from other groups in the United States. The U.S. Congress passed a law in 1924 declaring that Native Americans were U.S. citizens (Steinman, 2011), but not all Native Americans embrace U.S. citizenship. Many view themselves primarily or solely as citizens of their own Native nations. While the United States considers tribes to be domestic dependent nations (Venables, 2004), some of these nations hold a broader vision of their sovereign status. Native nations are governed by their own tribal governments and have the power to set and enforce laws, much as states can, yet erosion of sovereignty has left them subject to the authority of the federal government. Some Indigenous governments, such as the Haudenosaunee Confederacy, offer passports and reserve rights such as the ability to declare war, although such assertions of sovereignty are not necessarily recognized by the United States or other countries. Nonetheless, the United States recognizes that partial sovereignty is retained by Native nations.

The sovereign status of tribal nations and the government-to-government relationship between tribal nations and the United States has led to a distinct policy context that must be understood by human service providers. The federal government continues to operate specific agencies such as the Indian Health Service (IHS), the Office of Indian Education, and the Bureau of Indian Affairs that have no parallel for other ethnic populations in the United States. Likewise, there are specific policies that apply only to Native Americans such as the Indian Child Welfare Act (ICWA). This Act affirms the right of tribes to assume jurisdiction in cases where children who are tribal members or are eligible for membership are at risk of being removed from their families. ICWA also establishes different standards for removal and placement preferences (Weaver & White, 1999).

The understanding that Native Americans are members of distinct political bodies rather than an ethnic or racial group is affirmed by historical and contemporary jurisprudence and policies (Steinman, 2011). The United States, however, has ambivalent and conflicting perspectives on Indigenous sovereignty. Tribal nationhood has been both affirmed and undermined by Supreme Court rulings and acts of Congress. Tribal members have been included in U.S. citizenship yet retain citizenship in tribal nations. The political and legal status of Native Americans within the United States evokes strong feelings in many, with some Native people vehemently asserting sovereignty claims while others fully embrace being American. These different perspectives reflect the ambiguous and uneven incorporation of Native Americans into the United States (Steinman, 2011).

Sovereignty, or the ability to self-govern, is reflected in the fact that all Native nations have their own governments with the ability to pass and enforce laws including the ability to define criteria for citizenship within each Native nation. Many Native nations offer social and health services to their citizens. Sovereignty, however, has been significantly eroded by colonization. Most reservation territories maintain legal authority over their citizens while they are within reservation boundaries, yet they have little or no authority over non-Natives within their borders and are still subject to federal authority. Additionally, most Native governments are heavily dependent on federal funding to operate their social and health services and in many cases the governments themselves. Indeed, the legal and policy context for Native Americans is a murky mix of sovereignty and colonization, the balance of which is subject to constant reinterpretation by the U.S. Congress and Supreme Court.

## ACCESS TO SYSTEMS OF CARE

Because of their unique status as Indigenous Peoples, Native Americans have access to some social and health services not available to others. Native Americans may have access to services through their specific nations and/or may have access to federal programs such as the IHS. In spite of what would appear to be greater availability of services, Native Americans experience a lack of adequate healthcare (Blankenau, Comer, Nitzke, & Stabler, 2010; Browne et al., 2016).

The IHS is a federal program that provides health and some human services for Native Americans. Dependence on the U.S. government for healthcare is an outgrowth of colonization (Blankenau et al., 2010). As the United States made treaties with Indigenous nations, it established ongoing trust obligations. Federal provision of healthcare was often used as a bargaining chip for land successions. The devastating diseases introduced by Europeans rendered provision of healthcare highly important to Native nations (Blankenau et al., 2010).

The obligation to provide healthcare to Native people has never been fulfilled in a responsible manner. Federal studies have found Native people have less access and inferior healthcare than others in the United States (Blankenau et al., 2010). Health services are fragmented and the IHS is chronically underfunded, thus perpetuating health disparities (Lane & Simmons, 2011; Tiedt & Brown, 2014; Whitney, 2017). In 2016, the IHS spent $1,297 per Native American per year compared with an average of $6,973 spent per inmate in the federal prison system (Whitney, 2017). In a related problem, 19.3% of Native Americans lacked health insurance compared to 8.7% of the general population (U.S. Census Bureau, 2019). This lack of insurance is compounded by the limited resources of many tribes, which affects their ability to provide adequate services under their own auspices (Blankenau et al., 2010). The Patient Protection and Affordable Care Act (ACA) did contain provisions to ensure access to care for Native Americans, thus improving insurance coverage over previous years, but at the time of this writing, there were multiple efforts to repeal or erode pieces of the Act. It is likely that many Native Americans will continue to lack insurance coverage.

Access to services is often limited by discrimination. Approximately 25% of Native Americans report facing discrimination at doctor's offices and health clinics (Whitney, 2017). Stereotypes influence beliefs about who is credible and deserving of care (Browne et al., 2016). Fears of facing discrimination in healthcare settings can lead Native Americans to avoid seeking treatment (Moghaddam, Momper, & Fong, 2013), thus perpetuating health disparities (Tiedt & Brown, 2014). Native people may also receive services under different auspices than those used by others. For example, Native youth are more likely to receive mental health treatment through juvenile justice systems and inpatient settings than non-Native youth (Bigfoot & Schmidt, 2010). Under such circumstances, services are less likely to be voluntary and may not be welcomed or productive.

When examining access to systems of care, it is important to differentiate between urban and reservation-based populations. Urban populations are less likely than their reservation-based peers to have access to Native-specific services. Moving to cities has sometimes resulted in increased employment and educational opportunities, yet it has also meant decreased access to healthcare (Castor et al., 2006). Federal funding streams typically target tribal governments while only 1% of IHS funds support urban healthcare, even though the majority of Native people do not live on reservations (Castor et al., 2006; Duran, 2005). A lack of culturally appropriate mental health and substance misuse services in urban areas is associated with youth drug use and elevated risk for HIV (Pearce et al., 2015).

Reservation-based populations also face challenges in accessing social and health services. Most reservations are rural. Often IHS and tribal social services are the only available options and services may be very limited. For example, the IHS human service delivery system on reservations is limited to acute, crisis-oriented outpatient services that do not meet the needs of people struggling with persistent mental illness (Yurkovich & Lattergrass, 2008). Lack of transportation may also be a barrier to accessing services as populations may be spread over great distances on larger reservations. It is also important to note that access to services varies significantly between reservations, and there may be very different experiences, even for tribes located near each other (Blankenau et al., 2010).

Across the United States, Native American women have less protection from violence committed on tribal territories since tribal nations have little to no jurisdiction over perpetrators who are not tribal citizens. The 2019 reauthorization of the Violence Against Women Act being debated at the time of this writing would expand tribal jurisdiction over non-Native people accused of stalking, sexual assault, sex trafficking, or child abuse committed against tribal citizens on tribal territories (Friends Committee on National Legislation, 2019). As it stands now, the intersection of gender and Indigeneity creates substantial vulnerability to violence.

Service access is particularly limited in some areas such as Alaska. This is due not only to remote locations but to the legal framework of the Alaska Native Claims Settlement Act that has eroded sovereignty far more than in the continental United States. Following this Act, much of the traditional territories of Indigenous Peoples in Alaska were no longer considered to be *Indian Country*; therefore, tribal jurisdiction and protections available on reservations in other parts of the United States do not apply. In this context, gender and Indigenous status intersect and lead to substantial vulnerability for Native women. Indigenous women in Alaska experience sexual assault at 12 times the rate of non-Native women and domestic violence rates are 10 times higher than in the lower 48 states (American Indian Law and Order Commission, 2015).

## STRUGGLES AND RESILIENCE: THE PSYCHOSOCIAL RISKS AND NEEDS OF NATIVE AMERICANS

Native families experience significant stressors. Struggles in the lives of many contemporary Native Americans include trauma, health, mental health, substance misuse, and an environment mired in poverty and violence. While it is important for helping professionals to be aware of the prevalence of these concerns, it is also important to understand the strengths and resilience that Indigenous Peoples continue to display in the face of these assaults.

### Trauma

Trauma is a significant factor in the lives of many Native Americans. The genocide conducted against Indigenous Peoples as this continent was colonized left a painful legacy with traumatic memories passed to succeeding generations. This trauma is often the result of specific historical events and federal policies (Bigfoot & Schmidt, 2010). Attacks on Indigenous cultures and ways of life can result in cultural trauma. Likewise, the contemporary circumstances of many Native people are mired in poverty and violence, which compounds preexisting trauma. For Indigenous Peoples, trauma can be historical, intergenerational, cultural, and contemporary (Bigfoot & Braden, 2009). As noted earlier, poverty is a significant concern among Native Americans. Service providers must understand that socioeconomic factors and Indigenous status are intertwined, both identities being associated with elevated risks for trauma and its physical and mental health sequelae.

Colonization, genocide, acculturative stress, cultural bereavement, and racism have resulted in historical trauma that is cumulative, unresolved, and ongoing as well as historical (Brave Heart, Chase, Elkins, & Altshul, 2011). The rate of posttraumatic stress disorder (PTSD) is 22% for Native Americans, compared to 8% in the general population (Beauchamp, 2004; Brave Heart, 2004). Native youth have the same rate of PTSD as do combat veterans returning from Iraq and Afghanistan (American Indian Law and Order Commission, 2015). The traumatic events that Native people experienced in the past have an impact on contemporary health issues, thus contributing to health disparities (Beauchamp, 2004; Brave Heart, 2004).

The genocide perpetrated against Native Americans deliberately destroyed Indigenous cultures as well as directly killing Native people. Specific and deliberate efforts were made to undermine the roles of women and elders as part of the colonization process (Byers, 2010; Smyer & Clark, 2011). An intersectional analysis of boarding schools reveals that not only were they used to promote assimilation into settler societies, they specifically taught and enforced gender norms expected in those societies; norms that were vastly different from most Indigenous societies where women held considerable esteem and power. Colonization attacked the fabric of Indigenous societies, which affected the essence of communities and their members. Culturally based attacks included prohibiting the speaking of Native languages, banning spiritual practices, and relocating individuals or whole communities (Dunbar-Ortiz, 2014).

The significant presence of trauma in the lives of Native people has implications for contemporary service use. This is true across generations, but examining the experience of elders provides a particularly clear example. When looking at the intersection of age and Indigenous status, service providers must be aware that many Native American elders are boarding school survivors and come from a generation where language, cultural practices, and spiritual expressions were undermined or outlawed. Their experiences often make it difficult for them to trust service providers and systems. They may well harbor significant anger, fear, and grief; all factors that make forming a trusting connection with service providers difficult (Smyer & Clark, 2011).

### Health, Mental Health, and Substance Misuse

Health can be defined as being in balance or maintaining equilibrium. Being healthy means having a sense of harmony, and not being out of control in the spiritual, cognitive, emotional, and physical domains (Yurkovich & Lattergrass, 2008). This definition of health is more akin to wellness and differs from a Western definition of health as the absence of illness. Health statistics reveal that Indigenous populations are significantly out of balance.

Native Americans have some of the poorest health and social indicators of all people within the boundaries of the United States (Cho et al., 2014; Jernigan, Duran, Ahn, & Winkleby, 2010; McQuaid, Bombay, McInnis, Matheson, &

Anisman, 2015; Sarche, Tafoya, Croy, & Hill, 2017; Tsosie et al., 2011). Changes in traditional lifestyles of Native Americans have led to changes in eating habits and activity levels that impact health (Coble & Rhodes, 2006). Native Americans suffer from obesity more than any other population in the United States and often struggle with related health issues such as diabetes (Cho et al., 2014; Sarche et al., 2017). Diabetes has increased rapidly in recent decades and is a risk factor for cardiovascular disease, currently the number one killer of Native Americans (Berry, Samos, Storti, & Grey, 2009). Smoking rates for Native American youth and adults are the highest in the nation (Jernigan et al., 2010).

Urbanization has placed Native people at increasing risk for a host of biopsychosocial problems (Evans-Campbell, Lindhorst, Huang, & Walters, 2006). Among Native American women in New York City, 64.5% reported experiencing a period of depression and 50.9% reported a history of dysphoria (Evans-Campbell et al., 2006). It is important to note that there are links between poverty and risks for biopsychosocial problems that affect the well-being of Native Americans.

Significant trauma histories and subsequent social and health problems provide a context in which high rates of substance use fester. Native Americans have the highest rates of alcohol, marijuana, cocaine, and hallucinogen use in the United States and the second highest rates of methamphetamine misuse behind Native Hawaiians (Dickerson et al., 2011). High rates of substance use coexist with high rates of trauma and suicide. Native Americans who misuse substances also experience higher rates of psychiatric problems, higher rates of sexual and physical abuse, and more chronic medical problems than non-Natives (Dickerson et al., 2011). Trauma, substance misuse, and violence are all intertwined with gender and class. Human service providers must recognize the various aspects of Native American people's identity that influence risk and protective factors.

Age is also an important dimension of an individual's identity that is relevant to many aspects of well-being. Native American adolescents have high rates of mental health problems (La Fromboise, Albright, & Harris, 2010; Tsethlikai, Peyton, & O'Brien, 2007). Alcohol and drug use also begins earlier for Native youth than for their non-Native peers (Heavyrunner-Rioux & Hollist, 2010; Nalls, Mullis, & Mullis, 2009). In part, this may be attributed to self-medication for high rates of depression (Nalls et al., 2009). Reservation-based youth report the most high-risk behavior (Heavyrunner-Rioux & Hollist, 2010).

### Violence, Poverty, and Environmental Issues

Poverty and socioeconomic disadvantage are significant factors for many Native people (Mauer, 2017). Many Native people experience financial hardship, which increases stress and compounds the risk of exposure to crime and violence (Bigfoot & Braden, 2009). It is also important to recognize connections between humans, all other beings, and the environment. What affects the well-being of one affects the well-being of the others. Destruction of the natural environment reflects and exacerbates disadvantage in Indigenous communities.

Native grandparent caregivers raise children within a context of lower socioeconomic status and a multitude of social and health disparities. This group also has much lower service use (Byers, 2010). Among the Cherokee Nation of

Oklahoma, 64.3% of all grandparents are caregivers; for the Muskogee Creek Nation the percentage is 58.9%. Part of the necessity for caregiving is the absence of mothers, as Oklahoma is the state with the highest percentage of incarcerated females—10.6% of the state's female population (Byers, 2010). Cyclical detention and incarceration have also been identified as issues in the Baltimore Native community (Johnson, Gryczynski, & Wiechelt, 2007).

The violent crime rate for Native Americans age 12 and older is 2.5 times that of the population as a whole, with youth experiencing violence up to 10 times the rates of their peers (American Indian Law and Order Commission, 2015). Native Americans also have the highest rates of intimate partner violence of any group in the country (Burnette & Figley, 2017). A study of Native American women in New York City found 65.5% have experienced interpersonal violence and most experienced sexual assault (Evans-Campbell et al., 2006). In spite of the traditional respect accorded to elders, abuse is a growing problem for older Native people, with financial abuse being the most common followed by neglect and psychological abuse (Smyer & Clark, 2011). Straying from traditional cultural values is a factor leading to the abuse of elders. It is important to emphasize that high rates of violence are rooted in and perpetuated by colonial structures and cannot be adequately explained by individual or cultural factors.

The social environment of Native youth often exposes them to poverty, violence, drugs, alcohol, and prejudice. Negative school and neighborhood environments have a detrimental impact on Native youth. Lack of neighborhood safety, particularly crime and drug sales, is a strong predictor of depression and use of alcohol and drugs (Johnston-Goodstar & VeLure Roholt, 2017; Nalls et al., 2009). The current climate of racism and oppression experienced by Native people contributes to health disparities (Northridge, Stover, Rosenthal, & Sherard, 2003; Yurkovich & Lattergrass, 2008).

In addition to destructive factors in their neighborhoods, traditional Native youth constantly face prejudice and oppression from peers and schools (Robbins, 2010). Rather than serving as safe, supportive learning environments, school policies and administrators may reinforce and institutionalize microaggressions and biases (Johnston-Goodstar & VeLure Roholt, 2017). For example, the Wiyot Tribe of California has sued their local school district charging teachers with touching students' hair and other microaggressions (Clarren, 2017). Many Native students experience racism from their teachers every year including reinforcing perspectives that Native Americans have no contemporary contributions to knowledge or society, thus undermining students' sense of agency and competence (Cerecer, 2013).

A study of Native youth living on reservations found the biggest issue facing students was being judged harshly by members of the majority White culture. In contemporary society, discrimination, prejudice, and exposure to oppression are inevitable (Feinstein, Driving-Hawk, & Baartman, 2009). Contemporary poverty and racism compound the effects of historical trauma (Bigfoot & Schmidt, 2010).

In spite of significant challenges, Native people are working to improve their environments. Indigenous resilience is evident in positive trends in business ownership, home ownership, and educational attainment. Native people have made significant strides in working toward economic viability while maintaining cultural integrity (Grandbois & Sanders, 2009). There has also been significant activism confronting environmental racism and protecting the environment. The well-being of the natural world is intertwined with the well-being of all living beings. Supporting macro-level well-being is essential to individual wellness.

## ASSESSMENT

When working with Native families, it is important to begin with the basic question: What constitutes a family? Traditionally, the nuclear family is not the norm in Indigenous societies. Households are often multigenerational, and families may maintain connections to ancestors as well as generations yet unborn. It is not uncommon for Native families to contain people who are not related by blood, but nevertheless are considered family members (Smyer & Clark, 2011). Multigenerational households can be a source of strength and resources but can also present challenges.

Many Native American cultures have a sense of existing within the context of seven generations. This may be defined as seven generations preceding and seven generations following the present generation, or three generations before, three after, with the current generation nestled in the middle. Either way, there is a sense that the current generation is interdependent within a larger Indigenous context. Earlier generations had a responsibility to think ahead and plan for the present day. Because of their foresight, Indigenous Peoples have retained some of their land, culture, languages, and sovereignty. The current generation, in turn, bears a responsibility to plan for the future to ensure that it will be possible for subsequent generations to exist as distinct, Indigenous Peoples. The strong cultural value placed on the seven generations is often incorporated in prevention messages that resonate with Native people. For example, it is crucial that Native women not drink or use drugs during pregnancy because this can harm generations to come.

In the Indigenous cultural context, family may be defined broadly. Some traditional teachings of the Haudensaunee Peoples emphasize that spirits of children exist prior to conception. In a way, these are "pre-birth" family members. These spirit beings come from the Creator and can choose a family. Prospective parents have a responsibility to prepare their lives socially and economically for 2 years before a pregnancy. This traditional way of thinking provides an optimum environment for a baby. Likewise, strength and resources can be drawn from those who have passed on. A strong legacy of survival passed down from the ancestors encourages resilience in contemporary Native people (Grandbois & Sanders, 2009).

Extended family networks and clan systems are still viable parts of the lives of many Native Americans. Clans are groups of related individuals and may be named for an animal or feature of the natural world (i.e., Beaver clan). Clan leaders typically have responsibility for the well-being of clan members and may serve as counselors, mediators, or spokespersons when needed. There are often reciprocal relationships between clans. For example, following the death of a member of one clan, members of another clan are vested with responsibilities related to the funeral and burial, thus providing support and space for bereavement of those most directly affected by this loss.

Traditionally, a high value is placed on group connections as part of an interdependent society. "Resilience is embedded not only in their culture and close inter- and intrapersonal relationships, such as tiospaye and clanship [extended family networks], but also in the Oneness and sense of connection they feel with all of life" (Grandbois & Sanders, 2009, p. 575). This group orientation and extended family networks can be protective factors when the nuclear family is dysfunctional. In other words, members of the extended family and clan are poised to take on responsibilities such as caring for children or elders when other household members are not able to do so. As an example of this, Native women raise their grandchildren at a higher rate than any other ethnic group (Byers, 2010).

The strong sense of connection to others is often a positive source of support. For example, elders' resilience can be nurtured through families, relatives, and tribal communities. Likewise, youth resiliency is affected by support from family or peers, but strain in these systems can also have an impact (Feinstein et al., 2009). If family or peer networks are dysfunctional, this can have a strong negative influence.

Group cohesiveness is supported by an emphasis on the values of respect and responsibility. Members of Indigenous communities typically have particular role expectations that contribute to the well-being of the community. Likewise, the emphasis placed on respect for all beings (human and otherwise) contributes to the well-being of the family, community, and environment. Differential stature in Native communities may be based on factors such as age and community roles. For example, older women in Native cultures have a special stature based on their age and role as caregivers (Byers, 2010). In this case, the intersection of age and gender often results in an elevated status for Indigenous women within their societies, quite different than how older women are perceived and treated in more mainstream contexts.

While many Native Americans, including some in urban areas, firmly espouse traditional values and cultures, this is not true for all Native people. Some Native people know little of Indigenous values or choose to live their lives more aligned with dominant society standards or those of other cultural groups. Helping professionals must determine the level of connection that an Indigenous person maintains to his or her culture as part of the assessment process and determine whether culturally grounded interventions are appropriate. While some assessment tools attempt to measure cultural attachment, it is not necessary to use such instruments and in fact, many such tools are based on outdated theories of cultural identity. Rather, helping professionals can include a line of questioning about connection to culture as part of the larger assessment process.

The concept of balance is helpful for anchoring an assessment for Indigenous clients grounded in their culture. Balance is a defining aspect of Indigenous health and wellness (Rybak & Decker-Fitts, 2009). Many Native cultures place great importance on the medicine wheel or a comparable circle. The medicine wheel is a circle divided into quadrants. While there are tribal variations in the details, typically the quadrants are associated with four colors, directions, life stages, and races of people, among other things.

From a health and wellness perspective, the medicine wheel quadrants represent mind, body, spirit, and heart. If there is an imbalance in any aspect of the circle, it affects all others. For example, diabetes may originate as a medical disorder (body), but it also affects other areas of life (mind, spirit, and heart). Recognizing these connections across areas of a client's life is important. Using the concept of balance and the medicine wheel as part of the assessment will help identify how the client sees the problem and determine how to target an intervention in a culturally meaningful way. It is important to note, however, that the medicine wheel framework, while important to many, does not resonate with all Native people. Some come from traditions where other circular concepts are meaningful. Others may not connect to Indigenous concepts.

While maintenance of cultural traditions can be sustaining for many Native people, environmental contaminants make continuance of some traditional practices problematic. Native people may find themselves in a bind when practices that support traditional cultures and ways of life now pose health risks. For example, traditional seafoods nurture cultural identity for the Swinomish and are associated with community cohesion, knowledge transmission, ceremonial use, and food security. Unfortunately, in contemporary times, pollution has tainted the seafood they depend on. In this case, although the seafood is contaminated, it may be more harmful to the Swinomish to avoid its consumption based on their holistic conceptualization of health (Donatuto, Satterfield, & Gregory, 2011).

While there are abundant risk factors associated with being Native American, resilience is evident in those confronted with daily traumas associated with poverty and a chronic lack of resources. Survival, tenacity, and resilience are embedded characteristics of Native cultures (Grandbois & Sanders, 2009). In the traditional way of thinking, the current generation has a pact with the ancestors and must survive for the sake of the future. As part of the assessment process, helping professionals can look at effective coping mechanisms, resilience, and strengths.

There are several things to keep in mind when conducting an assessment with Native clients:

- Cultural identity must be assessed, as there is substantial variation in how Native people do or do not connect with Indigenous cultures.
- Historical trauma is an intergenerational phenomenon that plays a role in the contemporary well-being of some Native people.
- Contemporary racism, oppression, and violence are common experiences for many Native people and can compound historical trauma.
- Poverty and limited access to resources is a common experience and an additional situational stress that can compound trauma.
- Many strengths can be found in Indigenous traditions including cultural values, clans/extended networks, and spirituality.

## TREATMENT APPROACHES

While there are a variety of intervention approaches available for social and health problems, few have been developed or adapted for Native Americans. Today's push for evidence-based practice poses a particular bind for helping professionals working with Native people. Because of their small population numbers and the diversity among Native groups, few interventions have been tested and documented for effectiveness with Native Americans. In fact, the mandate that many Native-serving agencies have from their funding sources to use evidence-based models has forced them to use treatment approaches that have been proven effective for others but are of unproven merit for Native people. These models typically do not take into account Indigenous values and may be ineffective or harmful with Native clients, particularly clients from traditional cultural orientations. In such cases, the true spirit of evidence-based practice is lost and cultural incompetence triumphs (Nebelkopf et al., 2011).

As an alternative, some Native scholars, notably Terry Cross, former executive director of the National Indian Child Welfare Association, call for practice-based evidence. In this way of promoting quality services, researchers are encouraged to examine the interventions that appear effective with Native clients, thereby gathering evidence from practice and identifying effective models that may be replicated in other Native settings. This is a viable alternative to the more heavy-handed imposition of models developed for others on Native people (Nebelkopf et al., 2011). As a general principle, interventions grounded in social learning and cognitive behavioral theories are often compatible with Native cultural values. Cognitive behavioral therapy principles are complementary to many traditional teachings and healing methods (Bigfoot & Schmidt, 2010).

There are a number of Native-specific models developed and implemented at the grassroots level in Native communities. The Don't Forget Us program is an example of substance misuse, hepatitis, and HIV prevention services tailored for urban Native Americans delivered in four weekly sessions (Wiechelt, Gryczynski, & Johnson, 2009). While many Native-specific programs have yet to receive empirical evaluation, several have been described in the scholarly literature. For example, *Honoring Children: Mending the Circle* is a trauma-focused, cognitive behavioral therapy designed to facilitate children's healing from trauma. This intervention is compatible with Indigenous values and concepts of well-being. This framework is built on a circle, a conceptual scheme that resonates in many Native traditions and is appropriate for people with a strong Native cultural affiliation. *Honoring the Children: Mending the Circle* is one of a series of interventions that are adaptations of evidence-based treatments developed by the Indian Country Child Trauma Center at the University of Oklahoma Health Sciences Center including *Honoring Children: Making Relatives* (parenting techniques), *Honoring Children: Respectful Ways* (promoting children's self-respect and respect for others), and *Honoring Children: Honoring the Future* (suicide prevention) (Bigfoot & Braden, 2009).

Like the medicine wheel discussed in the "Assessment" section, the interventions described are based on a circular design. Other groups have also found this type of foundation to be helpful in interventions. For example, the *Circle of Wellness* model is an effective intervention for Native people with persistent mental illness (Yurkovich & Lattergrass, 2008).

Many Native people participate in traditional Indigenous healing practices instead of or in addition to Western ways of helping. This has been documented in urban populations as well as with reservation dwellers. In a study of Native American women in New York City, 60.7% have utilized mental health counseling and 67.9% have utilized traditional healing (Evans-Campbell et al., 2006). Sometimes a blended approach is most helpful. For example, a combination of Western and traditional healing may be appropriate for Native veterans struggling with PTSD (Shore, Orton, & Manson, 2009).

When possible, culturally grounded interventions should be based on the culture of the participants rather than a generic, pan-Indian model. The *Healthy Living in Two Worlds* project is a wellness intervention developed for urban Haudenosaunee (also known as Iroquois) youth. This prevention initiative educates youth and promotes healthy lifestyles with a particular focus on mitigating the health risk factors of recreational tobacco use, unhealthy dietary practices, and lack of physical activities (Weaver, 2010; Weaver & Jackson, 2010).

There are several treatment recommendations that can enhance the effectiveness of interventions with Native American clients:

- Recognize how racism permeates society, including shaping service providers' perceptions of Native Americans, then actively work to let go of biases, and truly listen to the life stories and strengths of Native clients.
- Strengthen healthy social networks and promote positive role models including strengthening communities to support individual well-being.
- Interventions that incorporate circular ways of understanding life are likely to resonate with culturally grounded Native clients.
- Interventions must recognize that life stresses such as racism and poverty often exacerbate other conditions such as mental illness and substance misuse.
- Seek out interventions proven effective with Native populations rather than assuming evidence-based practice modeled on other populations will be effective.
- Given the extensive trauma experienced by many Native people, interventions that acknowledge grief and loss while promoting healing may be appropriate.
- Be aware that clients may also participate in traditional healing processes and these can be therapeutic.
- Colonization and racism affect health and social well-being, thus, helping professionals must incorporate social justice concepts as integral components in their work.

## CASE VIGNETTE

Molly Jamieson is a 64-year-old widowed Cayuga grandmother who has been caring for her three grandchildren since her daughter, the children's mother, was incarcerated 3 years ago. Molly has only a small pension from her previous work in a school cafeteria and is not financially able to make needed home repairs. Her diabetes has become more severe in recent years, affecting her vision and putting her at risk for amputation. Two of her three grandchildren have begun skipping school regularly and school officials have expressed concern that the children are not adequately dressed for winter. The oldest child has been spending time with other youth who have dropped out of school and are suspected gang members. The school social worker has been meeting with colleagues to determine how they might assist the family and whether their concerns should be raised with other community agencies or authorities.

## CONCLUSION

Native Americans are a young and growing population. Poverty, racism, and trauma are common factors in the lives of many Native people and these provide a context for significant social and health disparities. It is also important to recognize the resilience and tenacity that have allowed Native people to survive as distinct cultural and political groups in spite of centuries of colonization. Helping professionals can play an important role in assisting Native clients to access needed services and nurture their resilience. Professionals can also bring a strong grounding in social justice to combat many of the struggles that affect Indigenous Peoples. In these ways, helping professionals have an important role to play in assisting Native people to improve their lives and the lives of generations to come.

## DISCUSSION QUESTIONS

1. When you look at Molly Jamieson's family, do you see strengths or deficits? Critically reflect on your ideas of what a family should look like. Where do your attitudes and beliefs come from? How might they influence your work with this family?
2. How will you identify the root of the problem and determine areas for intervention?
3. Reflect on what you have learned about Native American families. How might issues related to trauma play a role in the life circumstances of this family?
4. How can you engage with this family in ways that are validating, reach for their strengths, and offer appropriate supports?

## REFERENCES

American Indian Law and Order Commission. (2015). *A Roadmap for Making Native America Safer.* Retrieved from http://www.aisc.ucla.edu

Beauchamp, S. (2004). Mandan and Hidatsa families and children: Surviving historical assault. In E. Nebelkopf & M. Phillips (Eds.), *Healing and mental health for Native Americans: Speaking in red* (pp. 65–73). Walnut Creek, CA: Altamira Press.

Berry, D., Samos. M., Storti, S., & Grey, M. (2009). Listening to concerns about type 2 diabetes in a Native American community. *Journal of Cultural Diversity, 16*(2), 56–63.

Bigfoot, D. S., & Braden, J. (2009). Adapting evidence-based treatments for use with American Indian and Native Alaskan children and youth. *Child Law Practice, 28*(5), 76–78.

Bigfoot, D. S., & Schmidt, S. R. (2010). Honoring children, mending the circle: Cultural adaptation of trauma-focused cognitive-behavioral therapy for American Indian and Alaska Native children. *Journal of Clinical Psychology: In Session, 66*(8), 847–856. doi:10.1002/jclp.20707

Blankenau, J., Comer, J., Nitzke, J., & Stabler, W. (2010). The role of tribal experiences in shaping Native American health. *Social Work in Public Health, 25*(5), 423–437. doi:10.1080/19371918.2010.498699

Brave Heart, M. Y. H. (2004). The historical trauma response among Natives and its relationship to substance abuse: A Lakota illustration. In E. Nebelkopf & M. Phillips (Eds.), *Healing and mental health for Native Americans: Speaking in red* (pp. 7–31). Walnut Creek, CA: Altamira Press.

Brave Heart, M. Y. H., Chase, J., Elkins, J., & Altshul, D. B. (2011). Historical trauma among Indigenous Peoples of the Americas: Concepts, research, and clinical considerations. *Journal of Psychoactive Drugs, 43*(4), 282–290. doi:10.1080/02791072.2011.628913

Browne, A. J., Varcoe, C., Lavoie, J., Smye, V., Wong, S. T., Krause, M., . . . Fridkin, A. (2016). Enhancing health care equity with Indigenous populations: Evidence-based strategies from an ethnographic study. *BMC Health Services Research*, 16, 1–17. doi:10.1186/s12913-016-1707-9

Burnette, C. E. & Figley, C. R. (2017). Historical oppression, resilience, and transcendence: Can a holistic framework help explain violence experienced by Indigenous People? *Social Work*, 62(1), 15–23.

Byers, L. (2010). Native American grandmothers: Cultural tradition and contemporary necessity. *Journal of Ethnic and Cultural Diversity in Social Work*, 19(4), 305–316. doi:10.1080/15313204.2010.523653

Castor, M. L., Smyser, M. S., Taualii, M. M., Park, A. N., Lawson, S. A., & Forquera, R. A. (2006). A nationwide population-based study identifying health disparities between American Indians/Alaska Natives and the general populations living in select urban counties. *American Journal of Public Health*, 96(8), 1478–1484. doi:10.2105/AJPH.2004.053942

Cerecer, P. D. Q. (2013). Independence, dominance, and power: (Re)examining the impact of school policies on the academic development of Indigenous youth. *Theory into Practice*, 52, 196–202. doi:10.1080/00405841.2013.804313

Cho, P., Geiss, L. S., Burrows, N. R., Roberts, D. L., Bullock, A. K., & Toedt, M. E. (2014). Diabetes-related mortality among American Indians and Alaska Natives, 1990-2009. *American Journal of Public Health*, 104(S3), 496–503. doi:10.2105/AJPH.2014.301968

Clarren, R. (2017). Left behind: How punitive discipline, inadequate curriculums, and declining federal funding put Native American students at risk. *The Nation*, 305(4), 12–25.

Coble, J. D., & Rhodes, R. E. (2006). Physical activity and Native Americans: A review. *American Journal of Preventive Medicine*, 31(1), 36–46. doi:10.1016/j.amepre.2006.03.004

Dickerson, D. L., Spear, S., Marinelli-Casey, P., Rawson, R., Li, L., & Hser, Y. (2011). American Indian/Alaska Natives and substance abuse treatment outcomes: Positive signs and continuing challenges, *Journal of Addictive Diseases*, 30(1), 63–74. doi:10.1080/10550887.2010.531665

Donatuto, J. L., Satterfield, T. A., & Gregory, R. (2011). Poisoning the body to nourish the soul: Prioritizing health risks and impacts in a Native American community. *Health, Risk, and Society*, 13(2), 103–127. doi:10.1080/13698575.2011.556186

Dunbar-Ortiz, R. (2014). *An Indigenous People's History of the United States*. Boston, MA: Beacon Press.

Duran, B. (2005). American Indian/Alaska Native health policy. *American Journal of Public Health*, 95(5), 758. doi:10.2105/AJPH.95.5.758

Evans-Campbell, T., Lindhorst, T., Huang, B., & Walters, K. (2006). Interpersonal violence in the lives of urban American Indian and Alaska Native women; Implications for health, mental health, and help-seeking. *American Journal of Public Health*, 95(8), 1416–1422. doi:10.2105/AJPH.2004.054213

Feinstein, S., Driving-Hawk, C., & Baartman, J. (2009). Resiliency and Native American teenagers. *Reclaiming Children and Youth Journal*, 18(2), 12–17.

Friends Committee on National Legislation. (2019). *Native American Legislative Update, April 2019*. Retrieved from https://fcnl.actionkit.com

Grandbois, D. M., & Sanders, G. F. (2009). The resilience of Native American elders. *Issues in Mental Health Nursing*, 30, 569–580. doi:10.1080/01612840902916151

Heavyrunner-Rioux, A. R., & Hollist, D. R. (2010). Community, family, and peer influences on alcohol, marijuana, and illicit drug use among a sample of Native American youth: An analysis of predictive factors. *Journal of Ethnicity in Substance Abuse*, 9(4), 260–283. doi:10.1080/15332640.2010.522893

Jernigan, V. B. B., Duran, B., Ahn, D., & Winkleby, M. (2010). Changing patterns in health behaviors and risk factors related to cardiovascular disease among American Indians and Alaska Natives. *American Journal of Public Health*, 100(4), 677–683. doi:10.2105/AJPH.2009.164285

Johnson, J. L., Gryczynski, J., & Wiechelt, S. A. (2007). HIV/AIDS, substance abuse, and hepatitis prevention needs of Native Americans living in Baltimore: In their own words. *AIDS Education and Prevention, 19*(6), 531–544. doi:10.1521/aeap.2007.19.6.531

Johnston-Goodstar, K., & VeLure Roholt, R. (2017). "Our kids aren't dropping out, they're being pushed out": Native American students and racial microaggressions in schools. *Journal of Ethnic and Cultural Diversity in Social Work, 26*(1–2), 30–47. doi:10.1080/15313204.2016.1263818

La Fromboise, T. D., Albright, K., & Harris, A. (2010). Patterns of hopelessness among American Indian adolescents: Relationships by level of acculturation and residence. *Cultural Diversity and Ethnic Minority Psychology, 16*(1), 68–76.

Lane, D. C., & Simmons, J. (2011). American Indian youth substance abuse: Community-driven interventions. *Mount Sinai Journal of Medicine, 78*, 362–372. doi:10.1002/msj.20262

Macartney, S., Bishaw, A., & Fontenot, K. (2013). Poverty rates for selected detailed race and Hispanic groups by place and state: 2007-2011. Report number ACSBR/11-17. U.S. Census Bureau.

Mauer, K. W. (2017). Indian country poverty: Place-based poverty on American Indian territories, 2006-2010. *Rural Sociology, 82*(3), 473–498. doi:10.1111/ruso.12130

McQuaid, R. J., Bombay, A., McInnis, O. A., Matheson, K., & Anisman, H. (2015). Childhood adversity, perceived discrimination, and coping strategies in relation to depressive symptoms among First Nations adults in Canada: The moderating role of unsupportive social interactions from ingroup and outgroup members. *Cultural Diversity and Ethnic Minority Psychology, 21*(3), 326–336. doi:10.1037/a0037541

Moghaddam, J. F., Momper, S. L., & Fong, T. (2013). Discrimination and participation in traditional healing for American Indians and Alaska Natives. *Journal of Community Health, 38*, 1115–1123. doi:10.1007/s10900-013-9721-x

Nalls, A. M., Mullis, R. L., & Mullis, A. K. (2009). American Indian youths' perceptions of their environment and their reports of depressive symptoms and alcohol/marijuana use. *Adolescence, 44*(176), 965–978.

Nebelkopf, E., King, K., Wright, S., Schweigman, K., Lucero, E., Habte-Michael, T. & Cervantes, T. (2011). Growing roots: Native American evidence-based practices. *Journal of Psychoactive Drugs, 43*(4), 263–268. doi:10.1080/02791072.2011.628909

Norris, T., Vines, P. L., & Hoeffel, E. M. (2012). The American Indian and Alaska Native Population: 2010. Report number C2010BR-10. U.S. Census Bureau.

Northridge, M. E., Stover, G. N., Rosenthal, J. E., & Sherard, D. (2003). Environmental equity and health: Understanding complexity and moving forward. *American Journal of Public Health, 93*(2), 209–214. doi:10.2105/AJPH.93.2.209

Pearce, M. E., Jongbloed, K. A., Richardson, C. G., Henderson, E. W., Pooyak, S. D., Oviedo-Joekes, E., . . . Spittal, P. M. (2015). The Cedar Project: Resilience in the face of HIV vulnerability within a cohort study involving young Indigenous people who use drugs in three Canadian cities. *BMC Public Health, 15*(1), 1–12. doi:10.1186/s12889-015-2417-7

Robbins, R. (2010). Striving to remain a Native American in my America: Resistance to past and present injustices (Letter to my son on the day of his second piercing). *Journal for Social Action in Counseling and Psychology, 2*(2), 17–28.

Rybak, C., & Decker-Fitts, A. (2009). Understanding Native American healing practices. *Counseling Psychology Quarterly, 22*(3), 333–342. doi:10.1080/09515070903270900

Salazar, M. (2018). *Federal and state recognized tribes*. National Conference of State Legislatures. Retrieved from www.ncsl.org/research/state-tribal-institute/list-of-federal-and-state-recognized-tribes.aspx

Sarche, M., Tafoya, G., Croy, C. D., & Hill, K. (2017). American Indian and Alaska Native boys: Early childhood risk and resilience amidst context and culture. *Infant Mental Health Journal, 38*(1), 115–127. doi:10.1002/imhj.21613

Shore, J. H., Orton, H., & Manson, S. M. (2009). Trauma-related nightmares among American Indian veterans: Views from the dream catcher. *American Indian Alaska Native Mental Health Research: The Journal of the National Center, 16*(1), 25–38. doi:10.5820/aian.1601.2009.25

Smyer, T., & Clark. M. C. (2011). A cultural paradox: Elder abuse in the Native American community. *Home Health Care Management and Practice, 23*(3), 201–206. doi:10.1177/1084822310396971

Steinman, E. (2011). Sovereigns and citizens? The contested status of American Indian tribal nations and their members. *Citizenship Studies, 15*(1), 57–74. doi:10.1080/13621025.2011.534927

Tiedt, J. A., & Brown, L. A. (2014). Allostatic load: The relationship between chronic stress and diabetes in Native Americans. *Journal of Theory Construction & Testing, 18*(1), 22–27.

Tsethlikai, M., Peyton, V., & O'Brien, M., (2007). Exploring maternal social perceptions and child aggression among urban American Indians. *American Indian and Alaska Native Mental Health Research: The Journal of the National Center, 14*(1), 63–84. doi:10.5820/aian.1401.2007.67

Tsosie, U., Nannauck, S., Buchwald, D., Russo, J., Trusz, S. G., Foy, H., & Zatzick, D. (2011). Staying connected: A feasibility study linking American Indian and Alaska Native trauma survivors to their tribal communities. *Psychiatry, 74*(4), 349–361. doi:10.1521/psyc.2011.74.4.349

U.S. Census Bureau. (2019). *American Indian and Alaska Native Heritage Month: November 2018*. Retrieved from https://www.census.gov

Venables, R. W. (2004). *American Indian history: Five centuries of conflict and coexistence*. Santa Fe, NM: Clear Light Publishing.

Weaver, H. N. (2010). The Healthy Living in Two Worlds project: An inclusive model of curriculum development. *Journal of Indigenous Voices in Social Work, 1*(1), 1–18.

Weaver, H. N., & Jackson, K. F. (2010). Healthy Living in Two Worlds: Testing a wellness curriculum for urban native youth. *Child and Adolescent Social Work Journal, 27*(3), 231–244. doi:10.1007/s10560-010-0197-6

Weaver, H. N., & White, B. J. (1999). Protecting the future of Indigenous children and nations: An examination of the Indian Child Welfare Act. *Journal of Health and Social Policy, 10*(4), 35–50. doi:10.1300/J045v10n04_03

Wiechelt, S. A., Gryczynski, & Johnson, J. L. (2009). Designing HIV prevention interventions for urban American Indians: Evolution of the Don't Forget Us program. *Health and Social Work, 34*(4), 301–304. doi:10.1093/hsw/34.4.301

Whitney, E. (2017). Native Americans feel invisible in the U.S. health care system. *You, Me, and Them: Experiencing Discrimination in America.* Morning Edition, National Public Radio.

Yurkovich, E. E., & Lattergrass, I. (2008). Defining health and unhealthiness: Perceptions held by Native American Indians with persistent mental illness. *Mental Health, Religion & Culture, 11*(5), 437–459. doi:10.1080/13674670701473751

# 15

# Practice With Arab American Families

WAHIBA ABU-RAS AND SAMEENA AZHAR

## INTRODUCTION

Providing quality social services and healthcare in the United States requires the recognition of a population that is increasingly diverse in their ethnic and cultural backgrounds (Hammoud, White, & Fetters, 2005). The Arab American population in the United States is one such ethnic minority population that requires unique attention. The number of Arab Americans has rapidly increased in recent years from just 850,000 people with Arab ancestry in 1990 to 1.5 million people in 2010, representing a 76% increase (U.S. Census Bureau, 2013). Similarly, the number of Arab families in the United States has increased from 268,000 households in 1990 to 511,000 households in 2010, representing a 91% increase (U.S. Census Bureau, 2013). Other sources estimate the Arab population to be even larger, numbering 3.7 million people (Arab American Institute, 2018; Zogby, 2001). Exact numbers of the Arab American community are difficult to determine as individuals may be reluctant to identify themselves as Arabs on official government records because they suspect that such information might be used against them.

The Arab American community consists of many subcultures that are diverse in ethnicities, religious practices, political histories, social affiliations, migration experiences, and acculturation processes. In order for social workers to effectively assist individuals and families from Arab backgrounds, we must recognize the diversity within these communities and not assume that all Arab Americans share monolithic social histories (Azhar, 2019). It is also important to identify the protective factors that Arab American communities share in terms of their family support, religious beliefs, educational values, resiliency, and collectivist culture. In the current political climate, Arab Americans additionally face social and political oppression, discrimination, negative stereotypes, and prejudice. This chapter highlights both the strengths of Arab American families and the challenges they face, as well as outlines recommendations for clinical social work practice.

## SOCIODEMOGRAPHICS OF ARAB AMERICAN FAMILIES

The term *Arab* refers to those who consider Arabic their native language or who identify as being of Arab descent (Abraham & Abraham, 1983; U.S. Census Bureau, 2003). *Arab American* refers to Arabs who have immigrated to the United States from the Arab world (Abraham & Abraham, 1983), stretching from North Africa to the Arabian Gulf (Suleiman, 1999). Arab Americans have ancestral, cultural, ethnic, linguistic, familial, or heritage ties to one of 22 countries within the Arab league and where Arabic is the main spoken language (Abuelezam, El-Sayed, & Galea, 2018; El-Sayed & Galea, 2009). These countries include Algeria, Bahrain, Comoros, Djibouti, Egypt, Iraq, Jordan, Kuwait, Lebanon, Libya, Mauritania, Morocco, Oman, Palestine, Qatar, Saudi Arabia, Somalia, Sudan, Syria, Tunisia, United Arab Emirates, and Yemen (Council on Foreign Relations, 2014). Other countries in South Asia and Central Asia/Eastern Europe, such as Afghanistan, Pakistan, Turkey, and Kazakhstan, are often erroneously included in the Arab world as the majority of individuals in these other countries are also Muslim.

Apart from earlier groups of Arabs who had been brought to the United States involuntarily as slaves during colonial times (Austin, 2012), Arab American emigration to the United States occurred in three waves (El-Sayed & Galea, 2009). The first and largest wave (1880–1931) consisted of 212,825 immigrants from the Ottoman Empire, approximately 50% of whom were largely poor, unskilled, and illiterate in Arabic and English (Abraham & Abraham, 1983; Indiana Historical Society, 2010; Naff, 1983; Suleiman, 1987, 1994). These immigrants largely came from Mount Lebanon and Greater Syria around the turn of the century (Abu-Laban & Suleiman, 1989; Khater, 2001; Shakir, 1997). Their relative ethnic invisibility, due to their small numbers and successful assimilation, made them part of the "hidden minority" (Abraham & Abraham, 1983). During the late 1940s and early 1950s, due to political changes both in the Arab world and in American foreign policy, many of these Arab immigrants became socially isolated from mainstream American society. In the 1940s, the U.S. Census Bureau decided that Arab Americans were to be treated like European immigrants, leading the federal government to later classify Arabs under the racial category of "White" (Office of Management and Budget [OMB], 1995). The 2000 Census added the classification "Arab ancestry" to collect additional information regarding people from the Middle East and North Africa (Naber, 2008).

The second wave of Arab immigration (early 1950s to mid-1960s) largely consisted of those escaping political instability, for example, Palestinians displaced by the 1948 Arab–Israeli war. This wave was largely comprised of Sunni Muslims, who were students and highly educated professionals (Suleiman, 1999). They tended to settle where jobs were available. Those with less education tended to settle in urban centers in the East and the Midwest while highly skilled professionals tended to settle in the new suburbs and rural towns on the peripheries of industrial cities (Abraham & Abraham, 1983).

The third wave (1970s to 1980s) mainly consisted of asylees and refugees who established Arabic language schools, mosques, and charities—institutions that helped stimulate ethnopolitical consciousness (Abraham & Abraham, 1983; David, 2007). While the Arab community in the United States is largely taken to be recent immigrants, actually more than half of Arab Americans today are third-, fourth-, and fifth-generation immigrants (Hammoud et al., 2005).

While most Arab immigrants share a common language and culture, the Arab American community varies by immigrants' ethnicity, religion, nation of origin, extended family, and period of arrival (David, 2007). Arab immigrants also differ in terms of their assimilation to an American lifestyle and in their feelings of "foreignness" to the United States. According to the most recent census, many male Arab Americans feel that they do not belong here or are not made to feel part of the country (U.S. Census Bureau, 2010). About 31% of Arab Americans were born in the United States and 55% of those born abroad are naturalized citizens (Arab American Institute Foundation [AAIF], 2009). Around 38% arrived before 1990; 34% arrived after 2000; and 28% between 1990 and 2000 (AAIF, 2009). The average length of residency in the United States for men is between 18 and 32 years and for women 6–27 years (El-Badry, 1994; U.S. Census Bureau, 2013) although others have lived here for over 45 years (Abu-Ras & Abu-Bader, 2008, 2009).

Arab Americans live in all 50 states, but two thirds are concentrated in 10 states; one third of the total live in California, New York, and Michigan. About 94% of Arab Americans live in metropolitan areas. Los Angeles, Detroit, New York/New Jersey, Chicago and Washington, DC, are the top five metropolitan areas of Arab American concentration (AAI, 2020).

The notion of being Arab and being Muslim is often conflated (Laird, Amer, Barnett, & Barnes, 2007). However, most Arab Americans are not Muslim and the majority of Muslims in America are not Arab. Contrary to popular depictions, the vast majority of Arabs in the United States (77%) are actually Christian (Arab American Institute [AAI], 2018). As such, many prefer to identify themselves by their Christian sect, rather than as Arabs, such as the Chaldeans and Assyrian Christians of Iraq, the Maronites of Lebanon, and the Coptic Christians of Egypt. The vast majority of Arab Americans (about 89%) are high school graduates (Zogby, 2001). Over 46% have bachelor's degrees and another 19% have graduate degrees (AAI, 2007). About 70% who are over the age of and older are bilingual (AAI, 2007). Approximately 79% work in the private sector while 12% are government employees. The median household income of Arab American families is $59,012, which is only slightly above the median income for the general American population, which is $52,029 (AAI, 2007). Finally, married households are more common among Arabs than among the general population (Brittingham & De La Cruz, 2005).

## PSYCHOSOCIAL RISKS AND NEEDS

Many Arab Americans who have recently immigrated have had stressful experiences with migration (Aroian & Norris, 2003), which can in turn lead to mental health issues (Blair, 2000; Hinton, Tiet, Tran, & Chesney, 1997; Kuo & Tsai, 1986) ranging from social isolation and adjustment limitations (Carlson & Rosser-Hogan, 1991) to anxiety and depression (Abu-Ras & Abu-Bader, 2008; Blair, 2000; Hinton et al., 1997). Arab immigrants are at heightened risk for the development of post-traumatic stress disorder (PTSD), attention deficit and hyperactivity disorders, and depression (Weine & Laub, 1995; Nasser-McMillian & Hakim-Larson, 2003).

Migrants from countries that are politically unstable or more culturally different from the United States are more likely to exhibit mental health problems than those from more politically stable or culturally similar countries (Aroian & Norris, 2003; Khawaja, 2007; Knox & Britt, 2002). Many recent Arab Americans came to the United States as political refugees who have endured torture, abuse, displacement, and war (Pew Research Center, 2007), making them more susceptible to anxiety, mistrust, and the development of mental health issues. For example, in a study of Arab Americans receiving healthcare, Iraqi immigrants who arrived in the United States in the 1990s after the Persian Gulf War had elevated diagnoses of PTSD compared to other Arab clients (Jamil et al., 2002). Many immigrant Arabs may also feel socially alienated or may be mistrusting of their new environment (Abu-Ras & Abu-Bader, 2009).

Anti-Arab sentiment sharply increased in the early 2000s and was largely fueled by racial discrimination following 9/11. Prior to the terrorist attacks of 2001, Arab American writers used a trope of invisibility to characterize their experiences in the United States (Naber, 2008). The 9/11 attacks also uniquely traumatized Arab Americans as their communities were quickly subjected to increased suspicion, hate crimes (American-Arab Anti-Discrimination Committee [ADC], 2002; American Civil Liberties Union [ACLU], 2002; Singh, 2002), and heightened inquiries by the Federal Bureau of Investigation (FBI, 2006). This caused many Arab Americans to feel unwelcome in America as they were treated as inferior citizens (Gavrilos, 2002) or suspected to be terrorists. Hate crimes increased by 1,700% in the year after 9/11 (Singh, 2002). As a result, many Arab Americans felt anxious and concerned for their safety (Abu-Ras & Abu-Bader, 2008, 2009; Abu-Ras & Suárez, 2009). Additionally, for some Arab Americans, the trauma experienced by the 9/11 attacks revived earlier experiences of trauma and discrimination in their home countries. Increasing numbers of Arab Americans have sought psychological counseling from religious leaders, mosques, and churches for mental health concerns, marital problems, partner abuse, divorce, emotional and personality growth, and the promotion of inner consciousness (Abu-Ras, 2003, 2007; Abu-Ras, Gheith, & Courns, 2008; Ali, Milstein, & Marzuk, 2005; Al-Radi, 1999).

Post-9/11 government surveillance policies targeting the community, such as racially profiling Arab Americans for detention and deportation, contributed to a pervasive sense of insecurity and vulnerability within Arab communities (Abu-Ras & Abu-Bader, 2008, 2009; ADC, 2002). The post-9/11 backlash left many Arab Americans with a "sense of the indelibility" of the event and that their lives had reached an irreversible turning point (Abu-Ras, Senzai, & Laird, 2013). Many reported feeling unsafe due to discrimination and hate crimes (Abu-Ras & Suárez, 2009). Studies addressing the prevalence of post-9/11 mental health issues among Arab Americans (Abu-Ras & Abu-Bader, 2008, 2009; Amer & Hovey, 2007;

Amer & Hovey, 2011) also demonstrate that anxiety, PTSD, and depression can be passed down from parents to children (Sack, Clark, & Seely, 1996), which can cause intergenerational experiences of trauma.

While all immigrants are at heightened risk for substance abuse, Arab Americans remain under-represented in publicly funded substance abuse treatment (Arfken, Kubiak, & Farrag, 2008). This may be because alcohol and drug use are highly stigmatized and less available in Arab countries (Michalak & Trocki, 2006), leading Arab Americans to be less accepting of drug consumption and treatment (United Nations Office on Drugs and Crime, 2008). Therefore, stigma regarding substance abuse can be a cultural barrier to seeking treatment (Link, Yang, Phelan, & Collins, 2004) for Arab Americans.

## ACCESS TO MENTAL HEALTH SERVICES FOR ARAB AMERICANS

Existing mental health services in the United States are largely geared toward people who speak English as their native language. Though this is beginning to change with the increasing availability of social services in Spanish, particularly in certain parts of the country, mental health services are still not adequately set up to deal with ethnic minority groups' unique cultural influences and beliefs (Abu-Ras, 2003). Additionally, many Arab Americans also face cultural stigma that is associated with accessing mental healthcare (Gorkin & Othman, 1994). Due to the limited services targeted toward Arab Americans, many members of the Arab American community are at higher risk for the development of mental health problems (Abu-Ras & Abu-Bader, 2008, 2009; Abu-Ras & Suárez, 2009; Abu-Ras et al., 2008). Few social workers in the United States have familiarity with the Arabic language or Islamic culture and values (Abu-Ras & Abu-Bader, 2008). Additional services that target this minority group may not have been established due to a lack of resources, discrimination, a fear of negative societal reactions, or professional backlash (Abu-Ras & Abu-Bader, 2008).

Prior to 9/11, mental health and social services specifically targeting the Arab American community were virtually nonexistent. Many mental health services were created to address the wider community trauma of the terrorist event. Following 9/11, community members may be more reluctant to access mental health services because of fears that this could adversely impact their citizenship or immigration status. Many Arab Americans often instead turn to their religious leaders or family elders for mental health support. A study examining mental health settings for Muslims in New York City found that Muslim religious leaders, *imams*, played a major role in providing mental health services after 9/11 (Abu-Ras et al., 2008), although these leaders were not always adequately trained to address such issues (Abu-Ras, 2011a, 2011b).

In the current political climate, immigrants also face discrimination and frequent anti-immigrant attitudes and policies. For Arab Americans, such views are based on historical representations of Arab and Muslim societies as barbaric deviations from a modern and rational Europe (Said, 1978), images that trace back to tropes from the Medieval Crusades, which saw Islamic values as categorically distinct from Western democratic values (Huntington, 1993). In the current political climate, discrimination against Arab Americans has become endemic for mainstream America and is often confounded with notions of patriotism or nationalism (Salaita, 2005). Arabs who share physical, linguistic, or cultural similarities with suspected terrorists are often demonized. Biases against people who are seen to be Muslim, including Sikh Americans and South Asian Americans, have become manifest in the form of racial discrimination and harassment (Abu-Ras & Suárez, 2009).

Discrimination against Arab Americans often varies according to the extent that one appears to be "foreign," that is, having darker skin; sporting a beard; or wearing a hijab, an abayaah, or a kufi (Abu-Ras, Senzai, & Laird, 2013). Similarly, in the only known probability sample survey of Muslims in the United States, conducted by Pew Research Center in 2007 and 2011, women wearing hijab had a much lower likelihood of employment than non-Muslim women or non-veiling Muslim women (Abdelhadi, 2019). In a report on discrimination suits filed by Arab and Muslim Americans by the Council on American-Islamic Relations, it was found that 37% of people had been denied religious accommodations, 13% had experienced job termination, 8% had experienced verbal abuse, 8% had experienced unequal treatment, 7% had experienced denial of employment, and 5% had experienced denial of access to public facilities (Council on American-Islamic Relations [CAIR], 2001). Half of these incidents occurred in the workplace while 15% occurred in schools. The victim's perceived ethnic origin was associated with 25% of these discrimination cases and 18% were associated with Muslims praying (CAIR, 2001). In a study conducted in the Detroit metropolitan area, several individuals out of a sample of 34 Arab American nurses reported patient intimidation and rejection following 9/11 (Kulwicki, Khalifa, & Moore, 2008). Similarly, the Institute for Social Policy and Understanding found that Muslims are the most likely group to report experiencing religious discrimination (62%) with Muslim women reporting higher levels of discrimination (68%) than men (55%) (Institute for Social Policy and Understanding [ISPU], 2019). Certain anti-Muslim activists have even called for interning Muslim Americans who do not demonstrate "sufficient" loyalty to the United States (Ali, Liu, & Humedian, 2004; Nasser-McMillan & Hakim-Larson, 2003).

Arab and Muslim Americans also suffer from a relative lack of social support. Arab culture is largely collectivist in nature and places a high value on the strength of social support systems. As such, Arab Americans may be less likely to seek out assistance from individuals who may be perceived as outsiders, including social workers and mental health professionals. Additionally, they may be impeded by linguistic or cultural barriers to treatment. As a minority population, their ability to form strong social support systems may also be hindered by mistrust of Americans and feelings of "otherness." While this may conversely help for the formation of tightly knit communities, this lack of social support may ultimately harm mental health (Abu-Ras & Suárez, 2009).

Following 9/11, Arab and Muslim Americans have been subject to a range of social policies that have directly impacted their presence in the United States. One of these social policies was the National Security Entry-Exit Registration System (NSEERS). In 2002, the Department of Justice created a "special registration" process for individuals from 25 countries, initiating a system of discriminatory profiling of individuals from nations with predominantly Muslim populations (Penn State Law Immigrants' Rights Clinic and Rights Working Group, 2012). Following the creation of the USA Patriot Act, more than 80,000 men underwent call-in registration and thousands were subjected to interrogations; over 1,200 Muslims of Arab and South Asian heritage were detained (Singh, 2002); over 8,000 individuals were investigated; international students were monitored; and 16% of the 130,000 individuals who registered under the Immigration and Naturalization Service alien registration process on the basis of national origin and ethnicity were deported (ADC, 2002; Eggen, 2003).

In more recent years, anti-Muslim sentiment has become increasingly apparent in American politics. While on the election trail on November 7, 2015, then presidential candidate Donald J. Trump called for a "total and complete shutdown of Muslims entering the United States until our country's representatives can figure out what the hell is going on" (Johnson, 2015). On January 27, 2017, United States President Trump issued Executive Order 13769, titled "Protecting the Nation from Foreign Terrorist Entry into the United States," popularly known as the Muslim travel ban. The executive order lowered the number of refugees to be admitted into the United States in 2017 to just 50,000, suspended the U.S. Refugee Admissions Program for 120 days, suspended the entry of Syrian refugees indefinitely, and directed the suspension of visas for travelers from the countries of Iran, Iraq, Libya, Somalia, Sudan, Syria, and Yemen. Following the passing of the Muslim travel ban, more than 700 travelers were detained and up to 60,000 visas were provisionally revoked. In effect, the Muslim travel ban imposed blunt sanctions in the form of near categorical bans against Arabs and Muslims from particular countries (Panduranga, Patel, & Price, 2017). Except for the occasions in which it was blocked by federal courts, it was in effect until March 6, 2017, when it was replaced by Executive Order 13780 (Department of Homeland Security [DHS], 2018). Despite the fact that District Courts in Hawaii and Maryland judged that the executive order was likely motivated by anti-Muslim sentiment and therefore breached the Establishment Cause of the U.S. Constitution, the Supreme Court upheld the most recent version of the travel ban on June 26, 2018 (Liptak & Shear, 2018). The public treatment of United States Representatives Ilhan Omar and Rashid Tlaib also reflect increasing anti-Muslim sentiment from the President and others (Holmes, 2019).

Long-held Orientalist images have portrayed Arab Americans as a dangerous, emotionally volatile, and backward race (Said, 1978). Since 9/11, Arabs have been labeled as terrorists, hijackers, and extremists (Abu-Ras & Abu-Bader, 2008; Gavrilos, 2002). Discrimination against Arab and Muslim Americans is also thought to be linked to a general Western perception of Arabs as enemies of Christianity (Abu-Laban, 1988; Haddad, 1997; Suleiman, 1996) and modernity. Issues with racial identification and citizenship have traumatized many members of the Arab American population (Suleiman, 1987), negatively affecting the quality of life for Arab and Muslim Americans (Haddad, 1997). These experiences also have an impact on the likelihood of Arab Americans to seek out social services and mental health assistance. For example, the post-9/11 political climate has deterred battered Arab immigrant women from contacting police as they fear harassment and state-enforced backlash (Abu-Ras, 2007; Abu-Ras & Abu-Bader, 2008).

Multiple studies have supported the prevalence of anti-Arab and anti-Muslim sentiments in the United States. Lipset and Schneider (1977) found a pattern of "negative, close to racist" attitudes toward Muslims. Slade (1981) discovered that "Arabs remain one of the few ethnic groups who can still be slandered with impunity in America" (p. 148). Jarrar's (1983) study of 43 high-school social studies textbooks showed that Arabs were characterized as "primitive, backward, desert-dwelling, nomadic, war-loving, terrorist and full of hatred" (pp. 387–388). Various forms of hate crimes, including vandalism, threats, attacks, and discrimination, derive from ongoing and pervasive anti-Muslim and anti-Arab sentiments (Abu-Ras & Abu-Bader, 2008, 2009; Abu-Ras & Suárez, 2009; Abu-Ras, 2011a; Abu-Ras 2011b; Akram, 2002; Bushman and Bonacci, 2004; Cainkar, 2004, 2006, 2009). Such sentiments not only present serious challenges to the development of a positive ethnic self-identity (Jackson, 1997; Suleiman, 1988) but can also lead to biases and mistaken assumptions by social workers. This can significantly compromise the effectiveness of social services intended for Arab Americans. Nonetheless, issues specific to Arab communities have received little attention in the counseling and mental health literature (Erickson & Al-Tamimi, 2001). In cumulative effect, these social policies, experiences of discrimination and hate crimes have led many Arab Americans to express a constant sense of insecurity and vulnerability within the United States (ADC, 2002).

## Community-Specific Clinical Assessment

There are several community-specific psychological, social, cultural, spiritual, and political aspects that should be considered by social workers and service providers serving Arab American communities. One challenge can be the reluctance of Arab American communities to access social and mental health services (Abudabbeh, 1996; Abu-Ras, 2007; Kulwicki, 1996) as it is generally perceived that individual, couple, and family problems should be addressed within the home. Studies of battered Arab American immigrant women revealed that mental health and social services related to partner abuse were the least frequently used form of social intervention (Budman, Lipson, & Meleis, 1992; Gorkin, Massalha, & Yatziv, 1985). Participants were far more likely to turn to family, legal, or medical services as these were seen as less intrusive to a woman's private life.

Additionally, Arab clients with mental health problems commonly expressed their presenting problems in terms of physical complaints as these were seen as being more legitimate reasons for accessing help (Budman et al., 1992; Gorkin et al., 1985). Somatic presentations of mental health problems may be explained as a result of cultural stress, a heightened awareness of the mind–body connection, or the lack of concepts or terminology in Arabic to describe mental states as distinct from physical symptoms (Meleis, 1982). Such conceptualizations of mental health may be due to the individual's association of mental health intervention as being labeled insane or crazy, connotations that carry considerable social stigma (Gorkin et al., 1985; Kulwicki, 1996). *In another study, Arab American* clients specifically asked not to disclose to anyone that they had sought out counseling and worried that other community members would see them at the service site (Abu-Ras, 2007).

Arabs tend to be emotionally expressive, are likely to talk openly about pain and sorrow, and are likely to publicly weep at funerals (Nobles & Sciarra, 2000). In reference to seeking mental health assistance, Arabs tend to have less experience and are less comfortable with Western counseling approaches (Jackson, 1997). When confronted with mental health problems, many Arabs instead seek the advice of a family member, parent, or elder (Abudabbeh, 1996; Jackson, 1997), rather than getting professional help. Arab Americans tend not to discuss individual or family problems with non-family members, including social workers (Jackson, 1997). Doing so may be seen as a threat to group honor or a betrayal of the family (Abudabbeh & Nydell, 1993). For example, many immigrant Arab women remain in abusive marriages rather than face the consequences of the dishonor of violating family privacy by seeking help, which may help perpetuate violence (Abu-Ras, 2003, 2007).

Regarding gender roles, many Arabs link family shame and honor with the reputation and sexual behavior of women. Given traditional understandings of women's sexual purity and subordination to men, premarital sex, flirting, filing for divorce, challenging men's authority, criticizing one's husband, and dressing in ways that are seen to be sexually provocative may be viewed as acts that shame the family (Glazer & Abu-Ras, 1994). Despite women's increased role in the labor force, greater access to education, and higher levels of financial independence, rigid gender roles regarding the place of women as nurturers, caretakers and household keepers may still persist. While some Arab Americans feel that female domesticity is fundamental for preserving ethnicity and reproducing Arab culture (Cainkar, 1996), others have more readily disregarded patriarchal systems (Haddad & Smith, 1996). Though gender roles within Arab American communities may differ from mainstream American society, social workers and mental health providers should appreciate these differences and respect the positions that Arab women actively take in their communities.

Newer Arab American immigrant women may become more socially isolated in a foreign county as they miss the social circles and family support systems they may have had in their home countries. Others may face difficulties integrating or interacting with mainstream American society due to linguistic and cultural barriers (Aboul-Enein & Ahoul-Enein, 2010). These limitations may impact their ability to have a stable support system, affect their help-seeking behaviors, accelerate their social isolation, and decrease their interaction with others.

In counseling, many Arab Americans may view the mental health provider as an expert and expect them to offer detailed advice and give explicit directions for intervention (Gorkin et al., 1985). This may be due to cultural practices of seeking advice from elders, adherence to a hierarchical social structure, or early socialization experiences that foster respect for authority by displaying careful listening (Abudabbeh, 1996). Consequently, many Arab Americans turn over authority to someone they consider more knowledgeable for important family and life decisions. They may even view this act of advice giving to be a measure of how much the authority figure cares for them (Meleis, 1982). Therefore, social workers need to clearly explain their professional role and the social worker–client relationship, as well as address clients' expectations in therapy. This will be particularly true if the social worker is significantly younger than their client or is not of the same gender.

Another cultural aspect that may affect this relationship is a less structured orientation to time. Arab Americans may be more focused on the present situation, as opposed to future circumstances. Meleis (1982) described Arab Americans as being less concerned with whatever else was scheduled for the day because other events could be rescheduled or dealt with at a later time. Therefore, expecting clients to be comfortable with considering the hypothetical consequences of future decisions may be challenging as one's fate is largely seen to be under the control of divine will.

## Strengths and Resources

Family support and strong family values are among the Arab American community's most important sources of strength (Ajrouch, 2000). As Abudabbeh (1997) stated:

> There are today many signs of strain on the Arab family system due to factors such as industrialization, urbanization, war and conflict, and Westernization. Despite these pressures, the family remains the individual's main system of emotional and concrete support throughout the Arab world and for Arabs living elsewhere. (p. 118)

Many Arab societies tend to be collectivist and therefore discourage individuation (Abudabbeh, 1996; Almeida, 1996). Arabs tend to consider enhancing family honor (over individual success) as an important goal for family members (Nydell, 1987). They also tend to view the family as crucial to their social organization and collective identity (Abudabbeh & Nydell, 1993; Naff, 1983; Soliman, 1986). Therefore, many Arab Americans are more concerned for their family's well-being over their individual well-being. Considering one's personal needs may cause confusion or even guilt at having betrayed one's family (Gorkin et al., 1985).

Another key strength in personal well-being is the usage of religion, which can provide a framework for dealing with emotional hardship (Ellison & Levin, 1998). During difficult times, faith and religion can be a strong source of support for minority communities. Although there is little research on Muslim religiosity and health, a shared religion may influence how Arab Muslims perceive, evaluate, and seek help for their illnesses in ways that can both hinder and promote health (Laird, de Marrais, & Barnes, 2007). Since 9/11, many religious leaders have become involved in counseling Arab Americans (Flannelly, Roberts, & Weaver, 2005). Although the majority of Arab Americans are Christian, many Arab Americans still uphold Muslim values because the majority of Arabs in their home countries practice Islam (Loza, 2001). Additionally, Arab American Muslims may feel more isolated from American society and less likely to have a sense of belonging as compared to their Christian counterparts (Faragallah, Schumm, & Webb, 1997). They are also more likely to retain traditional family roles and cultural traditions—both constructs that are intertwined with religious values. Living in a pluralistic American society which may devalue the importance of religion may lead to less satisfaction with the quality of life in the United States.

Religion may serve as a source of coping for Arab communities. Social networks within religious spaces often emerge from immigrants' attempt to recreate a familiar world (Hattar-Pollara & Meleis, 1995; Maloof, 1981). Abudabbeh and Hamid (2001) suggest that religious or social networks at places of worship can help acculturate Arab Americans by substituting for one's extended family. Arab cultures tend to value the character traits of magnanimity, generosity, and hospitality (Nydell, 1987). As the pursuit of family honor encourages hard work, thrift, and conservatism, the goals of educational attainment and economic advancement are highly sought. Conversely, individuals are strongly encouraged to avoid criminal or indigent behavior (Naff, 1983) as such behaviors are seen to reflect badly not only on the individual or the family, but on the Arab American community at large.

Issues regarding shame and dishonor to the family may be compounded for Arabs who identify as lesbian, gay, bisexual, transgender, or queer. Queer Arab Americans may experience identity conflicts between their religious, racial, or ethnic identities and their queer identity. While orthodox Christian and Islamic interpretations have historically considered homosexuality to be a sin, deriving from the Biblical story of God's punishment to Lot (Jamal, 2001), contemporary interpretations of the Quran, known as *ijtihad*, may allow for alternative understandings of the religion's tolerance for gender or sexual nonconformity. While there is still no approximation for the numbers of queer Arabs or Muslims in the United States, an online support and discussion group, known as Al-Fatiha, exists for Muslim Americans who identify as queer (Minwalla, Rosser, Feldman, & Varga, 2005). Al-Fatiha can be considered part of a broader contemporary social movement of progressive Muslims, who define themselves as feminist, anti-racist, and anti-violent. What becomes problematic for Arab individuals who identify strongly with their faith is that in popular representations of organized religion, the proclamation of one's queer identity may also entail the implicit rejection of one's religious, ethnic or racial identity. As Jasbir Puar (2007) argues, there is a merging of nationalist views with queer identities, a process now termed homonationalism. This new homonormativity combines with Orientalist imaginings of "Muslim sexuality," which sees the queer Muslim as a failed man, sexually repressed, a polygamist, while all the while still being a terrorist. For social workers seeing Arab clients who may be grappling with issues regarding gender and sexuality, extreme sensitivity should be taken to not only validate the individual's process of questioning, even if this process be closeted from their families, but to also reassure clients that "coming out" need not entail the rejection of one's religious, racial or ethnic identities.

## TREATMENT APPROACHES AND PRACTICE IMPLICATIONS

Given the multiple factors that may affect Arab Americans' access to systems of clinical care, treatment strategies should be sensitive to engage members of this population group in the therapeutic helping process. While there is little research on effective social service and mental health interventions for Arab Americans, a few general suggestions can be made. Before using any intervention approach, social workers are strongly encouraged to assess the resources available to their Arab clients, their social environments, and the impacts of these factors on their clients' well-being. It is also important to assess the person's strengths and the level of their connectedness to family. It is also key to assess the individual's religious beliefs and how these beliefs may influence their attitudes toward help-seeking and mental health. Finally, social workers may need to assess the impact of 9/11 on the individual's identity and mental health. In assessing Arab individuals and families, social workers should pay extra attention to certain behaviors, such as anger, frustration, feelings of inferiority, shame, guilt, and acceptance toward mainstream American culture. Clinical countertransference may be inadvertently expressed by therapists who may use certain words to describe their client, such as "you" or "them" versus referring to themselves or other Americans as "we" or "us." The therapist/social worker should take care to demonstrate empathy, tolerance, and understanding in order to build trust.

Some Arab clients may initially hesitate to disclose their issues to someone who is not a family member or friend (Abu-Ras, 2007; Amer & Hovey, 2005). They may ask about the clinician's motivations and may desire to discuss their cultural mistrust of psychologists (Ali et al., 2004) or social workers, who may be seen to be representatives of discriminatory state mechanisms. A general distrust of a clinician's ability to maintain client confidentiality is also a recurring issue (Nasser-McMillan & Hakim-Larson, 2003). This can be especially detrimental for female Arab Americans, given the social stigma associated with exposing family matters to strangers (Abu-Ras, 2003, 2007). Clients therefore need to be reassured about social worker–client confidentiality in order to help clients feel more comfortable.

Given the cultural proclivity for hierarchical interactions with healthcare providers and other figures of authority (Al-Issa, Al Zubaidi, Bakal, & Fung, 2000), clients may expect the social worker to take a directive approach to the treatment process. As insight-oriented or client-directed psychotherapy may be resisted (Al-Abdul-Jabbar & Al-Issa, 2000; Nasser-McMillan & Hakim-Larson, 2003), it could be useful for the social worker to assume a more advisory role. Social worker disclosure of emotions and consolation of clients are also believed to strengthen the client–social worker relationship (Al-Abdul-Jabbar & Al-Issa, 2000; Nobles & Sciarra, 2000). These approaches allow Arab clients to learn from the social worker while fostering a safe environment for change.

### Psychoeducational Interventions

Because the stigma many Arab Americans experience toward both mental illness and the utilization of mental health services, a psychoeducational approach may be a preferred intervention. This approach helps Arab clients, as well as clients from other ethnic backgrounds, to identify barriers to learning about emotional response and other psychological processes associated with ongoing stress and stigma (Lukens et al., 2004). To be more effective in using the psychoeducational intervention model, social workers and therapists need to bear in mind that this treatment modality is not only intended to educate clients about mental health issues, but is also a tool to learn about their clients' perceptions, attitudes, belief systems, and cultural values. Mental health providers working with Arab or Muslim Americans must be trained on culturally specific issues, such as the importance of the month of Ramadan in Arab Muslim communities.

Sue, Arredondo, and McDavis (1992) outlined three domains in which social worker attitudes, knowledge, and skills are crucial to providing competent services: (a) awareness of their own assumptions, values, biases and awareness of negative stereotypes about Arabs and Muslims; (b) understanding of clients' worldviews by providing a safe environment for them to discuss discrimination, hate crimes, and stereotypes, as well as their attitudes toward seeking therapy; and (c) the use of culturally appropriate interventions while avoiding group counseling as feelings of fear, guilt, and shame may limit their effectiveness (Ali et al., 2004; Nasser-McMillian & Hakim-Larson, 2003).

A psychoeducational approach could also be used with the wider Arab American community, especially when traumas threaten the community's existence or purpose and may involve the death of community members (Williams, Zinner, & Ellis, 1999). Using the psychoeducational model, social workers may build on multiple psychosocial stress factors, including past trauma exposure, culture and spirituality, immigration status, and available avenues for support (Lukens et al., 2004). Immediately after the 9/11 attack, a strength-based psychoeducational approach was developed by HOPE-NY (Lukens et al., 2004). This model was adapted for members of diverse New York City communities faced with the overwhelming trauma of the 9/11 tragedy. The model includes four major principles: (a) building a collaborative community of care across and within systems (individual, family, community, structural, and provider), (b) attending to culturally relevant processes, context, and content, (c) disseminating information as a step toward personal and community empowerment, and (d) fostering resilience in the context of ongoing community trauma.

A psychoeducational intervention should be integrated into non-stigmatizing treatment settings, such as community centers or mosques, to minimize the stigma associated with mental health services and their facilities (Abu-Ras, 2007). Disseminating language-appropriate information and promoting psychosocial knowledge and education are essential to identifying severe stress reactions. These interventions will also enhance individual and community recovery. Psychosocial interventions may allow social workers to brief clients on mental health, help them develop a fundamental understanding of therapy, and engage them in longer term care. Such approaches may enable clients to better accept their mental health issues and cope with these issues with greater success. In addition, social workers could integrate Islam's spiritual and religious teachings into their psychotherapeutic interventions.

## Empowerment Approaches

An effective approach to working with Arab American clients is ensuring that their strengths and assets are highlighted. McWhirter (1998) outlined a useful treatment model: collaboration, context, critical consciousness, competence, and community. In sum, the social worker must identify the problem, attempt to understand how/why it arose, and help the client realize how their unique strengths can be used for personal empowerment (Ali et al., 2004). An empowerment model can help the client appreciate their own resources and recognize the mental health provider's attempts to provide culturally competent care.

When applying an empowerment model to Arab clients, social workers may initially explore the individual's identity (e.g., age, race, religion, gender, sexual orientation) in order to ease their anxiety and help both parties better understand the client's concerns. The mental health provider could then build on the ethical values considered central to the client's cultural and religious belief systems in order to help foster values, such as strength and resilience (Abraham, 1995; Abudabbeh, 1996; Erickson & Al-Tamimi, 2001; Jackson, 1997).

Rates of acculturation will considerably influence the patterns of how Arab culture is transferred and experienced in the new country (Al-Krenawi & Graham, 2003). Second-generation Arab Americans are likely to have differing notions of ethnic identity, acculturation, and religiosity than their parents. Mental health providers may encourage Arab Americans born in the United States to explore their sense of belonging to the Arab community, as well as mainstream American culture, emphasizing that healthy psychological acculturation strategies differ for different subgroups of an ethnic population. For example, second-generation and early immigrant Christian Arab Americans were found to have retained their cultural values and practices while still participating in mainstream American culture (Amer & Hovey, 2007). Mental health providers should encourage their clients to explore and negotiate the challenges and benefits of both cultures in the shaping of a healthy bicultural identity (Amer & Hovey, 2007).

## Faith-Based Coping

Religion is integral to many Arab Americans and may be a central component of their identity (Abudabbeh, 1996; Abudabbeh & Nydell, 1993), perhaps trumping other differentiating factors like nationality, occupation and marital status (Naff, 1983). As previously stated, in their home countries, the majority of Arabs are Muslims; however, in the United States, the majority of Arabs are Christians.

The Islamic faith follows the same monotheistic tradition as Judaism and Christianity, including a belief in the Ten Commandments, and the teachings of Abraham, Moses and Jesus (Jackson, 1997). The word *Allah* is the Arabic word for God and Muslims believe that Muhammad is the last prophet. Although religion and spirituality have been incorporated into other cognitive therapy models to treat mental health disorders among Christian and Jewish populations, limited attention has been paid to utilizing such an approach with Muslim clients (Hamdan, 2008). Social workers may suggest that Arab Muslim clients use Islamic tenets to cope with trauma, such as praying or reciting/reading specific Quranic passages (Abu-Ras et al., 2008).

Social workers may also wish to undertake a religious psychotherapy intervention. According to Islamic thought, one's mental and spiritual development is in a constant state of evolution that moves from self-gratification toward inner peace and self-assuredness (Mohit, 2001). Imams have used this Islamic therapeutic process, which combines elements of cognitive, behavioral, and psychodynamic therapy, to treat Muslim clients (Abu-Ras et al., 2008). Traditional Islamic teachings explain mental illness as a defective relationship with God, a divine punishment, or the result of God's will (Al-Krenawi, 1996; Al-Krenawi & Graham, 1999). Many Arab Muslims perceive mental illness as part of human suffering and often view mental illness as a means of atoning for previous sins. Some may believe that the reward for overcoming issues like anxiety and depression could be doubled if suffering is endured with patience and prayer. In the face of such tests, and to promote personal healing and growth, ritual acts of devotion, like prayer, fasting, repentance, and reciting the Quran, may be part of the healing process.

However, a faith-based approach should be used with caution, particularly when trauma is linked with clients' struggles with their religious identity (Hedayat-Diba, 2000). For example, the assessment of suicidal ideation may be particularly difficult for devout Muslim clients as Islam forbids suicide. Therefore, a social worker might rephrase crisis assessment by assessing for suicidality in a passive manner, such as asking "Do you wish that God would let you die?" (Hedayat-Diba, 2000) instead of asking, "Do you think about committing suicide?" Similarly, queer Arabs may find religious identification to also be problematic as many orthodox Muslim American groups openly reject homosexuality and gender nonconformity (Rayside, 2011).

## Family Support and Family Therapy

The maintenance of family unity is a strongly held value within Arab American culture. Paying attention to family dynamics is crucial in the planning and implementation of treatment. Learning about the status of the client within the family will determine the level of their independence, individualistic views of the worlds around them, and the level of support the client may need to cope with their issues. More attention may need to be focused on intrafamilial conflicts. Family functioning and social support are coping resources that could ease anxiety and depression. Clinicians should also pay attention to clients' comfortability with working with someone who may be of the same or opposite gender to themselves.

As Arab culture is built around the extended family system, social workers are strongly advised to advocate a multisystem intervention approach involving relatives, community members, religious leaders, and medical and social service providers, if this is appropriate. Family therapy may be an effective intervention in this regard (Amer & Hovey, 2005). Unlike psychodynamic traditions which often emphasize the primacy of individualistic needs (Al-Krenawi & Graham, 2003), the value of family within the context of a collectivist worldview dictates the inclusion of family members in the effective delivery of services and the fulfillment of life satisfaction. Family therapy could also help family members support each other and provide each other with feelings of belonging, especially if they are experiencing social isolation (Abudabbeh, 1996). Social workers working with predominantly Arab American populations have reported that including family members can alleviate client concerns and facilitate the development of trust in the social worker (Nasser-McMillan & Hakim-Larson, 2003).

However, as this inclusion process can be challenging, it should fully be the client's decision to include family in their treatment. Including the family may be especially pertinent when counseling Arab American women as child care may be difficult to arrange for women who are mothers (Nasser-McMillan & Hakim-Larson, 2003). Moreover, for women who do not have independent income, it may be difficult to convince their spouses that therapy is a needed usage of time or money (Nobles & Sciarra, 2000). Engaging a male spouse in the therapeutic process may reduce these concerns, thereby making it easier for women to attend therapeutic sessions. This may also be part of the natural course of therapy in collectivist cultures as issues confronting Arab American women will also affect their families (Abu-Baker, 2006). However, if an Arab woman's mental health issues are based on her dissatisfaction with her partner or are related to intimate partner violence, family engagement would not be warranted (Abu-Baker, 2006). In sum, social workers need to assess whether including family members will help their client's psychological well-being.

## CONCLUSION

Historically, culture has had major influences on the development of individual identities, families, ethnic groups, communities, and nations. Barnett (1988) argues that we should judge the human rights aspects of a cultural practice relatively in terms of the context in which the practice is embedded and respect cultural diversity. In the field of social work, researchers tend to place emphasis on how culture affect people's attitudes, belief systems, social interactions, and access to social and mental health services. Furthermore, these differences determine and shape our understanding of the ways to best assist people from different cultures.

Culture is a vital aspect to understanding and serving families from minority ethnic groups. The Arab American community is a minority group that is among those most misunderstood, misrepresented, and negatively perceived by mass media and mainstream American society. Such views do not only affect the ability of Arab immigrants to cope with mental health issues, family crises, and political challenges, but can also lead to prejudice, bias, and faulty assumptions on the part of social workers and others who serve them.

This chapter has highlighted important similarities, differences, and false assumptions associated with Arab culture. It is essential to understand the culture of Arab American immigrants, their strengths and needs, their cultural attitudes toward mental health services, and the post-9/11 anti-Arab political climate before choosing an appropriate intervention approach. Based on these issues, social workers need to take into consideration the diverse cultural values held within the Arab community while practicing within mainstream American health delivery systems. Additionally, providers must educate themselves on Arabic culture and Islamic values. Finally, it is imperative that clinicians explore other appropriate approaches when dealing with Arab individuals, families, and communities that reflect on their experiences, such as linkages to immigration services or partnering with an imam for counseling.

To reduce the psychosocial stress resulting from the current anti-Arab political climate, it is important to consider not only the social roots of these stressors but also the ways in which cultural and faith institutions might assist in shaping the social construction of mental illness. Religion and spirituality play an important role in the way that Arab and Muslim individuals, families, and communities understand and cope with mental health issues. For example, some communities may perceive mental illness to be the result of *al-junin*, or being possessed by spirits or *jinns* (Al-Krenawi & Graham, 2003). It is important to not discount such cultural beliefs, but work with clients on addressing mental health within such an understanding of mental illness. Using spiritual or religious teachings may also be effective with some Muslim clients as the Quran and the Hadith are generally considered a way of life among Muslims.

The overall implications of this chapter, for both research and social work practice, is the importance of recognizing the diversity within Arab cultures and ethnic groups, their religious and political affiliations, and gendered mechanisms for coping with psychosocial stressors. The community's cumulative and historical impact of trauma as a result of political instability and war in their home countries, as well as contemporary racial harassment, discrimination and hate crimes in the United States, should also be appreciated.

## REFERENCES

Abdelhadi, E. (2019). The Hijab and Muslim women's employment in the United States. *Research in Social Stratification and Mobility, 61*, 26–37. doi:10.1016/j.rssm.2019.01.006

Aboul-Enein, B. H., & Ahoul-Enein, F. H. (2010). The cultural gap delivering health care services to Arab American populations in the United States. *Journal of Cultural Diversity, 17*(1).

Abraham, N. (1995). Arab Americans. In R. J. Vecoli, J. Galens, A. Sheets, & R. V. Young (Eds.), *Gale encyclopedia of multicultural America* (Vol. 1, pp. 84–98). New York, NY: Gale Research.

Abraham, S., & Abraham, N. (1983). *Arabs in the new world: Studies on Arab American communities.* Detroit, MI: Wayne State University Press.

Abu-Baker, K. (2006). Aram/Muslim families in the United States. In Dawiry, M. A. (Ed.), *Counseling and psychotherapy with Arabs and Muslims: A culturally sensitive approach* (pp. 29–46). New York, NY: Teacher College Press.

Abudabbeh, N. (1996). Arab families. In M. McGoldrick, J. Giordano, & J. K. Pearce (Eds.), *Ethnicity and family therapy* (2nd ed., pp. 333–346). New York, NY: Guilford Press.

Abudabbeh, N. (1997). Counseling Arab-American families. In U. P. Gielen & A. L. Comunian (Eds.), *The family and family therapy: An international perspective* (pp. 115–126). Trieste, Italy: Edizioni LINT.

Abudabbeh, N., & Hamid, A. (2001). Substance use among Arabs and Arab Americans. In Straussner, S. L. A. (Ed.), *Ethnocultural factors in substance abuse treatment* (pp. 275–290). New York, NY: Guilford Press.

Abudabbeh, N., & Nydell, M. (1993). Transcultural counseling and Arab Americans. In J. McFadden (Ed.), *Transcultural counseling: Bilateral and international perspectives* (pp. 262–284). Alexandria, VA: American Counseling Association.

Abuelezam, N. N., El-Sayed, A. M., & Galea, S. (2018). The health of Arab Americans in the United States: An updated comprehensive literature review. *Frontiers in Public Health, 6*, 262. doi:10.3389/fpubh.2018.00262

Abu-Laban, S. (1988). The coexistence of cohorts: Identity and adaptation among Arab-American Muslims, *Arab Study Quarterly, 11*(8 & 9), 45–63.

Abu-Laban, B., & Suleiman M. (1989). *Arab Americans: Continuity and change.* Belmont, MA: Association of Arab-American University Graduates, Inc.

Abu-Ras, W. (2003). Barriers to services for Arab immigrant battered women in a Detroit suburb. *Journal of Social Work Research and Evaluation: An International Publication, 4*(1), 49–66.

Abu-Ras, W. (2007). Cultural beliefs and utilization of services by Arab immigrant battered women. *Violence Against Women, 13*(10), 1002–1028. doi:10.1177/1077801207306019

Abu-Ras, W. (2011a). Muslim chaplain's role as perceived by directors and chaplains of New York City hospitals and health care settings. *Journal of Muslim Mental Health, 6*(1), 21–43. doi:10.3998/jmmh.10381607.0006.103

Abu-Ras, W. (2011b). Chaplaincy and spiritual care services: The case for Muslim patients. *Topics in Integrative Health Care: An International Journal, 2*(2), 1–16.

Abu-Ras, W. (2013). American Muslim physicians' public role post-9/11 and minority community empowerment: Serving the underserved. *Journal of Immigrant & Refugee Studies, 11*(1), 1–23. doi:10.1080/15562948.2013.759012

Abu-Ras, W., & Abu-Bader, S. (2008). The impact of 9/11 on the Arab-American well-being. *Journal of Muslim Mental Health, 3*(2), 217–239. doi:10.1080/15564900802487634

Abu-Ras, W., & Abu-Bader, S. (2009). Risk factors for posttraumatic stress disorder (PTSD): The case of Arab- & Muslim-Americans, post-9/11. *Journal of Immigrant & Refugee Studies, 7*(4), 393–418. doi:10.1080/15562940903379068

Abu-Ras, W., Gheith, A., & Cournos, F. (2008). Religion and Imam's role in mental health promotion: A study at 22 mosques in New York City's Muslim community. *Journal of Muslim Mental Health, 3*(2), 155–176. doi:10.1080/15564900802487576

Abu-Ras, W., Senzai, F., & Laird, L. (2013). Muslim physicians' experiences post 9/11: Cultural trauma and the formation of Islamic identity. *Traumatology, 19*(1), 11–19. doi:10.1177/1534765612441975

Abu-Ras, W., & Suárez, Z. E. (2009). Muslim men and women's perception of discrimination, hate crimes, and PTSD symptoms post 9/11. *Traumatology, 15*(3), 48–63. doi:10.1177/1534765609342281

Ajrouch, K. J. (2000). Place, age, and culture: Community living and ethnic identity among Lebanese American adolescents. *Small Group Research, 31*(4), 447–469. doi:10.1177/104649640003100404

Akram, S. M. (2002). The aftermath of 9/11, 2001: The targeting of Arabs and Muslims in America. *Arab Studies Quarterly, 24*, 61–118.

Al-Abdul-Jabbar, J., & Al-Issa, I. (2000). Psychotherapy in Islamic society. In I. Al-Issa (Ed.), *Al-Junun: Mental illness in the Islamic world* (pp. 277–293). Madison, CT: International Universities Press.

Ali, S. R., Liu, M. W., & Humedian, M. (2004). Islam 101: Understanding the religion and therapy implications. *Professional Psychology: Research and Practice, 35*(6), 635–642. doi:10.1037/0735-7028.35.6.635

Ali, O., Milstein, G., & Marzuk, P. (2005). The imam's role in meeting the counseling needs of Muslim communities in the United States. *Psychiatric Services, 56*, 202–205. doi:10.1176/appi.ps.56.2.202

Al-Issa, I., Al Zubaidi, A., Bakal, D., & Fung, T. S. (2000). Beck Anxiety Inventory symptoms in Arab college students. *Arab Journal of Psychiatry, 11*, 41–47.

Al-Krenawi, A. (1996). *A study of dual use of modern and traditional mental health systems by the Bedouin of the Negev.* Unpublished doctoral dissertation, University of Toronto, Toronto, Ontario, Canada.

Al-Krenawi, A., & Graham, J. R. (1999). Social work and Koranic mental health healers. *International Social Work, 42*, 53–65. doi:10.1177/002087289904200106

Al-Krenawi, A., & Graham, J. R. (2003). Principles of social work practice in the Muslim Arab world. *Arab Studies Quarterly, 25*, 75–91.

Almeida, R. (1996). Hindu, Christian, and Muslim families. In M. McGoldrick, J. Giordano, & J. K. Pearce (Eds.), *Ethnicity and family therapy* (2nd ed., pp. 395–423). New York, NY: Guilford Press.

Al-Radi, O. (1999). *The role of the mosque in mental health.* Paper presented at the Sixth International Congress of WIAMH, Tuzla, Bosnia and Herezegovina.

Amer, M. M., & Hovey J. D. (2005). Examination of the impact of acculturation, stress, and religiosity on mental health variables for second generation Arab Americans. *Ethnicity & Disease, 15*(1 Suppl 1): S1, 111–112.

Amer, M. M., & Hovey, J. D. (2007). Socio-demographic differences in acculturation and mental health for a sample of 2nd generation/early immigrant Arab Americans. *Journal of Immigrant Minority Health, 9*, 335–347. doi:10.1007/s10903-007-9045-y

Amer, M. M., & Hovey, J. D. (2011). Anxiety and depression in a post-September 11 sample of Arabs in the USA. *Society for Psychiatry and Epidemiology, 47*(3), 409–418. doi:10.1007/s00127-011-0341-4

American-Arab Anti-Discrimination Committee. (2003). Report on Anti-Arab hate crimes and discrimination. Washington, DC: Author. Retrieved from https://www.mbda.gov/sites/mbda.gov/files/migrated/files-attachments/September_11_Backlash.pdf

American Civil Liberties Union. (2002). *International civil liberties report*. Retrieved http://www.aclu.org/FilesPDFs/iclr2002.pdf

Arab American Institute. (2018). *Demographics*. Retrieved from https://www.aaiusa.org/demographics

Arab American Institute Foundation. (2009). *Quick facts about Arab Americans*. Retrieved from http://www.aaiusa.org/demographics

Arfken, C., Kubiak, S. P., & Farrag, M. (2008). Arab Americans in publicly financed alcohol/other drug abuse treatment. *Alcoholism Treatment Quarterly, 26*(3), 229–240. doi:10.1080/07347320802071547

Aroian, K. J., & Norris, A. E. (2003). Depression trajectories in relatively recent immigrants. *Comprehensive Psychiatry, 44*(5), 420–427. doi:10.1016/S0010-440X(03)00103-2

Austin, A. D. (2012). *African Muslims in antebellum America: Transatlantic stories and spiritual struggles*. New York, NY: Routledge Press.

Azhar, S. (2019). Islamic Processes for Managing Grief, Loss and Death. In B. Counselman-Carpenter, & A. Redcay (Eds.), *Working with grief and traumatic loss: Theory, practice, personal self-care and reflection for clinicians*. San Diego, CA: Cognella.

Barnett, C. R. (1988). Is there a scientific basis in anthropology for the ethics of human rights? In T. E. Downing & G. Kushner (Eds.), *Human rights and anthropology*. Cambridge: Cultural Survival.

Blair, R. G. (2000). Risk factors associated with PTSD and major depression among Cambodian refugees in Utah. *Health and Social Work, 25*, 23–30. doi:10.1093/hsw/25.1.23

Brittingham, A., & De La Cruz, P. (2005). *We the people of Arab ancestry in the United States: Census 2000 Special Reports*. Retrieved from http://www.census.gov/prod/2005pubs/censr-21.pdf

Budman, C. L., Lipson, J. G., & Meleis, A. I. (1992). The cultural consultant in mental health care: The case of an Arab adolescent. *American Journal of Orthopsychiatry, 62*(3), 359–370. doi:10.1037/h0079347

Bushman, B. J., & Bonacci, A. M. (2004). You've got mail: Using e-mail to examine the effect of prejudiced attitudes on discrimination against Arabs. *Journal of Social Experimental Psychology, 40*, 753–759. doi:10.1016/j.jesp.2004.02.001

Cainkar, L. (1996). Immigrant Palestinian women evaluate their lives. In B. C. Aswad & B. Bilge (Eds.), *Family and gender among American Muslims: Issues facing Middle Eastern immigrants and their descendants* (pp. 41–58). Philadelphia: Temple University Press.

Cainkar, L. (2004). The impact of the September 11 attacks and their aftermath on Arab and Muslim community in the United States. *Global Security and Cooperation Quarterly, Social Science Research Council, 13*. Retrieved from http://www.ssrc.org

Cainkar, L. (2006). The social construction of difference and the Arab American experience. *Journal of American Ethnic History, 25*(2–3), 243–278.

Cainkar, L. (2009). *Homeland insecurity: The Arab American and Muslim American experience after 9/11*. New York, NY: Russell Sage.

Camarota, S. A. (2002). *Immigrants from the Middle East: A Profile of the Foreign-born Population from Pakistan to Morocco*. Center for Immigration Studies. Retrieved from https://cis.org/Report/Immigrants-Middle-East

Carlson, E. B., & Rosser-Hogan, R. (1991). Trauma experiences, posttraumatic stress, dissociation, and depression in Cambodian refugees. *American Journal of Psychiatry, 148*, 1548–1551. doi:10.1176/ajp.148.11.1548

Council on American-Islamic Relations. (2001). The Status of Muslim Civil Rights in the United States. Washington, DC. Retrieved from https://www.swissinfo.ch/media/cms/files/swissinfo/2002/08/arabic.pdf

Council on Foreign Relations. (2014). *The Arab League*. Retrieved from https://www.cfr.org/backgrounder/arab-league

David, G. C. (2007). The creation of "Arab American": Political activism and ethnic (dis)unity 1. *Critical Sociology 33*, 833–862. doi:10.1163/156916307X230340

Department of Homeland Security. (2018). *Executive Order 13780: Protecting the Nation From Foreign Terrorist Entry Into the United States*. Initial Section 11 Report. Retrieved from https://www.dhs.gov/sites/default/files/publications/Executive%20Order%2013780%20Section%2011%20Report%20-%20Final.pdf

Eggen, D. (2003, December 19). Tapes show abuse of 9/11 detainees: Justice Department examines videos prison officials said were destroyed. *The Washington Post*, p. A01.

El-Badry, S. (1994). The Arab Americans. *American Demographics, 1994*, 22–30.

Ellison, C. G., & Levin, J. S. (1998). The religion-health connection: Evidence, theory, and future directions. *Health Education and Behavior, 25*(6), 700–720. doi:10.1177/109019819802500603

El-Sayed, A. M., & Galea, S. (2009). The health of Arab-Americans living in the United States: a systematic review of the literature. *BMC Public Health, 9*(1), 272. doi:10.1186/1471-2458-9-272

Erickson, C. D., & Al-Tamimi, N. R. (2001). Providing mental health services to Arab Americans: Recommendations and considerations. *Cultural Diversity and Ethnic Minority Psychology, 7*(4), 308–327. doi:10.1037/1099-9809.7.4.308

Faragallah, M. H., Schumm, W. R., & Webb, F. J. (1997). Acculturation of Arab-American immigrants: An exploratory study. *Journal of Comparative Family Studies, 28*, 182–203.

Federal Bureau of Investigation. (2006). *Hate crimes in the United States, 2006 report*. Retrieved from http://www.fbi.gov/ucr/hc2006/abouthcs.htm

Flannelly, K. J., Roberts, S. B., & Weaver, A. J. (2005). Correlates of compassion fatigue and burnout in chaplains and other clergy who responded to the September 11th attacks in New York City. *The Journal of Pastoral Care & Counseling, 59*(3): 213–224. doi:10.1177/154230500505900304

Gavrilos, D. (2002). Arab Americans in a nation's imagined community: How news constructed Arab American reactions to the Gulf War. *Journal of Communication Inquiry, 26*(4), 426–445. doi:10.1177/019685902236900

Glazer, I., & Abu-Ras, W. (1994). On aggression, human rights, and hegemonic discourse: The case of a murder for family honor in Israel. *Sex Roles, 30*(3–4), 269–288. doi:10.1007/BF01420994

Gorkin, M., Massalha, S., & Yatziv, G. (1985). Psychotherapy of Israeli-Arab patients: Some cultural considerations. *Journal of Psychoanalytic Anthropology, 8*, 215–230.

Gorkin, M., & Othman, R. (1994). Traditional psychotherapeutic healing and healers in the Palestinian community. *Israel Journal of Psychiatry and Related Sciences, 31*, 221–231.

Haddad, Y. Y. (1997). Make some room for Muslims? In W. H. Conser, Jr., & S. B. Twiss (Eds.), *Religious diversity and American religion history* (pp. 218–261). Athens: University of Georgia Press.

Haddad, Y. Y., & Smith, J. I. (1996). Islamic values among American Muslims. In B. C. Aswad & B. Bilge (Eds.), *Family and gender among American Muslims: Issues facing Middle Eastern immigrants and their descendants* (pp. 19–40). Philadelphia, PA: Temple University Press.

Hamdan, A. (2008). Cognitive restructuring: An Islamic perspective. *Journal of Muslim Mental Health, 3*, 99–116. doi:10.1080/15564900802035268

Hammoud, M. M., White, C. B., & Fetters, M. D. (2005). Opening cultural doors: Providing culturally sensitive healthcare to Arab American and American Muslim patients. *American Journal of Obstetrics and Gynecology, 193*(4), 1307–1311. doi:10.1016/j.ajog.2005.06.065

Hattar-Pollara, M., & Meleis, A. I. (1995). The stress of immigration and the daily lived experiences of Jordanian immigrant women in the United States. *Western Journal of Nursing Research, 17*(5), 521–539. doi:10.1177/019394599501700505

Hedayat-Diba, Z. (2000). Psychotherapy with Muslims. In P. S. Richards & A. E. Bergin (Eds.), *Handbook of psychotherapy and religious diversity* (p. 518). Washington, DC: American Psychological Association.

Hinton, W. L., Tiet, Q., Tran, C. G., & Chesney, M. (1997). Predictors of depression among refugees from Vietnam: A longitudinal study of new arrivals. *Journal of Nervous and Mental Disease, 185*, 39–45. doi:10.1097/00005053-199701000-00007

Holmes, O. (2019). Israel bars entry to US politicians Ilhan Omar and Rashida Tlaib. *The Guardian.* Retrieved from https://www.theguardian.com/world/2019/aug/15/israel-netanyahu-ilhan-omar-rashida-tlaib-visit

Huntington, S. (1993). The clash of civilizations. *Foreign affairs, 72*(3), 22–49.

Institute for Social Policy and Understanding. (2019). *American Muslim Poll 2019: Key Findings.* Retrieved from https://www.ispu.org/american-muslim-poll-2019-key-findings

Jackson, M. (1997). Counseling Arab Americans. In C. Lee (Ed.), *Multicultural issues in counseling: New approaches to diversity* (2nd ed., pp. 333–349). Alexandria, VA: American Counseling Association.

Jamal, A. (2001). The Story of Lot and the Quran's perception of the morality of same-sex sexuality. *Journal of Homosexuality, 41*(1), 1–88.

Jamil, H., Hakim-Larson, J., Farrag, M., Kafaji, T., Duqum, I., & Jamil, L. H. (2002). A retrospective study of Arab American mental health clients: Trauma and the Iraqi refugees. *American Journal of Orthopsychiatry, 72*(3), 355–361. doi:10.1037/0002-9432.72.3.355

Jarrar, S. (1983). *Education in the Arab world.* New York, NY: Praeger.

Johnson, J. (2015, Dec. 7). Trump Calls for "Total and Complete Shutdown of Muslims Entering the United States." *Washington Post.* Retrieved from https://www.washingtonpost.com/news/post-politics/wp/2015/12/07/donald-trump-calls-for-total-and-complete-shutdown-of-muslims-entering-the-united-states/

Khater, A. F. (2001). *Inventing home: Emigration, gender, and the middle class in Lebanon, 1870-1920.* Berkeley: University of California Press.

Khawaja, N. G. (2007). An investigation of the psychological distress of Muslim migrants in Australia. *Journal of Muslim Mental Health, 2*, 39–56. doi:10.1080/15564900701238526

Knox, S. A., & Britt, H. (2002). A comparison of general practice encounters with patients from English-speaking and non-English speaking backgrounds. *Medical Journal of Australia, 177*, 98–101. doi:10.5694/j.1326-5377.2002.tb04681.x

Kulwicki, A. (1996). Health issues among Arab Muslim families. In B. Aswad & B. Bilge (Eds.), *Family and gender among American Muslims: Issues facing Middle Eastern immigrants and their descendants* (pp. 187–207). Philadelphia, PA: Temple University Press.

Kulwicki, A., Khalifa, R., & Moore, G. (2008). The effects of September 11 on Arab American nurses in metropolitan Detroit. *Journal of Transcultural Nursing, 19*(2), 134–139. doi:10.1177/1043659607313071

Kuo, W. H., & Tsai, Y. (1986). Social networking, hardiness and immigrant's mental health. *Journal of Health and Social Behavior, 27*, 133–149. doi:10.2307/2136312

Laird, L. D., Amer, M. M., Barnett, E. D., & Barnes, L. L. (2007). Muslim patients and health disparities in the UK and the US. *Archives of Disease in Childhood, 92*(10), 922–926. doi:10.1136/adc.2006.104364

Laird, L. D., de Marrais, J., & Barnes, L. L. (2007). Portraying Islam and Muslims in MEDLINE: A content analysis. *Social Science and Medicine, 65*(12), 2425–2439. doi:10.1016/j.socscimed.2007.07.029

Link, B. G., Yang, L. H., Phelan, J. C., & Collins, P. Y. (2004). Measuring mental illness stigma. *Schizophrenia Bulletin, 30*(3), 511–541. doi:10.1093/oxfordjournals.schbul.a007098

Lipset, S. M., & Schneider, W. (1977, November). Carter vs. Israel: What the polls reveal. *Commentary,* p. 22.

Liptak, A., & Shear, M. D. (2018). Trump's Travel Ban Is Upheld by Supreme Court. *New York Times.* Retrieved from https://www.nytimes.com/2018/06/26/us/politics/supreme-court-trump-travel-ban.html

Loza, N. (2001). *Insanity on the Nile: The history of psychiatry in Pharaonic Egypt.* Paper presented at the Second Biennial National Conference on Arab American Health Issues, Dearborn, MI.

Lukens, E., O'Neill, P., Thorning, H., Waterman-Cecutti, J., Gubiseh- Ayala, D., Abu-Ras, W., . . . Chen, T. (2004). Building resiliency and cultural collaboration Post September 11th: A group model of brief integrative psychoeducation for diverse communities. *Traumatology, 10*(2), 107–129. doi:10.1177/153476560401000204

Maloof, P. S. (1981). Fieldwork and the folk health sector in the Washington, D.C. metropolitan area. *Anthropological Quarterly, 54*(2), 68–75. doi:10.2307/3318009

McWhirter, E. H. (1998). An empowerment model of counsellor education. *Canadian Journal of Counselling, 32*(1), 12–26.

Meleis, A. I. (1982). Effect of modernization on Kuwaiti women. *Social Science & Medicine, 16*(9), 965–970. doi:10.1016/0277-9536(82)90364-1

Michalak, L., & Trocki, K. (2006). Alcohol and Islam: an overview. *Contemporary Drug Problems, 33*(4), 523–562. doi:10.1177/009145090603300401

Minwalla, O., Rosser, B. S., Feldman, J., & Varga, C. (2005). Identity experience among progressive gay Muslims in North America: A qualitative study within Al-Fatiha. *Culture, Health & Sexuality, 7*(2), 113–128. doi:10.1080/13691050412331321294

Mohit, A. (2001). Mental health and psychiatry in the Middle East: Historic development. *Eastern Mediterranean Health Journal, 7*(3), 336–347.

Naber, N. (2008). Introduction: Arab Americans and U.S. Racial Formations. In A. A. Jamal, N. Naber, & N. C. Naber (Eds.), *Race and Arab Americans before and after 9/11: From invisible citizens to visible subjects*. Syracuse, NY: Syracuse University Press.

Naff, A. (1983). Arabs in America: A historical overview. In S. Abraham & N. Abraham (Eds.), *Arabs in the new world: Studies on Arab American communities* (pp. 8–12). Detroit, MI: Wayne State University Press.

Nasser-McMillan, S. C., & Hakim-Larson, J. (2003). Counseling considerations among Arab Americans. *Journal of Counseling & Development, 81*, 150–159. doi:10.1002/j.1556-6678.2003.tb00236.x

Nobles, A. Y., & Sciarra, D. T. (2000). Cultural determinants in the treatment of Arab Americans: A primer for mainstream therapists. *American Journal of Orthopsychiatry, 70*(2), 182–191. doi:10.1037/h0087734

Nydell, M. K. (1987). *Understanding Arabs: A guide for Westerners*. Yarmouth: Intercultural Press.

Office of Management and Budget. (1995). *Standard for the Classification of Federal Data on Race and Ethnicity*. Washington, DC: Office of Information and Regulatory Affairs. Retrieved from https://obamawhitehouse.archives.gov/omb/fedreg_race-ethnicity

Panduranga, H., Patel, F., & Price, M. W. (2017). *Extreme vetting & the Muslim ban*. New York, NY: New York University Brennan Center for Justice.

Penn State Law Immigrants' Rights Clinic and Rights Working Group. (2012). *The NSEERS Effect: A Decade of Racial Profiling, Fear, and Secrecy*. Center for Immigrants' Rights Clinic Publications. Book 11. Retrieved from http://elibrary.law.psu.edu/irc_pubs/11

Pew Research Center. (2007). *Muslim-Americans: Middle class and mostly mainstream*. Washington, DC: Author.

Puar, J. K. (2007). *Terrorist assemblages: Homonationalism in queer times*. Durham, NC: Duke University Press.

Rayside, D. (2011). *Faith, politics, and sexual diversity in Canada and the United States*. Vancouver, BC, CAN: UBC Press.

Sack, W. H., Clarke, G. N., & Seeley, J. (1996). Multiple forms of stress in Cambodian adolescent refugees. *Child Development, 67*(1), 107–116. doi:10.2307/1131689

Said, E. W. (1978). *Orientalism*. New York, NY: Pantheon Press.

Salaita, S. (2005). Ethnic identity and imperative patriotism: Arab Americans before and after 9/11. *College Literature, 32*, 146–168. doi:10.1353/lit.2005.0033

Shakir, E. (1997). *Bint Arab: Arab and Arab American Women in the United States*. Wetport, CT: Praeger Publishers.

Singh, A. (Ed.). (2002). *We are not the enemy: Hate crimes against Arabs, Muslims, and those perceived to be Arab or Muslim after 9/11* (Vol. 14). New York, NY: Human Rights Watch.

Slade, S. (1981). The image of the Arab in America: Analysis of a poll on American attitudes. *Middle East Journal, 35,* 147–150.

Soliman, A. M. (1986). Status, rationale and development of counseling in the Arab countries: views of participants in a counseling conference. *International Journal for the Advancement of Counseling, 10*(2), 131–141. doi:10.1007/BF00156467

Sue, D., Arredondo, P. M., & McDavis, R. J. (1992). Multicultural counseling competencies and standards: A call to the profession. *Journal of Counseling & Development, 70,* 477–483. doi:10.1002/j.1556-6676.1992.tb01642.x

Suleiman, M. (1987). Early Arab-Americans: the search for identity. In E. Hooglund (Ed.), *Crossing the water.* Washington, DC: Smithsonian Institution Press.

Suleiman, M. W. (1988). *The Arabs in the mind of America.* Brattleboro: Amana Books.

Suleiman, M. W. (1994). Arab-Americans and the political process. In E. McCarus (Ed.), *The development of Arab-American identity.* Ann Arbor: University of Michigan Press.

Suleiman, M. W. (1996). The Arab-American Left. In P. Buhle & D. Georgakas (Eds.), *The immigrant left in the United States.* New York, NY: State University of New York Press.

Suleiman, M. W. (1999). Islam, Muslims, and Arabs in America: the other of the other of the other. *Journal of Muslim Minority Affairs, 19*(1), 33–47. doi:10.1080/13602009908716423

United Nations Office on Drugs and Crime. (2008). *World Drug Report.* Bernan. New York, NY: United Nations.

U.S. Census Bureau. (2000). *U.S. Department of Commerce, Economics, and Statistics Administration.* Retrieved from http://www.Census.gov

U.S. Census Bureau. (2003). *The Arab Population: 2000. Census 2000 Brief.* Washington, DC: U.S. Department of Commerce.

U.S. Census Bureau. (2013). *Arab Households in the United States: 2006-2010.* Retrieved from https://www.census.gov/library/publications/2013/acs/acsbr10-20.html

Weine, S., & Laub, D. (1995). Narrative constructions of historical realities in testimony with Bosnian survivors of "ethnic cleansing." *Psychiatry: Interpersonal and Biological Processes, 58*(3), 246–260. doi:10.1080/00332747.1995.11024729

Williams, M., Zinner, E. S., & Ellis, R. R. (1999). The connection between grief and trauma: An overview. In M. Williams, E. S. Zinner, & R. R. Ellis (Eds.), *When a community weeps: Case studies in group survivorship* (pp. 3–17). Philadelphia, PA: Brunner/Mazel.

Zogby, J. (2001). *What ethnic Americans really think: The Zogby culture polls.* Washington, DC: Zogby International.

# 16

# Practice With Lesbian, Gay, Bisexual, and Transgender People and Their Families

GERALD P. MALLON

*"Are you out to your family?"*
*How did your family deal with your being bisexual?"*
*"Do your children know that you are gay?"*
*What was it like for your ex when you transitioned?"*

## INTRODUCTION

All of the above are questions that almost inevitably arise in the process of getting to know a lesbian, gay, bisexual, or transgender person. Families supply physical and emotional sustenance, connect us with our pasts, and provide a context within which we learn about the world, including attitudes and mores of our society (Goldberg & Allen, 2012). A LGBT person's family is very important. Although some radical right ideologues erroneously promote the belief that an LGBT identity is a threat to the family, as if it were intrinsically antithetic to the idea of family life, nothing, could be further from the truth. LGBT people need to be part of their families as much as any other individual. Given the stigmatizing status that lesbian, gay, bisexual, and transgender identity continues to hold for many in Western society, the family is one place where a LGBT person most needs to feel accepted. Most LGBT people hope that their family will continue to love and care for them after they disclose their sexual orientation and/or gender identity expression. For many, this is the case, but sadly, for others acceptance by one's family is not forthcoming.

Utilizing an ecological perspective of practice to work with LGBT people and families offers a broad conceptual lens for viewing family functioning and needs. Germain (2013) who led the development of this perspective, noted that "practice is directed toward improving the transactions between people and their environments in order to enhance adaptive capacities and improve environments for all who function within them" (Germain, 2013, p. 17). As such, practitioners need to seek to influence the direction of change in both the person and the environment. With respect to LGBT people within a family context, changing the environment means educating families and assisting them in dealing with heterocentric attitudes.

Consider the following example:

> Damond is a 16-year-old, Trinidadian youngster who has been sent to the United States to live with an aunt after his mother has been psychiatrically hospitalized. His aunt is a single mother, has lupus, works full-time, and has three other children to support in her home. Damond is depressed because of his mother's illness. He is feeling isolated by his separation from his mother and the difficult acclimation to a new country and culture. In addition, Damond is dealing, in silence, with his own emerging gay identity.
>
> While cleaning Damond's room one afternoon, his aunt finds a letter that he wrote to a boy in school. Enraged, confused, and armed only with her religious and cultural notions about a gay or lesbian identity, even worrying that Damond's gay identity might be contagious and put her own children at risk, she tells him that he is sick and needs help.

From this brief sketch, one can begin to see how and why this family is in crisis. There are numerous stresses in this environment. The economy requires that the aunt works to support her family despite her chronic illness; the young man is grieving over his mother's illness, his own relocation to a new environment, and dealing in silence with his own emerging gay identity. Add to this case the cultural factors, in that some cultures have particularly negative views of individuals (even family members) who are LGBT and the fact that the young man was "found out" and did not choose to disclose his orientation, and it is easy to see how this young person may become the target of his family's anger. As this example suggests, many personal, family, and environmental factors converge and interact with each other to influence the family. In other words, as Pecora, Whittaker, Maluccio, & Barth (2012, p. 68) so eloquently said, "Human behavior is not solely a function of the person or the environment, but of the complex interaction between them."

All too often, despite the increasing emphasis on family-centered practice there is a tendency for practitioners to see LGBT people primarily, if not solely, as individuals who are "gay," "lesbian," "bisexual," or "transgender" rather than as members of a family of origin and as possible creators of their own family systems, families of choice (Weston, 1997), or biological families. By not acknowledging that "human beings can be understood and helped only in the context of the intimate and powerful human systems of which they are a part," of which the family is one of the most important (Pecora et al., 2012, p. 63), practitioners miss out on many important opportunities for fostering more positive relationships between LGBT people and their families.

This chapter, based on the author's analysis of the existing literature, qualitative data analysis from interviews conducted with LGBT people and their families, and more than 44 years of clinical practice with individuals and their families, examines the experience of LGBT people and their families through an ecological lens. Such a perspective creates a framework where individuals and environments are understood as a unit, in the context of their relationship to one another (Germain, 2013). As such, this chapter examines the primary reciprocal exchanges and transactions that LGBT people and their families face as they confront the unique person: environmental tasks involved in a society that assumes all of its members are heterosexual and oriented to the gender in which they were born. The focus of this chapter is limited to an analysis of LGBT people within the context of their family system. As such the author explores the following areas: demographic issues; psychosocial risks and psychosocial needs of LGBT people; the clinical assessment issues of working with an individual where sexual orientation and/or gender identity expression is the presenting issue; and recommendations for intervening with this population. Recommendations for practice with LGBT people and their families are presented in the conclusion of the chapter. Issues pertaining to LGBT families created through adoption, foster care, alterative insemination, and surrogacy are not addressed, as they have been addressed elsewhere (Mallon, 2017d).

## DEMOGRAPHIC PROFILE

Although there are many stereotypes of LGBT people, and these are images that the popular media continues to perpetuate about LGBT people, the reality is that LGBT people are part of every race, culture, ethnic group, body type, religious, and socioeconomic affiliation and family in the United States, and internationally as well.

Since LGBT people are socialized to hide their sexual orientation and/or gender identity expression, most are a part of an invisible population. In addition, in many areas of the United States (mostly outside of urban areas, although urban areas can also be unsafe), it is still unsafe for most LGBT people to live openly and acknowledge their sexual orientation and/or gender identity expression. Individuals who are socialized to hide or who have real or perceived reasons to fear for their safety do not come forward to be counted. In fact, although there is an increasing awareness about LGBT people, mainly from media representations of the population, it is safe to assume that most LGBT people in the United States remain closeted and do not live as "out" or "openly" as LGBT people.

## PSYCHOSOCIAL RISKS/PSYCHOSOCIAL NEEDS OF LGBT PEOPLE

LGBT people experience environmental and psychological stresses that are more elevated than most of their heterosexual counterparts not necessarily because of their gay, lesbian, bisexual, or transgender orientation, but due in large part to the negative societal response to their sexual orientation and/or gender identity expression. Such conditions are unique to their membership in what remains in

American society as a stigmatized and marginalized population (Haines, Boyer, Giovanazzi, & Galupo, 2018).

As such, LGBT people may most commonly experience difficulties in the following areas:

Accessing systems of care (health, mental health, social services) (Appleby, 2013; Bolderston & Ralph, 2016; Hunter & Mallon, 1998; Israel, Tarver, & Shaffer 2001; Lev, 2013; Winter, Elze, Saltzburg, & Rosenwald, 2015) that are affirming of and sensitive to the needs of LGBT clients.

Mental health illness that is unique to their situation—especially anxiety-related disorders and mood disorders (Fredriksen-Goldsen et al., 2014; Jones & Hill, 2008; Weitzman, 2006). Lesbian and gay youth, according to some studies (Garofalo, Wolf, Wissow, Woods, & Goodman, 1999; Hatzenbuehler & Keyes, 2013; Mustanski & Liu, 2013; Plöderl et al., 2013; Stone et al., 2014), are up to three times more likely to attempt suicide than their heterosexual counterparts. Trans and nonbinary may face many other challenges (Clark, Veale, Townsend, Frohard-Dourlent, & Saewyc, 2018; Lev, 2013; Nealy, 2017).

Substance abuse is generally thought to be elevated in the LGBT communities, since much of the initial coming out process (at least until the advent of Internet dating apps) may have centered on the "bar" scene (Klein, 2014; Kus, 2014).

The effect of trauma—psychological, political, and vicarious—are often reported by LGBT people as issues of concern since living within the context of a "false sense of self" and hiding or monitoring one's behaviors, mannerisms, speech, and life can be very debilitating and lead to maladaptive responses (Bradford, 2004; Ka'ahumanu & Hutchins, 2015; Molina et al., 2015). Politically, LGBT people are frequently the subjects of "moral" debates by politicians (Congress & Gonzalez, 2012) for many LGBT people who are tired of politicians who attempt to make their lives illegal or immoral. The issue of coming out alone—since this is a process and not a one-time event—is an exhausting transaction that can lead to trauma (Aranda et al., 2015). LGBT people who are parents and have children may experience vicarious traumatization in watching their children struggle with homophobic comments or reactions from peers or their community (Mallon, 2012; 2017a; 2017b).

Although it is a common myth that all LGBT people are economically advantaged, many LGBT people experience economic poverty (Badgett, Durso, & Schneebaum, 2013), inadequate housing or threat of losing one's housing, and unemployment (Israel, 2005; Worthen, 2013 see www.aclu.org). The literature is replete with evidence that LGBT people experience high levels of oppression and exploitation (Watson & Miller, 2012) and incidence of community violence and discrimination on multiple levels (Meyer, 2003).

Racism is also an issue for LGBT people to contend with, both from inside the LGBT communities, and from outside the LGBT communities (Aranda et al., 2015; Diaz, 2013; Elder, Morrow, & Brooks, 2015; Herdt, 2013; Walters, 2013).

## CLINICAL ASSESSMENT FOR FAMILIES WHERE SEXUAL ORIENTATION AND/OR GENDER IDENTITY EXPRESSION IS AN ISSUE

Although not all people will need counseling because someone in the family has identified as gay, lesbian, bisexual, or trans, some families will come to the attention of a social services agency for a variety of reasons and services which might not at initial assessment seem to be pertaining to issues of sexual orientation and/or gender identity expression (Chu, Leino, Pflum, & Sue, 2016; Diamond et al., 2013; O'Dell, 2000; Oswald, 2002a, 2002b).

The following actual case example illustrates the relevance of these dimensions. A young couple, Betsy and Clark, sought help from a family service agency. Initially, they identified concerns with the behavior of their 9-year-old son Todd who was attending an after-school program. The after-school center staff reported that he was hitting other children, unable to relax during quiet time, and had frequent temper tantrums. Betsy and Clark were concerned that the center might refuse continued service, affecting their ability to maintain their employment. The helping professional engaged with Betsy and Clark to assess Todd's behaviors, the tensions within the marital relationship, and both parents' satisfaction with their lives. Clark was struggling with a worsening depression that he attributed to a growing remoteness between himself and Betsy, a detachment he couldn't explain. Several times Betsy mentioned being unable to be herself in the relationship and alluded to a secret that she couldn't share. Through a skillful series of individual and joint discussions, the helping professional was able to help Betsy acknowledge the reality of her lesbian sexual orientation and share this with Clark. With the secret out, the helping professional, Betsy, and Clark began to identify and work together on the many decisions that each faced individually and as parents to Todd. In reflecting upon their initial call to this particular family service agency, Betsy noted having seen a brochure in Todd's pediatrician's office describing the agency's service, including a group on parenting issues for lesbian and gay parents. Once connected to the agency, Betsy had experienced the helping professional as open in her ongoing assessment of the range of possible sources of Betsy's expressed ability to "be herself" in her relationship with Clark.

The following case example explores issues of and/or gender identity expression from a different family-centered perspective.

Shamir, a 15-year-old Pakistani male is sitting in his bedroom in the apartment which he shares with his mother, father, and three younger brothers, reading a very personal letter that a boy in school wrote to him. He has already read this letter several times, but like many adolescents venturing into the world of relationships, he is re-reading it because it is a special letter to him. When his mother yells to him from the kitchen that he has a phone call, he puts the letter down on his bed and leaves his room to get the phone. During the time that he is on the phone, his 9-year-old brother enters his room and begins to read the letter that Shamir has left on the bed. The younger sibling, realizing that its contents are questionable, shows the letter to his mother.

When Shamir returns from his phone call, finding his letter missing, he begins to panic. Shamir knows that it will be obvious to anyone who reads the letter that he is gay. Up to this point, Shamir has been successful at keeping his identity a secret. But now his secret is out in the open—he is angry that he didn't have an opportunity to come out on his own terms—he has been found out—and there is a big difference! When he sees his mother's face, he knows that she has read the letter, but she says nothing to him. When he approaches her, she backs away and says, "We'll talk about this when your father gets home and when all of your brothers are asleep."

The next few hours are filled with dread and isolation for Shamir. What's going to happen? What is his father going to do? He's not prepared for this, and he's terrified of the repercussions. What Shamir doesn't know is that his mother and father feel the same way—this is not the way things are supposed to be; they are not prepared for this. No one ever told them about the prospect of having a son who was gay. Should they send him for therapy? Should they send him away to protect the other boys? Should they even tell anybody about this?

For the helping professional experienced in working with family systems, the situation in the above vignette presents the ideal opportunity for an intervention. A crisis has occurred, the family is in turmoil, and everyone is poised for something to happen. Family members are confused, frightened, shame-filled, unprepared, and angry. They can act in a reckless manner, lashing out at the individual who has disclosed or they might fall into a conspiracy of silence and become completely paralyzed and numbed by the circumstances. Professionals who have spent years with families, or even those who have recently entered the field, know that what happens next is not always predictable. When the situation involves an issue of sexual orientation and/or gender identity expression in the family, one can almost guarantee that there will be a great deal of ambivalence in this process. Coming out in the context of a family system can yield unpredictable outcomes.

## THE COMING OUT PROCESS WITHIN A FAMILY

Coming out, a distinctively LGBT phenomenon (Corrigan, Kosyluk & Rüsch, 2013; Firestein, 2007; Lev, 2013; Patterson, 2013; Patterson & D'Augelli, 2013; Pistella et al., 2016; Savage & Miller, 2011; Trussell, Xing, & Oswald, 2015), is defined as a developmental process through which LGBT people recognize their sexual orientation and/or gender identity expression and integrate this knowledge into their personal and social lives (Stein & Cohen, 2013). Although several theorists have written about coming out from a uniquely adolescent experience (Grafsky & Gary, 2018; Isay, 2010; Mallon, 2017a, 2017b; Savin-Williams, 2009), developmentally, the coming out process can eventuate at any stage of an individual's life. Therefore, it is important to consider the consequences of a person coming out in the context of his or her family, as a child, as an adolescent, as an unmarried young adult, as a married adult, as a parent, or as a grandparent.

The events that mark coming out and the pace of this process vary from person to person. Consequently, some people move through the process smoothly, accepting their sexuality or their gender fit, making social contacts, and finding a good fit within their environments. Others are unnerved by their sexuality, vacillating in their conviction, hiding in their uneasiness, and struggling to find the right fit.

Although the experience of an adolescent coming out is qualitatively different from that of a parent or an adult who comes out, there are several conditions, broadly conceived that all family members share. Earlier literature (Legate, Ryan, & Weinstein, 2012) focused primarily on the negative consequences of disclosure, and indeed there can be many, but a range of responses to a family member's disclosure is perhaps a more appropriate characterization (Schmitz & Tyler, 2018). The following description by Rothberg and Weinstein (1996) captures many of the salient aspects of this experience:

> When a family member comes out there are a multitude of responses. At one end of the spectrum is acceptance . . . but rarely, if ever, is this announcement celebrated. Take for example, the announcement a heterosexual person makes to his or her family of origin of an engagement to marry. This is usually met with a joyous response, a ritual party and many gifts. Most LGBT people do not receive this response. Instead, the coming out announcement is often met with negative responses which can range from mild disapproval to complete non-acceptance and disassociation. These responses, though usually accepted, cause considerable stress and pain for the lesbian and gay person seeking approval. (p. 81)

## RELIGIOUS FACTORS

Some families, particularly families with strong religious convictions, may openly condemn an LGBT identity, unaware that one of their own family members is lesbian, gay, bisexual, or trans (DeYoung, 2015; Gnuse, 2015; Page, Lindahl, & Malik, 2013).

Blumenfeld and Raymond (1993) note that families with strong religious convictions often support their views of their religion even against a family member. Personal biases, particularly cultural or religious biases that view a LGBT identity negatively, can make "coming out" to one's family a painful experience. This distress is manifest by this young person's narrative:

> Everybody in the family knew that I was bisexual. The only person that couldn't deal with me being bi was my mother. Everyone else that I thought was going to have a hard time, didn't. My mother is a devout Baptist and she has a very hard time with my being bi. She has said that she hated me and to this very day she tells me that it is against God's will and it's against His proposition and when the day comes for Him to take over the world again I'm going to suffer. She always says that she doesn't want me to suffer because I am her son, but she doesn't realize that she is making me suffer because of the ways that she acts toward me.

Helping professionals must be aware of the strong anti-LGBT sentiment held by many religious groups and the impact that this has on family members for whom sexual orientation and/or gender identity expression is an issue. The Bible has historically been erroneously used as a weapon against LGBT people causing a great deal of distress in many families of faith. Several excellent resources (Durso & Meyer, 2013; Good, 2015; Goodwill, 2000; Griffin, Wirth, & Wirth, 2016; Hubbard, 2013; Lease & Schulman, 2003; McNeill, 2015) exist that provide practitioners with an alternative LGBT affirming perspective.

## CULTURAL FACTORS

Race and cultural ethnicity can also play important roles in the disclosure process. People of color, many of whom have experienced significant stress related to oppression and racism based on skin color or ethnicity may experience even greater difficulty coming out within the family context as some may view a lesbian, gay, or bisexual orientation and/or gender identity expression as one more oppressed status to add to one's plate (Balsam, Molina, Beadnell, Simoni, & Walters, 2011; Colon, 2001; Hatzenbuehler & Pachankis, 2016; Omi & Winant, 2014; Poon, 2004).

People of color who are LGBT confront a tricultural experience. They experience membership in their ethnic or racial community and in the larger society. In addition, they are not born into the LGBT communities. Many become aware of their difference in adolescence and not only must deal with the stigma within their own cultural/racial community but must also find a supportive LGBT community to which they can relate. The LGBT community is often a microcosm of the larger society, and many may confront racism there, as in the larger society. To sustain oneself in three distinct communities requires an enormous effort and can also produce stress for the adolescent (Feinstein, Wadsworth, Davila, & Goldfried, 2014; Harbeck, 2014; Leong, 2014; Poon, 2004; Toomey, Ryan, Diaz, Card, & Russell, 2010). The reality is that LGBT people are part of every race, culture, ethnic grouping, class, and extended family.

## EMOTIONAL FACTORS

If the LGBT identified individual chooses to come out voluntarily, then he, she, or they have had time to prepare for the event. Some individuals may have role-played their coming out process with a supportive friend or therapist; others may have written a letter or planned the event after experiencing positive disclosure events with several other trusted confidants. The truth, however, is that in most cases, even if the individual has had time to prepare for this event, the actual moment of disclosure catches most families off guard. Families have frequently not had this period of time to prepare and are often shocked by the disclosure, but in truth, there is a range of emotions expressed by families addressing issues of disclosure by a LGBT child (Eriksen, 2017; Owens-Reid & Russo, 2014). Jean Baker (2014) psychologist and mother of two gay sons, expresses the range of her feelings as a parent when she writes:

> I still recall the night so vividly. Gary was helping me with dinner, which he occasionally did. He had just gotten a new haircut and immediately I hated it. I still don't know why, because it had never occurred to me that Gary might be gay, but for some reason I said to him, "With that haircut people will think you're gay." He hesitated for a moment and then, looking directly at me he said, "I think maybe I am."

> I stared at my son, totally speechless, stunned, momentarily unable to react. Then I started crying and found myself talking incoherently about the tragedy of being gay. . . . I rambled on senselessly about homosexuality as an adolescent phase, something people can grow out of, something that may be just a rebellion . . . Knowing what I know about homosexuality and having examined my own feelings

and attitudes, I think my reactions that night were deplorable. My son deserved to hear immediately that I respected him for his honesty and his courage. What he heard instead was that his mother thought being homosexual was a tragedy.

As I think about my reactions that first night and during subsequent days and nights, I am still ashamed of what I learned about myself as a mother dealing with a son's homosexuality. Instead of thinking first about how I could help my son cope with what he might have to face in a society so condemning of homosexuals, I focused on how I felt. Though I didn't want to admit it, I was concerned about the prejudice and stigma I myself might have to face. (pp. 41–43)

Feelings surrounding the initial disclosure can range from shame, to guilt, to embarrassment, or even complete disassociation.

Acceptance is also a possible reaction, one which is increasing for many LGBT people, but one that is still not the experience by most LGBT people who seek the assistance of helping professionals.

## MANAGING DISCLOSURE TO OTHERS

Deciding how to manage the disclosure of a LGBT orientation to the family is an important consideration at this point. The family that reacts extremely negatively to the disclosure, that is, a child who is thrown out of the home by parents or a spouse who is told to leave their home by their partner, may require outside intervention to assist them in dealing with the disclosure which should be viewed as a crisis situation. Who to tell and who not to tell, and how to address the disclosure within the context of the family are other issues that families must eventually discuss. Getting through the initial crisis of disclosure, however, should be the primary focus of the intervention.

Being "found out" as illustrated in Shamir's case presented earlier in this chapter, precipitates a somewhat different type of crisis which may also require immediate intervention. In the sections that follow, we explore the possibilities of a child or adolescent's coming out in his or her family system.

## WHEN A CHILD COMES OUT WITHIN THE FAMILY SYSTEM

Although disclosure can occur at any point in the developmental process, for the purposes of this section, I will specifically address the issues as they pertain to a child or adolescent who comes out or is found out by their family.

Although one of the primary tasks of adolescence is to move away from one's family toward independence, families are still extremely important economic and emotional systems for them. Lack of accurate information about LGBT identity and fears about individuals who identify as LGBT lead many families to panic about how to manage the disclosure of a family member.

The following two case examples illustrate several points with respect to the coming out process for adolescents.

## YUAN IS FOUND OUT

Yuan Fong is a Chinese American, 18-year-old senior in a public high school in a large West Coast city. He resides with his parents who are Chinese born in an apartment with an older brother, age 20, and two younger siblings, ages 12 and 10. Yuan is the captain of the football team, well-liked by his peers and by teachers. He is a very handsome young man. Yuan has dated a few girls, but he is so into his football career that it leaves little time for anything else. Yuan has been aware of his feelings for guys for some time and has been trying to repress these feelings. Recently, however, he met a guy named Tommy whom he really likes, and Yuan's feelings have become more difficult to repress. Tommy and Yuan begin to see each other, first as friends, and then their friendship blossoms into a romance.

One evening, while talking to Tommy on the phone, Mrs. Fong overhears their conversation. It seems to her that Yuan is speaking to Tommy like she would expect him to speak to a girl that he was dating. When Yuan hangs up the phone his mother confronts him about what she heard. Yuan blows it off and laughs, blaming her interpretation on her imperfect English, but he knows that this is not the case. He is in a panic because he knows that his mother will not let this go.

Mrs. Fong becomes hypervigilant about Yuan and begins to search in his room while he is at school for clues. She finds letters that Tommy has written to Yuan and then when she finds a small card from an LGBT youth group she takes it as confirmation that her son Yuan is gay. Mrs. Fong shares this information with her husband who chastises her for snooping in their son's room. But they are both upset and unprepared for how they should deal with this new information which changes their notion of their family.

When Yuan arrives home from football practice, both Mr. and Mrs. Fong ask to speak with him. They tell him what they have found and ask him if he is gay? Yuan, fearful and caught off guard, is unsure of how to respond, but it seems like there is no way out. Even though he is pretty sure that he is gay, Yuan tells them, "I think I am bisexual," rationalizing that being half gay is easier that being totally gay. Mr. and Mrs. Fong ask if he has ever been sexually abused by someone, they ask if he is just going through a phase, and insist that he is going to see their family doctor. Although they do not say it out loud, Mr. and Mrs. Fong are also concerned about how this will affect their two younger children. Yuan has on occasion baby-sat when they went out, and they wonder if Yuan might molest the younger children. This family is obviously in a crisis state.

## ROBIN COMES OUT

Robin is a 17-year-old Caucasian who lives with her mother, father, and two younger sisters on a small family-run farm in the Midwest.

Robin is an average student, in the 11th grade in a public high school. Robin has a very close friend named Patsy who is a year older and attends the same school. After an initial period of confusion, Robin and Patsy realize that they have strong feelings for one another and that their feelings are "more than just a phase." Although neither of them identify as lesbian at first, in time, they first come to label their identity as gay, and then later are comfortable calling themselves lesbian.

Robin has always been close to her family and has always been helpful around the farm. Not wanting to lie to her parents, Robin decides that she should tell her parents how she feels about Patsy. She plans the event, making sure that it is an evening when her sisters are already in bed and asks her parents to sit with her in her bedroom. She starts by telling her family that what she needs to tell them is not an easy thing to tell, but that she loves them and wants them to know her for who she really is. They seem puzzled thinking that they already know their daughter quite well. She explains that since she was little, about 6 or 7, she has always liked other girls, not boys. She tells that at first she thought the feelings would go away, but they didn't. At this point, her mother and father are completely aghast about what she is trying to tell them. Robin makes it clear and says, "Mom, Dad, I still like girls and I have come to understand lately that I am a lesbian."

Robin's parents are without words. They are completely unprepared for having a lesbian daughter. They suggest therapy, they ask if she is sure and suggest that it still might be a phase, and they also ask if it is her way of rebelling against them. She answers no to all of their queries. Robin's parents are in shock, confused, embarrassed, and unsure of what to do. Robin's disclosure has created an imbroglio for the family that all are unprepared to deal with.

Like many families, these families had little accurate information about LGBT people and as a consequence relied mostly on myths as their primary source of information. At first both families believed that their family member's differentness might be an adolescent phase. Both families suggested that their young person should attempt to change their sexual orientation and/or gender identity expression via therapy. Additionally, although it was almost too frightening to mention, the families expressed fears about the possible molestation of younger siblings by their LGBT child. These families, like most families who have had to deal with an unexpected disclosure, are clearly in a state of shock. Consequently, they are unprepared as their teens are growing up LGBT in a heterosexual world. Most parents never allow themselves to think that they might have a child who is LGBT. Parents are also aware of the shame and secrecy surrounding LGBT identity and as such are unsure of what their child's disclosure will mean for them and for the other family members (Baiocco et al., 2016; Diamond et al., 2013; Perrin-Wallqvist, & Lindblom, 2015; Saltzburg, 2004).

In some cases, though not in Yuan's or Robin's case, the disclosure of a LGBT identity can lead to an array of abusive responses from family members. In other instances, a LGBT disclosure can lead to youths' expulsion from their home leading to out-of-home placement. In many families, the crisis of disclosure is resolved after the initial reaction of shock and the family moves forward. When a parent comes out in a family context, however, the issues are quite different.

## WHEN A PARENT COMES OUT WITHIN THE FAMILY SYSTEM

When a parent or a spouse comes out or is found out by family members, there are unique and distinctive repercussions. As observed in the previous case examples, lack of accurate information about LBGT identity and fears about individuals who identify as LGBT lead many families to panic about how to manage the disclosure of a family member. The issues of shame and stigma serve to further complicate these issues (Tasker & Delvoye, 2018). The following two case examples illustrate several points with respect to the coming out process for family members. A dad discloses his bisexual identity to his son in the first case example; a husband is unexpectedly "found out" by his wife as a trans person in the second scenario.

## A BI DAD'S DISCLOSURE

> Pete, a Caucasian, sixth grade child, attending a private elementary school, resides in a large suburban environment in a small condo with his dad, Brendan, aged 36, and Jamie his "uncle." Pete was 10 when his dad decided to tell him that Uncle Jamie, who had lived with the family for eight of Pete's 10 years, was really his life partner.
>
> Brendan decided to disclose his bisexual orientation to Pete because he felt that he was getting older and he wanted him to know the truth about his dad. He didn't want anyone to make fun of Pete or for him to find out that he was bisexual before he had the opportunity to tell him. Brendan planned the disclosure and sat with Pete privately in their kitchen to tell him. Jaime, although not initially involved in the disclosure, joined them after Brendan and told Pete.
>
> At first, Pete was shocked and denied that his dad or Uncle Jaime, with whom he had an excellent relationship, were bisexuals. Pete said that he didn't want to talk about it. Although he didn't say it at the time, he was embarrassed that his friends and teachers in school would find out about his dad and that he would be treated differently. After the initial disclosure, Pete began to distance himself from his Dad and Uncle Jaime. When Brendan checked in to see how things were going with him, Pete simply replied that things were "fine."
>
> But things were not fine. Pete began to have problems in school (prior to the disclosure Pete was an A student) and on two occasions, Pete's dad received notices from school notifying him that Pete had gotten into trouble in the classroom.
>
> Noting this marked change in behavior, the helping professional at the school phoned Pete's dad and asked him to come into school for a conference.

## ALEX AND LINDA

Alex, a 35-year-old Latino, has been married to Linda, a 31-year-old Latina for 8 years. They have two children, Pedro, age 6 and Isabel, age 4. They live in a small house in a suburb of a large southern city, which is comprised primarily of working-class Latinos like themselves. Although they have been married for 8 years, Alex has always known since he was a teenager that he is "different." When he married, he thought that his feelings about himself would change, but they did not. He never discussed these feelings with Linda, but some part of him always thought that she knew that he always felt like a woman inside, not a man. Although Alex never talked openly about his trans identity, he did occasionally read a trans magazine called *Tapestry* and visited trans web sites on his computer.

One evening, when Alex arrived home after work, Linda met him at the door and asked for an explanation about the *Tapestry* magazines she had in her hand and the visits to the web sites on transgender people that she found in files in the computer. Alex initially denied that the magazines were his and denied visiting the web sites but after a while he acknowledged that the magazines were his and that he had many times visited the web sites for trans people. Linda told Alex that he had to leave their home immediately. She screamed that he had exposed her and her children to all kinds of things and that he had lied to all of them. Alex did not know where to turn. His family lived in Venezuela and he did not have a close family support system except for Linda and his children. Alex pleaded with Linda to go with him to see someone—a marriage or family therapist. Linda refused, telling him that he was disgusting and told him to leave their home immediately.

Alex was confused, now estranged from his partner and his children, and feeling completely dejected. Alex went to the home of a coworker to ask if he could stay overnight. In the morning, he went to visit his parish priest to ask for counseling. The priest referred him to a family center in the community. Linda was devastated, ashamed, and told no one about her separation from Alex, except her sister.

Although the issues of disclosure for a parent coming out to their child are far different than for a wife who finds out that her husband is exploring a transgender identity are very different, both case examples reflect the level of denial, shock, and confusion that some family members experience in this process. In the first case, Brendan has clearly thought out his disclosure and it seems that he will work with his son to process this new information. In the second case, Linda and Alex have definitely not planned the disclosure and the consequences of his being found out seem to be, at this juncture, quite weighty for him and his family. Most families bring themselves out of a crisis without professional help, others will need support during the disclosure of a LGBT identity of a family member so that the family may remain intact and its members may grow through the experience (Elze, 2012; Mallon, 2012; Trahan, & Goodrich, 2015). Others will need assistance. The benefits of a family support and family counseling have particular relevance in each of these four cases (Madsen, 2013; Moore & Stambolis-Ruhstorfer, 2013; Winter et al., 2015).

## TREATMENT CONSIDERATIONS WITH FAMILIES WHERE SEXUAL ORIENTATION AND/OR GENDER IDENTITY EXPRESSION IS THE ISSUE

Family-centered services often call for crisis intervention services at least in the initial phases of the disclosure process. Families experiencing high stress, such as where there has been a disclosure of sexual orientation and/or gender identity expression, may find that their regular coping mechanisms have broken down, leaving them open to change in either a positive or negative direction. The family member's increased vulnerability under these conditions can serve as a catalyst to seeking help to resolve their immediate issues (Kwon, 2013; LaSala, 2013; Strydom, 2014). If professionals trained in family preservation techniques can be available and gently encouraging, the pressure families feel can motivate them to change and to share their concerns. The immediate goal of this intervention is clearly to move the family out of crisis and to restore the family to at least the level of functioning that existed before the crisis (Combrinck, 2015; Strydom, 2014). Many family preservation professionals go well beyond that goal, increasing families' skill levels and resources so that they function better after the crisis than they did before.

Utilizing a family-centered approach (Maluccio, Pine, & Tracy, 2013) for working with families, the following sections suggest some intervention guidelines for practitioners.

## INTERVENTION

Addressing issues of sexual orientation and/or gender identity expression disclosure requires professionals to first explore their own personal, cultural, and religious biases about people who are LGBT oriented. Although many professionals might believe that they are non-biased in their approach to LGBT people, all professionals must first examine their own bias and be comfortable dealing with issues which are seen by most in Western society as "sensitive." Although most professionals receive little, if any, formal training on dealing with issues of and/or gender identity expression in child welfare, there are several books within the past decade that provide a wonderful overview of the issues confronting LGBT people in human services settings (Alessi, 2013; Hunter & Hickerson, 2003; Inch, 2016; Mallon, 2017b; Mallon & Hess, 2014; Morrow & Messinger, 2006; van Wormer & Wells, 2000) which can be helpful for professional development.

## INITIAL PREPARATIONS

Keeping people safe is one of the primary goals of this intervention. Workers should be aware that issues of sexual orientation and/or gender identity expression can frequently lead to violence within the family system. Being able to predict the potential for violence is an essential skill for workers to possess.

Preparing for the initial meeting by gathering information, for example by talking to the referring worker (if the case has been referred) or by gathering information directly from the family members by calling them to schedule an interview, can assist in forming a positive relationship that might make things easier when the worker arrives at the home. In some situations, as in Alex and Linda's case, it might be a good idea to schedule the initial meeting outside the family's home, say in a public, structured environment such as a restaurant or in a private meeting space in a community center. When situations are potentially volatile, meeting in a public place or a safe space can make it easier for family members to retain control.

## THE INITIAL MEETING

Whenever possible, the initial meeting should take place in the home of the family. In three of the four cases presented herein, this would be advisable. Meeting clients on their own turf, in their home is an integral part of the philosophy of family preservation (Combrinck, 2015). Professionals should be conscious of being considerate and careful with all family members. In cases when a disclosure of sexual orientation and/or gender identity expression is involved, family members might view the person who has come out or been found out as the only person who needs to be spoken with.

In some cases, family members should be met with one at a time. This is particularly true for the family members who are most upset, pessimistic, or uncooperative. In most cases, they should also be talked with first. This individual needs to feel important and understood. De-escalating this family member and gaining his or her confidence can be helpful in supporting the process and encouraging other family members to participate. Engaging in active listening techniques using "I" statements (Kinney, Haapala, & Booth, 1991: Chapter 4); permitting the professional to share their own feelings about the situation; notifying family members of the consequences of their actions; calling for a time out; seeking the assistance of a supervisor, if necessary; reconvening at a neutral location or actually leaving the home if the situation escalates to a point where police intervention is necessary are all options that professionals may need to consider and act upon during their initial visit.

## SUBSEQUENT CONTACTS

The first session is usually the most fragile one. The family who has had a member disclose their sexual orientation and/or gender identity expression is, as noted, in a crisis mode. Family members in crisis feel vulnerable and anxious. Some may be angry, and others mistrustful. Many families feel secretive about disclosing family business to a stranger, especially when it pertains to a sensitive issue like one's gender expression or sexual orientation and/or gender identity expression. The goal in the first session is usually to calm everyone down and begin unfolding the narrative. Establishing trust and forming a partnership between family members and the professional are the next steps.

## ASSESSING STRENGTHS AND PROBLEMS AND FORMULATING GOALS

In subsequent sessions, the professional will need to assist the family in organizing information about their "crisis." Workers should work with family members to minimize blame and labeling and instead focus on generating options for change. This may be facilitated by working with the family to reach consensus about the fact that their family member is in one way not as they thought he or she was, but at the same time, still the same person that they have always been. Assisting family members with shaping less negative interpretations about a LGBT identity is an important place to begin. Helping families to define problems in terms of their own skill deficits by settings goals, making small steps, prioritizing issues of concern for the family, and being realistic with family members can lead families back toward homeostasis. As means toward addressing issues of accountability, utilizing standardized outcome measures to test the veracity of clinical interventions with clients has increasingly become a significant aspect of practice (Epstein & Buhovac, 2014; Wampold & Imel, 2015).

## HELPING FAMILIES LEARN

One of the most dominant elements that is apparent in each of the case vignettes is the lack of accurate and relevant information about LGBT individuals. The myths and misconceptions which guide families are graphically present in their initial concerns about molestation, about the need for therap, and about the possibility of changing one's sexual orientation and/or gender identity expression. Changing family's notions about LGBT family members is not always a smooth or easy process. A great deal of the worry that families have about LGBT people is based on irrational fear and shame. The disclosure of a LGBT orientation within a family context spreads the societal stigmatization of homosexuality to all family members. Goffman called this phenomenon "courtesy stigma" (Goffman, 1963).

Although they caution about developing realistic expectations for all families, Kinney et al. (1991) posit that there are several ways to facilitate learning with clients: (a) direct instruction; (b) modeling; and (c) learning from one another. These strategies can be useful in helping families affected by issues of gender expression or sexual orientation and/or gender identity expression as highlighted below.

## DIRECT INSTRUCTION

The helping professional who engages a family with issues of sexual orientation and/or gender identity expression must be prepared to present and provide a great deal of direct instruction with family members. Providing families with accurate and relevant information about their child or their family member's orientation is an essential part of this process. Bibliotherapy, providing families with reading material, is an integral component of this strategy. Although finding this information is not the problem that it once was (as there is a plethora of information available, especially online), workers may have to access this information by visiting a local LGBT bookstore or order them via the Internet, as the books are frequently not carried in mainstream bookstores. Increasing the family's knowledge about sexual orientation and/or gender identity expression (Baker, 2014; Griffin et al., 2016; Israel, 2005; Lev, 2013; Pillemer & McCartney, 2013; Vela, 2015; Walsh, 2015) and knowing about resources that support families, like Parents and Friends of Lesbians and Gays (Mallon, 2017c) are important ways to strengthen and support the families of LGBT people. Furnishing young people with literature, especially work written by LGBT young people for LGBT young people, is one of the most beneficial techniques that can be employed (see Chrisler, Smischney, & Villarruel, 2014; Fuss, 2013; Miceli, 2013; Moore & Rosenthal, 2007; Savin-Williams, 2009). Videos and guest speakers can and should be also be utilized in this process. Such information is useful in assisting the LGBT-oriented youngster in abolishing myths and stereotypes and correcting misconceptions about their identity. This information can also help educate non-LGBT teens about their LGBT peers (Miceli, 2013).

During the past decade, many high schools and colleges have housed lesbian, gay and straight alliances (see www.glsen.org) and many cities have LGBT community centers (see www.lgbtcenters.org).

These and other community-based organizations that might be house LGBT friendly programs in mainstreamed community centers are important referral sources for practitioners and as such practitioners should know how to locate these organizations and be prepared to visit them.

The Internet has liberated many LGBT people from their extreme isolation, supplying them limitless opportunities to communicate with other LGBT people in chat rooms and on bulletin boards, most LGBT adolescents have little access to information about their emerging identity and few adult role models from whom to learn. In recent years the Internet has grown exponentially. Its growth has permitted thousands of LGBT people who may not be able to openly visit libraries or bookstores, or who may live in geographically isolated areas to gain information and connect with others.

Although there is a very limited body of literature which focuses on the impact of disclosure on the non-gay spouses of LGBT people (Buxton, 2000, 2005; Klein, 2014; Strock, 2008), there is an excellent website, known as the Straight Spouses Network located at www. straightspouse.org, that offers valuable support to the partners of LGBT spouses. Klein and Schwartz (2001) also provide guidance on the topic from a bisexual perspective. Patterson and Farr (2015), Bigner (2013), and Tasker (2013) have all addressed issues of parental disclosure to their children. An excellent web site which addresses the concerns of the children of lesbian and gay parents (Children of Lesbian and Gay Parents Everywhere—COLAGE) is located at www.colage.org. Garner (2004) and Snow (2004) both address these issues in their books.

Although published sources can be purchased at LGBT bookstores in larger metropolitan areas, these sources and many others not mentioned here can also be ordered via the Internet.

## MODELING

Modeling the behaviors ourselves to show clients how to do them is a very useful strategy for working with families who are dealing with issues of sexual orientation and/or gender identity expression. The LGBT adolescent who comes out or the family who is affected by a disclosure by family members might benefit from attending a support group with other individuals who share their experience. Individuals and family members, anxious about attending a support group for the first time, might very much benefit from a professional who agrees to accompany the client to the session. Accompanying the client to purchase books about LGBT topics at the bookstore or assist them in identifying appropriate online resources, or attending a LGBT run function with clients can be other ways for workers to model acceptance for the client. Linking clients to religious leaders in their communities and of their faith who have an affirming stance about LGBT individuals can also be a useful modeling experience for family members.

## LEARNING FROM OTHERS

Families can also learn from one another by connecting with other families where sexual orientation and/or gender identity expression is an issue. If connections with other families cannot be made in person because of geographic distance, the Internet, on-line groups, and "Skype-type" platforms can be useful substitutes. There are many sites that include opportunities for LGBT individuals and families affected by issues of sexual orientation and/or gender identity expression to communicate with one another. It is the responsibility of the helping professional working with the family to identify and access resources for support within the community where families live. Workers need to be aware of these resources and visit them prior to making such referrals to clients.

Helping professionals must also be prepared to assist families in overcoming barriers that will inevitably occur while assisting them in the learning process. Acknowledging, validating, and rewarding small signs that family members are considering new options and beginning to try them is also an important task for workers.

## SOLVING PROBLEMS

Helping professionals trained in problem resolution strategies must incorporate issues of sexual orientation and/or gender identity expression into such designs. Professionals must focus on listening to and helping families to clarify what is causing them the most discomfort. Intervening with clients to assist them in intrapersonal problems can occur via direct interventions, cognitive strategies, values clarifications, and behavioral strategies are all methods suggested by Madsen (2013). Most families dealing with issues of sexual orientation and/or gender identity expression may need help controlling and clarifying their own emotions. Assisting families to develop effective communication skills and problem-solving strategies is a major focus of a family preservation model which can be effective with LGBT children, youth, and families.

## CONCLUSION

All family-centered services, notwithstanding issues of sexual orientation and/or gender identity expression, maintain the position that families are best treated when their own families are meaningfully engaged in the process. Viewed ecologically, both assessment and intervention with families must focus primarily on the goodness of fit (Gitterman & Germain, 2008) between the LGBT individual and those other systems with which he or she is in transaction, the most central of which in this case is the family. Many of the issues that surface when a family member discloses or is dealing with aspects of sexual orientation and/or gender identity expression, can be best dealt with by a competent helping professional trained in family systems. Such issues must be viewed as deficits within the environment, dysfunctional transactions among environmental systems, or as a lack of individual or family coping skills or strategies (Dorfman, 2013). Providing education and intensive training effort for family-centered practitioners (Browning & Pasley, 2015; Mallon, 2012) that would help them feel competent about broadly addressing issues of sexual orientation and/or gender identity expression could provide support for families in crisis and prevent unnecessary family disruption. Family-centered practitioners must also be prepared to serve as advocates for their clients, including an LGBT child or adolescent; a parent who identifies as LGBT; or for a couple where one of the partners identifies as other than heterosexually oriented.

Family-centered social practitioners working with the primary goal of keeping families together can deliver these services within the context of the client's natural environment—their community. Programs like the Homebuilders model (Roberts, 2014) have opportunities to help families grappling with issues of sexual orientation and/or gender identity expression. Community-based family and children's services centers also provide many opportunities for addressing issues of sexual orientation and/or gender identity expression within the family system. These approaches also have relevance for other situations where spouses or parents come out as LGBT. Working with family systems in their communities makes helping professionals in a family-centered programs ideally situated to see what is really going on in a family's natural environment. By being located in the home or in the community, the worker is able to make an accurate assessment and design an intervention that will support and preserve the family system. With a greater awareness of issues of sexual orientation and/or gender identity expression, family-centered practitioners can educate parents, ease the distress experienced by couples where one partner is LGBT and the other is heterosexual, as well as model and shape new behaviors that can transform lives for LGBT people.

## REFERENCES

Alessi, E. J. (2013). Acknowledging the impact of social forces on sexual minority clients: Introduction to the special issue on clinical practice with LGBTQ populations. *Clinical Social Work Journal, 41*(3), 223–227. doi:10.1007/s10615-013-0458-x

Appleby, G. A. (2013). Social work practice with gay men and lesbians within organizations. In G. P. Mallon (Ed.), *Foundations of social work practice with lesbian and gay people* (pp. 249–270). New York, NY: Routledge.

Aranda, F., Matthews, A. K., Hughes, T. L., Muramatsu, N., Wilsnack, S. C., Johnson, T. P., & Riley, B. B. (2015). Coming out in color: Racial/ethnic differences in the relationship between level of sexual identity disclosure and depression among lesbians. *Cultural Diversity and Ethnic Minority Psychology, 21*(2), 247. doi:10.1037/a0037644

Badgett, M. V., Durso, L. E., & Schneebaum, A. (2013). *New patterns of poverty in the lesbian, gay, and bisexual community.* Los Angeles, CA: The Williams Institute.

Baiocco, R., Fontanesi, L., Santamaria, F., Ioverno, S., Baumgartner, E., & Laghi, F. (2016). Coming out during adolescence: Perceived parents' reactions and internalized sexual stigma. *Journal of Health Psychology, 1*(8), 1809–1813. doi:10.1177/1359105314564019

Baker, J. M. (2014). *Family secrets: Gay sons; a mother's story.* New York, NY: Routledge.

Balsam, K. F., Molina, Y., Beadnell, B., Simoni, J., & Walters, K. (2011). Measuring multiple minority stress: The LGBT People of Color Macroaggressions Scale. *Cultural Diversity and Ethnic Minority Psychology, 17*(2), 163. doi:10.1037/a0023244

Bigner, J. J. (2013). *An introduction to GLBT family studies.* New York, NY: Routledge.

Blumenfeld, W., & Raymond, D. (Eds.). (1993). *Looking at lesbian and gay life.* Boston, MA: Beacon Press.

Bolderston, A., & Ralph, S. (2016). Improving the health care experiences of lesbian, gay, bisexual and transgender patients. *Radiography, 22*(3), e207–e211. doi:10.1016/j.radi.2016.04.011

Bradford, M. (2004). The bisexual experience: Living in a dichotomous culture. *Journal of Bisexuality, 4*(1/2), 7–23. doi:10.1300/J159v04n01_02

Browning, S., & Pasley, K. (Eds.). (2015). *Contemporary families: translating research into practice.* New York, NY: Routledge.

Buxton, A. P. (2000). Writing our own script: How bisexual men and their heterosexual wives maintain their marriages after disclosure. *Journal of Bisexuality, 1*(2–3), 155–189. doi:10.1300/J159v01n02_06

Buxton, A. P. (2005). A family matter: When a spouse comes out as gay, lesbian, or bisexual. *Journal of GLBT Family Studies, 1*(2), 49–70. doi:10.1300/J461v01n02_04

Chrisler, A., Smischney, T. M., & Villarruel, F. A. (2014). *Promoting Positive Development of Lesbian, Gay, Bisexual, and Transgender Youth.* Minneapolis, MN: The Military REACH Team. University of Minnesota.

Chu, J., Leino, A., Pflum, S., & Sue, S. (2016). A model for the theoretical basis of cultural competency to guide psychotherapy. *Professional Psychology: Research and Practice, 47*(1), 18–29.

Clark, B. A., Veale, J. F., Townsend, M., Frohard-Dourlent, H., & Saewyc, E. (2018). Non-binary youth: Access to gender-affirming primary health care. *International Journal of Transgenderism, 19*(2), 158–169. doi:10.1080/15532739.2017.1394954

Colon, E. (2001). An ethnographic study of six Latino gay and bisexual men. *Journal of Gay & Lesbian Social Services, 12*(3/4), 77–99. doi:10.1300/J041v12n03_06

Combrinck, J. M. (2015). *Family preservation services: Experiences of families at risk* (Doctoral dissertation, University of Pretoria).

Congress, E. P., & Gonzalez, M. J. (Eds.). (2012). *Multicultural perspectives in social work practice with families.* New York, NY: Springer Publishing Company.

Corrigan, P. W., Kosyluk, K. A., & Rüsch, N. (2013). Reducing self-stigma by coming out proud. *American Journal of Public Health, 103*(5), 794–800. doi:10.2105/AJPH.2012.301037

DeYoung, K. (2015). *What does the Bible really teach about homosexuality?* Meadville, PA: Crossway.

Diamond, G. M., Diamond, G. S., Levy, S., Closs, C., Ladipo, T., & Siqueland, L. (2013). Attachment-based family therapy for suicidal lesbian, gay, and bisexual adolescents: A treatment development study and open trial with preliminary findings. *Psychotherapy*, 49(1), 62–71. doi:10.1037/a0026247

Diaz, R. M. (2013). *Latino gay men and HIV: Culture, sexuality, and risk behavior*. New York, NY: Routledge.

Dorfman, R. A. (2013). *Clinical social work: Definition, practice and vision*. New York, NY: Routledge.

Durso, L. E., & Meyer, I. H. (2013). Patterns and predictors of disclosure of sexual orientation to healthcare providers among lesbians, gay men, and bisexuals. *Sexuality Research and Social Policy*, 10(1), 35–42. doi:10.1007/s13178-012-0105-2

Elder, W. B., Morrow, S. L., & Brooks, G. R. (2015). Sexual self-schemas of gay men: A qualitative investigation. *The Counseling Psychologist*, 43(7), 942–969. doi:10.1177/0011000015606222

Elze, D. E. (2012). *In-home services for families of LGBTQ youth*. Des Moines, IA: National Resource Center for In-Home Services.

Epstein, M. J., & Buhovac, A. R. (2014). *Making sustainability work: Best practices in managing and measuring corporate social, environmental, and economic impacts*. Oakland, CA: Berrett-Koehler Publishers.

Eriksen, T. (2017). *Unconditional: A guide to loving and supporting your LGBTQ child*. Coral Gables, FL: Mango Press.

Firestein, B. A. (2007). *Becoming visible: Counseling bisexuals across the lifespan*. New York, NY: Columbia University Press.

Feinstein, B. A., Wadsworth, L. P., Davila, J., & Goldfried, M. R. (2014). Do parental acceptance and family support moderate associations between dimensions of minority stress and depressive symptoms among lesbians and gay men? *Professional Psychology: Research and Practice*, 45(4), 239. doi:10.1037/a0035393

Fredriksen-Goldsen, K. I., Simoni, J. M., Kim, H. J., Lehavot, K., Walters, K. L., Yang, J., & Muraco, A. (2014). The health equity promotion model: Reconceptualization of lesbian, gay, bisexual, and transgender (LGBT) health disparities. *American Journal of Orthopsychiatry*, 84(6), 653. doi:10.1037/ort0000030

Fuss, D. (2013). *Inside/out: Lesbian theories, gay theories*. New York, NY: Routledge.

Garner, A. (2004). *Families like mine: Children of gay parents tell it like it is*. New York, NY: HarperCollins.

Garofalo, R., Wolf, C., Wissow, L. S., Woods, W. R., & Goodman, E. (1999). Sexual orientation and the risk of suicide attempts among a representative sample of youth. *Archives of Pediatric Adolescent Medicine*, 153, 487–493. doi:10.1001/archpedi.153.5.487

Germain, C. B. (2013). *Social work practice*. New York, NY: Columbia University Press.

Gitterman, A., & Germain, C. B. (2008). *The life model of social work practice: Advances in theory and practice*. New York, NY: Columbia University Press.

Gnuse, R. K. (2015). *Trajectories of justice: What the Bible says about slaves, women, and homosexuality*. Eugene, OR: Wipf and Stock Publishers.

Goffman, E. (1963). *Stigma: Notes of the management of a spoiled identity*. Englewood Cliffs, NJ: Prentice-Hall.

Goldberg, A. E., & Allen, K. R. (Eds.). (2012). *LGBT-parent families: Innovations in research and implications for practice*. New York, NY: Springer Science & Business Media.

Good, D. (2015). Reading strategies for biblical passages on same-sex relations. *Theology & Sexuality*, 7, 70–82. doi:10.1177/135583589700400706

Goodwill, K. A. (2000). Religion and the spiritual needs of gay Mormon men. *Journal of Gay & Lesbian Social Services*, 11(4), 23–38. doi:10.1300/J041v11n04_02

Grafsky, E. L., & Gary, E. A. (2018). What sexual minority youths want in a program to assist with disclosure to their family. *Journal of Gay & Lesbian Social Services, 30*(2), 172–191. doi:10.1080/10538720.2018.1444526

Griffin, C. W., Wirth, M. J., & Wirth, A. G. (2016). *Beyond acceptance: Parents of lesbians and gays talk about their experiences.* New York, NY: St. Martin's Griffin.

Haines, K. M., Boyer, C. R., Giovanazzi, C., & Galupo, M. P. (2018). Not a real family: Microaggressions directed toward LGBTQ families. *Journal of Homosexuality, 65*(9), 1138–1151. doi:10.1080/00918369.2017.1406217

Harbeck, K. M. (2014). *Coming out of the classroom closet: Gay and lesbian students, teachers, and curricula.* New York, NY: Routledge.

Hatzenbuehler, M. L., & Keyes, K. M. (2013). Inclusive anti-bullying policies and reduced risk of suicide attempts in lesbian and gay youth. *Journal of Adolescent Health, 53*(1), S21–S26. doi:10.1016/j.jadohealth.2012.08.010

Hatzenbuehler, M. L., & Pachankis, J. E. (2016). Stigma and minority stress as social determinants of health among lesbian, gay, bisexual, and transgender youth: Research evidence and clinical implications. *Pediatric Clinics of North America, 12*(5), 2220–2229. doi:10.1016/j.pcl.2016.07.003

Herdt, G. (2013). *Gay and lesbian youth.* New York, NY: Routledge.

Hubbard, P. (2013). *Love into light: The Gospel, the homosexual and the Church.* Greenville, SC: Ambassador International.

Hunter, S., & Hickerson, J. (2003). *Affirmative practices: Understanding and working with LGBT people.* Washington, DC: NASW.

Hunter, J., & Mallon, G. P. (1998). Social work practice with lesbian and gay people within communities. In G. P. Mallon (Ed.), *Foundations of social work practice with lesbian and gay people,* (pp. 229–248). New York, NY: Routledge.

Inch, E. (2016). Are you ready? Qualifying social work students' perception of their preparedness to work competently with service users from sexual and gender minority communities. *Social Work Education, 36*(5), 1–18. doi:10.1080/02615479.2016.1237628

Isay, R. (2010). *Being homosexual: Gay men and their development.* New York, NY: Vintage.

Israel, G. E. (2005). Translove: Transgender people and their families. *Journal of Gay and Lesbian Family Studies, 1*(1), 53–67. doi:10.1300/J461v01n01_05

Israel, G. E., Tarver, D. E., & Shaffer, J. D. (2001). *Transgender care: Recommended guidelines, practical information, and personal accounts.* Philadelphia, PA: Temple University Press.

Jones, B. E., & Hill, M. J. (Eds.). (2008). *Mental health issues in lesbian, gay, bisexual, and transgender communities* (Vol. 21). Arlington, VA: American Psychiatric Pub.

Ka'ahumanu, L., & Hutchins, L. (2015). *Bi any other name: Bisexual people speak out.* New York, NY: Riverdale Avenue Books LLC.

Kinney, J., Haapala, D., & Booth, C. (1991). *Keeping families together: The homebuilders model.* Hawthorne, NY: Aldine de Gruyter.

Klein, F. (2014). *The bisexual option.* New York, NY: Routledge.

Klein, F., & Schwartz, T. (2001). *Bisexual and gay husbands: Their stories, their words.* Binghamton, NY: Harrington Park Press.

Kus, R. J. (2014). *Addiction and recovery in gay and lesbian people.* New York, NY: Routledge.

Kwon, P. (2013). Resilience in lesbian, gay, and bisexual individuals. *Personality and Social Psychology Review, 17*(4), 371–383. doi:10.1177/1088868313490248

LaSala, M. C. (2013). Out of the darkness: Three waves of family research and the emergence of family therapy for lesbian and gay people. *Clinical Social Work Journal, 41*(3), 267–276. doi:10.1007/s10615-012-0434-x

Lease, S. H., & Shulman, J. L. (2003). A preliminary investigation of the role of religion for family members of lesbian, gay male, or bisexual male and female individuals. *Counseling and Values, 47*(3), 195–209. doi:10.1002/j.2161-007X.2003.tb00266.x

Legate, N., Ryan, R. M., & Weinstein, N. (2012). Is coming out always a "good thing"? Exploring the relations of autonomy support, outness, and wellness for lesbian, gay, and bisexual individuals. *Social Psychological and Personality Science, 3*(2), 145–152. doi:10.1177/1948550611411929

Leong, R. (2014). *Asian American sexualities: Dimensions of the gay and lesbian experience.* New York, NY: Routledge.

Lev, A. I. (2013). *Transgender emergence: Therapeutic guidelines for working with gender-variant people and their families.* New York, NY: Routledge.

Madsen, W. C. (2013). *Collaborative therapy with multi-stressed families.* New York, NY: Guilford Press.

Mallon, G. P. (2012). Practice with families where gender or sexual orientation is an issue: Lesbian, gay, bisexual, and trans individuals and their families. In E. Congress & M. Gonzalez (Eds.), *Multicultural perspectives in social work practice with families* (pp. 205–220). New York, NY: Springer Publishing Company.

Mallon, G. P. (2017a). Knowledge for practice with LGBT people. In G. P. Mallon (Ed.), *Social work practice with lesbian, gay, bisexual and transgender people* (3rd ed., pp. 1–24). New York, NY: Routledge.

Mallon, G. P. (Ed.). (2017b). *Social work practice with lesbian, gay, bisexual, and transgender people* (3rd ed.). New York, NY: Routledge.

Mallon, G. P. (2017c). Social work practice with LGBT people within families. In G. P. Mallon (Ed.), *Social work practice with lesbian, gay, bisexual, and transgender people* (3rd ed., pp. 239–266). New York, NY: Routledge.

Mallon, G. P. (2017d). Social work practice with LGBT parents and their children. In G. P. Mallon (Ed.), *Social work practice with lesbian, gay, bisexual, and transgender people* (3rd ed., pp. 267–310). New York, NY: Routledge.

Mallon, G. P., & Hess, P. M. (2014). *Child welfare for the twenty-first century: A handbook of practices, policies, & programs.* New York, NY: Columbia University Press.

Maluccio, A. N., Pine, B. A., & Tracy, E. M. (2013). *Social work practice with families and children.* New York, NY: Columbia University Press.

McNeill, J. J. (2015). *The church and the homosexual.* Boston, MA: Beacon Press.

Meyer, I. H. (2003). Prejudice, social stress and mental health in lesbian, gay, and bisexual populations: Conceptual issues and research evidence. *Psychological Bulletin, 129,* 674–697. doi:10.1037/0033-2909.129.5.674

Miceli, M. (2013). *Standing out, standing together: The social and political impact of gay-straight alliances.* New York, NY: Routledge.

Molina, Y., Marquez, J. H., Logan, D. E., Leeson, C. J., Balsam, K. F., & Kaysen, D. L. (2015). Current intimate relationship status, depression, and alcohol use among bisexual women: The mediating roles of bisexual-specific minority stressors. *Sex Roles, 73*(1–2), 43–57. doi:10.1007/s11199-015-0483-z

Moore, S. M., & Rosenthal, D. A. (2007). *Sexuality in adolescence: Current trends.* New York, NY: Routledge.

Moore, M. R., & Stambolis-Ruhstorfer, M. (2013). LGBT sexuality and families at the start of the twenty-first century. *Annual Review of Sociology, 39,* 491–507. doi:10.1146/annurev-soc-071312-145643

Morrow, D. F., & Messinger, L. (2006). *Sexual orientation and gender expression in social work practice: Working with gay, lesbian, bisexual, and transgender people.* New York, NY: Columbia University Press.

Mustanski, B., & Liu, R. T. (2013). A longitudinal study of predictors of suicide attempts among lesbian, gay, bisexual, and transgender youth. *Archives of Sexual Behavior, 42*(3), 437–448. doi:10.1007/s10508-012-0013-9

Nealy, E. (2017). *Transgender children and youth: Cultivating pride and joy with families in transition.* New York, NY: W.W. Norton & Co.

O'Dell, S. (2000). Psychotherapy with gay and lesbian families: Opportunities for cultural inclusion and clinical challenge. *Clinical Social Work Journal, 28*(2), 171–182. doi:10.1023/A:1005154217642

Omi, M., & Winant, H. (2014). *Racial formation in the United States.* New York, NY: Routledge.

Oswald, R. F. (2002a). Inclusion and belonging in the family rituals of gay and lesbian people. *Journal of Family Psychology, 16*(4), 428–436. doi:10.1037/0893-3200.16.4.428

Oswald, R. F. (2002b). Resilience within the family networks of lesbians and gay men: Intentionality and redefinition. *Journal of Marriage and Family, 64*(2), 374–383. doi:10.1111/j.1741-3737.2002.00374.x

Owens-Reid, D., & Russo, K. (2014). *This is a book for parents of gay kids: A question & answer guide to everyday life.* San Francisco, CA: Chronical Books.

Page, M. J., Lindahl, K. M., & Malik, N. M. (2013). The role of religion and stress in sexual identity and mental health among lesbian, gay, and bisexual youth. *Journal of Research on Adolescence, 23*(4), 665–677. doi:10.1111/jora.12025

Parents and Friends of Lesbians and Gays. (1997). *Beyond the Bible: Parents, families and friends talk about religion and homosexuality.* Washington, DC: Author.

Patterson, C. J. (2013). Family lives of lesbian and gay adults. In G. W. Peterson & K. R Bush (Eds.), *Handbook of marriage and the family* (pp. 659–681). New York, NY: Springer Publishing Company.

Patterson, C. J., & D'Augelli, A. R. (2013). *Handbook of psychology and sexual orientation.* New York, NY: Oxford University Press.

Patterson, C. J., & Farr, R. H. (2015). Children of lesbian and gay parents: Reflections on the research–policy interface. In K. Durkin & H. R. Schaffer (Ed.), *The Wiley handbook of developmental psychology in practice: Implementation and impact* (pp. 121–142). Hoboken, NJ: Wiley.

Pecora, P. J., Whittaker, J. K., Maluccio, A. N., & Barth, R. P. (2012). *The child welfare challenge: Policy, practice, and research.* New York, NY: Aldine Transaction.

Perrin-Wallqvist, R., & Lindblom, J. (2015). Coming out as gay: A phenomenological study about adolescents disclosing their homosexuality to their parents. *Social Behavior and Personality: An International Journal, 43*(3), 467–480. doi:10.2224/sbp.2015.43.3.467

Pillemer, K. & McCartney, K. (Eds.) (2013). *Parent child relations throughout life.* Hillsdale, NJ: Lawrence Erlbaum.

Pistella, J., Salvati, M., Ioverno, S., Laghi, F., & Baiocco, R. (2016). Coming-out to family members and internalized sexual stigma in bisexual, lesbian and gay people. *Journal of Child and Family Studies, 25*(5), 1–8. doi:10.1007/s10826-016-0528-0

Plöderl, M., Wagenmakers, E. J., Tremblay, P., Ramsay, R., Kralovec, K., Fartacek, C., & Fartacek, R. (2013). Suicide risk and sexual orientation: A critical review. *Archives of Sexual Behavior, 42*(5), 715–727. doi:10.1007/s10508-012-0056-y

Poon, M. K. (2004). A missing voice: Asians in contemporary gay and lesbian social service literature. *Journal of Gay & Lesbian Social Services, 17*(3), 87–106. doi:10.1300/J041v17n03_05

Roberts, M. C. (2014). *Model programs in child and family mental health.* New York, NY: Routledge.

Rothberg, B., & Weinstein, D. L. (1996). A primer on lesbian and gay families. In M. Shernoff (Ed.), *Human services for gay people: Clinical and community practice* (pp. 55–68). New York, NY: Harrington Park.

Saltzburg, S. (2004). Learning that an adolescent child is gay or lesbian: The parent experience. *Social Work, 49*(1), 109–118. doi:10.1093/sw/49.1.109

Savage, D., & Miller, T. (Eds.). (2011). *It gets better: Coming out, overcoming bullying, and creating a life worth living.* New York, NY: Penguin.

Savin-Williams, R. C. (2009). *The new gay teenager* (Vol. 3). Cambridge, MA: Harvard University Press.

Schmitz, R. M., & Tyler, K. A. (2018). The complexity of family reactions to identity among homeless and college lesbian, gay, bisexual, transgender, and queer young adults. *Archives of Sexual Behavior, 47*(4), 1195–1207. doi:10.1007/s10508-017-1014-5

Snow, J. (2004). *How it feels to have a gay or lesbian parent*. New York, NY: Harrington Park Press.

Stein, T. S., & Cohen, C. J. (Eds.). (2013). *Contemporary perspectives on psychotherapy with lesbians and gay men*. New York, NY: Springer Science & Business Media.

Stone, D. M., Luo, F., Ouyang, L., Lippy, C., Hertz, M. F., & Crosby, A. E. (2014). Sexual orientation and suicide ideation, plans, attempts, and medically serious attempts: Evidence from local youth risk behavior surveys, 2001–2009. *American Journal of Public Health, 104*(2), 262–271. doi:10.2105/AJPH.2013.301383

Strock, C. (2008). *Married women who love women*. New York, NY: Routledge.

Strydom, M. (2014). Community based family support services for families at-risk: Services rendered by child and family welfare organisations. *Social Work/Maatskaplike Werk, 49*(4), 501–518. doi:10.15270/49-4-41

Tasker, F. (2013). Lesbian and gay parenting post-heterosexual divorce and separation. In A. E. Goldberg and K.R. Allen (Eds.), *LGBT-Parent Families* (pp. 3–20). New York, NY: Springer Publishing Company.

Tasker, F., & Delvoye, M. (2018). Maps of family relationships drawn by women engaged in bisexual motherhood: defining family membership. *Journal of Family Issues, 39*(18), 4248–4274. doi:10.1177/0192513X18810958

Toomey, R. B., Ryan, C., Diaz, R. M., Card, N. A., & Russell, S. T. (2010). Gender-nonconforming lesbian, gay, bisexual, and transgender youth: School victimization and young adult psychosocial adjustment. *Developmental Psychology, 46*(6), 1580–1589. doi:10.1037/a0020705

Trahan, D. P., & Goodrich, K. M. (2015). "You think you know me, but you have no idea": Dynamics in African American families following a son's or daughter's disclosure as LGBT. *The Family Journal, 23*(2), 147–157. doi:10.1177/1066480715573423

Trussell, D. E., Xing, T. M., & Oswald, A. G. (2015). Family leisure and the coming out process for LGB young people and their parents. *Annals of Leisure Research, 18*(3), 323–341. doi:10.1080/11745398.2015.1075224

van Wormer, K., & Wells, J. (2000). *Social work with lesbians, gays, and bisexuals: A strengths perspective*. New York, NY: Allyn & Bacon.

Vela, C. A. (2015). *Experiences of LGBTQ adolescents and their parents with secondary school counselors: A qualitative study* (Doctoral dissertation, Texas A&M University-Corpus Christi).

Walsh, F. (2015). *Strengthening family resilience*. New York, NY: Guilford Publications.

Walters, K. L. (2008). Negotiating conflicts in allegiances among lesbian and gays of color: Reconciling divided selves and communities. In G. P. Mallon (Ed.), *Foundations of social work practice with lesbian and gay people* (pp. 47–98). New York, NY: Routledge.

Wampold, B. E., & Imel, Z. E. (2015). *The great psychotherapy debate: The evidence for what makes psychotherapy work*. New York, NY: Routledge.

Watson, S., & Miller, T. (2012). LGBT oppression. *Multicultural Education, 19*(4), 2.

Weitzman, G. (2006). Therapy with clients who are bisexual and polyamorous. *Journal of Bisexuality, 6*(1/2), 137–164. doi:10.1300/J159v06n01_08

Weston, K. (1997). *Families we choose: Lesbians, gays, kinship*. New York, NY: Columbia University Press.

Winter, E. A., Elze, D. E., Saltzburg, S., & Rosenwald, M. (2015). Social services for LGBT young people in the United States: are we there yet? In J. Fish & K. Karban (Eds.), *Lesbian, gay, bisexual and trans health inequalities: International perspectives in social work* (pp. 113–130). doi:10.1332/policypress/9781447309673.003.0006

Worthen, M. G. (2013). An argument for separate analyses of attitudes toward lesbian, gay, bisexual men, bisexual women, MtF and FtM transgender individuals. *Sex Roles, 68*(11–12), 703–723. doi:10.1007/s11199-012-0155-1

# Part V

## Physical and Mental Health Issues With Multicultural Families

# 17

# Health Beliefs, Care, and Access of Individuals and Families From Diverse Backgrounds

ELAINE P. CONGRESS

## INTRODUCTION

Health issues and care impact all people. This chapter takes an intersectional approach in looking at people from diverse cultural and ethnic backgrounds, as well as other intersectional factors such as social-economic status, education, age, immigrant status, and gender that impact on their health issues and access.

In considering health, we must first look at the increasing number of immigrants in the United States. Over 44 million people in the United States are foreign born (Batalova & Alperin, 2018), and an additional 36 million have one foreign-born parent (U.S. Census Bureau, 2018). While many immigrants live in urban centers such as New York, Los Angeles, or Miami, an increasing number of immigrants live in smaller cities, suburban, and rural areas (Chang-Muy & Congress, 2016). Immigrants and refugees are a very diverse population coming from over 140 different countries and speaking 150 languages (Castillo, 2015). While immigrants come from many countries, Mexico (29%), China (5%), India (5%), Philippines (4%), El Salvador (3%), Vietnam (3%), Cuba (3%), Korea (3%), Dominican Republic (2%), and Guatemala (2%) have sent the most immigrants (Center for Immigration Studies, 2012).

In looking at the health issues for people from different cultures and ethnicities, we need to individualize and avoid assumptions that all people from a particular country or culture have similar health problems. An intersectional approach is very helpful in looking at the health issues for different people who come from the same country. For example, a Mexican undocumented 26-year-old woman with limited education who migrated last week and works in the kitchen of a restaurant is very different than a 56-year-old Mexican man who immigrated on a work visa 20 years ago and is now employed in an administrative position in a tech company. Their health issues and health access may be very different.

## HEALTH AS A HUMAN RIGHT

Promoting good health for all people is an international issue. The United Nations has developed 17 Sustainable Goals to work on achieving by 2030. SDG#3 focuses on promoting good health and well-being, which includes both physical and mental health. The 17 Sustainable Goals apply to all countries, including developed countries such as the United States as well as developing countries.

Goals are generalities and therefore SDG#3 like the other Sustainable Goals have different targets that address specific issues such as maternal mortality, childhood mortality, communicable diseases such as AIDS and water-borne illnesses, substance abuse, traffic accidents, and reproductive health. These targets are further broken down into 24 indicators. Has the United States been able to achieve its targets? In a major NIH study of 17 developed countries, the United States fared poorly in many health areas as they had high rates of maternal mortality, infant mortality, heart and lung disease, sexually transmitted infections, adolescent pregnancies, injuries, and homicides.

In terms of maternal mortality, the United States has a three times higher rate than other developed countries (see Figure 17.1). Life expectancy was at

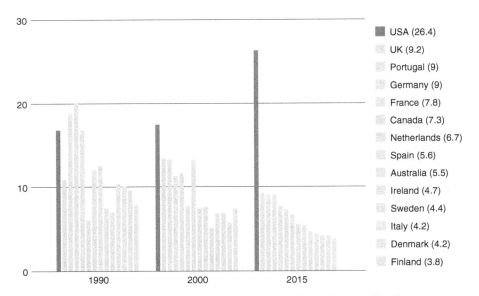

Figure 17.1 *Maternal mortality continues to rise in the United States. (Deaths per 100,000 live births.)*

Source: Data from GBD 2015 Maternal Mortality Collaborators. (2016). Global, regional, and national levels of maternal mortality, 1990–2015: A systematic analysis for the Global Burden of Disease Study 2015. *Lancet, 388*(10053), 1775–1812. doi:10.1016/S0140-6736(16)31470-2

least 4 years less than that of the highest-ranking developed countries (National Institutes of Health [NIH], 2013), and recently, life expectancy in this country has decreased even more (see Figure 17.2).

What is life expectancy for different ethnic groups? Non-Hispanic Whites still have a higher life expectancy than non-Hispanic Blacks—78.8 years versus 75.2 years. Hispanics, at 81.8 years, have the highest life expectancy of the three demographic groups (Achenbach, 2016). It is well known that there are many challenges to good health and well-being and that social determinants of health affect health outcomes in the United States as well as around the world. For many years, cultural differences in health beliefs has been seen as important for those who work with immigrants (Congress & Lyons, 1992), but it is of increased importance now with more people entering the United States.

Since there are social determinants that impact on health, one would expect that Hispanics who often are poorer and have less education would have lower life expectancy, not higher life expectancy. One explanation is that cultural factors such as close social and family networks of the Hispanic population serve as protective factors that counteract the negative effects of poverty, lack of education, and preventive care (Arias, 2019). In terms of life expectancy, data are mostly available on Whites, Hispanics, and Blacks but not easily accessible on Native American or Asian populations.

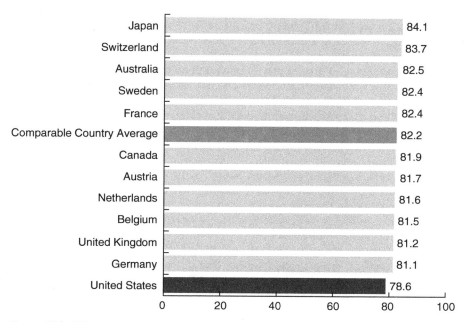

Figure 17.2 *Life expectancy at birth in years, 2016 or nearest year.*

Note: Data for Canada and France are for 2015.

Source: Reproduced with permission from Kaiser Family Foundation analysis of 2018 OECD data: "ECD Health Data: Health status: Health status indicators, OECD Health Statistics (database).

## HEALTH ACCESS AND CARE

A major target included under SDG#3 is universal healthcare to all. This certainly is not the reality in the United States and a major difference between the United States and other developed countries. At the time that this chapter was written, the Patient Protection and Affordable Care Act (aka Affordable Care Act [ACA]) continues as the major health plan in the United States. While the plan expanded healthcare to many who were previously excluded, it is still much tied to employment. All businesses with over 50 employees are required to provide health insurance. Those who work in organizations with less than 50 employees or who are not employed at all may not be able to purchase very expensive healthcare. The undocumented may experience further challenges in accessing affordable healthcare (Ku, 2006).

In *Healthy People 2020* (Office of Disease Prevention and Health Promotion [ODPHP], 2019), the CDC defined social determinants of health "as conditions in the environments in which people live, learn, work, play, worship, and age that affect a wide range of health, functioning, and quality-of-life outcomes and risks." Conditions are further defined as social, economic, and physical (Congress, 2017). Kennedy and colleagues (2015) looked at health outcomes and mortality for racial and ethnic minorities in several major areas including heart disease and stroke, cancer, HIV, AIDS, respiratory diseases, diabetes, maternal and child health, and mental health and found that poorer minorities usually had poorer outcomes.

Heart disease and cancer are the major causes of death in the United States (Kochanek, Xu, Murphy, Minino, & Kung, 2011). The mortality rates for each of these diseases are much higher among those from immigrant and/or non-White backgrounds. A major reason from higher death rates due to cardiovascular illness among these populations is linked to differences in care. Differences in cardiovascular care contribute to greater mortality among ethnic and racial minorities (U.S. Institute of Medicine [IOM] Committee on Understanding and Eliminating Racial and Ethnic Disparities in Health Care, 2003). Often, poor non-White people are less likely to have regular medical exams and, even when problems are detected, because of financial and work challenges they are less likely to receive follow up care.

While racial/ethnic differences in the diagnosis and treatment of cancer may be less well documented than with cardiovascular illnesses, there is some evidence that certain ethnic minorities have higher rates of cancer than Whites (Ward et al., 2008). Moreover, ethnic minorities are often diagnosed with cancer at a later stage, when the disease is less treatable. This may be particularly true for immigrants with limited healthcare access who often do not have access to or benefit from early diagnostic care.

People of color have the highest rates of HIV/AIDS and subsequent death due to the disease than Whites. The likelihood of death within 3 years of receiving an HIV diagnosis is much greater than for White populations (Hall, McDavid, Ling, & Sloggett, 2006). See Chapter 19, "HIV/AIDS and Latino Families: Practice Considerations," for a more detailed discussion about HIV/AIDS.

## IMPACT OF IMMIGRANT STATUS

A major factor that influences access to healthcare is immigration status. Some immigrants came when they were children and have lived in the United States for most of their lives. Others that are undocumented do not have the necessary documents to remain in the United States. DACA (Deferred Action for Childhood Arrivals) has been a federal government policy that provided adolescents and young adults a way to move toward citizenship (Chang, 2016), and at the time this chapter was written remains as a policy that positively affects young people's access to healthcare (Shear & Yee, 2017). Legalizing young peoples' status has enabled many to access healthcare through insurance (if they work for an employer with over 50 employees) or to receive Medicaid if they are not employed and within Medicaid standards.

Other immigrants are recent arrivals and may have initially come as visitors, students, or with work permits. See Chapter 7, "Legal Issues in Practice With Immigrants and Refugees," for a fuller discussion about different legal categories in the United States. These immigrants may receive temporary health benefits from their schools or employers. While some stay only for a short time, such as international students, others remain in the United States after their status has changed and enter the ranks of the undocumented. They are not covered by health insurance and thus their access to healthcare may be very limited and only provided when they are seen on an emergency basis. Often undocumented people have to rely exclusively on emergency departments for healthcare where hospitals are guided by the Hippocratic principle that all who are ill are entitled to receive care. Some states have special health programs for vulnerable populations like children and pregnant women. Although the undocumented may receive the most attention in public media, they are certainly not the majority of immigrants as most immigrants are either naturalized citizens or may be "green card holders" waiting to apply for citizenship (Passel & Cohn, 2016).

## HEALTH OF IMMIGRANTS—A LONGITUDINAL APPROACH

What is the health of those from different cultural backgrounds? Health is one of the topics addressed in the culturagram (see Chapter 1, :Using the *Culturagram* and an Intersectional Approach in Practice With Culturally Diverse Families," for further discussion), but to explore this issue more closely, especially for the foreign-born, a longitudinal approach is helpful. This author developed the Cultural Health Assessment Tool (CHAT) for looking at the health of immigrants at three points: (1) in country of origin, (2) in transit to the United States, and (3) in their current situation (Congress, 2016) (see Figure 17.3).

First, it is important to assess the health of the individual before migrating to the United States. Did the immigrant suffer any food or water deprivation? Was there exposure to different infectious diseases because of lack of sanitation or immunization? It is well documented that there is a much higher risk of people succumbing to childhood diseases in developing countries. Those who survive may have recurring health conditions throughout their lives. Climate change and global warming have been seen as contributing to the increase of insect bearing diseases as well as life threatening weather changes (European Commission Joint Research Centre, 2018). Some immigrants especially those from the Middle East or Africa may have spent years in refugee camps with inadequate sanitation, food, and water supplies.

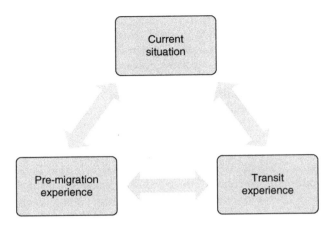

Figure 17.3 *Cultural Health Assessment Tool (CHAT).*

Source: Adapted from Heyman, J., & Congress, E. P. (2018). *Health and social work: Practice, policy, and research.* New York, NY: Springer Publishing Company.

The second part of the CHAT involves the transit experience. Access by air may only be available to those who have a visa and legal right to migrate and thus usually these immigrants with higher income and more education are able to travel this way. As poor undocumented people begin the migration process, there may be many health challenges along the way. These immigrants who come by land or sea, usually from the United States' southern border, may be challenged by illegal desert crossings with limited water and extreme heat or by dangerous, unsafe water trips. Some who are detained may spend months in detention camps where there is inadequate access to healthcare. A number of immigrant deaths in border camps have been well documented in the media (Human Rights Watch, 2018).

The third part of the CHAT analysis explores the health of immigrants after their relocation in the United States. Poor immigrants face many challenges to their health. Those who settle in rural areas may be exposed to dangerous chemicals and working conditions on farms (National Center for Farmworker Health, 2016). In urban environments, those who work on construction sites may have dangerous assignments and if they "work off the books" are not covered by union and government safety rules (Congress, 2017).

Inadequate income may lead to homelessness and lack of nutritious food. In poor neighborhoods, there are many food deserts with few resources for fruits and vegetables. Healthy foods that are available are often much more expensive than cheaper carbohydrates. Even schools which are available to all have recently cut back on lunch programs for poorer students. Other issues that may detrimentally affect the health of recently arrived poor immigrants and their families are the lack of available exercise opportunities for themselves and their families. Those who came from a rural environment may have walked each day and children can easily access safe outside play areas. In poorer immigrant communities, parks and outdoor recreational activities may not be that easily available

(Radford & Krogstad, 2019). Another major challenge that many immigrants face who migrate from the south is the sudden transition to a colder climate. Often, a poorer family may not be able to afford to buy the heavy clothing required in the North, and for many recently arrived immigrants, the first winter brings many health challenges with recurrent upper respiratory infections.

The Healthy Immigrant Effect (Kennedy et al., 2015) proposes that, despite health challenges in the country of origin and in transit, many immigrants arrive healthier than native-born Americans and become sicker the longer they remain. It has been noted that many Hispanics have a greater risk of developing diabetes and high blood pressure once they arrive (Koya & Egede, 2007; Misra & Ganda, 2007). The cause has been attributed to a change of diet and exercise in that many immigrants now eat more carbohydrates than previously because of easy access and affordability. Limited income of many Hispanics can definitely affect accessibility to healthy foods. While this has been seen to be particularly true of Latinx immigrants, increased risk for diabetes is also seen to affect other ethnic populations such as Arab-Americans (Bertran, Pinelli, Masri, Sills, & Jaber, 2018), Asian Indians (Deol, 1970), and Chinese Americans (Ho, Tran, & Chesla, 2015). Medication adherence may also differ among different cultural groups (Jin & Acharya, 2016).

Access to healthcare differs greatly depending on immigrant status and location (Krogstad & Lopez, 2014). As stated previously, those who are undocumented often have to rely only on emergency department care (Xu & Borders, 2008). Then health problems that could have been more easily treated at the beginning of the disease become more acute. Even those who are documented may have difficulty accessing healthcare. While those who work in organizations with over 50 employees have obligatory healthcare, many immigrants work in smaller businesses. Hispanics in general, and even those with legal status, are less likely to have access to healthcare (Livingston, Minushkim, & Cohn, 2008).

Why are immigrants less likely to be able to access healthcare? In addition to the policy aspects of healthcare that limit access to affordable healthcare to those who are employed in larger organizations, lack of education about available healthcare, nonavailability of information in languages they can understand, and alternative healthcare options may play a role (Congress, 2018). Many immigrants have been raised in countries with minimal focus on prevention. Doctors were only seen when one was very sick and not on a regular basis. The need for a healthy diet and a smoke-free environment were not stressed. Preventive measures such as childhood immunizations, Pap smears, mammograms, and prostate tests were not well known or available. This is most apparent with immigrants that come from poorer socioeconomic backgrounds with limited education, while more educated, richer immigrants may have learned more about preventive care in their countries of origin. Cultural factors certainly influence immigrant and refugee women's beliefs about their health (Birkhead, Kennedy, Callister, & Paredes Miyamoto, 2011). Some may not know about or pursue preventive and early intervention health measures such as mammograms and Pap smears.

While children of immigrants now attend schools that teach about healthy life practices, adult migrants did not benefit from learning about preventive health measures. Even when there is messaging about healthy practices, it is often in English which many immigrants do not understand. Although there has been effort in the health field to increase the number of bilingual staff, there are still serious gaps, especially given the multiplicity of languages. Finally, while immigrants who live in urban areas may have many healthcare options in rural areas, doctors and other medical personnel may be many miles away (Rosenblatt & Hart, 2000). There may be additional environmental risks for women and their children when they are exposed to dangerous work conditions on farms (National Center for Farmworker Health, 2016).

There are age differences in terms of health beliefs, practice, and accessibility. More and more families are mixed in that parents were not born and raised in the United States, but their children are. This certainly impacts on the way that children receive and utilize healthcare (Desai et al., 2016). Also seniors from different cultural backgrounds often have differing views about strokes (Chang et al., 2018), as well as Alzheimer's (Sayegh & Knight, 2012).

It is important to consider the enormous stresses families encounter in the process of acculturation due to sudden and radical shifts in family dynamics. Parents in a recently migrated family often are aligned with the culture of the country of origin, while their offspring are likely to adapt to the dominant culture more rapidly. This often leads to intergenerational conflicts (Carteret, 2010) in terms of health beliefs and practices.

## FOCUS ON PREVENTION

In the United States, there is a major focus on prevention at all ages, but especially for children. Before birth, pregnant women attend prenatal clinics, babies beginning at birth regularly attend well baby clinics, children receive immunizations, and all are influenced by public media messages about healthy eating and lifestyles. This may be very strange for a recently arrived poor immigrant who was raised in a country with very limited health facilities and with beliefs that medical treatment was only sought when one was very ill. Sometimes the lack of focus on prevention may have very negative consequences as this case example illustrates.

One night Carmen with her very sick 2-year-old son appeared in the emergency department of a large public hospital. After noting that the child's temperature was 103 degrees, the doctor immediately asked where the child's immunization records were. The mother responded that she had never brought the child to a doctor before because he had not been sick. The doctor immediately called the social worker to discuss if this mother should be reported to child welfare because of medical neglect (Heyman & Congress, 2018). This case example illustrates cultural differences in health beliefs around prevention and healthcare. An interesting ethical dilemma arises about whether this is an example of medical neglect as the mother failed to bring her child for preventive care which is seen as expected in American society.

## OTHER HEALTHCARE PROVIDERS

In addition to varied views on prevention, members of an immigrant family may pursue different health providers. For example, a Latino woman may first consult a spiritualist for a physical problem rather than a doctor or other healthcare professional. An Asian immigrant may be concerned about eating the proper amount of hot and cold foods, as well as seek acupuncture for a recurring health problem. This may be challenging for the helping professional who works for a medical establishment and/or is convinced that the American system of medicine that involves oral medications, x-rays, blood tests, and surgery is the best way to deal with a medical problem. It is interesting to note that many different cultural medical practices such as acupuncture have become more readily accepted (Congress, 2013). A common belief is that adult immigrants are more traditional than their school-age children in pursuing the health beliefs they had when they migrated to the United States. There is some evidence, however, that college students who were not born in the United States retained some of their traditional beliefs (Rothstein & Rajapaksa, 2003).

Health literacy and self-management of chronic diseases may vary among different populations (Shaw, Armin, Torres, Orzech, & Vivian, 2012). To work more effectively with immigrants from different backgrounds, it behooves clinicians to learn more about the specific cultural beliefs of their clients (Ross, Timura, & Maupin, 2012), especially the Muslim populations that may be very unfamiliar to them (Consumer Health Beliefs, 2011).

## MENTAL HEALTH/BEHAVIORAL HEALTH

Mental health continues to be an area where ethnic minorities receive less treatment than Whites. Explanations about the absence of mental healthcare include the lack of health insurance to cover costs, reliance on cultural beliefs about mental health and its treatment, and distrust of formal mental health services and service providers. Hispanics are less likely to pursue mental health treatment than either Whites or African Americans (Wells, Klap, Koike, & Sherbourne, 2001). Many immigrants come from countries where mental health treatment does not exist and/or there is a stigma associated with mental illness (Congress, 2004).

In the United States, traditionally there has been a sharp division between physical and mental health. Different funding paths have contributed to this division, but there are current efforts to have a more integrative approach (Stanhope, Heyman, Amarante, & Doherty, 2018). For many immigrants, physical and mental issues have not been defined separately (Stanek, 2014). For example, a Latino woman who complained about *dolor de cabeza* was not referring to a physical headache but rather anxious feelings related to a low income and problems with her adolescent son.

With many poor, there has been a stigma related to mental illness. Mental health problems may not be recognized or if so, hidden. Having a *loco* (Spanish translation of crazy) family member might be kept hidden in a poor Hispanic or Asian family as it is a source of strain and embarrassment. There may also be ignorance about mental illness as this brief case example about an Asian family indicates.

A 19-year-old Asian girl, Wing Sue, came into a community mental health clinic to ask about her mother. She reported that she and her parents had emigrated from China when she was 5 years old. Her father worked long hours in the kitchen in a restaurant in Chinatown. Her mother never left their small apartment and spent most of her days in a dark room. Wing Sue had heard that this sometimes happened to women during menopause, but this seems to have been of at least 10 years' duration. In college, Wing Sue was enrolled in a psychopathology class, and she became increasingly concerned that her mother was clinically depressed.

Not only beliefs about healthcare but also access to physical and mental healthcare may affect families from varied cultural and socioeconomic backgrounds in a different way. The following case example, adapted from a previous chapter by the author that appeared in the *Handbook of Public Health Social Work* (2004), illustrates some of these issues.

## CASE VIGNETTE

Carmen Perez, a 35-year-old Latina woman, met with the hospital social worker to discuss discharge plans for her 60-year-old mother, Rosa, who had been hospitalized for the last two days following a trip to the emergency department. The emergency department physician diagnosed Rosa's condition as chronic kidney disease, which may result in Rosa needing to go on dialysis. Additional tests have been ordered to determine the seriousness of her condition. Rosa does not want to return to the hospital and says that the spiritualist can provide the care that she needs.

In exploring more about family and social-economic issues, the social worker learned that Carmen was having increasing conflicts with her 16-year-old son, Juan Jr., who had begun to cut school and stay out late at night. Her 14-year-old daughter, Lucia, had gained 50 pounds over the past 2 years and now weighed 200 pounds. Recently, Lucia had become very depressed, tearful, and did not want to go to school. Last week Carmen found that Lucia had hidden two bottles of aspirin in her room. In contrast to her two older children, who presented many problems, Carmen described her 12-year-old daughter, Maria, as "an angel." Maria is very quiet, helpful with household chores, and often accompanied Carmen and Rosa to different medical appointments. Maria goes to school regularly without any complaints, and earns passing grades, but does not socialize with other children.

Carmen also has some health problems of her own. Because of excessive vaginal bleeding, she had recently gone to the emergency department. Carmen had initially asked Juan Jr. to accompany her as no interpreter might be available. Using her teenage son to interpret especially with this type of problem was very difficult and fortunately a bilingual attendant was found to interpret.

Carmen learned that she needed more tests and possible surgery. Carmen is not eligible for Medicaid and does not have funds for follow-up treatment.

Carmen indicated Juan Jr. was the source of much family conflict as he believed he did not have to respect Pablo, Carmen's boyfriend, who is not Juan's father. Juan complained that his mother and stepfather were "dumb" because they did not speak English. He felt that his parents did not understand how difficult his school experiences were and believed that teachers favor lighter skin Latinos. Juan has much darker skin than others in his family.

At age 20, Mrs. Perez moved to the United States from Mexico with her husband, Juan Sr. She states that they were very poor in Mexico and had heard there were better job opportunities in the United States. At the time, Juan Jr. was 2 and Carmen was pregnant with Lucia. One year later, Juan Sr. died in an automobile accident on a visit back to Mexico. Shortly afterward, Carmen met Pablo, who had come to New York from Guatemala to visit a terminally ill relative. After she became pregnant with Maria, Juan and Carmen began to live together. Pablo indicated that he was very fearful of returning to Guatemala, stating that several people in his village had been killed in gang violence.

Many immigrant families have mixed legal status as does this family. Lucia and Maria were born here, so they are American citizens and thus eligible for Medicaid to cover their health needs. Carmen reports that Maria is a model child, but there are some signs that Maria may have some mental health issues. It is unusual for a 12-year-old girl to choose to stay at home all the time rather than socialize with her friends.

The other family members are undocumented, and thus, they may be severely limited in terms of their access to healthcare. Lucia is very overweight and may be clinically depressed and suicidal. Carmen may have a serious gynecological problem, but it is difficult for her to access care. Because of government crackdowns on undocumented people, this family is very anxious even to seek medical care for fear of being apprehended and deported. In addition to affecting their access to healthcare, an undocumented status also makes it difficult for either Pablo or Carmen to secure regular employment. They both most work at "off the books" jobs without any guaranteed minimum wage and other government work protections. Recently, however, Carmen has been able to work more regularly in cleaning homes and taking care of the elderly. With a cultural belief that men should be the primary breadwinner, this shift in role has increased family conflict between Pablo and Carmen.

Carmen is very close to her mother, Rosa, who came to live with the family 9 years ago. Rosa has not been able to help recently because of her health problems. Rosa, who does not have health insurance, first consulted a spiritualist to help her with her health concerns before she went to the emergency department with a severe backache and fatigue. Pablo has no relatives in New York, but has several friends at the social club in his neighborhood. Recently, he has started to stay out late with his friends and often he arrives home drunk and says he can do whatever he wants.

This Latino family has numerous physical and mental health problems. In terms of health issues, the grandmother, Rosa, has serious kidney problems and may need dialysis, while Carmen has gynecological problems that require further investigation and possible surgery. Lucia is extremely overweight and is at risk for diabetes and has expressed some suicidal thoughts. Suicide among Latina adolescents is rising and a suicide assessment risk is indicated. (See Chapter 22, "Culture, Intersectionality, and Suicide," for a longer discussion about suicide risk.) Pablo needs treatment for alcohol abuse, even though he is still in denial about his alcohol problems. There also are family issues in that Juan Jr. does not respect the man who is not his father. Rosa, Carmen, and Pablo are all undocumented immigrants and unemployed. Consequently, they are able to access only emergency treatment. Juan Jr. is also undocumented, but he may be eligible to stay under DACA and can receive medical treatment if he lives in a state that provides healthcare services to children and adolescents regardless of immigration status. Lucia and Maria are U.S. citizens because of their birthplace, and Carmen could apply for healthcare benefits for them. In the current immigration environment, the parents may be fearful, however, that if their undocumented immigrant status is discovered they will be deported and the two youngest children placed by Child Protective Services.

Cultural issues are very relevant in understanding the needs of this family. The grandmother consulted a spiritualist before seeking medical treatment only on an emergency basis. With a possible life-threatening disease, should the clinician insist that Rosa follow up with Western medical assessment and treatment rather than continuing to pursue care from a spiritualist? Discrimination, racism, and sexism are also evident in this case example. Juan Jr. feels discriminated against because he is the darkest in his family, as well as at school. Also, neither parent is able to work regularly because they are undocumented immigrants. It has been easier for Carmen to find undocumented work as a domestic or child care worker. The fact that she is the one who has brought income into the family, rather than Pablo, has led to increased conflict in Carmen and Pablo's relationship.

## Discussions Questions

1. From a micro-practice perspective, how should the clinician worker assess and develop appropriate interventions for individual family members as well as this family as a whole?
2. What macro practice and policy issues impact on this family? What resources should the clinician seek? What is the best way to intervene?
3. Do you think it is better to work with each member individually or as a family? Why?
4. This family has multiple physical and mental health issues. What would you address first and why?

## REFERENCES

Achenbach, J. (2016, June 3). Life expectancy is up sharply for blacks and Hispanics; whites are lagging. The Washington Post. Retrieved from https://www.washingtonpost.com/news/to-your-health/wp/2016/06/03/big-gains-for-black-hispanic-longevity-in-u-s-since-2000-white-gains-much-smaller/?noredirect=on

Arias, E. (2019). *Hispanic paradox, CDC National Center for Health Statistics report*. Retrieved from https://www.nytimes.com/2010/10/19/health/research/19aging.html

Batalova, J. B. J., & Alperin, E. (2018, August 1). *Immigrants in the U.S. with the fastest-growing foreign-born populations*. Retrieved from https://www.migrationpolicy.org/article/immigrants-us-states-fastest-growing-foreign-born-populations

Bertran, E. A., Pinelli, N. R., Masri, D. E., Sills, S. J., & Jaber, L. (2018). Self-disclosure among men and women of Arab descent: Implications for group-based health education. *American Journal of Educational Research, 6*(3), 196–200. doi:10.12691/education-6-3-6

Birkhead, A. C., & Kennedy, H. P., Callister, L. C., & Paredes Miyamoto, T. (2011). Navigating a new health culture: Experiences of immigrant Hispanic women. *Journal of Immigrant and Minority Health, 13*, 1168–1174. doi:10.1007/s10903-010-9369-x

Carteret, M. M. (2010, November 2). *Cultural differences in family dynamics*. Retrieved from https://www.dimensionsofculture.com/2010/11/culture-and-family-dynamics

Castillo, J. (2015). *At least 350 languages spoken in U.S. homes*. Retrieved from http://www.cnbc.com/2015/11/04/at-least-350-languages-spoken-in-us-homes-new-report.html

Center for Immigration Studies. (2012). *Profile of America's foreign-born populations; Table 5*. Retrieved from http://cis.org/2012-profile-of-americas-foreign-born-population#3

Chang, F. (2016). Legal classifications of immigrants. In F. Chang-Muy & E. Congress (Eds.), *Social work with immigrants and refugees: Legal issues, clinical skills, and advocacy* (2nd ed., pp. 43–66). New York, NY: Springer Publishing Company.

Chang, E., Choi, S., Kwon, I., Araiza, D., Moore, M., Trejo, L., & Sarkisian, C. (2018). Characterizing beliefs about stroke and walking for exercise among seniors from four racial/ethnic minority communities. *Journal of Cross-Cultural Gerontology, 33*, 387–410. doi:10.1007/s10823-018-9356-6

Chang-Muy, F., & Congress, E. (Eds.). (2016). *Social work with immigrants and refugees: Legal issues, clinical skills, and advocacy* (2nd ed.). New York, NY: Springer Publishing Company.

Congress, E. (2004). Cultural and ethnic issues in working with culturally diverse patients and their families: Use of the culturagram to promote cultural competency in health care settings. *Social Work in Health Care, 39*(3/4), 249–262. doi:10.1300/J010v39n03_03

Congress, E. (2013). Immigrants and health care. In R. Keefe (Ed.), *Handbook for public health social work* (pp. 103–121). New York, NY: Springer Publishing Company.

Congress, E. (2016). Introduction: Legal and social work issues with immigrants. In F. Chang-Muy & E. Congress (Eds.), *Social work with immigrants and refugees: Legal issues, clinical skills, and advocacy* (2nd ed., pp. 3–41). New York, NY: Springer Publishing Company.

Congress, E. (2017). Immigrants and refugees in cities: Issues, challenges, and interventions for social workers. *Urban Social Work, 1*(1), 20–35. doi:10.1891/2474-8684.1.1.20

Congress, E. (2018). Health for immigrants and refugees. In J. Heyman & E. Congress (Eds.), *Health and social work: Practice, policy and research* (pp. 235–250). New York, NY: Springer Publishing Company.

Congress, E., & Lyons, B. P. (1992). Cultural differences in health beliefs: Implications for social work practice in health care settings. *Social Work in Health Care, 17*(3), 81–96.

Consumer Health Beliefs. (2011, August 11). *Religious beliefs shape health care attitudes among U.S. Muslims*. Retrieved from https://www.uchicagomedicine.org/forefront/news/2011/august/religious-beliefs-shape-health-care-attitudes-among-us-muslims

Deol, H. (1970, January 1). *The lived experience of South Asian women with gestational diabetes mellitus*. Retrieved from https://open.library.ubc.ca/cIRcle/collections/ubctheses/24/items/1.0166607

Desai, N. R., Ross, J. S., Kwon, J. Y., Herrin, J., Dharmarajan, K., Bernheim, S. M., . . . Horwitz, L. I. (2016, December 27). *Association between hospital penalty status under the hospital readmission reduction program and readmission rates for target and nontarget conditions*. Retrieved from https://www.ncbi.nlm.nih.gov/pubmed/28027367

European Commission Joint Research Centre. (2018). Climate change promotes the spread of mosquito and tick-borne viruses. Retrieved from https://www.sciencedaily.com/releases/2018/03/180316111311.htm

Hall, H., McDavid, K., Ling, Q., & Sloggett, A. (2006). Determinants of progression to AIDS or death after HIV diagnosis, United States, 1996 to 2001. *Annals of Epidemiology, 16*(11), 824–833. doi:10.1016/j.annepidem.2006.01.009

Heyman, J., & Congress, E. P. (2018). *Health and social work: Practice, policy, and research*. New York, NY: Springer Publishing Company.

Ho, E. Y., Tran, H., & Chesla, C. A. (2015). Assessing the cultural in culturally sensitive printed patient-education materials for Chinese Americans with type 2 diabetes. *Health Communication, 30*(1), 39–49. doi:10.1080/10410236.2013.835216

Human Rights Watch. (2018, June 21). *U.S.: Poor medical care, deaths, in immigrant detention*. Retrieved from https://www.hrw.org/news/2018/06/20/us-poor-medical-care-deaths-immigrant-detention

Institute of Medicine (US) Committee on Understanding and Eliminating Racial and Ethnic Disparities in Health Care. (2003). *Unequal treatment: Confronting racial and ethnic disparities in health care.* Retrieved from https://www.ncbi.nlm.nih.gov/pubmed/25032386

Jin, L., & Acharya, L. (2016). Cultural beliefs underlying medication adherence in people of Chinese descent in the United States. *Health Communication, 31*(5), 513–521. doi:10.1080/10410236.2014.974121

Kennedy, S., Kidd, M., McDonald, J., & Biddle, N. (2015). The healthy immigrant effect: Patterns and evidence from four countries. *Journal of International Migration and Integration, 16*(2), 317–332. doi:10.1007/s12134-014-0340-x

Kochanek, K. D., Xu, J., Murphy, S. L., Minico, A. M., & Kung, H.-C. (2011). Deaths: Preliminary data for 2009. *National Vital Statistics Reports, 59,* 1–51.

Koya, D. L., & Egede, L. E. (2007). Association between length of residence and cardiovascular disease risk factors among an ethnically diverse group of United States immigrants. *Journal of General Internal Medicine, 22*(6), 841–846. doi:10.1007/s11606-007-0163-y

Krogstad, J., & Lopez, H. (2014). *Hispanic immigrants more likely to lack health insurance than U.S. born.* Retrieved from http://www.pewresearch.org/fact-tank/2014/09/26/higher-share-of-hispanic-immigrants-than-u-s-born-lack-health-insurance

Ku, L. (2006). *Why immigrants lack health care and health insurance.* Washington, DC: Migration Policy Institute. Retrieved from https://www.migrationpolicy.org/article/why-immigrants-lack-adequate-access-health-care-and-health-insurance

Livingston, G., Minushkim, S., & Cohn, D. (2008). *Hispanics and health care in the United States.* Washington, DC: Pew Research Center. Retrieved from https://www.pewresearch.org/hispanic/2008/08/13/hispanics-and-health-care-in-the-united-states-access-information-and-knowledge

Misra, A., & Ganda, O. (2007). Migration and its impact on adiposity and type 2 diabetes. *Nutrition, 23,* 696–708. doi:10.1016/j.nut.2007.06.008

National Center for Farmworker Health. (2016). *Women in the fields: Las Mujeres en los Campos.* Retrieved from http://www.ncfh.org/ncfh-blog/-women-in-the-fields-las-mujeres-en-los-campos

National Institutes of Health. (2013). *U.S. health in international perspective: Shorter lives, poorer health.* Retrieved from https://www.nap.edu/resource/13497/dbasse_080620.pdf

Office of Disease Prevention and Health Promotion. (2019). *Social determinants of health.* Retrieved from https://www.healthypeople.gov/2020/topics-objectives/topic/social-determinants-of-health

Passel, J., & Cohn, D. (2016). *Overall number of unauthorized immigrants holds steady since 2009.* Washington, DC: Pew Research Center. Retrieved from https://www.pewresearch.org/hispanic/2016/09/20/overall-number-of-u-s-unauthorized-immigrants-holds-steady-since-2009/

Radford, J., & Krogstad, J. M. (2019). *Recently arrived U.S. immigrants, growing in number, differ from long-term residents.* Retrieved from https://www.pewresearch.org/fact-tank/2019/06/03/recently-arrived-u-s-immigrants-growing-in-number-differ-from-long-term-residents/

Rosenblatt, R. A., & Hart, L. G. (2000). Physicians and rural America. *The Western Journal of Medicine, 173*(5), 348–351. doi:10.1136/ewjm.173.5.348

Ross, N., Timura, C., & Maupin, J. (2012). The case of curers, noncurers, and biomedical experts in Pichatara, Mexico. *Medical Anthropology Quarterly International Journal for the Analysis of Health, 26*(20), 159–181. Retrieved from https://anthrosource.onlinelibrary.wiley.com/doi/10.1111/j.1548-1387.2012.01199.x

Rothstein, W. G., & Rajapska, S. (2003). *Health beliefs of college students born in the United States, China, and India.* Retrieved from https://www.tandfonline.com/doi/abs/10.1080/07448480309596350

Sayegh, P., & Knight, B. G. (2013). Cross-cultural differences in dementia: The sociocultural health belief model. *International Psychogeriatrics, 25,* 1–14. doi:10.1017/S104161021200213X

Shaw, S., Armin, J., Torres, C. H., Orzech, K., & Vivian, J. (2012). Chronic disease self-management and health literacy in four ethnic groups. *Journal of Health Communication, 17*(S3), 67–81. doi:10.1080/10810730.2012.712623

Shear, M., & Yee, V. (2017, June 17). Dreamers to stay in U.S. for now, but their long-term fate is unclear. *The New York Times,* A17.

Stanek, M. (2014). *Promoting physical and behavioral health integration: Considerations for aligning federal and state policy.* National Academy for Promotion of State Health Policy. Retrieved from https://www.integration.samhsa.gov/news/Promoting_Integration.pdf

Stanhope, V., Heyman, J., Amaranate, J. C., & Doherty, M. (2018). Integrated behavioral health care. In J. Heyman & E. Congress (Eds.), *Health and social work: Practice, policy and research* (pp. 105–124), New York, NY: Springer Publishing Company.

U.S. Census Bureau. (2018, March 6). *Data.* Retrieved from https://www.census.gov/programs-surveys/cps/data-detail.html

Ward, E., Jemel, A., Cokkinides, V., Singh, G., Cardinez, C., Ghafoor, A., & Thun, M. (2008). Cancer disparities by race/ethnicity and socioeconomic status. *CA: A Cancer Journal for Clinicians, 54*(2), 67–118. doi:10.3322/canjclin.54.2.78

Wells, K., & Klap, R., Koike, A., & Sherbourne, C. (2001). Ethnic disparities in unmet need for alcoholism, drug abuse, and mental health care. *The American Journal of Psychiatry, 158*(12), 2027–2032. doi:10.1176/appi.ajp.158.12.2027

Xu, K. T., & Borders, T. (2008). Does being an immigrant make a difference in seeking physician services? *Journal of Health Care for the Poor and Underserved, 19*(2), 380–390. doi:10.1353/hpu.0.0001

# 18

# Spirituality and Culturally Diverse Families: The Intersection of Culture, Religion, and Spirituality

ZULEMA E. SUÁREZ AND EDITH A. LEWIS

## INTRODUCTION

Since the United States is the most religious and religiously diverse of Western nations (Fuller, 2001; Lugo, Stencel, Green, Smith, Cox, & Pond, 2008; Pew Research Center, 2015), and given the vast diversity within and between families nationally and worldwide, writing about religion and spirituality in culturally diverse families is daunting. Moreover, there has been a religious resurgence worldwide (Derezotes, 2009), and many of the immigrants coming to this country have diverse religious traditions and practices (Jasso, Massey, Rosenzweig, & Smith, 2003; Lugo et al., 2008; Pew Research Center, 2015) that counterbalance the secularization and religious alienation of predominantly White Americans. Hence, the increasing complexity of our society (Hess, Maton, & Pargament, 2014; Pargament, 2001) and emerging issues like religiously inspired terrorism and globalization require that social workers have knowledge of the cultural, spiritual, and religious dimensions of people's lives (Canda & Furman, 2010; Derezotes, 2009; Hodge, 2003). While it is unrealistic to write about such vast practices, cultural and religious worldviews, and religious and spiritual trends in the United States, how these vary according to intersecting social identities can inform and guide social work with families.

We begin by providing an overview of contemporary religious trends in the United States and how these vary according to age, sex, and socioeconomic status to show its increasing diversity and the shifts that are taking place in people's religious and spiritual identification. Following this demographic context, we examine the interrelation between ethnicity, religion, education, and religious and spiritual identification. To better understand some recent changes in the spiritual lives of Americans in the United States, we review the distinction between religion and spirituality; once used interchangeably, these terms have different meanings in today's world. From there, we explore religious and cultural worldviews, their interrelationship, and how these influence our feelings and behaviors. Finally, we discuss implications for practice with ethnically diverse families and communities and provide a case example.

Before proceeding, bear in mind an important caveat while reading this chapter: We are only providing a high level overview of religions in the United States since we are lumping several denominations under umbrella terms; yet, religions often encompass different movements that result in vast differences within and between denominations. For example, Christianity consists of four groups: Evangelical, Catholic, Mainline Protestant, and Orthodox (Lugo et al., 2008; Pew Research Center, 2015), Judaism consists of four (Orthodox, Conservative, Secular Humanist, and Reformed), and Islam consists of Sunni, Shia, and other groups.

## RELIGIOUS TRENDS IN THE UNITED STATES

Although U.S. American adults are "far more religious" than those in other wealthy Western countries, and the United States has more Christians than any other country in the world, with seven of ten identifying with this faith tradition, contemporary religious and spiritual trends reveal a changing and increasingly diverse and complex society. According to a Pew survey , America's Changing Landscape (2015, the overall number of people who identify as Christian is declining (from 78.4% in 2007 to 70.6% in 2014), a trend observed across age groups, race, and ethnicity (whites, blacks, and LatinXs), across educational levels, and across males and females. This decrease in identification with an organized religion coincides with an increase in the number of people identifying as spiritual but are not affiliated with a religion (from 16.1% to 22.8%), also known as "spiritual but not religious," as unaffiliated, or "Nones" (Barna, 2017; Fuller, 2001; Lugo et al., 2008; Pew Research Center, 2015).

A survey by Barna (2017) takes a closer look at this growing segment of the population, including a subgroup they identify as those who "Love Jesus but Not the Church," which make up one-tenth of the population and is growing (up from 7% in 2004). According to the study, this group is mostly female (61%), and four-fifths (80%) are between the ages of 33 and 70; they are mostly Gen-Xers (36%) and Boomers (44%), not Millennials (14%) or Elders (6%). Because older adults are the most likely to attend church regularly, they are underrepresented in this group, and Millennials are most likely to be unchurched and the least likely to either identify as Christian or to claim faith as very important to their life. The percentage of Americans who are religiously unaffiliated (spiritual-but-not religious, self-described atheists, agnostics or "nothing in particular") increased by more than six points, from 16.1% to 22.8%. It should be noted that the unaffiliated are almost parallel in size with Evangelical Christians, who are holding steady at (25.4%). However, this difference could be due to measurement error.

Another phenomenon taking place in the United States is the increase of mixed religion marriages (Lugo et al., 2008; Pew Research Center, 2015). Almost 39% of people who married since 2010 were in mixed religion households, compared with 19% in 1960, which may be due to the growth of the unaffiliated population. Approximately one-in-five of survey participants are either unaffiliated and married a Christian spouse or vice versa. Finally, Americans who identify with non-Christian faiths also has gradually risen from 4.7% in 2007 to 5.9% in 2014, especially among Muslims and Hindus; even though these groups are small to begin with, this may also account for intermarriage rates.

In this section, we saw that although the United States is an overwhelmingly Christian country, this is quickly changing due to an increase in the number of people with no religious identification and a smaller increase in non-Christian groups. However, while traditional, or mainline, Christian churches are losing membership, the Evangelical movement has stayed constant and those without religious affiliation ("Nones") are increasing (Pew Research Center, 2015). Given these changes, it may not be surprising that the rate of mixed religion couples has increased. Next, we look at the relationships between race, ethnicity, education, and religious identification.

## RACE, ETHNICITY, AGE, GENDER, AND RELIGIOUS IDENTIFICATION

Although the role of race and ethnicity has been key in the establishment of religions and/or denominations in this country (e.g., the Puritans, the African Methodist Episcopal (AME) church, Mormons, the Amish), social scientists often confused the external status of race with the internal or self-ascribed status of ethnicity. We make this distinction clear at the outset, as the literature on this topic is better understood within the context of the definitions of race and ethnicity used by researchers.

There is a strong interconnection between race, ethnicity, and religious affiliation (Canda & Furman, 2010; Kim, 2011; Pew Research Center, 2015). For example, there are close associations between ethnicity and religious beliefs in groups like the Amish, Mormons, Jews, American Hindus, and Buddhists (Pew Research Center, 2015). Because of the close link between culture and religion, these groups may intentionally or unconsciously maintain a boundary between themselves and outsiders. According to Kim, theorists agree that since ethnicity and religion provide people with meaning, identity, and community, congregations that combine both ethnicity and religion "have a stronger basis for meaning construction and cohesion" (p. 10). So, notwithstanding overt racism and ethnocentrism, people self-select into more homogenous congregations, especially if they are immigrants or have a strong ethnic identity (Pew Research Center, 2015). This explains, according to social scientists and theologians, persistent segregation by religion that renders Sunday morning service—the most segregated hour in the United States (Kim, 2011; Kosmin & Keysar, 2008).

Given the interrelationship between race and religion, it is not surprising that several denominations traditionally embraced in the United States are predominantly White (Pew Research Center, 2015). According to the National Congregations Study (Chaves & Anderson, 2014), about eight in ten U.S. congregants still attend services at congregations that are at least 80% racially or ethnically homogeneous. However, this trend is also changing, as one out of five congregants in the survey were worshiping in congregations without a racial or ethnic dominant group. As the number of primarily White Christians flee to the "unaffiliated" group, denominations have become more racially and ethnically diverse, especially with the constant influx of immigrants (Pew Research Center, 2015). The weakening relationship between ethnicity and religion is especially evident among LatinXs whose presence has grown in evangelical Protestant, mainline Protestant, and Catholic religions (about a third are Catholic). As a result of these changes, 41% of Catholics (up from 35% in 2007), 24% of evangelical Protestants (up from 19%), and 14% of mainline Protestants (up from 9%) are racial and ethnic minorities (Pew Research Center, 2015).

Despite the prominence of race and ethnicity, other variables impact what researchers call "the changing religious landscape" of the United States. Young adults (18–39 years old) throughout the world are considerably less likely than older adults to identify with a religion, to engage in religious practices, and are more likely to be atheists, which has contributed to the "graying" and diminution of mainline congregations (Pew Research Center, 2018a). In the global survey by the Pew Foundation (2018a), only in two countries (Chad and Ghana) were young adults more likely to identify with a religious group.

Scholars have three theories that may explain this change (Pew Research Center, 2018). One theory is that as societies develop economically and young adults collectively worry less about daily survival, and tragic events become fewer, they have less need for religion; and, since education is linked to economic development, this may contribute to decreased religiosity. Finally, according to another theory, religious commitment varies according to life stage. Although young adults may start out as less religious than people who are older adults, they tend to become more religious as they become parents and begin to face their own mortality.

Finally, gender also characterizes the affiliated and non-affiliated (Pew Research Center, 2015). Women are more likely to affiliate with a religion than men. Since the last PEW Survey in 2007, more than half of nearly all Christian denominations are women. Specifically, about 75% of Jehovah's Witnesses are women, as are 59% of historically black Protestant congregants, over half (55%) of evangelical and mainline Protestant traditions, and 54% of Catholics and Mormons are also women.

On the other hand, men comprise most of the religiously unaffiliated group. Seventy-five percent of self-identified atheists are men, as are 62% of agnostics and 55% of those who identify their religion as "nothing in particular" and find religion as unimportant. Those who do not have a particular religion but say religion is at least somewhat important to them, however, are about equally women and men.

In this section, we saw that the relationships between race, ethnicity, and religion is so strong that, despite advances made in the Civil Rights Movement, churches in the United States are still primarily segregated. This relationship, however, is beginning to weaken. We also looked at the relationship between age, gender, and religious affiliation. As a result of societal changes, church participants are older while the "Nones" or unaffiliated are younger. Women are more likely to be affiliated while men are more likely to be atheists, agnostics, or unaffiliated.

## Religious Inclusion and Exclusion of LGBT

The attitudes and policies toward LGBT individuals varies across religious groups according sexual identification. According to The National Congregations Survey, between 2006 and 2012 (Chaves & Anderson, 2014), the percentage of congregations embracing openly gay or lesbian couples as full-fledged members increased from 37% to 48%; further, congregations were more likely (18% in 2006 vs. 26% in 2012) to allow openly gay and lesbian members as congregational leaders (Pew Research Center, 2015).

People who are transgender, however, are generally less accepted than people with other socially marginalized sexual identities, and the reception from religious groups has been mixed (Smith, 2017). In the United States, some denominations, like Reform Judaism, the United Church of Christ, Unitarian Universalist and Episcopal churches, have adopted official statements of full inclusion in the life of the church, including service as ordained ministers, while the Evangelical Lutheran Church in America (ELCA), Presbyterian Church (USA), and United Methodist Church have inclusion but do not have an official statement. Denominations with a mixed position include African Methodist Episcopal Church, Church of God (Cleveland, Tennessee), Presbyterian Church in America, and Roman Catholic Church. Finally, the Assemblies of God, Church of Jesus Christ of Latter Day Saints, The Lutheran Church Missouri Synod, and the Southern Baptist Convention have stated barriers to inclusion.

The mixed reception of LGBT people may explain why, according to the 2014 Pew Research Center survey (Pew Research Center, 2015; Schwadel & Sandstorm, 2019), LGBT adults are less religious than the general public in the United States; 41% identify as atheist, agnostic, or "nothing in particular" as compared to 22% of their straight adult counterparts (Schwadel & Sandstorm, 2019). According to LGBT Americans who responded to the Pew survey (Sandstorm, 2015), particular religious institutions, especially Islam (84%), the Mormon church (83%), the Catholic Church (79%), and evangelical churches (73%) are unreceptive of people like them. Their perception of the Jewish religion and mainline Protestant churches were mixed; while 47% and 44% of LGBT adults, respectively, perceived those religions as unfriendly, 10% described each of them as friendly while the remainder were neutral.

In this section, we see that LGBT groups have received a mixed reception from religious denominations—while few are open and welcoming, others may condemn them and bar them from full participation in the life of the church. This rejection or mixed reception of sexually marginalized communities may explain why LGBT individuals are less likely to be religious than their counterparts in the general population.

## Where Americans Find Meaning

Whether Americans find meaning in faith and religion varies according to socioeconomic class and religious identification. In two studies (one qualitative or open-ended and a survey) conducted by the Pew Foundation, Americans shared their sources of meaning (Pew Research Center, 2018b). Seven out of 10 respondents across demographic groups cited family as the most popular source of meaning and fulfillment when asked an open-ended question. However, people who were married were more likely to feel this way than unmarried people. Also, Americans with higher income and education were more likely to report friendship, good health, stability, and travel as sources of meaning and satisfaction.

Evangelical Christians were more likely to find meaning in faith than atheists, who found activities and finances as their primary sources of meaning. Historically Black Protestants, mainline Protestants, and Catholics also found meaning in faith but less so than evangelicals. It should be noted that atheists have higher levels of education, which correlates with money and activities over faith. Finally, people who are more politically conservative are more likely to identify religion as a source of life meaning than liberals who were more likely to find meaning in the arts and social and political causes. In sum, how and where people derive meaning in their lives varies according to religious, socioeconomic, and political identities.

## SPIRITUALITY VERSUS RELIGION

Although before the 20th century, the terms religious and spiritual were often interchangeable, they have assumed distinct meanings in contemporary society where modern intellectual and cultural forces have accentuated the difference between "private" and "public life" (Barna, 2017; Fuller, 2001). Moreover, the advent of scientific and biblical scholarship, and cultural relativism has challenged educated U.S. residents' blind loyalty to the traditions of established religious institutions, causing them to question existing orthodoxies (Borg, 2004; Fuller, 2001).

Since spirituality is difficult to define (Bergin & Richards, 2005; Canda & Furman, 2010), a composite of different definitions provides a working understanding of the concept. According to Canda and Furman (2010), "Spirituality refers to the fundamental aspects of what it is to be human—to search for a sense of meaning, purpose, and moral frameworks for relating with self, others, and the ultimate reality" (p. 37). Richards and Bergin (1997, p. 13) define spirituality as "those experiences, beliefs, and phenomena that pertain to the transcendent and existential aspects of life (i.e., God or a Higher Power, the purpose and meaning of life, suffering, good and evil, death, etc.)." Although spirituality may be expressed through religion or independently, today many associate spirituality with "private" or personal belief systems and religion with the public realm of institutional membership, participation in formal rituals, and adherence to official denomination doctrine. On the other hand, in recent years, the proliferation of global meditation events for world harmony challenges the assumption that spirituality is strictly a personal affair (Williams, 2004).

Richard and Bergin (1997) view religion as a subset of spirituality, suggesting:

> Religious expressions tend to be denominational, external, cognitive, behavioral, ritualistic, and public. Spiritual experiences tend to be universal, ecumenical, internal, affective, spontaneous, and private. It is possible to be religious without being spiritual and spiritual without being religious. (p. 13)

Although religion has to do with theistic beliefs, practices, and feelings often expressed institutionally, denominationally, and personally, this is not always the case. Research shows that many people attempt to integrate elements of religion and spirituality; people who identify as religious have a higher interest in church participation and commitment to orthodox beliefs (Barna, 2017; Fuller, 2001).

Hence, although the terms spiritual and religious are interrelated, they are different. Indeed, research shows that whether a person gravitates toward "subjective spirituality" as opposed to "tradition-oriented religiousness" is related to different personality dispositions (Saucier & Skrzypińska, 2006).

## SPIRITUAL, BUT NOT RELIGIOUS

This group consists of people who hold official membership in a church but attend sporadically and those who do not belong to a church but attend on special occasions and holidays. Finally, the third group is concerned with spiritual issues but choose not to practice within the context of organized religion. For example, a person may pray and read the Bible, living life according to their understanding of scripture, but not to belong to a religious institution. When viewed in total, this group is the fastest growing in this country (Lugo et al., 2008).

While the majority of research disaggregates religious affiliation, there may be a fourth relationship between religiosity and spirituality. For more than 50 years, there have been groups of individuals who have formed institutions in which aspects of multiple faith traditions are practiced simultaneously (Fetsch, 2014). These "interfaith" groups have developed a body of thought linking religious and spiritual ideals as practiced by multiple religions. Over the last two decades, they have developed formal scholarly training leading to recognized certifications, for example, as ordained Interfaith Ministers. Along with this formal training, these groups have developed and been successful in disseminating magazines and books for audiences in several countries, including the United States. Traditional Native American religious practices might also be included in these numbers. Although they differ in terms of practices, beliefs, and practitioners, these religious practices have been instrumental in the development of other religious theories such as creation or feminist theologies.

### Worldview and Values

Whether one chooses to express one's spirituality intrinsically or extrinsically, through organized religion, the cultural life of all societies is shaped and directed by worldviews—beliefs about the universe and the nature of reality that provide answers about the meaning of life and about the most daunting questions about the human condition (Richards & Bergin, 1997, p. 51). Whether or not we are aware of our worldviews, they influence our behavior, our conceptions of nature, of our place in the world, and our interpersonal relationships. Worldviews also include affective-cognitive elements that are inextricably bound and vary on a continuum from explicit to implicit (Papajohn & Spiegel, 1975). Indeed, in many societies, members do not always draw a clear line between their culture and way of life and Western researchers' concept of religion. For example, although some Koreans may be Christian, culturally, their family lives are often influenced by Confucianism (Kim, 1997; Kim & Ryu, 2005). Hence, to understand families culturally and spiritually, awareness of the existence of diverse worldviews is essential. Although cultural and spiritual-religious worldviews are interrelated, anthropologists and social scientists have approached these separately (see Bergin & Richards, 2005).

## RELIGIOUS WORLDVIEWS

According to Dilthey (as cited in Bergin & Richards, 2005), although there are a variety of religious belief systems in the world, these can be subsumed into fewer than three major types in their existential and metaphysical questions. Following, we briefly summarize naturalism, idealism of freedom, and objective idealism.

Naturalism posits reality as a physical system accessible only through the five senses. The "good life" is the pursuit of happiness and power, and the idea of mechanistic determinism tends to override freedom of will. Rationalism, positivism, existentialism, Marxism, and secular humanism are provided as examples of this worldview. The United States, as a secular industrialized country that has placed its faith in science and technology, adheres to a naturalist view. However, given the overwhelming number of Christians in this country, and the influence of religious worldviews in our public debates, it becomes questionable whether we are a Christian rather than a secular society. Despite the separation of church and state in the United States, the motto "In God We Trust" is printed on all its currency. Positivism (i.e., if it cannot be seen or measured, it does not exist) may explain the reverence in our society and universities for science and empirical research that validate our physical reality. Others argue that every experience in the world cannot be accessed through the five senses and that there is an "inner life" for all matter (Guadalupe & Lum, 2005; Zukav, 1999). Each of these experiences evinces the diversity in this worldview.

The Kantian notion of idealism of freedom takes a subjective view of reality in which human beings have free will, and is grounded in a transcendental spiritual realm (Allison, 1996). The "good life" is defined as obedience to conscience or divine will and upholds moral freedom. As Mahatma Gandhi and Rev. Dr. Martin Luther King Jr. demonstrated with their practice of *satyagraha* (nonviolence), people facing injustice can either respond in kind, or exercise their moral freedom by choosing to love their enemies to bring about the change they sought (McGreal, 1995). Western, or monotheistic, world religions like Judaism, Christianity, Islam, Zoroastrianism, and Sikhism exemplify this worldview.

Finally, objective idealism avoids the dualism in idealism of freedom by proclaiming the unity and divinity of all that is and uniting determinism and indeterminism (Almeder, 1980). In this worldview, dichotomies in thinking (black or white, we are either dead or alive) are absent. Things are not seen as opposites of each other but as part of a whole that encompasses reality. For example, in this belief system, we cannot understand white without understanding black and how they interact with each other, nor can we know life without knowing death, as exemplified by the popular Yin and Yang symbol. Eastern religions, such as Buddhism, Hinduism, Jainism, Shintoism, Confucianism, and Taoism are examples of this worldview.

The ability of religions and people to recognize the similarities they have with one another is only possible when the "other's" divinity can be recognized (Derezotes, 2009). Although according to Dilthey (cited in Bergin & Richards, 2010), naturalism, idealism of freedom, and objective idealism have traditionally rivaled each other in providing alternative answers to the major questions of life, many people combine elements of these three types to form their own unique worldview that draws upon and transcends the prevailing view of the major religions.

## CULTURAL WORLDVIEWS

As spirituality is concerned with finding the meaning and purpose of life, the suffering that befalls us, and moral and interpersonal frameworks for relating to others, cultural value systems also include moral standards and mores for living, as well as motivation and patterns of interpersonal behavior (Guadalupe & Lum, 2005; Papajohn & Spiegel, 1975). Cultural anthropologists and social psychologists have synthesized the variations in existential judgments and systems of belief, such as those found in various religious orientations, philosophies, and science with other cultural patterns to give us a better understanding of unique and universal cultural patterns (Chatters, Taylor, Jackson, & Lincoln, 2008; Cohen & Hill, 2007; Mattis et al., 2001). Although the generalizations based on observations of one culture cannot be universally applied, some scholars argue that there is a fundamental universality to human problems, and societies have found similar answers for some of these existential challenges (Guadalupe & Lum, 2005; Papajohn & Spiegel, 1975).

Building on the work of Kluckhohn and Strodbeck (1961), Papajohn and Spiegel (1975) present a classification for understanding people's worldviews across cultures. This model of value orientations has three underlying assumptions. First, the number of existential problems to which all people must find solutions is finite since we all must die, and live in families and communities, no matter what our ethnic and racial backgrounds are. Second, although there is variability in people's responses to these problems, there is a limited, non-random range of possible solutions. For example, since death is universal, we all must grieve. How that happens may be different within and between ethnic groups. This was evident when one of the authors ran an immediate loss group for Dominican women. Whereas people from rural areas included the community in their mourning rituals, the urban women in the group were more private and resented opening their homes for community members to mourn with them. Third, although there will be a dominant profile of value orientations composed of the most highly valued orientations, there will also be variant orientations that are universal. Hence, although as noted earlier, the naturalist worldview is dominant in Western countries like the United States, numerous values may also permeate our personal and public lives. Social workers must be aware of these constructions of spirituality and religiosity, both for themselves as well as those with whom they are engaged in services (Guadalupe & Lum, 2005).

According to Papajohn and Spiegel's model, four major problems have challenged people across places and times. What is the modality of activity (activity orientation)? What is the relationship of humans to nature (human nature orientation)? What is the modality of human relationships (relational orientation)? What is the relationship of humans to nature (human nature orientation)? The responses to these questions are complex and reflect all the value orientations simultaneously. Hence, the authors caution the reader from literally interpreting these tendencies. For the sake of definition, however, we examine these orientations separately.

The activity orientation question refers to humans' mode of self-expression in activity and includes at least three possibilities: being, being-in-becoming, and doing. Cultures with a being orientation prefer spontaneous expression of impulses and desires. This does not mean, however, that people are not censored from acting on aggressive or negative impulses since all societies have a moral code, although these may vary. People with this orientation tend to live in the present instead of planning or anticipating the future. Being present requires attention to the overt and covert experiences of the current moment or situation. The focus of activity is not development, but the "is-ness" of the personality and the spontaneous expression of the "is-ness." For example, a person with this orientation may be late to a class if they bump into a friend they have not seen in a while along the way, since the chance of encounter may override the planned event. This is not to say that the person does not value the planned activity; however, the person is just being spontaneous. Some non-Western societies such as India or Latin American countries are considered to have a dominant "being" orientation. Thich Nhat Hanh's body of work on mindfulness is an example of a "being" orientation.

Although the being-in-becoming, like the being orientation, is concerned with what the human being is instead of what they can accomplish, the idea of development is paramount. Hence, within the being-in-becoming orientation, activity strives to develop a more integrated and whole personality. People who identify as "spiritual but not religious" view spirituality as a journey of spiritual growth and development (Fuller, 2001). Hence, they will read extensively and will attend workshops and retreats that will enhance their growth. While secular in its orientation and not affiliated with a religious or spiritual tradition, Byron Katies's work of "Loving What Is" contains strategies consistent with a being-in-becoming orientation.

The doing preference characterizes American society, according to Papajohn and Spiegel (1975). This orientation stresses activity that is goal-oriented and leads to measurable accomplishments. The more we do, the more we will achieve. This is important because an individual's worth in this society is determined primarily on their past and future accomplishments more so than by their virtues. Consistent with the naturalist value for measuring, degrees and stock portfolios gain significance over kindness and compassion, the abstract concepts that cannot easily be quantified. Hence, for the most part, the pursuit of money and status is revered above personal and spiritual development. This value is in contrast to Confucianism (objective idealism worldview) that holds that inner virtue and proper conduct is the path to personal and social harmony (Bergin & Richards, 2005).

The second human problem, according to this conceptual framework, addresses interpersonal relationships (Papajohn & Spiegel, 1975). This orientation also has three subdivisions: lineal, collateral, and individualistic. Although all societies pay attention to all three principles in relationships, it is a matter of emphasis. In Shintoism, as an example of a lineal and objective idealism worldview, "loyalty and fulfilling one's duty to family, ancestors, and traditions are important" (Richards & Bergin, 1997, p. 70).

Collateral relationship patterns consist of a network of horizontal extended relationships consisting of large family systems that include blood and fictive kin since humans do not stand alone, but are part of a web (Papajohn & Spiegel, 1975). Therefore, children are trained to depend on the family network and to be obedient. Family loyalty is exchanged for caretaking throughout the person's life. Latin American families tend to nurture collateral relationships.

Individualism is a dominant U.S. middle-class value (Papajohn & Spiegel, 1975). From early on, children are raised to be independent and to exercise self-control. They are also trained to experience separation from the family as normal by, for example, going to day care and summer camp (Papajohn & Spiegel, 1975). Under this value orientation, adults make decisions based on their individual self-interest as opposed to considering the needs of the extended family network. This value is consistent with a naturalist worldview.

Of interest in the present economic period, however, is the extent to which this individualistic worldview can survive. With the number of economic blows facing formerly middle income families, adult children moving back to their parents' homes, and the rise of a young adult population, sociologists refer to as "emerging adulthood" (Arnett, 2004; Burn & Szoeke, 2016; Tanner & Arnett, 2016), and the numbers of health disparities leaving grandparents raising their grandchildren (Hayslip Jr., Fruhauf, & Dolbin-MacNab, 2017), rugged individualism may be waning. The number of religious organizations now engaged in providing food and shelter, the use of small and large groups to identify methods of support to the unemployed workers with families, and the incorporation of worldwide "days of prayer" or "global meditations" may represent a shift in the persistent idealism of individuality in the country.

Three preferences characterize human beings' place in time, the third existential problem. All societies deal with a past, present, and future, but they vary greatly according to which dimension they make dominant. Earlier, we said that cultures with a being orientation value spontaneity and living in the present. Since values and religious worldviews are interrelated, this time orientation is also evident in religious thought. For example, most North American Christians, according to Marcus Borg (2004), a Lutheran theologian, "see[s] the Christian life as centered in believing now for the sake of salvation later—believing in God, the Bible, and Jesus as a way to heaven" (p. xiii); "[a]n emerging paradigm with God that transforms life in the present" (p. 15). Hence, rewards come from being in relationship with God in the present, not from the afterlife (the future). As a relatively young country, the United States emphasizes a future orientation that will bring bigger and better things.

The fourth human problem is human being's relationship with nature. The three-point range in this orientation is subjugation-to-nature, harmony-with-nature, and mastery-over-nature. Eurocentric scholars with a doing orientation often misinterpret the subjugation-to-nature orientation to mean that people who adhere to this orientation are fatalistic about climate changes, illness, and death—implying passivity before the forces of nature and giving up without a fight. Our interpretation is different. We see subjugation-to-nature orientation as knowing when to surrender to forces greater than we are when things are beyond our control. In Taoism, this is known as we-wei—principle of passive action meaning that one should not resist, confront, or defy (Bergin & Richards, 2005). Ironically, in the U.S. culture, we try to outwit nature via medical technology and meteorology and we have allowed the medical community to medicalize natural changes in our bodies, such as menopause, aging, and dying. The hospice movement is a response to this medicalization, as are strategies of healing that integrate holistic methods with Western medicine.

The harmony-with-nature orientation does not separate humans from nature as they both are seen as being part of the same whole (objective idealism). This orientation is more characteristic of Eastern, many African, South or Central American countries, and of Native American people who see humans as being one with the natural environment. For example, Native American shamans see the Earth as a living organism, a belief common among many tribes, and encourage their clients' connections to natural forces (Krippner & Welch, 1992: Schwartz, 2015). The Asian religion, Shintoism, views spirituality "as feelings of appreciation and closeness to nature and enjoyment of life" (Bergin & Richards, 2005, p. 70). To Native Americans and women who practice women's spirituality, the Earth Mother is sacred and should not be exploited or pillaged (Spretnak, 1982; Starhawk, 1990). Jains follow the principle of *ahimsa* (non-violence) and apply this to all humans, animals, and plants. This knowledge may help us to better understand why Julia Butterfly Hill lived in a giant redwood tree named Luna for 2 years to protect it from the ax and to raise consciousness about saving these magnificent trees (Fitzgerald, 2002).

Mastery-over-nature, a third way of conceptualizing this relationship, is consistent with a naturalist worldview. According to this view, human beings can overcome and exploit natural forces, confident that the resources used can be replenished, or that alternatives for them can be discovered and utilized. This orientation is dominant in industrialized countries like the United States and is evinced by our destruction and exploitation of the natural environment for material and scientific gains. Since as a country, we do not share a harmony-with-nature view, we will cut down forests to build housing developments and shopping malls, and ignore climate changes due to pollutants, as well as defiling grounds that are sacred to people who have a harmony-with-nature orientation.

The fifth common human problem deals with innate human nature. Are human beings evil (neutral or a mixture of both)? Whether these are changeable or unchangeable increases this threshold classification to six possibilities. Human beings can be considered evil and unalterable or evil but redeemable. According to Bergin and Richards (2005), many Christians see humans as being evil because of the fall of Adam and Eve, but as alterable through God's grace. Hindus see humans as being divine, while Shintoism sees them as inherently good and unalterable. This may explain why Hinduism does not provide a binding moral code for its followers. Other societies see humans as being good and corruptible since they have free will (some Christians, some Muslims, Sikhs, and followers of Zoroastrianism, to name a few). Others view humans as an unalterable mixture of good and evil. Since religions, for the most part, provide a way out of our state of suffering and imperfection, this may be a secular value. Finally, some hold that humans are a mixture of both good and evil but this is subject to influence. In other words, we are a mixture of light (good) and darkness (innocent misunderstanding, or evil). According to Pema Chödrön (see Chödrön, 2010), a Western Buddhist monk, the Buddha taught that:

> There is a kind of innocent misunderstanding that we all share, something that can be turned around, corrected, and seen through, as if we were in a dark room and someone showed us where the light switch was. It isn't sin that we are in a dark room. (1991, p. 13)

In the preceding section, we examined the importance of religious and cultural worldviews in human behavior. Although people do not generally distinguish between their way of life and their worldviews, awareness and knowledge of these can help us contextualize the feelings and behaviors of people who are different from us.

As seen in this chapter, spirituality and religiosity are sufficiently complex topics for professionals working in social services. These complexities are amplified when one considers the role of other social group memberships such as ethnicity, race, economic class, gender expression/identity, and or physical and mental abilities. Recognizing and integrating the intersections of these various social group memberships may often determine the effectiveness of our interventions. The following case study serves as an illustration of how to work intersectionally with persons for whom religion and or spirituality are an issue.

## CASE STUDY

### Finding, Losing, and Regaining a Spiritual Home

Imani was born into a very religious middle class Protestant family of Ghanaian descent. Her parents held leadership positions in her church and, from the time she entered preschool, she was given religious texts to memorize and speeches highlighting various religious holidays to recite. She was active in her parents' religious organization, observed all of the rituals and traditions it utilized, and was a member of several youth groups. Because she was a woman, she could not hope to become a minister in the religious body because women were predetermined to hold subordinate places in the denomination. She could, however, sing in the various choirs and was known for her ability to interpret the meanings of sacred songs.

Among Imani's earliest childhood memories, however, was a feeling that she was not comfortable with the dresses, ribbons and lace she was forced to wear. When she expressed disdain for being a female, she was regaled with religious texts about the ways women and men were separate beings with distinct roles and life responsibilities. By the time she was 12, Imani knew that to discuss her feelings with her parents was a precursor to punishment so she entered into a silence that would last for 8 years.

By age 18, Imani could no longer ignore the feeling that she had been born into the wrong body and was, in fact, male. By then, Imani had entered college, and sought out courses in human sexuality. Attending a predominantly religious college, however, made access to these resources limited, and Imani decided to drop out of college, a decision that her parents vehemently disapproved. As a result, they refused to acknowledge or interact with Imani. This type of extrusion is not uncommon among families of adolescents who are G/L/B/T or questioning. Imani was not only cut off from family members but also from her religious congregation. She felt lost without her supports and was unsure where else to turn.

At her job, Imani met an older coworker who was also a PFlag member. Over time, their friendship gave Imani an adult role model with whom she could share her struggles with being forced to live out a female gender identity. Gifty, the coworker, sensing an opportunity to support Imani, introduced Imani to members of the PFlag community, who, in turn, introduced Imani to other young people who had similar experiences. Hearing their stories and receiving their support helped Imani to feel validated and able to want to take a proactive approach to being both a person of color and a transgender person. Imani embraced and explored this latter term, which brought her a great deal of comfort and well-being.

Imani was referred to an agency specializing in services to G/L/B/T/I youth and worked with them during the next eight months. Programmatic services included individualized and group therapy, health maintenance and referrals, and social gathering. Over time, Imani declared a name change to Tunde and began living as a man. For all of its comprehensive services, the organization did not, however, address Tunde's feelings of loss about their desire for a spiritual life. Tunde had come to an understanding that the gender identity change had not cut Tunde off from being loved and cared for by God. Tunde, moreover, missed singing and giving thanks in a corporate setting for the blessings experienced during in life.

Luckily, Tunde had a social worker who was able to introduce Tunde to two spiritual communities in the city. The first was a waystation for young people who had been persecuted by family, friends, and communities for their gender identify and/or expression. With this group, Tunde learned to release the sadness and embraced the joyfulness of being reunited with spirituality and religion. Through that waystation, Tunde was taken to an interfaith community, in which Tunde found their real home. People from many ethnic, racial, gender identities, and religious backgrounds attended the services. It was not unusual to find rituals from many traditions, all woven together and examined from a belief in how God or Creation is based on love. A typical service might begin with the blowing of a sheep's horn, followed by music and a guided meditation. Someone from the community would offer a set of reflections and those in attendance could participate in a brief period in each service about the main points gleaned from the reflections. Tunde joined a choir and soon became proficient in singing songs in many languages from many traditions.

When Tunde began the sexual reassignment surgical process, these two spiritual communities became Tunde's family and support network. They were the representatives to Tunde's multidisciplinary team overseeing the surgeries and Tunde's mental health. While Tunde's parents never accepted the change, other family members did, and Tunde's biological and fictive kin networks combined to become a large supportive extended family.

## CONCLUSION

In this chapter, we highlight intersectionalities to consider when acknowledging the role of spiritual or religious traditions in the lives of families. Using Papajohn and Spiegel's (1975) conceptual framework and religion surveys (Barna, 2017; Pew Research Center, 2015), we have identified the following "lessons" of importance for this work.

There are as many intrareligious differences as there are interreligious differences. Given the large number of Christian denominations, Jewish, and Muslim, not to mention other less well-known traditions in the United States, we cannot make assumptions about the religious beliefs or practices of clients. Instead we must think of combinations and permutation of religiosity and spirituality (Canda & Furman, 2010). For example, among Christians, Lutherans may belong to the Missouri Synod, Wisconsin Synod, or Evangelical Lutheran Church in American (ELCA). The differences among these groups are so vast that the Wisconsin and Missouri Synods do not welcome ELCA Lutherans to the communion table, while the ELCA and the Episcopal Church of the United States have formed an alliance to recognize and share the sacraments with one another. Therefore, we need to learn from clients about their Christian affiliation and/or any other traditions and interfaith practices due to mixed marriages or the syncretization of different traditions, and be cautious about not imposing our understanding of the requirements of orthodox traditions on our clients, even with those who are nominally in the same religion as we are. One way to accomplish this is to directly engage others at the time of intake or initial discussions with an exploration of their belief systems and how these influence their lives and decision-making processes.

Workers can engage the number of people who are disenfranchised from organized religion to explore the beliefs of people who are spiritual but do not affiliate to one particular religion or are atheists and agnostics by exploring what gives them meaning in life. For example, although they may not find comfort in God, they may do so in Nature, and this can be integrated into any treatment plan.

Given the changing "religious landscape in the United States, we need to bear in mind that just because a client does not indicate a religious preference on an intake form, it does not mean the individual is not spiritual, perhaps having an orientation like the "spiritual but not religious," or adhering to at least one major religious category such as Christian, combined with other traditions such as Buddhism or Jainism (Canda & Furman, 2010; Fetsch, 2014; Freedman, 2009). Since multiple orientations would not be represented in a standard agency intake form, social workers should ask the people they work with about their spiritual tradition or choice to refrain from engagement with spiritual or religious practices.

Although the United States is still numerically Christian from primarily Protestant and Catholic denominations, the number of non-Christians and those who do not identify with a religion is rapidly growing. Given current anti-Muslim sentiment, and that most Evangelicals are disproportionately drawn from minority groups (Pew Research Center, 2015), like women and the poor, and others who have been denied power, we must attend to issues of religious freedom and social justice (Canda & Furman, 2010; Hodge, 2003). We need to be clear about the ways in which religious freedom (including the freedom to not affiliate with a particular tradition) and social justice issues are being ignored in our public social lives, and how as social workers we may be contributing to the oppression of these groups, as for example, the case of people who are transgender or LGB. Of utmost importance is to understand the ways in which our own subjective and objective orientations about spirituality and religiosity influence our lives.

We must also bring forth into the public limelight the needs of religious minorities, highlighting the strengths of their different traditions. For example, in many parts of the country, it is not uncommon to see Muslim workers bring their prayer mats to the workplace, find a quiet place in the building, and do their daily prayers. In cities like Detroit, Michigan, the presence of large numbers of Muslims have influenced change so that their religious needs are being recognized and positively addressed. It is now not uncommon to find spaces devoted to spiritual or religious practice within airports, larger corporations, or hospitals. The Peace Alliance Foundation (formerly the World Renaissance Alliance), an umbrella organization made up of several spiritual traditions, has organized prayer circles throughout the country for citizens to gather with their neighbors and to identify ways to individually and collectively work toward peace nationally and in the world. The alliance, built around a 12-step model, is another current example of the way religious and spiritual traditions are beginning to blend for the purposes of social justice.

Because people differ in their ways of understanding themselves and others, partly because of their socialized ways of viewing human behavior, it is useful to stop and determine the differences and similarities between the client and the worker when attempting to address religion and spirituality in practice. Using the Papajohn and Spiegel (1975) and the Dilthey typologies, the social worker can generate useful dialogue, leading participants to using mutually understandable terminology in their communication. In cases where this knowledge may be essential, such as counseling services provided by a particular religious or spiritual body, making a grid of these typologies and asking consumers to use checkmarks to identify their worldviews about these positions may be helpful. Social workers can also use these grids to communicate clearly with those seeking the services their agencies can or cannot provide.

Finally, given the rise in mixed religion families, couples can benefit from acknowledging the differences in their spiritual and religious traditions so that conflicts can be managed effectively by helping them to honor the richness of the different traditions. McGoldrick, Giordano, and Garcia-Preto (2005), in their work across ethnic backgrounds, identify the conflicts that may arise for mixed ethnicity families over values and beliefs, when to celebrate a holiday, childrearing practices, and how to mourn their dead. By helping mixed religion (and sometimes mixed ethnicity) couples harmoniously acknowledge and determine methods to live out their different traditions, social workers can help them gain insight about these conflicts without judgment. From that exploration, new ways of integrating both sides of a couple's tradition can be established and shared with other members of the extended family.

## DISCUSSION POINTS

Why did Tunde's case have a positive outcome?

1. Someone in Imani/Tunde's community recognized a need and made a referral. Lay people, or those with professional backgrounds, can do this quite readily.
2. Programs and services existed that would allow Tunde to work effectively with Tunde's own intersections of ethnicity, gender identity, and economics after Tunde had to leave the parental home.
3. Social workers recognized and built in all aspects of Tunde's life, including the desire to continue engagement in spiritual and religious activities. This was done over years but allowed a solid base Tunde could return to as their needs changed.
4. Over time, all of Tunde's psycho-social, mental, physical, and spiritual needs were united, resulting in a person whose intersectionality could be integrated rather than fracture.

## REFERENCES

Allison, H. E. (1996). *Idealism and freedom: Essays on Kant's theoretical and practical philosophy.* Cambridge: Cambridge University Press.

Almeder, R. F. (1980). *The philosophy of Charles S. Peirce: A critical introduction.* Totowa, NJ: Rowman and Littlefield.

Arnett, J. J. (2004). *Emerging adulthood: The winding road from the late teens through the twenties.* New York, NY: Oxford University Press.

Barna. (2017, March 17). *Research releases: Meet those who "Love Jesus but not the Church".* Retrieved from https://www.barna.com/research/meet-love-jesus-not-church

Barna. (2017, April 6). *Research releases: Meet the "Spiritual but not religious."* Retrieved from https://www.barna.com/research/meet-spiritual-not-religious

Bergin, A. E., & Richards, P. S. (2005). *A spiritual strategy for counseling and psychotherapy.* New York, NY: American Psychological Association.

Borg, M. J. (2004). *The heart of Christianity: Rediscovering a life of faith.* San Francisco, CA: HarperOne.

Burn, K., & Szoeke, C. (2016). Boomerang families and failure-to-launch: Commentary on adult children living at home. *Maturitas, 83,* 9–12. doi:10.1016/j.maturitas.2015.09.004

Canda, E. R., & Furman, L. D. (2010). *Spiritual diversity in social work practice: The heart of helping.* New York, NY: Oxford University Press.

Chatters, L. M., Taylor, R. J., Jackson, J. S., & Lincoln, K. D. (2008). Religious coping among African Americans, Caribbean Blacks and non-Hispanic Whites. *Journal of Community Psychology, 36*(3), 371–386. Retrieved from http://hdl.handle.net/2027.42/58064

Chaves, M., & Anderson, S. L. (2014). Changing American congregations: Findings from the third wave of the National Congregations Study. *Journal for the Scientific Study of Religion, 53*(4), 676–686. doi:10.1111/jssr.12151

Chödrön, P. (2010). *The wisdom of no escape: And the path of loving-kindness.* Boston, MA: Shambhala Publications.

Cohen, A. B., & Hill, P. C. (2007). Religion as culture: Religious individualism and collectivism among American Catholics, Jews, and Protestants. *Journal of Personality, 75*(4), 709–742. doi:10.1111/j.1467-6494.2007.00454.x

Derezotes, D. (2009). Religious resurgence, human survival, and global religious social work. *Journal of Religion & Spirituality in Social Work: Social Thought, 28*(1–2), 63–81. doi:10.1080/15426430802643604

Fetsch, E. (2014). *Mixing and Matching: Who Practices Multiple Religions?* Public Religion Research Institute (PRRP). Retrieved from https://www.prri.org/spotlight/mixing-and-matching-a-look-at-who-practices-multiple-religions

Fitzgerald, D. (2002). *Julia Butterfly Hill: Saving the redwoods.* Millbrook, CT: Millbrook Press.

Freedman, S. G. (2009, December, 9). *Many Americans Mix Multiple Faiths.* Retrieved from https://www.nytimes.com/2013/07/13/us/a-religion-that-embraces-all-religions.html

Fuller, R. C. (2001). *Spiritual, but not religious: Understanding unchurched America.* New York, NY: Oxford University Press.

Guadalupe, K. L., & Lum, D. (2005). *Multidimensional contextual practice: Diversity and transcendence.* Belmont, CA: Thomson Brooks/Cole.

Hayslip Jr, B., Fruhauf, C. A., & Dolbin-MacNab, M. L. (2017). Grandparents raising grandchildren: What have we learned over the past decade?. *The Gerontologist, 59*(3), e152–e163. doi:10.1093/geront/gnx106

Hess, R. E., Maton, K. I., & Pargament, K. (2014). *Religion and prevention in mental health: Research, vision, and action.* New York, NY: Routledge.

Hodge, D. R. (2003). The challenge of spiritual diversity: Can social work facilitate an inclusive environment? *Families and Society, 84*(3), 348. doi:10.1606/1044-3894.117

Jasso, G., Massey, D. S., Rosenzweig, M. R., & Smith, J. P. (2003). Exploring the religious preferences of recent immigrants to the United States: Evidence from the New Immigrant Survey Pilot. In Y. Y. Haddad, J. I. Smith, & J. L. Esposito (Eds.). *Religion and Immigration: Christian, Jewish, and Muslim experiences in the United States* (pp. 217–253). Walnut Creek, CA: AltaMira Press.

Kim, S. C. (1997). Korean American families. *Working with Asian Americans: A guide for clinicians,* 125–135.

Kim, R. Y. (2011). Religion and ethnicity: Theoretical connections. *Religions, 2*(3), 312–329. doi:10.3390/rel2030312

Kim, B.-L. C., & Ryu, E. (2005). Korean Families. In M. McGoldrick, J. Giordano, & N. Garcia-Preto (Eds.), *Ethnicity and family therapy.* New York, NY: Guilford Press.

Kluckhohn, F. R., & Strodtbeck, F. L. (1961). *Variations in value orientations.* Oxford, UK: Row Petersen.

Kosmin, B., & Keysar, A. (2008). *American religious identification survey summary report.* Hartford, CT: Trinity College.

Krippner, S., & Welch, P. (1992). *Spiritual dimensions of healing.* New York, NY: Irvington Publishers.

Lugo, L., Stencel, S., Green, J., Smith, G., Cox, D., & Pond, A. (2008). *U.S. religious landscape survey.* Retrieved from https://www.pewresearch.org/wp-content/uploads/sites/7/2008/06/report2-religious-landscape-study-full.pdf

Mattis, J. S., Murray, Y. F., Hatcher, C. A., Hearn, K. D., Lawhon G. D., Murphy, E. J., & Washington, T. A. (2001). Religiosity, spirituality, and the subjective quality of African American men's friendships: An exploratory study. *Journal of Adult Development, 8*(4), 221–230. Retrieved from http://hdl.handle.net/2027.42/44637

McGoldrick, M., Giordano, J., & Garcia-Preto, N. (2005). *Ethnicity and family therapy.* New York, NY: Guilford Press.

McGreal, I. P. (1995). *Great thinkers of the Eastern world.* New York, NY: HarperCollins.

Papajohn, J., & Spiegel, J. P. (1975). *Transactions in families: A modern approach for resolving cultural and generational conflicts.* San Francisco, CA: Jossey-Bass.

Pargament, K. I. (2001). *The psychology of religion and coping: Theory, research, practice.* New York, NY: Guilford Press.

Pew Research Center. (May 12, 2015). *America's changing religious landscape.* Washington, DC: Author.

Pew Research Center. (June 13, 2018a). *The age gap in religion around the world.* Washington, DC: Author

Pew Research Center. (November 20, 2018b). *Where Americans find meaning in life.* Washington, DC: Author

Richards, P. S., & Bergin, A. E. (1997). *A spiritual strategy.* Washington, DC: American Psychological Association.

Sandstorm, A. (2015). Religious groups' policies on transgender members vary widely. Fact Tank: News in the Numbers. Retrieved from http://pewrsr.ch/1OxlONV

Saucier, G., & Skrzypińska, K. (2006). Spiritual but not religious? Evidence for two independent dispositions. *Journal of Personality, 74*(5), 1257–1292. doi:10.1111/j.1467-6494.2006.00409.x

Schwadel, P., & Sandstrom, A. (2019, May 24). *Lesbian, gay and bisexual Americans are less religious than straight adults by traditional measures.* Pew Foundation. Retrieved from https://www.pewresearch.org/fact-tank/2019/05/24/lesbian-gay-and-bisexual-americans-are-less-religious-than-straight-adults-by-traditional-measures

Schwartz, S. A. (2015). Two roads converge in a yellowing wood—shamanism, science, and climate change. *Explore: The Journal of Science and Healing, 11*(2), 85–88. doi:10.1016/j.explore.2014.12.006

Smith, G. (2017, November 27). *Views of transgender issues divide along religious lines.* Pew Foundation. Retrieved from https://www.pewresearch.org/fact-tank/2017/11/27/views-of-transgender-issues-divide-along-religious-lines

Spretnak, C. (1982). *The politics of women's spirituality: Essays on the rise of spiritual power within the feminist movement.* Sioux City, IA: Anchor Publishers.

Starhawk. (1990). *Truth or dare: Encounters with power, authority, and mystery.* New York, NY: HarperOne.

Tanner, J. L., & Arnett, J. J. (2016). The emergence of emerging adulthood: The new life stage between adolescence and young adulthood. In *Routledge handbook of youth and young adulthood* (pp. 50–56). New York, NY: Routledge.

Williams, B. J. (2004). GCP technical note: Global harmony revisited. *Global Consciousness Project exploratory analysis.* Retrieved from BJ Williams – noosphere.global-mind.org

Zukav, G. (1999). *The seat of the soul.* New York, NY: Simon and Schuster.

# 19

# HIV/AIDS and Latinx Families: Practice Considerations

CLAUDIA LUCIA MORENO

## INTRODUCTION

HIV/AIDS has changed from being a death sentence to being a long-term illness due to advances in medications. In spite of these medical advances, HIV/AIDS continues to be a threat to the Latinx community. The Latinx population is the largest minority group in the United States (U.S. Census Bureau, 2018). Social workers need to be adept at confronting the challenges of this rapid growth and diversity in the Latinx community to provide culturally relevant services for this emergent group. HIV/AIDS has been stigmatized since the beginning, as anyone who is sexually active or uses intravenous equipment can become infected. Social workers in any field of practice can encounter people with HIV/AIDS, not necessarily just in centers for HIV+ individuals. Stigma continues to be a big issue and people still conceal or do not know their HIV status.

HIV/AIDS presents challenges for social workers when practicing and providing services to infected individuals and their families. Social workers should be knowledgeable about the biology, medications, risk factors, and socio-cultural issues of HIV/AIDS. This requires that social workers be armed with awareness, knowledge, and skills about how to work effectively with this population. This requires knowing about the biology of HIV, current advances and discoveries, risk factors, gender norms, and the psychosocial and residual impact of being HIV infected, stigma, medical regimens for the treatment for HIV/AIDS, and belief systems, spirituality, and end-of-life. HIV/AIDS impacts not only individuals, but it affects families, friends, communities, settings, and society in general.

Latinx are the largest minority group in the United States and come from about 20 different countries with different histories and different journeys of immigration. The Latinx community is very diverse, and the information included in this chapter discusses the major Latinx groups. There are emergent Latinx groups and a dearth of research studies. This chapter focuses specifically on Latinx families, which is central in the Latinx culture. Families are considered essential for the functioning of the individual and of communities. HIV/AIDS infects individuals and affects the entire family system and communities.

## SCOPE AND SERIOUSNESS OF THE ISSUE

HIV was identified in 1980 as a retrovirus. There are two specific types of the HIV virus: HIV1 and HIV2. HIV1 is the most common of the virus types, and it has different subtypes. HIV2 is mostly found in West Africa, and in this region, HIV2 is rare (Kirchner, 2019). HIV is an immunodeficiency virus; when it enters the body it destroys specific blood cells that fight disease (T-cells or CD4 cells), leading to an incurable life-threatening condition. People can get HIV by contact with infected body fluids such as having unprotected sex (oral, anal, vaginal), sharing infected needles, and through breast milk. Infection via blood transfusions is now rare owing to the careful examination of blood supplies undertaken since 1985.

HIV causes AIDS. AIDS occurs when the T-cells are below 200. After the HIV virus enters the body, it can take from 3 to 6 months to be detected by specific HIV tests. This is what is called the window period. Tests can detect the antibodies of the HIV virus earlier, but if a person gets tested and is negative, it does not mean that is truly negative until the person uses protection for every sexual encounter or needle sharing for 3 to 6 months and then gets tested again. This will give a more adequate reading of the HIV status of the person.

People with very high viral loads transmit the virus rapidly. The amount of HIV presence in the body (viral load) varies from person to person, length of time living with HIV, and medications taken. Current antiretroviral medications can lower the viral load making HIV undetectable. Undetectable means no transmission. Antiretroviral medication has been responsible for lowering HIV transmission around the globe. The challenge is making people get tested to find out their HIV status and once infected to take their medications. This is called medication adherence. HIV medications can have awful and compromising side effects, but these medications have prolonged people's lives. HIV medications require a regular regimen, and missing dosages can lead to resistance and making the medication ineffective, increasing the viral load and leading to progression of HIV. People with HIV not only transmit the virus but also their resistance to medications and the viral load. Thus, a person receiving the virus not only gets HIV but also receives the transmitter's resistance to medications. Most of the transmission that occurs is male-to-male resulting in about 66% of the HIV/AIDS cases; heterosexual sex is the cause in about 24% of the cases (Centers for Disease Control and Prevention [CDC], 2017).

Currently we have a variety of medications on the market, and new medications are being developed. HIV can be prevented by these three methods:

1. By using condoms (female and male condoms).
2. By PreP (pre-exposure prophylaxis), which means that if a person wants to have unprotected sexual encounters with an infected partner, both the infected and non-infected person will have to take antiretroviral medication to reduce transmission of the virus.

3. By PEP (post-exposure prophylaxis) is also used when a HIV-negative person thinks that he or she has been exposed to the virus, and will have to take antiretroviral medication for a certain amount of time to reduce the likelihood of the virus reproducing.

Latinx have the second highest incidence of HIV infection and have the highest mortality rates due to AIDS (CDC, 2017). Latinx represent 26% of the HIV/AIDS diagnoses even though they represent 18% of the population. More Latinx men than women are infected. In 2016, 87% of the new HIV/AIDS diagnosis were men and 12% were Latinx women (CDC, 2017). Among Latinx men, 85% of HIV infections were attributed to male-to-male contact, while for Latinx women, 88% of the HIV infections were attributed to heterosexual contact.

Testing in the Latinx community remains a challenge; one in six of the Latinx population are unaware of their HIV status. By the time Latinx persons get tested for HIV, they do not have HIV but AIDS because testing has been delayed for many years. HIV is a silent virus that can remain in the body for many years without any serious symptoms. Undocumented Latinx individuals are less likely to get tested or receive HIV medical services (CDC, 2017). In 2015, only 50% of Latinx individuals with HIV were retained in HIV medical care and only 49% had a suppressed viral load (CDC, 2017).

Stigma, fear, and homophobia remain serious challenges in the community and interfere with testing, transmission, and care. HIV/AIDS still carry a huge amount of stigma within the Latinx population, and many people do not get tested for fear of knowing the results. HIV/AIDS continues to spread and affect many individuals and families.

## INTERSECTIONALITY AS A FRAME OF REFERENCE TO UNDERSTAND LATINX FAMILIES AFFECTED BY HIV/AIDS

Intersectionality is a framework used to conceptualize an individual or a group of people, not just in terms of race/ethnicity but the overlapping social inequality such as race, class, gender, identity, sexual orientation, religion, poverty, and other identities in healthcare outcomes (Cusick, 1999; Qiao, Li, & Stanton., 2001; Shaffer et al., 2001).

HIV/AIDS continues to be a threat for the lives of many Latinx people living in the United States. HIV does not only infect a person but affects the entire family. HIV/AIDS is experienced differently by different families. HIV/AIDS still is stigmatized, and responses are intersected in a psycho-cultural context that includes belief systems, gender norms, values, emotional patterns, social inequality, and perceived mode of transmissions. These factors impact how and when people get infected and obtain services. Living with HIV/AIDS is an empowerment and spiritual experience that can be a transformative experience for individuals.

### Social and Environmental Inequality

HIV is an epidemic intersecting at different levels of inequalities at the macro-structural, meso-institutional, and micro-interpersonal levels (Watkins-Hayes, 2014). These levels cannot be viewed separately from HIV factors that influence risk and include violence and level of empowerment, poverty, limited educational and job opportunities, discrimination, and immigration status (Moreno, 2007). There is a complex relationship between HIV and poverty. Poverty is a risk factor for being infected with HIV, and when people are infected with the HIV virus, the virus impacts their earning power. Poverty makes people live in dangerous places that impact on their risk of HIV infection (Latkin, Weeks, Galletty, & Albarracin, 2010). HIV is more prevalent in poverty-stricken neighborhoods resulting in HIV-stricken epidemics as defined by the United Nations Joint Program on HIV/AIDS (UNAIDS) (CDC, 2010). In order to obtain money, people get involved in HIV risky activities. Poverty fosters the spread of the illness due to lack of power and access to education, and basic HIV prevention. Poverty is not just about the lack of power, but it is also about the lack of decision-making. Individual risk is no longer viewed in a vacuum, and the concept of risky neighborhoods is emerging as structural risk factors for HIV. Latinx individuals in the United States represent 18% of the nation's population, and is the group with the greatest poverty rate in the nation—27.2% (U.S. Census Bureau, 2019).

Macro-structural factors are implicated in HIV risk and services. The intersectional social marginalization results in HIV risk and substance abuse coping strategies. Macro-structural factors related to HIV include poverty, neighborhoods, media, values, belief systems, gender inequality, and sexual oppression (Pardasani, Moreno, & Forge, 2010). Social norms at the macro level that influence risk include norms regarding drug use, same-sex behaviors, gender roles, and condom use (Latkin et al., 2010). Meso-institutional factors include lack of services, legal and healthcare policies, funding, and research. Micro-interpersonal factors include beliefs, lack of education, low income, substance abuse, values, number of sexual partners, level of personal empowerment, and agency (Moreno, 2007). All of these factors are important to understand HIV risk factors, services, and prevention.

Most HIV interventions adopted by the CDC focus specifically on individual behaviors without addressing how poverty, racism, gender inequality, and sexual oppression intermingle with HIV virus transmission; there are a handful of interventions that are taking the macro-structural factors into consideration (Lauby, Smith, Stark, & Person, 2000).

As mentioned, poverty increases the risk for HIV infection, and AIDS increases the likelihood of living in poverty (Whiteside, 2000). HIV compromises the immune system and impacts on income earning ability. Poverty also hinders access to services and exacerbates stress and poor health among Latinx individuals who are already HIV infected (Harris, Firestone, & Vega, 2005; Kalichman & Grebler, 2010). Latinx families who live in poverty might suffer from more psychosocial stressors when HIV enters their homes.

The Latinx community in the United States is the poorest compared to other groups. There are many new immigrants who come to this country, running away from violence, poverty, and corruption. New Latinx immigrants come with language barriers, limited job skills, and unawareness of HIV risk. As a result, some Latinx immigrants encounter HIV in neighborhoods that are infested with poverty, drugs, and high-risk sexual behavior. Some Latinx individuals find themselves in relationships that are riskier due to their economical dependency and immigration status. These macro-structural circumstances create conditions and exacerbate Latinx risk for HIV.

Historically, Latinx women and the LGBTQI community have been oppressed, marginalized, and disenfranchised and suffer from ethnic discrimination, homophobia, gender inequality, and power imbalances. These macro-level factors contribute to micro-level risk, health status, stressors, treatment access, and medication adherence, and it is also implicated in their ability to negotiate safer sex and self-care (Moreno, 2007).

There are some cultural factors that have been associated with HIV in the Latinx community that include language barriers, stigma, gender norms, and belief systems about risk and treatment. Language barriers hinder their ability to navigate and communicate with medical personnel and social services and other related services.

Being abused at any point in life and living in violent situations are surfacing as being related to HIV risk and has a tremendous impact on the care of an HIV-infected person. Women and the transgender community have a high incidence of trauma and violence directed at them (Moreno, 2007).

It is imperative to understand the intersectionality and the different levels of the socio-environmental context of HIV. HIV cannot be seen in a vacuum and attributed to the individual's behavior but it must be viewed with an understanding of how different macro-level, meso-level, and micro-level factors put people at risk, interfere with care, increase transmission, and interfere in the management of the condition. Intersectional interventions and practices are imperative when addressing HIV in families of color. Gender inequality, cultural factors, race/ethnicity, poverty, and violence interact to create a distinct set of challenges and conditions for lower income minorities with HIV/AIDS (Lekas, Siegel, & Schrimshaw, 2006).

## Micro-Level Factors

Micro-level factors are not only implicated to HIV risk but also to how Latinx families deal and perceive HIV transmission, infection, treatment, and prevention.

### Gender Violence

The literature is linking the overlapping relationship between gender-based violence and HIV infection—the same factors that put people at risk for partner violence are the same risk factors for HIV. Abused women have been found to have higher rates of unsafe sexual practices, and usually their sexual partners themselves have an array of unsafe sexual practices such as multiple sexual partners, unprotected encounters, transactional sex, histories of abuse, and substance abuse (Dunkle & Jewkes, 2007). Gender violence interferes with self-care and disclosure of HIV status. For Latinx families, gender violence minimizes their ability to negotiate safe sex and to receive care (Gonzalez-Guarda, Vasquez, Urrutia, Villarruel, & Peragallo, 2011; Moreno, 2007). One in three Latinx women have been abused in their life times, and 50% of them never report the abuse because of lack of confidence in the police and systems of care, guilt, cultural expectations, fear of deportation, and previous experiences with victimization (National Latino Alliance Network, 2019).

### Gender Scripts

Many Latinx individuals adhere to a tradition of an unequal power balance between men and women. Power is fundamental and affects many dimensions of a person's life (Cianelli, Ferrer, & McElmurry, 2008). Among Latinx, these power inequalities are characterized by the cultural scripts of *machismo* and *marianismo*. These cultural scripts are not unique to the Latinx community and can be found in other cultures.

*Machismo* describes a man's behavior in a restrictive way of hypermasculinity characterized by being dominant, virile, and independent. Machismo is being portrayed as having positive and negative characteristics. The positive characteristics of machismo are the cavalier, the breadwinner, the responsible and caring person for the wife and children. The negative characteristics of machismo are the domineering, intimidating, and controlling of women (Arciniega, Andreson, Tovar-Blank, & Tracy, 2008). *Marianismo* is the term used to describe some behaviors that are the opposite from *machismo*. The person that first used this term was Evelyn Stevens in 1973 to describe some gender structures present among many Latinx women. This is a gender norm that is oppressive and the name comes from the virgin Mary-Maria, which characterizes women in a similar behavior as the virgin Mary and performing an ideal role such as being passive, self-sacrificing, submissive, nurturing, docile, dependent, and chaste (Moreno, 2007). Although there are different levels of *machismo* and *marianismo*, not all Latinx men and women practice these traditions, but they still prevail in Latin America and still influence relationships and ultimately HIV risk behaviors and HIV treatment. For men, *machismo* can both be a risk factor and a protective factor—a risk factor when men are domineering and do not share power and decision-making, especially in the bedroom, related to sex and safety, having many sexual partners and many unprotected encounters, using drugs and alcohol, the more women they have the more of a man they are. The protective factor of *machismo* is the man who cares about his family and does not bring HIV to the household and uses protection with responsibility. A protective factor under a *marianista* tradition is that women are supposed to have only one sexual partner and take care of the family. This is a risk factor because women are not supposed to be knowledgeable about sex, and they are expected to accept infidelity for the sake of the family and because "that is the way men are." Men's infidelity is tolerated but when a woman is unfaithful, she is rejected and her behavior is not accepted by many because she does not fit the culturally prescribed gender roles. Some Latinx women with HIV experience more rejection from families compared to men with HIV (Moreno, 2007).

For some, Latinx, men with HIV are seen very differently than women with HIV. There is harsher judgment for women who are HIV positive and often are given labels of "slut" or "druggy." Latinx women with HIV have to withstand more labels and misjudgments from family members and friends, even though many of them neglect their own health and take care of their HIV-infected partners but no one takes care of them (Moreno, 2007).

Some researchers have suggested that *machismo* and *marianismo* affect the Latinx gays. Some gays are gendered when they do not conform to the prescribed roles. For Latinx LGBTI, the cultural gender expectations of masculinities and femininities are oppressive, damaging, and homophobic and can compromise disclosure, self-worth, and self-esteem for individuals who do not fit in those two systems (Asencio, 2011).

## Historical Trauma

This is a social construct that in recent years has emerged to help understand the psychological and physiological impact of historical oppression, colonization, cultural genocide, and rape in Indigenous communities in North America (Yellowbird, 2004). The application of historical trauma in communities from Latin America is emerging. The Latinx population has suffered more than 500 years of genocide, colonialism, and dominance, and these forms of oppression are still present in the lives of many Latinx today. The impact of these cultural genocides have resulted in economic, social, health, and political disparities that continue to have repercussions on the lives of Latinx around the world. In the field of HIV, it is important to keep in mind how historical trauma might be related to current traumas, distrust in the system, and helplessness.

## Immigration and Trauma

Latinos have immigrated into the United States for a variety of reasons. The southern border is the passage for many migrants from Mexico and Central and South America. Lately, migrants have arrived into the United States fleeing chaotic conditions back home such as extreme poverty, crime, insecurity, and political unrest. For many the journey into the United States can be traumatic because of many challenging conditions during the journey such as extreme weather conditions, food insecurity, rape, and death (Slack & Whiteford, 2011). The migration journey before, during, and after the dislocation can lead to psychological distress (Perez-Foster, 2001). Many migrants suffer family separation, leaving behind loved ones; for some at the border the separation of parents and children can be very traumatic. Latinx families in their new homes can experience poor living conditions, unemployment, insufficient supports, language barriers, and immigration persecution increasing their psychological stress and trauma. These situations can put someone at risk for HIV, and for those with HIV, it can exacerbate their medical condition and the way they seek and receive treatment.

## Familism

Familism is a concept that describes the importance of the family. Familism is a belief that the family unit (extended and nuclear) should come first before the individual's needs and family members should be interdependent and cooperative (Moreno, 2006). Families are highly regarded in the Latino community, and familism is one of the most fundamental aspects of the culture. Familism has been defined as having a strong family commitment, family support, familial honor, loyalty, and emotional closeness. Familism values family relationships, and there is a strong value placed on childbearing, females as central to keeping the family together, and a transmission of values, nurture, guidance, and support. Strong familiasm has been associated with lower HIV risk among women and a protective factor for mental health problems among Latinos (DeSantis, Gonzalez-Guarda, & Provencio-Vasquez, 2012). Because of the centrality of the family, some Latinx with HIV do not disclose their status to the family for fear of being rejected and because HIV can bring "shame" to the family unit. According to some studies, those Latinx who disclose their HIV status to the family have suffered rejection by family members (DeSantis et al., 2012). Rejection can interfere with self-worth and self-care for a person with HIV.

### Fatalismo

*Fatalismo* is a belief that an individual's health aliment or wellness is predetermined by a higher powerand it is beyond the individual's control. This is a cultural belief that is not unique to Latinx and is rooted in Catholicism where the person has no control over any human event, and everything is controlled by God's power. This cultural belief has implications for how a person perceives health as being beyond the person's control, and it is dependent on luck, fate, chance, or God. Illnesses, diseases, and accidents are perceived as "punishments" from God, and people have to make retributions for wrongdoings (Falicov, 1998). Many believe that there is more to human events that a person has no control over, a belief system that may inhibit healthcare utilization and also healthcare behaviors (Franklin et al., 2007). Fatalistic attitudes have been implicated in being involved in how people perceive HIV protection to self and others and also care. Fatalistic attitudes are not just embedded in religiosity but also in the context of poverty, discrimination, oppression, and other factors that influence people's views of self-efficacy and self-control. Many families with HIV/AIDS suffer from inadequate social, psychological, and emotional support systems. Fatalism need to be looked at from an intersectional point of view to understand how it can influence HIV prevention efforts and treatment and care for families affected with HIV/AIDS.

## Stigma and HIV/AIDS

HIV changed from being a death sentence to being a long-term illness. Stigma is considered one of the major barriers to combat the HIV epidemic and is related to prevention, testing, disclosure, and medical and social management of the condition. Researchers in the field of HIV/AIDS have identified stigma not just at the intrapersonal level but also at the family, organizational, and community levels (Pardisani, Moreno, & Forge, 2010). For people with HIV, stigma is felt as fear, anxiety, hostility, shame, and a threat to survival. HIV continues to be a condition highly stigmatized because of its history since HIV was first recognized as an illness in the gay community. This stigma toward people with HIV is related to homophobia. For many Latino gays, disclosing their HIV status is not just disclosing their condition to their families but also their sexual orientation.

Helping people infected with HIV to disclose their status is also helping them to deal with stigma. Some research studies suggest that Latinx have a low incidence of disclosing their HIV status to their families and disclosure depends on the quality of the relationship (Cusick, 1999). This fear of being stigmatized deters Latinos from seeking testing and treatment.

## Maternal Disclosure of HIV Status to Children

HIV transmission from mother to children has decreased a great deal. Maternal transmission was usually during birth and also through breastfeeding, which is called vertical transmission. Because of medical development and public health campaigns, vertical transmissions have decreased tremendously.

The literature suggests that women disclose more about their status to their romantic partners and close friends but find it difficult to disclose to their own children (Shaffer, Jones, Kotchick, & Forehand, 2001). When mothers disclose their HIV status, they are more likely to disclose when they are quite ill and in their final stages of the illness. Mothers tend to disclose more to older children and female children. In addition, the literature suggests that when a family member is HIV infected, the entire family experiences more stress and burden. Children of parents who are HIV positive undergo more stress and adjustment difficulties (Dorsey, Watts, Morse, Forehand, & Morse, 1999).

Disclosing HIV status to family and children can be very difficult because HIV brings a great deal of stigmatization and discrimination not only toward the mother but to the family. Latinx might find it difficult to disclose their HIV status to their own children because of the cultural value of *familismo*. HIV brings shame, and misconceptions about how people become infected. Some studies have found that maternal-headed single-parent families have lower rates of disclosure to children compared to two-parent Latinx families (Thompkins, 2007).

Because HIV/AIDS is still highly stigmatized, helping professionals should be informed about how the process of disclosure can be difficult to some Latinx families. Support to families who have a member who is HIV positive is necessary, and it is important to help them in the process of knowing about the condition, destigmatizing HIV, and educating them about the condition. This support should be tailored according to families and be culturally relevant with a process that includes issues of disclosure such as when to disclose, age-specific issues, relationships, and family context. Therapeutics helps in dealing with emotions and fears in a way that embraces cultural values and traditions.

## HELPING PROFESSIONS RESPONDING

Latinx families are affected by HIV/AIDS in many different ways. For Latinx, families play a central role in the emotional and nurturing development of the individual. HIV infects the individual but affects the nuclear family and the extended family, communities, and organizations. Families are better served by comprehensive services that are culturally tailored and delivered in a culturally responsive way. By using the intersectionality perspective, HIV/AIDS service delivery can involve different and complex systems. Individual interventions are not enough and service delivery requires structural interventions (Latkin, Weeks, Glassman, Galletty, & Albarracin, 2010). Poverty is related to HIV throughout the world. Often, people with HIV/AIDS are poor and their families are as well. HIV/AIDS brings many challenges for Latinx families, creating vicious cycle because before HIV, many families are poor, and after the infection, HIV further reduces income, diminishes opportunities, and for many immigrants changes their dream of reuniting with families and making a decent living (Moreno, 2007). Helping professionals can be more effective by integrating these complexities when helping families affected by HIV. Helping professionals can help families not only to understand HIV, but the medical and psychological challenges that it brings. Families will benefit from access to social support, comprehensive resources, skills to manage stigma, access to training, jobs, education, and ways of improving their situation. Helping professions can assist families not just in dealing with the medical challenges of HIV/AIDS but with the threats that poverty brings; for example, language barriers, underinsured or uninsured status, negotiating an unfamiliar socio-political system, a different culture, and for some dealing with challenges for being undocumented. Helping professionals can assist families in their journey with HIV/AIDS, teaching coping skills, mastery, and empowerment; offering psycho-educational services, family counseling, and ways to deal with stigma related to HIV, homophobia, and shame. Services for HIV affected families can include families to shape services, deliver services in a comprehensive way, not just to focus on the individual with HIV but also their romantic partners, families, organizations, and communities. Changes at the macro level include structural and policy interventions to better serve families affected by HIV/AIDS.

## Practice Principles Common to All Interventions

### Risk Factors

Families affected by HIV often have misinformation about the virus. Families need education to understand risk factors, transmission, and management of HIV not only to help their family member who is infected but also to make sure that HIV stops there. Regardless of the service setting, service providers should educate clients about HIV/AIDS, risk factors, how HIV is transmitted, medications, medication adherence, and what we can do to avoid getting HIV. Education about HIV is imperative because it can prevent infection and re-infection with the different strains of HIV. Anyone who is sexually active and/or is sharing needles can be at risk for HIV.

### Stigma and Confidentiality

Stigma is a factor that is prevalent in HIV/AIDS. As members of a minority group, many Latinx individuals have experienced discrimination, oppression, violence, and historical trauma. They have experienced a multitude of stigmas. Having a family member with HIV can exacerbate fear and shame and increase the stigma about HIV. According to studies, many Latinos have difficulties disclosing their HIV status to others. Families choose carefully who to disclose to (Cusick, 1999; Qiao, Li, & Stanton, 2013; Schaffer et al., 2001). Disclosing is a process, and service providers need to understand the totality of their experience. Clients might be juggling with other issues, not just the stigma of HIV, such as poverty, unemployment, mental health issues, drug abuse, and other external factors. It is imperative that service providers develop a relationship and establish *confianza* (trust) by building a relationship that is conducive to exploring how stigma comes from misinformation and might harm families. Finding ways to empower families to feel safe about when, where, and to whom they disclose their family member's status. Since HIV/AIDS is a condition that is highly stigmatized, clients need to be educated about the biology of HIV, health and nutritional factors, medical management, and especially about retroviral therapy whichi reduces the incidence of transmission. High levels of stigma have been associated with poor medication adherence, which in turn can lead to medication resistance, health problems, and eventually death. Service providers should explain to families about confidentiality and HIPAA guidelines, understanding and contextualizing the family's concerns about privacy, and provide support and guidance around difficult disclosure decisions.

### Assessment

Assessment is an ongoing process; service providers should be attuned to the entire process. Latinx people do not open up at the beginning of the relationship, and as *confianza* (trust) is developed, they will be more willing to share their inner feelings and concerns once this relationship has been developed. An individualized, contextual, culturally relevant, mutual, and ongoing assessment process that has a lens of strengths and needs is essential in working with families affected by HIV/AIDS. The literature demonstrates that providers who have preconceptions about patients based on group membership can misdiagnose culturally appropriate behaviors (Alegria & Woo, 2009). Symptom presentation varies across racial and ethnic groups, and, based on this information, an intersectionality lens to assess clients and families is important for an accurate assessment (Alegria & Woo, 2009).

Providers should assess families, and look for acculturation differences, cultural beliefs, religion, belief in supernatural powers, secrets, worldviews, cultural norms, and meanings regarding relationships, coupling, parenting, gender roles, caretaking roles, spirituality, immigration history, abuse, historical trauma, oppression, and patterns of communication. What they know about the illness and what HIV means to them should be explored (Moreno, 2007; Moreno, 2013).

Providers should be attuned to and be aware of the needs of each family as they differt. Families of the LGTB population might have different challenges compared to heterosexual families. Families of the LGTB community might be dealing not just with HIV/AIDS and its health issues but they might be dealing with the stigma of the illness and the stigma of having a family member in the LGTB group. Research shows that when families reject individuals because of their sexual orientation and gender expression, the person's health is compromised and risky behaviors increase (Ryann, Huebner, Diaz, & Sanchez 2009).

Medical advances in drug therapy have changed the landscape of HIV. People are not only living longer and living healthier lives, but these advances have also reduced the incidence of HIV transmission and have made HIV undetectable in their bodies. Many families affected by HIV/AIDS suffer from a variety of stressors; they might be dealing with their family member's medical challenges that include the management of health issues such as fatigue, anemia, digestive problems, bone problems, and fat misdistribution, which are side effects of the medications. On the other hand, families might be dealing with psychological challenges that include depression, dementia, isolation, fear, low self-esteem, and the awareness that death might come. Stigma persists among family members and the individual with HIV/AIDS might feel this rejection in many different ways. Providers need to be attuned to this dynamic and should provide psychoeducational services to families and inform them about HIV myths in transmission and proper medical management (Lichtenstein, Sturdevant, & Mujumdar, 2010). Empowering families to help their relatives with HIV/AIDS is imperative. Families eventually can organize, request, and shape services and resources for and become influential in creating better community services and social policy.

## Cultural Competence

Latinx are the largest minority group in the United States and the population will continue to grow in rapid numbers. This underscores the need for the providers who can work effectively with this emerging group. The literature suggests that when providers are culturally competent, they will provide better outcomes in therapy (Cardemil & Sarmiento, 2009). In working with Latinx families, it is imperative to have familiarity with cultural values, patterns, language, emotion expression, immigration journeys, and transnationality. Latinx individuals are very diverse and come from 20 different countries and have distinct service needs. Most models of cultural competence agree that a culturally competent provider must have three specific elements: (a) self-awareness, (b) knowledge acquisition, and (c) skill development (Smith & Montilla, 2006). Being aware of biases and pre-conceived notions is imperative and fundamental in cultural competency development. Negative stereotypes about Latinx and HIV/AIDS can get in the way when working with families and can result in misdiagnosis and poor matching of services (Alegria & Woo, 2009). Knowledge is needed about the diversity of Latinx, differential exposure to the U.S. culture, cultural values, belief systems, symptom representation, and the intersectionality of socio-economic status, language, gender norms, power and privilege, and family structure—as well as becoming knowledgeable about Latinx's worldviews. Such knowledge acquisition is a life-long process. It is imperative that providers become knowledgeable about all the different dimensions of Latinx families to personalize the treatment and to avoid a one-size-fits-all approach (Alegria & Woo, 2009; Smith & Montilla, 2006).

Cultural competence must address the unique experiences of the way that families of HIV-infected clients experience stigma, historical trauma, trauma, oppression, and discrimination. An intersectionality lens is needed to understand how socioeconomic status, immigration status, acculturation, sexual orientation and gender expression, geography, drug use, and health status affect Latino families (Werkmeister Rozas & Smith, 2009). Providers also need to be aware of the centrality of the family and the extended family and also the different definitions of family. People are connected by blood, adoption, relationship agreement, emotional links, and a strong sense of connectedness. Familism, which is the strong belief in family, is important to Latinx and a source of support, self-definition, care, guidance, and healing. When family ties are cut off, this can be the source of suffering, isolation, depression, perceived cultural incompatibilities and stress for many Latinx. Some studies have suggested that when *"familismo"* is too strong, this might deter the family from seeking outside services in order to keep the "problem" within the family (Cardemil & Sarmiento, 2009). When working with families affected by HIV/AIDS, it is important to explore the meaning of family and to work with clients with a family perspective in mind. Providers should embrace religious beliefs and spirituality, which are a means of coping under hardships and disadvantages. Many Latino families in the United States are *transnational*, living in the United States and coming from their home country gives them a "third identity" which means that *"no son de aqui ni son de alla"* (they are not from here and they are not from there). Transnationalism also means having two or three identities, two countries, and two or three cultures, and not having to pick one over the other one as in acculturation. When working with Latinx, the cultural value of *personalismo* is also important. *Personalismo* relates to *familismo*, which is a central cultural construct for Latinx; it refers to the importance of personal goodness, interpersonal interactions, and reciprocity that involve respect, honor, and courtesy (Werkmeister Rozas & Smith, 2009). One the relationship with the provider has been established, families might have a greater need of *personalismo* with the provider. *Respeto* refers to the cultural belief that everyone deserves to be treated with respect and courtesy, especially lines of authority within the family structure. *Espiritismo* refers to the belief that "spirits" of ancestors are present in a spiritual form to provide support and guidance, and also "punishment." For some Latinx, illnesses, this case HIV/AIDS, are thought to be caused by spiritual forces that causes physical and emotional suffering. Some families might attribute HIV to a punishment from God for being homosexual and having sexual relationships with many sexual partners. *Espiritismo* is also embedded in fatalistic attitudes that behavior cannot be changed. Providers must explore these belief systems and provide restructuring. Since every cultural value has protective and risk factors, providers should look for the positives of the cultural values to help families in a culturally embedded perspective and to enable families to cope with HIV/AIDS to deal with the acceptance of difference within the family.

## CASE VIGNETTE

Juan is a 30-year-old man who was born in El Salvador. He came to the United States about 2 years ago after planning the trip for several months. Juan started the journey going to different countries in Central America. Upon arriving in Mexico, he contacted several people upon the recommendation from some friends from his native hometown. In Mexico, he spent several weeks hiding from the police and waiting for the "coyotes" who will help him cross the border into the United States. While being in captivity, he was raped, and forced to perform sexual acts with both women and men by two of the "coyotes," he mentions that it was a brutal act and could not say anything otherwise he will be killed and his plans to come to the United States will end. Juan crossed the border via the desert; the journey almost killed him, because he suffered from hunger, thirst and at the border a bullet almost hit him. Civilians were shooting migrants randomly and killed a person who was crossing the border with the group. Juan relates this as very traumatic. Once they crossed the border, they went to a house to hide and recuperate from the journey. At the house, he suffered physical and verbal abuse along with the other migrants housed there. Once his family in New York was contacted and the payment was made, Juan was able to travel to New York to reunite with his family.

Juan met with this mother, two brothers, his sister, and brother in-law. Juan started working in the landscaping business after looking for a job for several weeks. The payment was low but he was able to help to pay for the rent and send money back home to support his wife and two children who stayed in El Salvador. Juan started having flashbacks of the torture and rape that he suffered during this journey to the United States. He became depressed and anxious but had to hide how he felt from his family. He never told anyone about the incident. After some months of being in the United States, Juan started sweating and having fever at night. He also felt like the beginning of a cold. These symptoms went away and Juan started to feel better. Two years after migrating from El Salvador, Juan ended up in the hospital with pneumonia. After several tests, the doctor ordered an HIV test. The test came back positive, not for HIV but for AIDS. The disease had progressed. Juan's family had a hard time dealing with Juan's diagnosis. Juan's life changed forever since the diagnosis; because of his health, Juan was too weak to work. Because of his legal status, Juan had to apply for services in hospitals that see patients regardless of their immigration status. Juan did not qualify for Medicaid services or rental assistance. Juan was forced to continue living with his family who were undocumented with a very low income. His family in El Salvador suffered economically since Juan was unable to send money to support his family.

A counselor was assigned by the hospital to help him deal with his depression, anxiety, PTSD, and also with his sexual orientation. Juan was dealing with having feelings toward men and was fearful of telling his family. Juan felt that his family would blame him for having HIV as a result of doing something against God. Juan was living a double life in El Salvador. Juan mentioned to the counselor that he had to get married and have a family but that he always felt attracted to men. Gays are not accepted in El Salvador and some are killed. Juan felt that by telling his family about this attraction to men, his wife and children will be rejected from the rest of the family and by the community.

Juan mentioned that when his family knew about his diagnosis, they behaved differently toward him. His family gives him coffee and food in paper goods. Juan is not allowed to kiss or hug his nieces and nephews. Juan feels rejected by his family and this attitude has been detrimental to his health.

## DISCUSSION QUESTIONS

1. What will be the first step that you as provider will take with Juan to help him?
2. Identify relevant medical, social, and cultural factors for this case.
3. From an intersectionality perspective identify the stressors that Juan presents.
4. As a provider, what are the cultural elements to keep in mind in working with Juan?
5. As a culturally competent provider, what belief systems and cultural elements do you need to know to initiate change for this client?
6. Provide a case formulation and treatment for this client.

## REFERENCES

Alegria, M., & Woo, M. (2009). Conceptual issues in Latino mental health. In F. Villaruel, G. Carlo, J. Grau, M. Azmitia, N. Cabrera, & T. Chahin (Eds.), *Handbook of U.S. Latino psychology: Developmental and community-based perspectives* (pp. 15–30). Los Angeles, CA: Sage.

Arciniega, G. M., Anderson, T. C., Tovar-Blank, Z. G., & Tracey, T. J. G. (2008). Toward a fuller conception of machismo: Development of a traditional machismo and caballerismo scale. *Journal of Counseling Psychology, 55*, 19–33. doi:10.1037/0022-0167.55.1.19

Asencio, M. (2011). Gender conformity in migrant Puerto Rican gay masculinities. *Gender & Society, 25*(3), 335–354. doi:10.1177/0891243211409214

Cardemil, E. V., & Sarmiento, I. A. (2009). Clinical approaches to working with Latino adults. In F. Villaruel, G. Carlo, J. Grau, M. Azmitia, N. Cabrera, & T. Chahin (Eds.), *Handbook of U.S. Latino psychology: Developmental and community-based perspectives* (pp. 329–345). Los Angeles, CA: Sage.

Centers for Disease Control and Prevention. (2010). Retrieved from http://www.cdc.gov/nchhstp/newsroom/povertyandhivpressrelease.html

Centers for Disease Control and Prevention. (2017). *Diagnosis of HIV infection in the United States and dependent areas, 2017*. Retrieved from https://www.cdc.gov/hiv/statistics/overview/ataglance.html

Centers for Disease Control and Prevention (2019, March). HIV and pregnant women, infants, and children. Retrived from https://www.cdc.gov/hiv/pdf/group/gender/pregnantwomen/cdc-hiv-pregnant-women.pdf

Centers for Disease Control and Prevention. (2020). HIV and Hispanics/Latinos. Retrieved from: https://www.cdc.gov/hiv/group/racialethnic/hispaniclatinos/index.html

Cianelli, R., Ferrer, L., & McElmurry, B. J. (2008). HIV prevention and low-income Chilean women: Machismo, marianismo and HIV misconceptions. *Culture, Health and Sexuality, 10*(3), 297–306.

Cusick, L (1999). The process of disclosing positive HIV status: Findings from qualitative research. *Culture, Health and Sexuality, 1*(1), 3–18.

DeSantis, J., Gonzalez-Guarda, R. M., & Provencio-Vasquez, E. (2012). Psychosocial and cultural correlates of depression among Hispanic men with HIV infection: A pilot study. *Journal of Psychiatric and Mental Health Nursing, 19*(10), 860–869. doi:10.1111/j.1365-2850.2011.01865.x

Dorsey, S., Watts, M., Morse, E., Forehand, R., & Morse, P. (1999). Children whose mothers are HIV infected: Who resides in the home and is there a relationship to child psychosocial adjustment? *Journal of Family Psychology, 13*(1), 103–117. doi:10.1037/0893-3200.13.1.103

Dunkle, K. L., & Jewkes, R. (2007). Effective HIV prevention requires gender-transformative work with men. *Sexually Transmitted Infections, 83*(3), 173–174. doi:10.1136/sti.2007.024950

Falicov, C. J. (1998). *Latino families in therapy: A guide to multicultural practice*. New York, NY: Guilford Press.

Franklin, M., Schlundt, D., McClellan, L., Kinebrew, T., Sheats, J., Bulue, R., . . . Hargraves, M. (2007). Religious fatalism and its association with health behavior outcomes. *American Journal of Health Behavior, 31*(6), 563–572. doi:10.5993/AJHB.31.6.1

Gonzalez-Guarda, R. M., Vasquez, E. P., Urrutia, M. T., Villarruel, A. M., & Peragallo, N. (2011). Hispanic women's experiences with substance abuse, intimate partner violence, and risk for HIV. *Journal of Transcultural Nursing, 22*(1), 46–54. doi:10.1177/1043659610387079.

Harris, R. J., Firestone, J. M., & Vega, W. A. (2005). The interaction of country of origin, acculturation, and gender role ideology on wife abuse. *Social Science Quarterly, 86*(2), 463–483. doi:10.1111/j.0038-4941.2005.00313.x

Kalichman, S., Grebler, T. (2010). Reducing number of sex partners: Do we really need special intervention for sexual concurrency? *AIDS Behavior, 14*, 987–990.

Kirchner, J. T. (2019). The origin, evolution, and epidemiology of HIV1 and HIV2 (p. 15-20). In *Fundamentals of HIV medicine for the HIV specialist. American Academy of HIV Medicine.* New York, NY: Oxford University Press.

Latkin, C., Weeks, M. R, Glassman, L., Galletty, C, & Albarracin, D. (2010). A dynamic social systems model for considering structural factors in HIV prevention and detection. *AIDS Behavior, 14*(suppl2), 222–238. doi:10.1007/s10461-010-9804-y

Lauby, J., Smith, P. Stark, M., & Person, B. (2000). A community-level HIV prevention intervention for inner-city women: Results of the women and infants demonstration projects. *American Journal of Public Health, 90*(2), 216–222. doi:10.2105/AJPH.90.2.216

Lekas, H. M., Siegel, K., & Schrimshaw, E. (2006). Continuities and discontinuities in the experiences of felt and enacted stigma among women with HIV/AIDS. *Qualitative Health Research, 16*(9), 1165–1190. doi:10.1177/1049732306292284

Lichtenstein, B., Sturdevant, M., & Mujumdar, A. (2010). Psychosocial stressors of families affected by HIV/AIDS: Implications for social work practice. *Journal of HIV/AIDS & Social Services, 9*, 130–152. doi:10.1080/15381501003795717

Moreno, C. L. (2006). Latino families: The use of culture as an informative perspective. In R. Fong, R. G. McRoy, & C. Ortiz-Hendricks (Eds.), *Intersecting child welfare, substance abuse, and family violence: Culturally competent approaches* (pp. 166–186). Washington, DC: CSWE.

Moreno, C. L. (2007). The relationship between culture, gender, structural factors, abuse, trauma, and HIV/AIDS for Latinas. *Qualitative Health Research, 17*(3), 340–352. doi:10.1177/1049732306297387

Moreno, C. L. (2013). Latino families affected by HIV/AIDS. In M. Gonzalez & E. Congress (Eds.), *Multicultural perspectives in working with families* (3rd ed.). New York, NY: Springer Publishing Company.

National Latino Alliance Network. (2019). *Thirty-one facts about violence in the Latino community.* Retrieved from http://www.nationallatinonetwork.org/learn-more/facts-and-statistics/references

Pardasani, M., Moreno, C. L., & Forge, N. R. (2010). Cultural competence in HIV. In C. Poindexter (Ed). *Social services and social action in the HIV pandemic: Principles, methods and populations.* Hoboken, NJ: Wiley.

Perez-Foster, R. M. (2001). When immigration is trauma: Guidelines for the individual and family clinician. *American Journal of Orthopsychiatry, 71*(2), 153–170.

Qiao, S., Li, X., & Stanton, B. (2013). Disclosure of parental HIV infection to children: A systematic review of global literature. *AIDS and Behavior, 17*(1), 369–389.

Ryan, C., Huebner, D., Diaz, R. M., & Sanchez, J. (2009). Family Rejection as a Predictor of Negative Health Outcomes in White and Latino Lesbian, Gay, and Bisexual Young Adults. *Pediatrics, 123*, 346–342.

Shaffer, A., Jones, D., Kotchick, B., & Forehand, R. (2001). Telling the children: Disclosure of maternal HIV infection and its effects on child psychosocial adjustment. *Journal of Child and Family Studies, 10*(33), 301–313.

Slack, J., & Whiteford, S. (2011). Violence and migration on the Arizona-Sonora border. *Human Organization, 70*(1), 11–21.

Smith, R., & Montilla, E. (2006). *Counseling and family therapy with Latino populations: Strategies that work.* New York, NY: Routledge.

Thompkins, T. (2007). Disclosure of HIV status to children: To tell or not to tell . . . that is the question. *Journal of Child and Family Studies, 16*(6), 773–788. doi:10.1007/s10826-006-9124-z

U.S. Census Bureau. (2018). *Hispanic heritage month 2018: Profile American facts and figures: CB18-FF.07, September 2018.* Retrieved from https://www.census.gov/content/dam/Census/library/visualizations/2018/comm/hispanic-fff-2018.pdf

U.S. Census Bureau. (2019). *Hispanic poverty rate hit an all-time low in 2017.* Retrieved from https://www.census.gov/library/stories/2019/02/hispanic-poverty-rate-hit-an-all-time-low-in-2017.html

Watkins-Hayes, C. (2014). Intersectionality and the sociology of HIV/AIDS: Past, present, and future research directions. *Annual Review of Sociology, 40,* 431–457. doi:10.1146/annurev-soc-071312-145621

Werkmeister Rozas, L., & Smith, E. (2009). Being on this boat: The provision of culturally competent mental health services to people living with HIV/AIDS. *Journal of HIV/AIDS & Social Services, 8,* 166–187. doi:10.1080/15381500903077911

Whiteside, A. (2000). Poverty and HIV/AIDS in Africa. *Third World Quarterly, 23*(2), 313–332. doi:10.1080/01436590220126667

Yellowbird, M. (2004). Toys of genocide: icons of American colonialism. *Wicazo Sa Review, 19*(2), 43.

# 20

# Substance Abuse

LINDA WHITE-RYAN AND JANNA HEYMAN

## INTRODUCTION

Substance abuse is a serious public health crisis in the United States, with approximately 19.7 million people over the age of 12 having a substance use disorder (Substance Abuse and Mental Health Services Administration [SAMHSA], 2018a). Substance use disorders (SUDs) are a significant health problem that has been historically affected by racial discrimination and oppression (Skewes & Blume, 2019). These data are significant, but they do not truly capture how the health of many individuals, families, and communities of all races, ethnicities, cultures, and socioeconomic status are adversely impacted. It is imperative for continuing research to develop evidence-based practices and policies that address this challenging health issue.

A recent study showed that only 4.0 million people received any type of treatment for SUDs, yet so many individuals and their families are affected (SAMHSA, 2018a). Furthermore, the health and healthcare costs associated with substance abuse is staggering, with approximately $740 billion annually in costs related to healthcare, crime, lost work (National Institute on Drug Abuse, 2017). The information for different ages, races, and ethnicities provides further data that are noteworthy. Data on the percentage of SUDs for individuals aged 12 and older indicates similar trends for Whites (7.7%), Blacks/African Americans (6.8%), and Hispanics (6.6%). However, for American Indians and Alaska Natives, the percentage is higher at 12.8%, while Native Hawaiian and Pacific Islanders represent 4.6%, and Asians having the lowest percentage at 3.8% (SAMHSA, 2018b).

When considering gender, males tend to abuse and participate in risky alcohol consumption more frequently than females (Hunter, Goodie, Oordt, & Dobmeyer, 2017). According to Hunter et al. (2017), "Although risky drinking behavior can occur in anyone, those falling in multiple risk categories— male, 18–25 years old, and American Indian or Alaska Native, White, Hispanic, Native Hawaiians or other Pacific Islander—may be at greatest risk" (p. 176). Also at greater risk for SUDs are lesbian, gay, bisexual, and transgender individuals when compared to heterosexual individuals (Lipsky et al., 2012).

The stage of adolescence can be a challenging transition period of the lifespan to navigate. Numerous changes take place during adolescence both physically and psychologically. The adolescent brain is affected negatively by consistent exposure to alcohol and the abuse of other drugs due to the neurocognitive changes happening during adolescent development (Siegel, 2013; Volkow, 2015). Scientific research has reported that the human brain is not fully developed until approximately the age of 26 (Volkow, Koob, & McLellan, 2016). Data with respect to age, as well as race and ethnicity, are important to understand because many youth are engaged in the use and abuse of mood-altering substances (Volkow et al., 2016). Alcohol use is extremely prevalent and is a significant problem among adolescents, with more than three in five high school students reporting having had at least one drink (Kann et al., 2018). Binge drinking among adolescents (five or more alcoholic beverages consumed in one sitting) is common among youth and is important to address. For example, in 2017, 1.3 million youth aged 12 to 17 reported binge alcohol use in the past month (SAMHSA, 2019). When comparisons were made to the national average, "past-month binge alcohol use was higher among non-Hispanic White youth and was lower among Hispanic youth and among non-Hispanic Black and Asian youth" (SAMHSA, 2019, p. 5). It is interesting to note that immigrant Hispanic youth may begin abusing alcohol due to sociocultural mechanisms such as difficulties with acculturation (Burrow-Sanchez, 2014; Burrow-Sanchez, Minami, & Hops, 2015; Lui & Zamboanga, 2018). It is important to understand that Latino youth are in need of effective treatments because, as compared to White youth (12.7%), they experience 14% higher rates of substance abuse (CASA, 2011).

While alcohol still remains the number one substance that adolescents in high school use and abuse, according to the 2018 Monitoring the Future (MTF) survey of drug use and attitudes among eighth, 10th, and 12th graders in hundreds of schools across the country, vaping is increasingly significant. The study found that 17.6% of eighth graders, 32.3% of 10th graders, and 37.3% of 12th graders reporting past-year vaping. Miech et al. (2019) stated that "increases in vaping in 2018 are the largest ever seen for any of the 30-day prevalence outcomes monitored by Monitoring the Future in the 44 years it has continuously tracked adolescent substance use" (pp. 528–529). While these data do not address the cultural differences, they point to the peer culture of use of vaping by many adolescents today. As vaping has increased, the use of cigarettes has declined with only 3.2% among youth aged 12 to 17 overall, and "among Hispanic youth, and among non-Hispanic White, Black, and American Indian or Alaska Native youth" (p. 1). Marijuana use has also declined among youth aged 12 to 17 (SAMHSA, 2019).

Substance abuse is not a problem that affects only the lives of young people. It also influences the lives of adults and older adults. There are significant racial/ethnic differences found in prevalence rates for binge drinking in adults. Bryant and Kim (2012) found that the most common rate of binge drinking was "among non-Hispanic Whites (11.9%), followed by Latinos (10.8%), American Indian/Alaska Natives (9.8%), Blacks (8.0%), and Asians (4.2%)" (p. 208). The abuse of opioids has created a current climate of fear and crisis in the United States. According to the CDC, between 1999 to 2017, more than 702,000 people have died from a drug overdose. Unfortunately one of the alarming statistics is that in 2017, more than 70,000 people died from drug overdoses, making it a leading cause of injury-related death in the United States. (Centers for Disease Control and Prevention, 2020). "Among the many health problems affected by racial discrimination and oppression, both historical and current, are substance use disorders" (Skewes & Blume, 2019, p. 88).

The number of adults aged 50 and older with alcohol and substance abuse problems are projected to double from 2.8 million to 5.7 million by the year 2020 (Wu & Blazer, 2011). Mattson, Lipari, Hays, and Van Horn (2017) stress that this growing problem contributes to older adults' use of emergency departments, falls, and other significant health concerns. Older adults are particularly vulnerable to developing substance use problems due to the physiological changes and psychological and social changes that take place during senescence. For example, many older adults are required to take multiple prescription medications and over-the-counter (OTC) medications. In the assessment of older adults, many with substance abuse issues and SUDs are "invisible" to healthcare providers and family members and fail to be identified (Han, Gfroerer, Colliver, & Penne, 2009; Oslin, 2006). Older adults may "take prescribed medication (sometimes not as prescribed) for physical and psychiatric problems, buy over-the-counter medication (which they may not take according to instructions), drink alcohol, smoke cigarettes, and use illicit drugs" (Crome & Crome, 2005, p. 343). Han et al. (2009) have estimated that 90% of older adults take prescription and OTC medications. They explain that when the medications are combined with alcohol, the interaction can produce dangerous consequences.

While data by race and age are not available, an estimated 11.4 million people misused opioids in 2017, including 11.1 million people who misused drugs to relieve pain and 886,000 heroin users (SAMHSA, 2018a). An earlier study by the Drug Abuse Warning Network (DAWN) reported 750,529 drug-related emergency department visits by adults aged 65 or older, where 105,982 visits involved illicit drug use, use of alcohol in combination with other substances, or non-medical use of pharmaceuticals (e.g., prescription medications, OTC remedies, dietary supplements) (Mattson et al., 2017).

This chapter highlights the importance of addressing the current public health crisis of substance abuse and SUDs with various population groups from different cultural backgrounds. Client-centered practice from an intersectional perspective with a special focus on families is emphasized. The importance of health practices and policies that decrease disparities in healthcare are important to the well-being of marginalized groups from different cultures is extremely important. Culture and its impact on perceptions, beliefs, and behaviors of different groups are critical to developing evidence-based treatments for substance abuse that are efficacious.

## INTERSECTIONALITY

An intersectional lens is crucial to providing competent services for substance abuse problems. It provides a lens that captures the complexity of different interrelated systems. The core of intersectionality is that it considers the impact of the overlapping of different systems and its contribution to oppression and discrimination (Crenshaw, 1991). Intersectionality addresses social justice inequities by promoting changes in the social ideas that create the marginalization of certain individuals by narrowly defining their identities (Chun, Lipsitz, & Shin, 2013). Kimberle Crenshaw (1989) originally coined the term "intersectionality" in a law review article. Crenshaw's work at that time focused on identifying the plight of Black and immigrant women in the workplace. Crenshaw (1991) stated, "My focus on the intersections of race and gender only highlights the need to account for multiple grounds of identity when considering how the social world is constructed" (p. 1245).

In regard to the public health problem of substance abuse, it is important to consider the significance of intersectionality. For example, individuals experiencing substance abuse problems who belong to a sexual minority group with differing social identities in race and gender (such as women) may experience more discrimination then that of White males (Mereish & Bradford, 2014). However, it is also true in general that those individuals with a diagnosis of a substance-related disorder experience more stigma as compared to those who do not have a substance-related disorder (Earnshaw, Smith, Cunningham, & Copenhaver, 2015). Heathcare professionals across all disciplines have an ethical responsibility to be aware of their own personal biases in order to provide culturally competent and responsive services to the clients and families they serve.

## MULTICULTURAL PRACTICE

Substance abuse treatment has made significant advances during the past 20 years. However, there remains a growing public health danger to individuals, families, and communities throughout the United States (Volkow et al., 2016). Currently, among most healthcare professionals substance-related disorders and addiction are considered a disease with significant consequences. Throughout history, there have been efforts to address the serious adverse health problems associated with substance abuse and addiction (Henninger & Sung, 2014).

One of the most notable contributions to help shift the perception of alcohol abuse as a moral failing to understanding it as a disease was made by Dr. Benjamin Rush in the nineteenth century (Henninger & Sung, 2014). Another important influence to the recovery of individuals suffering from problems with alcohol was the development of the self-help organization of Alcoholics Anonymous in 1935 (Lemanski, 2001). This self-help, peer-facilitated group was started by two men that both had serious and seemingly hopeless addictions to alcohol, Dr. Bob Smith and Bill Wilson. The contribution of these two men has had a tremendous influence on providing ongoing support for individuals throughout the world with severe alcohol use disorders.

Currently, a growing body of research placing importance on providing integrated models of treatment has been found to be state-of-the-art for those with SUDs, stressing the need for integrated behavioral health treatment (Hunter et al., 2017). Integrated behavioral health can address the many chronic health challenges faced by those individuals with substance-related disorders including diabetes, co-occurring mental health issues, hypertension, and other health problems (SAMHSA, 2019).

A focus on practice with clients that is collaborative, centered on the specific needs of the client and their families, and is culturally responsive with an emphasis on integrated care is most effective (Huey, Tilley, Jones, & Smith, 2014; Hunter et al., 2017). Healthcare practitioners across disciplines work with individuals with problems with substance abuse and SUDs. The significance of including family members whenever possible in assessment and treatment plans is substantial. Utilizing an intersectional approach in practice involves awareness on the part of the healthcare provider to understand that race, gender, socioeconomic status, and sexual orientation all interact and may contribute to oppression, discrimination, and power imbalances (Mereish & Bradford, 2014). In order to achieve successful outcomes when working with diverse populations, it is paramount to understand that the level of self-awareness providers have developed has a correlation to successful treatment. Self-awareness is directly linked with culturally competent services provision and the ability to work effectively with individuals and families from diverse cultural backgrounds (Lui & Zamboanga, 2018).

Ethical considerations regarding culture must guide practitioners' approaches to client-centered practice at all times. This includes informed consent, confidentiality, scope of practice, and competence (Runyan, Robinson, & Gould, 2013). The *Diagnostic and Statistical Manual of Mental Disorders, Fifth Edition* (DSM-5; American Psychiatric Association [APA], 2013) developed a section entitled "The Cultural Formulation Interview" that provides culturally sensitive information to guide practitioners in making clinical diagnoses (APA, 2013). This section of *DSM-5* was developed due to the expanding knowledge in the healthcare field regarding the essential need for culturally responsive approaches in working with individuals with mental health disorders (Dziegielewski, 2015; Zuckerman, 2019).

The widespread problem of substance abuse has a great deal of stigma attached to it. Individuals and families frequently experience feelings of shame associated with substance abuse creating a barrier to reaching out for treatment. The family is the most important basis for the growth and development of individuals (Lander, Howsare, & Byrne, 2013). Families affected by substance abuse and SUDs experience serious problems with feelings of shame and family dysfunction, and as well may have intersecting difficulties with sociocultural stress and substance abuse and may suffer from feelings of shame and alienation (Gilbert & Zemore, 2016). Sociocultural stress refers to bicultural stress (stress from trying to adapt to a new culture and continue to maintain the old culture) and perceived discrimination, and may lead to the abuse of alcohol. Multicultural families may have challenges that include substance abuse and feel powerless about finding solutions.

Treatment models that address family-based approaches to deal with substance abuse and substance-related disorders is critical when working with families from different cultures. Keeping in mind language needs when conducting assessments, and developing intervention plans increases the likelihood of effective outcomes. Providing psychoeducation to families about substance abuse while also respecting varying cultural differences opens the level of communication within the family system. This can assist families to understand the biological as well as mental implications of substance abuse.

Of special importance is the need to help both individuals and families to understand that the neurotransmitter dopamine is one of the key agents in the development of addiction (SAMHSA, 2015). The reward pathway is stimulated when dopamine is released in the brain and this in turn activates the reward center of the brain (Volkow, 2015). According to Volkow (2015), the "brain is hijacked" when there is consistent abuse of mood-altering drugs.

## SCREENING AND ASSESSMENT

Effective screening is the first step in making a diagnosis leading to development of an individualized treatment plan that addresses the needs of the individual (Dziegielewski, 2015; Zuckerman, 2019). Treatment providers conduct assessments in varied settings such as hospitals, community agencies, mental health clinics, schools, homeless shelters, and other healthcare settings. Screening, assessment, and diagnosis may be different for different cultures. According to Zuckerman (2019), when conducting assessments it is important to remember that "[c]ulture may include ethnicity, race, religion, social class, gender, age and similar categories" (p. 273). Culture touches all aspects of human behaviors, images of self, and the way in which an individual may respond to treatment (Zuckerman, 2019). According to Dziegielewski (2015), "during those times of emotional or psychological turmoil, human nature is such that all individuals regardless of age, strive for meaning in their lives using their cultural lens: their values, beliefs and experiences" (p. 57). When screening for possible substance use disorders it is critical to consider culture and to utilize an intersectional lens.

The model of Screening, Brief Intervention, and Referral to Treatment (SBIRT) provides a universal screening tool that is brief and easy to utilize to address public health problem of substance abuse (Mitchell, Grycyznski, O'Grady, & Schwartz, 2013; Ong-Flaherty, 2012). SBIRT is meant to identify the individuals who may be at risk for substance abuse issues, which makes it useful for screening of adolescents to identify if there are indicators of the possible risk of future substance abuse (Johnston, O'Malley, Bachman, & Schulenberg, 2012).

An extremely simple to use screening tool for alcohol use problems is the CAGE. The CAGE is the easiest screening instrument for possible alcohol problems. It contains four questions: (a) Have you ever felt you should cut down on your drinking? (b) Have people annoyed you by criticizing your drinking? (c) Have you ever felt bad or guilty about your drinking? (d) Have you ever had a drink first thing in the morning to get rid of your hangover or to steady your nerves? (Ewing, 1984; Mayfield, McLeod, & Hall, 1974). A positive score is two positive answers and the instrument is reported to have excellent validity and reliability (Ewing, 1984). Another instrument found to be effective for screening of alcohol problems is the Alcohol Use Disorders Identification Test (AUDIT). This instrument contains 10 questions and therefore is brief and easy to administer. The maximum score is 40 with a score of eight or higher indicating possible problem drinking (Fujii et al., 2016). The Drug Abuse Screening Test (DAST) is a 28-question self-report instrument that screens for drug abuse. The questions are yes/no with a one-point value. The range is from 0 to 28. A score of 6 indicates a possible problem, and a score of 12 indicates a substance use disorder (Yudko, Lozhkina, & Fouts, 2007).

The Michigan Alcoholism Screening Test is a longer screening instrument with a 24-item geriatric version (MAST-G) that includes elderly specific concerns (Blow et al., 1992). The cut-off score is five positive responses, and studies have found a comparable sensitivity and specificity to the CAGE in identifying alcohol problems in older adults (Menninger, 2002). A shorter version of 10 items from the MAST-G, known as the SMAST-G, is reported to be valid and reliable. The cut-off score is two. This instrument is more appropriate and sensitive for use with older adults (Blow et al., 1992).

The assessment process follows screening, and identifies and interprets all of the pertinent information needed to develop an accurate diagnosis. A complete medical history begins with history of the present complaint and moving on to the individual's developmental history. Family history is important in assessing the needs of the individual, especially in the case of possible SUDs or other co-occurring mental health disorders. It is vital in conducting an assessment for a substance-related issue to ask specific questions regarding the individual's history of using mood-altering substances, regarding onset, type of drugs used frequency, duration, and the progression of use (Dziegielewski, 2015; Zuckerman, 2019).

Co-occurring substance-related disorders may be present along with other mental health disorders; therefore, specific questions during the assessment about mental health history of both the individual and the family must be included. Family assessment is part of the overall picture. Family stressors are important to consider in both the social and cultural context of the family system. After the assessment process is completed, a formulation of the problem leads to developing a diagnosis based on the criteria included in the *DSM-5*. The diagnosis dictates the level of treatment indicated if the individual is determined to have a substance-related disorder.

## TREATMENT

State-of-the-art treatment approaches include the use of evidence-based practices to treat the public health crisis of substance-related problems. Motivational interviewing (MI), cognitive behavioral therapy (CBT), and harm reduction are among the most frequently utilized best practices found to be effective for substance abuse (Dziegielewski, 2015; Zuckerman, 2019).

According to Madson, Schumacher, Baer, and Martino (2016), evidence supporting the use of MI for the treatment of substance abuse and SUDs is substantial. MI is an evidence-based treatment with a great deal of support for use with substance abusers and individuals with substance-related disorders. It originated in the addictions field because William Miller found that confrontational methods did not seem to be effective. William Miller and Stephen Rollnick together developed MI in 1991. MI is a client-centered, directive method for enhancing intrinsic motivation to change by exploring and resolving ambivalence. Most models are designed for the action stage of treatment. However, this model views cycling through the stages of change several times as normal, not as failure. Interventions match the stage of the client and their readiness for change. Resistance is perceived in terms of the clinician not understanding the stage of readiness to change of the individual. The work between the individual and practitioner focuses on the process of change. This collaborative process involves shared decision-making. The major goal is to encourage change in the direction of health (DiClemente, 2018; Miller & Rollnick, 2013).

Another evidence-based approach for working with individuals with SUDs is CBT. CBT is grounded in the idea that dysfunctional thinking has an effect on the individual's mood (feelings) and behavior (Beck, 2011). Underlying beliefs and thought patterns are considered to contribute to certain behaviors. Changing those thoughts through CBT is helpful when dealing with dysfunctional and self-destructive behaviors. A main premise of CBT for use with individuals with substance abuse problems is that repeated use of substances is related to reinforcement of certain behaviors (both positive and negative) including the stimulation of the pleasure pathway of the brain. An important component of CBT when working with individuals with substance-related disorders is teaching individuals about behaviors, conditioning, triggers, and the phenomenon of drug craving. A focused education about cognitive skills such as using thought interruption to deal with urges is useful in preventing relapse (McHugh, Hearon, & Otto, 2010). Empirical evidence has shown CBT to be an efficacious treatment for those with SUDs. Analysis of dysfunctional beliefs and anticipation of the effects of substance use teach the individual about certain cues and triggers that may lead to relapse (McHugh et al., 2010).

A model that has caused some conflict among professionals is harm reduction. Many healthcare providers believe that abstinence from all mood-altering substances should be the goal of treatment. Proponents of the model of harm reduction believe that the most critical aspect of providing care for individuals with substance abuse problems who may not be ready to embrace models that include abstinence is safety from harm. Psychoeducation is an important component of treatment to educate individuals about the possible dangerous consequences of drug use in hopes to begin to reduce use. In harm reduction, drug use is not viewed as positive or negative. The individual with the substance-related problem is always given the right of self-determination and thought competent to make choices about using drugs and is approached with respect and a nonjudgmental attitude at all times (Marlatt, Larimer, & Witkiewitz, 2012). Education and treatment tactics include overdose education programs including information regarding naloxone to deal with overdose of opioids (Hawk, Vaca, & D'Onofrio, 2015; Volkow, 2015). The approach of harm reduction is a public health approach that is evidence-based and presents strategies to give support to substance abusers not ready to stop using and to keep them safe from harm.

Working with families from diverse cultures with an emphasis on understanding the family's cultural identity promotes engagement and a collaborative spirit of partnership between the family and treatment professional. Families with addiction have been referred to as having a family disease. This is because every member of the family system is affected. A family is a social system, in which each of its parts interact and communicate with other parts of the system in a fluid and dynamic exchange of energy. Families in which substance abuse exists can become systems that are bound in progressively debilitating processes of conflict, disorganization, and poor communication.

Family approaches that are evidence based include such models as brief strategic family therapy (BSFT) used for families where poor communication is identified and usually takes place over 12 to 14 sessions. The family communication style is addressed and negative interaction patterns are changed (Zimic & Jukic, 2012). Multisystemic therapy (MST) is a community-based type of therapy used to address families where a member such as an adolescent is experiencing substance abuse issues that are viewed within the family context (Henggeler, Schoenwald, Borduin, Rowland, & Cunningham, 2009). MST is effective in many situations where the substance use is affecting school performance, family discipline issues, and delinquent or criminal behavior. Research has shown that family influences including cultural values have a significant impact on the attitude of adolescents toward the use of substances (Burrow-Sanchez et al., 2015).

Pharmacology is an extremely important component of treatment for SUDs. First and foremost is the determination made for medical safety, which includes assessment of the need for possible medical detoxification (Volkow, 2015). Medical approaches that utilize medications as part of a treatment plan are critical to healing and support the recovery process both physically and mentally for individuals that have severe substance-related disorders (Volkow et al., 2016, Urschel, 2009). Substance abuse is a public health problem and treatment needs can be costly. For those fortunate enough to have insurance coverage for medical needs there remains a stigma and disparity for funding of substance use disorders when compared to other chronic medical illnesses (McLellan & Woodworth, 2014; Volkow, 2015). Unfortunately, there are health disparities that exist for those marginalized individuals who do not have access to adequate healthcare due to lack of resources. Policy advocacy needs to be part of addressing the public health emergency of substance abuse currently facing the nation. Developing policies that support healthcare reform and treatment are critical in addressing the major public health crisis of SUDs.

## CASE VIGNETTE

Sam is a 17-year-old Hispanic male going into his senior year of high school. He currently lives with his parents. Sam was referred to a mental health agency by a social worker at his high school. Sam had repeatedly been missing classes and was caught drinking alcohol and smoking marijuana on school premises. A bilingual clinician was assigned to work with Sam and his family. During the assessment, Sam reports that he does not think his behavior is "such a big deal." He had previously been involved in sports but states "I have no interest anymore." Information provided by his parents indicates they have noticed many changes in Sam during the past 10 months. Sam's parents do not speak much English and Sam used to be very helpful to them in assisting with paying bills and so on. However, they report that now he is not home much at all. Sam's grades in school have slipped. Sam's parents had hopes that he would be the first in the family to attend college. Sam was supposed to apply to college in his senior year. Sam was a good student up until about 10 months ago. At that time, he started to hang out with some young people in his neighborhood that appear to use drugs and get into trouble with the police according to Sam's parents. Sam has two siblings, a brother named Roderigo who is 13 and a sister named Luisa who is 11 with whom he reports he has a good relationship. Sam's parents seem distraught and Sam's father stated, "We had such high hopes for Sam and now we just don't know where to turn." The parents are in their mid-50s and both work at jobs that do not require them to speak English. The family is from Mexico and both sets of grandparents live with the family.

## CONCLUSION

Individuals of diverse cultures suffer from SUDs. These individuals and the families that love them face devastating adverse consequences. It is crucial for research to continue to develop best practices and policies that address the public health emergency that exists across all socioeconomic levels, races, genders, cultures, and so on.

Evidence-based practices that are culturally sensitive, and that address substance abuse problems of individuals, families, and communities are paramount to achieving successful outcomes. Education regarding the deleterious effects of substance abuse on the human brain are important in increasing awareness of all members of society.

Treatment approaches such as MI and CBT have been shown in numerous studies to be efficacious and in combination with medication-assisted therapy have brought hope to many individuals and families affected by substance abuse. Advances in healthcare include the integration of mental health, substance abuse, and primary care services and have proven to be an effective approach to caring for people with multiple needs.

Finally, the training and education of healthcare professionals in the importance of culturally relevant and sensitive treatment for SUDs is vital. Understanding substance abuse and recognizing each person and their cultural background and experience is valuable in making a difference in the lives of individuals, families, and communities with substance abuse issues.

## DISCUSSION QUESTIONS

1. What are some important points for working with Sam and his family using a multicultural perspective?
2. What are some evidence-based approaches and best practices for the treatment of Sam's substance abuse problems?
3. Should Sam's family be involved in treatment?

## REFERENCES

American Psychiatric Association. (2013). *Diagnostic and statistical manual of mental disorders* (5th ed.). Arlington, VA: Author.

Beck, J. S. (2011). *Cognitive behavior therapy: Basics and beyond* (2nd ed.). New York, NY: The Guilford Press.

Blow, F. C., Brower, K. J., Schulenberg, J. E., Demo-Dananberg, L. M., Young, K. J., & Beresford, T. P. (1992). The Michigan Alcoholism Screening Test, Geriatric Version (MAST-G): A new elderly specific screening instrument [Abstract]. *Alcoholism: Clinical and Experimental Research, 16,* 172.

Bryant, A. N., & Kim, G. (2012). Racial/ethnic differences in prevalence and correlates of binge drinking among older adults. *Aging and Mental Health, 16*(2), 208–217. doi:10.1080/13607863.2011.615735

Burrow-Sanchez, J. J. (2014). Measuring ethnic identity in Latino adolescents with substance use disorders. *Substance Use and Misuse, 49,* 982–986. doi:10.3109/10826084.2013.794839

Burrow-Sanchez, J. J, Minami, T., & Hops, H. (2015). Cultural accommodation of group substance abuse treatment for Latino adolescents: Results of an RCT. *Cultural Diversity and Ethnic Minority Psychology, 21*(4), 571–583. doi:10.1037/cdp0000023

CASA. (2011). *Adolescent substance use: America's #1 public health problem*. New York, NY: Columbia University Press.

Centers for Disease Control and Prevention. (2020). Opioid overdose. https://www.cdc.gov/drugoverdose/index.html

Chun, J. J., Lipsitz, G., & Shin, Y. (2013). Intersectionality as a social movement strategy: Asian immigrant women advocates. *Journal of Women in Culture and Society, 389*(41), 917–940. doi:10.1086/669575

Crenshaw, K. (1989). Demarginalizing the intersection of race and sex: A Black feminist critique of antidiscrimination doctrine, feminist theory and antiracist politics. *University of Chicago Legal Forum, 1989*, 139–167.

Crenshaw, K. (1991). Mapping the margins: Intersectionality, identity politics, and violence against women of color. In M. A. Finemane & R. Mykitiuk (Eds.), *The public nature of private violence* (pp. 93–118). New York, NY: Routledge.

Crome, I., & Crome, P. (2005). "At your age what does it matter": Myths and realities about older people who use substances. *Drug Education, Prevention & Policy, 12*(5), 343–347. doi:10.1080/09687630500221473

DiClemente, C. C. (2018). *Addiction and change: How addictions develop and addicted people change* (2nd ed.). New York, NY: The Guilford Press.

Dziegielewski, S. (2015). *DSM-5 in action* (3rd ed.). Hoboken, NJ: John Wiley & Sons, Inc.

Earnshaw, V. A., Smith, L. R., Cunningham, C. O., & Copenhaver, M. M. (2015). Intersectionality of internalized HIV stigma: Implications for depressive symptoms. *Journal of Health Psychology, 20*(8), 1083–1089. doi:10.1177/1359105313507964

Ewing, J. A. (1984). Detecting alcoholism: The CAGE questionnaire. *JAMA, 252*, 1905–1907. doi:10.1001/jama.1984.03350140051025

Fujii, H., Nishimoto, N., Yamaguchi, S., Kurai, O., Miyano, M., Ueda, W., & Okawa, K. (2016). The Alcohol Use Disorders Identification Test for Consumption (AUDIT-C) is more useful than pre-existing laboratory tests for predicting hazardous drinking: A cross-sectional study. *BMC Public Health, 16*(1), 379. doi:10.1186/s12889-016-3053-6

Gilbert, P. A., & Zemore, S. E. (2016). Discrimination and drinking: A systematic review of the evidence. *Social Science & Medicine, 161*, 178–194. doi:10.1016/j.socscimed.2016.06.009

Han, B., Gfroerer, J. C., Colliver, J. D., & Penne, M. A. (2009). Substance use disorder among older adults in the United States in 2020. *Addiction, 104*(1), 88–96. doi:10.1111/j.1360-0443.2008.02411.x

Hawk, K. F., Vaca, F. E., & D'Onofrio, G. (2015). Reducing fatal opioid overdose: Prevention, treatment and harm reduction strategies. *The Yale Journal of Biology and Medicine, 88*(3), 235–245.

Henggeler, S. W., Schoenwald, S. K., Borduin, C. M., Rowland, M. D., & Cunningham, P. B. (2009). *Multisystemic therapy for antisocial behavior in children and adolescents* (2nd ed.). New York, NY: The Guildford Press.

Henninger, A., & Sung, H. E. (2014). History of substance abuse treatment. In Bruinsma G., & Weisburd D. (Eds). *Encyclopedia of criminology and criminal justice.* (pp. 2257–2269). New York, NY: Springer Publishing Company.

Huey, S. J., Tilley, J. L., Jones, E. O., & Smith, C. A. (2014). The contribution of cultural competence to evidence-based care for ethnically diverse populations. *Annual Review of Clinical Psychology, 10*, 305–338. doi:10.1146/annurev-clinpsy-032813-153729

Hunter, C. L., Goodie, J. L., Oordt, A. C., & Dobmeyer. A. C. (2017). *Integrated behavioral health primary care: Step-by-step guidance for assessment and intervention* (2nd ed.). Washington, DC: American Psychological Association.

Johnston, L. D., O'Malley, P. M., Bachman, J. G., & Schulenberg, J. E. (2012). *Monitoring the future national results on adolescent drug use: Overview of key findings, 2011.* Ann Arbor, MI: Institute for Social Research, The University of Michigan

Kann, L., McManus, T., Harris, W. A., Shanklin, S. L., Flint, K. H., Queens, B., . . . Ethier, K. A. (2018). Youth Risk Behavior Surveillance – United States, 2017. *Surveillance Summaries, 67*(8), 1–114. Retrieved from https://www.cdc.gov/mmwr/volumes/67/ss/ss6708a1.htm?s_cid=hy-yrbs2017-mmwr

Lander, L., Howsare, J., & Byrne, M. (2013). The impact of substance use disorders on families and children: From theory to practice. *Social Work in Public Health, 28*(3–4), 194–205. doi:10.1080/19371918.2013.759005

Lemanski, M. (2001). *History of addiction and recovery in the United States.* Tucson, AZ: Sharp Press.

Lipsky, S., Krupski, A., Roy-Byrne, P., Huber, A., Lucenko, B. A., & Mancuso, D. (2012). Impact of sexual orientation and co-occurring disorders on chemical dependency treatment outcomes. *Journal of Studies on Alcohol and Drugs, 73*, 401–412. doi:10.15288/jsad.2012.73.401

Lui, P. P., & Zamboanga, B. L. (2018). Acculturation and alcohol use among Asian Americans: A meta-analytic review. *Psychology of Addictive Behaviors, 32*, 173–180. doi:10.1037/adb0000340

Madson, M. B., Schumacher, J. A., Baer, J. S., & Martino, S. (2016). Motivational interviewing for substance use: Mapping out the next generation of research. *Journal of Substance Abuse Treatment, 65*, 1–5. doi:10.1016/j.jsat.2016.02.003

Marlatt, G. A., Larimer, M. E., & Witkiewitz, K. (Eds.). (2012). *Harm reduction: Pragmatic strategies for managing high-risk behaviors.* New York, NY: The Guilford Press.

Mattson, M., Lipari, R. N., Hays, C., & Van Horn, S. L. (2017). *A day in the life of older adults: Substance use facts.* Rockville, MD: The CBHSQ Report: Center for Behavioral Health Statistics and Quality, Substance Abuse and Mental Health Services Administration.

Mayfield, G., McLeod, P., & Hall, C. (1974). The CAGE questionnaire: Validation of a new screening instrument. *American Journal of Psychiatry, 131*, 1121–1123.

McHugh, R. K., Hearon, B. A., & Otto, M. W. (2010). Cognitive behavioral therapy for substance use disorders. *Psychiatric Clinics of North America, 33*(3), 511–525. doi:10.1016/j.psc.2010.04.012

McLellan, A. T., & Woodworth, A. M. (2014). The Affordable Care Act and treatment for "substance use disorders:" Implications of ending segregated behavioral healthcare. *Journal of Substance Abuse Treatment, 46*(5), 541–545. doi:10.1016/j.jsat.2014.02.001

Menninger, J. A. (2002). Assessment and treatment of alcoholism and substance related disorders in the elderly. *Bulletin of the Menninger Clinic, 66*(2), 166–184. doi:10.1521/bumc.66.2.166.23364

Mereish, E., & Bradford, J. (2014). Intersecting identities and substance use problems: Sexual orientation, gender, race, and lifetime substance use problems. *Journal of Studies on Alcohol and Drugs, 75*, 179–188. doi:10.15288/jsad.2014.75.179

Miech, R. A., Johnston, L. D., O'Malley, P. M., Bachman, J. G., Schulenberg, J. E., & Patrick, M. E. (2019). *Monitoring the future national survey results on drug use, 1975–2018: Volume I, Secondary school students.* Ann Arbor, MI: Institute for Social Research, The University of Michigan. Retrieved from http://monitoringthefuture.org/pubs.html#monographs

Miller, W. R., & Rollnick, S. (2013). *Motivational interviewing: Helping people change* (3rd ed.). New York, NY: The Guilford Press.

Mitchell, S. G., Gryczynski, J., O'Grady, K. E., & Schwartz, R. P. (2013). SBIRT for adolescent drug and alcohol use: Current status and future directions. *Journal of Substance Abuse Treatment, 44*(5), 463–472. doi:10.1016/j.jsat.2012.11.005

National Institute on Drug Abuse. (2017). *Trends and statistics.* Retrieved from https://www.drugabuse.gov/related-topics/trends-statistics

Ong-Flaherty, C. (2012). Screening, brief intervention, and referral to treatment: A nursing perspective. *Journal of Emergency Nursing, 38*(1), 54–56. doi:10.1016/j.jen.2011.09.009

Oslin, D. W. (2006). The changing face of substance misuse in older adults. *Psychiatric Times, 23*(13), 41–48.

Runyan, C., Robinson, P., & Gould, D. A. (2013). Ethical issues facing providers in collaborative primary care settings: Do current guidelines suffice to guide the future of team based, primary care? *Families, Systems & Health, 31*, 1–8. doi:10.1037/a0031895

Siegel, D. (2013). *Brainstorm: The purpose of the teenage brain.* New York, NY: Penguin Publishing.

Skewes. M. C., & Blume, A. W. (2019). Understanding the link between racial trauma and substance use among American Indians. *American Psychologist, 72*(1), 88–100. doi:10.1037/amp0000331

Substance Abuse and Mental Health Services Administration. (2015). *Alcohol.* Retrieved from https://www.samhsa.gov/atod/alcohol

Substance Abuse and Mental Health Services Administration. (2018a). *Key substance use and mental health indicators in the United States: Results from the 2017 National Survey on Drug Use and Health* (HHS Publication No. SMA 18-5068, NSDUH Series H-53). Rockville, MD: Center for Behavioral Health Statistics and Quality, Substance Abuse and Mental Health Services Administration. Retrieved from https://www.samhsa.gov/data

Substance Abuse and Mental Health Services Administration. (2018b). *Results from the 2017 National Survey on Drug Use and Health: Detailed Tables.* Retrieved from https://www.samhsa.gov/data/sites/default/files/cbhsq-reports/NSDUHDetailedTabs2018R2/NSDUHDetailedTabs2018.pdf

Substance Abuse and Mental Health Services Administration. (2019). *Behavioral health barometer: United States, Volume 5: Indicators as measured through the 2017 National Survey on Drug Use and Health and the National Survey of Substance Abuse Treatment Services.* HHS Publication No. SMA–19–Baro-17-US. Rockville, MD: Substance Abuse and Mental Health Services Administration, Retrieved from https://www.samhsa.gov/data/sites/default/files/cbhsq-reports/National-BH-BarometerVolume5.pdf

Urschel, H. (2009). *Healing the addicted brain: The revolutionary, science-based alcoholism and addiction recovery program.* Naperville, IL: Sourcebooks, Inc.

Volkow, N. (2015). *Principles of drug addiction treatment: A research based guide* (3rd ed.). National Institutes of Health, National Institute on Drug Abuse. Retrieved from https://www.drugabuse.gov/sites/default/files/podat_1.pdf

Volkow, N., Koob, G. F., & McLellan, A. T. (2016). Neurobiological advances from the brain disease model of addiction. *New England Journal of Medicine, 374*(4), 363–371. doi:10.1056/NEJMra1511480

Wu, L. T., & Blazer, D. G. (2011). Illicit and nonmedical drug use among older adults: A review. *Journal of Aging and Health, 23*(3), 481–504. doi:10.1177/0898264310386224

Yudko, E., Lozhkina, O., & Fouts, A. (2007). A comprehensive review of the psychometric properties of the Drug Abuse Screening Test. *Journal of Substance Abuse Treatment, 32*(2), 189–198. doi:10.1016/j.jsat.2006.08.002

Zimic, J., & Jukic, V. (2012). Familial risk factors favoring drug addiction onset. *Journal of Psychoactive Drugs, 44*(2), 173–185. doi:10.1080/02791072.2012.685408

Zuckerman, E. L. (2019). *Clinician's thesaurus: The guide to conducting interviews and writing psychological reports* (8th ed.). New York, NY: The Guilford Press.

# 21

# Practice With Immigrant Victims of Domestic Violence

PATRICIA BROWNELL, ZSUZSANNA MONIKA FEHER, AND DENISE GOSSELIN

## INTRODUCTION

Since the 1970s, social workers, along with lawyers, grassroots advocates, and progressive government officials and lawmakers, have sought legislative, regulatory, and procedural remedies to protect the safety and well-being of women who are domestic violence victims (Dziegielewski & Swartz, 2007). While domestic violence can affect all women regardless of socioeconomic and citizenship status, domestic violence victims without citizenship remain particularly vulnerable to continued abuse and exploitation, disadvantage in child custody contests, and deportation (Ibrahim, 2018). This chapter focuses primarily on domestic violence and social work practice with low-income immigrant women, particularly those who are undocumented.

Impressive social and legal remedies were achieved for victims of domestic violence in the beginning of the women's movement. However, legislative and regulatory changes were critically needed for domestic violence victims with immigrant and refugee status to ensure their ability to access needed social welfare services and public benefits such as income support, healthcare, employment, education, housing, and personal social services. In addition, social workers were challenged to develop new models of intervention and practice that addressed the needs of immigrant domestic violence victims.

Domestic violence has been a concern of social workers and social reformers since the early days of the social work profession. In the late 19th century, the social response was to attempt to remove children from families where there was wife battering (Brace, 1872). The social work profession began with charity organization and settlement house workers assisting poor urban immigrants (Gordon, 1988). This mission to assist people of diverse cultures obtain needed resources, services, and opportunities remain with the profession today, as reflected in the National Association of Social Workers (NASW) Code of Ethics (NASW, 2008).

The NASW Code of Ethics provides guidance for the professional social worker to practice in a culturally competent manner. Section 1.05 of the code is entitled Cultural Competency and Social Diversity. This section defines culturally competent social work practice as social workers' understanding culture and its function in human behavior and society, having a knowledge base about their clients' culture, demonstrating competence in the provision of services that are sensitive to clients' culture and differences among people and cultural groups, and understanding cultural diversity and oppression (NASW, 2008).

Cultural awareness is defined as an understanding that an individual has different cultures, defined as races, religions, gender, ages, and physical disabilities (Fong, McRoy, & Hendricks, 2006). Domestic violence is a significant social problem in the United States. It is essential for social workers to detect and address domestic violence given its prevalence and consequences. Education and training for social workers should address the impact on race, ethnicity, culture, and immigration status: This enhances the ability of practitioner to offer more culturally responsive services (Danis, 2003).

## DEMOGRAPHIC PROFILE OF IMMIGRATION IN THE UNITED STATES

According to a Pew Research Center analysis of the U.S. Census Bureau's American Community Survey, more than 14 million people, approximately 14% of the U.S. population, was born in another country in 2017 (Connor & Budiman, 2019).

Since 1965, the number of immigrants living in the United States has more than quadrupled—the U.S. foreign-born population reached a record 44.4 million in 2017. According to the Pew Research Center estimates based on augmented U.S. Census Bureau data, the foreign-born population in the United States in 2017 comprised the following: lawful immigrants 35.2 million (77%), from which naturalized citizens were 20.7 million (45%) and lawful permanent residents 12.3 million (27%), temporary permanent residents 2.2 million (5%) and unauthorized immigrants 10.5 million (23%) (Radford, 2019).

More than a million immigrants arrive to the United States every year. In 2017, most immigrants came from India (126,000), Mexico (124,000), China (121,000), and Cuba (41,000). Looking at race and ethnicities, fewer people came from Latin America and since 2010 more Asian people arrived than Hispanics. By 2055, Asian Americans will be the largest immigrant group in the United States (Radford, 2019).

Each year, thousands of immigrant women who are married to United States citizens or lawful permanent residents (LPR) enter the United States (Raj & Silverman, 2002). The vulnerability of interpersonal violence victims/survivors depends on their age, gender, physical, intellectual, and emotional states, socioeconomic standing, and lack of social support (Davies, Todahl, & Reichard, 2017). Providing trauma-sensitive services is essential for social workers to work with all victims of domestic violence.

For battered immigrant women, immigrant status, lack of support, the language barrier, and low economic status add significant obstacles to their ability to terminate an abusive relationship (Orloff, 2001; Raj & Silverman, 2002; Romkens, 2001; Rothwell, 2001).

## DEFINITIONS

### Domestic Violence

Domestic violence is defined as a social problem in which one's property, health, or life are endangered or harmed as a result of intentional behavior by another family member or significant other (Barker, 2003). Domestic violence is defined and interpreted differently in individual state statutes and penal codes. For example, the State of Massachusetts defines domestic violence as actual or attempted physical harm, fear of imminent serious physical harm, or nonconsensual sex perpetrated by a current or former spouse, boyfriend, girlfriend, or fiancé, a current or former roommate or housemate, a blood relative, a current or former relative by marriage, or a person with whom the victim has had a child. This definition may vary from state to state.

In the United States, more than one in three (36.4% or 43.6 million) women and about one in three (33.6% or 37.3 million) men experienced contact sexual violence, physical violence, and/or stalking by an intimate partner during their lifetime (Smith et al., 2018). Domestic violence also has severely affected children. Over 15 million U.S. children live in families in which partner violence occurred at least once in the past year, and 7 million children live in families in which severe partner violence occurred (McDonald, Jouriles, Ramisetty-Mikler, Caetano, & Green, 2006). Domestic violence is believed to be more prevalent among immigrant women than among women who are U.S. citizens, and the majority of immigrants in the United States are women with children (Erez & Globokar, 2009).

### Immigration Status

Immigration status, coupled with gender and race, may place women and their children at increased risk of being trapped in an abusive situation because of their vulnerability within a family relationship and their social isolation within their communities (Zarza, Ponsoda, & Carrillo, 2009).

While male immigrants may also be victims of violence, including domestic abuse, the focus of this chapter is on immigrant women victims of domestic violence. Terms related to immigration and refugee status are defined here. An immigrant is a noncitizen who was born in a country other than the United States and remains in the United States with or without lawful admission for temporary or permanent resident status, as defined by the U.S. government. Immigrants with documentation that enables them to remain in the United States pending citizenship proceedings have qualified immigrant status. Others may have entered the United States with work, student, or other temporary visas or permits; these may have current or expired status (Chang-Muy, 2009).

Immigrants without any formal immigrant status or history of formal immigrant status are referred to as nondocumented immigrants. According to the U.S. Department of Homeland Security (DHS), a refugee is a person outside their country of nationality, who is unable/unwilling to return to their country of nationality, because of persecution/a well-founded fear of persecution on account of race, religion, nationality, membership in a particular social group, or political opinion; and an asylee is a person who meets the definition of refugee and is already present in the United States or is seeking admission at a port of entry (DHS, 2019). For the purposes of this discussion, noncitizen domestic violence victims are identified as immigrants regardless of their immigration status, unless otherwise specified.

## Domestic Violence and Immigration

Domestic violence advocates have broadened the definition of domestic violence for battered immigrant women. Categories of domestic violence and abuse related to immigrant women include emotional abuse, economic abuse, sexual abuse, use of coercion and threats, using children, using citizenship or residency privilege, intimidation, isolation and minimizing, blaming, and denying the abusive acts. Battering is also defined as the use of coercive behavior (physical, sexual, or psychological) by a man against his intimate cohabitating partner to force the partner to do what the man wants regardless of the partner's own needs or desires, rights, or best interests (Dziegielewski & Swartz, 2007).

Advocates argue that these categories of abuse have special potency for immigrant women, because perpetrators can lie about immigration status as a form of emotional abuse, threaten to report any paid work to the Immigration and Naturalization Service (now the Bureau of Citizenship and Immigration Services or BCIS) as a form of financial abuse, threaten to report the woman to the government if she refuses sex, threaten to report her or her children to the BCIS, fail to file papers to legalize her immigration status, hide or destroy important papers such as passports, not allow her to learn English, and try to convince her that she is a burden and the source of blame for the abuse. It should be noted again here that the INS has been renamed the Bureau of Citizenship and Immigration Services (BCIS) and is part of the U.S. Department of Homeland Security (Carey, 2003).

Not every woman married to a U.S. citizen or lawful permanent resident is sponsored for legal status by her spouse. In abusive relationships, spouses who are citizens or lawful permanent residents may not file immigration documents on behalf of their spouses (Dutton, Orloff, & Hass, 2000). Several studies have shown that women whose status depends on their spouse are at higher risk of becoming victims of domestic violence than others (Kwong, 2002; Orloff, 2001, 2003). Constant fear of deportation bars immigrant women from terminating abusive relationships. The abusers often use their victims' immigration status to control them (Romkens, 2001; Sitowski, 2001).

Using an intersectionality framework for understanding social inequities, social identities, and domestic violence, Erez, Adelman, and Gregory (2009) analyze the relationship between immigration and domestic violence based on interviews with 137 immigrant women in the United States from 35 countries. According to this study, immigration shapes how women understand domestic violence, their access to resources, and their responses to domestic violence. It found observed dynamics of structural intersectionality for immigrant women as national origin and citizenship status form another layer of identity politics and marginalization in relation to domestic violence.

## RISKS AND NEEDS OF IMMIGRANT DOMESTIC VIOLENCE VICTIMS

Battered immigrant women experience economic, social, and legal problems that are unique to their legal and cultural status in the United States. In the United States, there is pride in diversity and multiculturalism (Sue, 2006). However, new refugees, immigrants, and other minority groups often face misunderstanding and confusion when American traditional values conflict with their beliefs and customs. Immigrants may also experience conflicts with civil and criminal justice systems.

Patriarchy and belief in fate may make women feel that they cannot control violence, and women from war-torn countries may not recognize familial violence. Recent immigrants face multiple stressors, including pressures to assimilate. Conflicts between batterers who attempt to enforce traditional gender roles and their victims who want to take advantage of educational opportunities can escalate into domestic violence. Pressures on victims to present their ethnic immigrant community in a positive light by not reporting or speaking out about the abuse, and dependence on their batterers because of their immigration status, are also salient factors (Mills, 1998).

Barriers to protective services for immigrant domestic violence victims include those of gender, cultural norms, and fear of deportation. When people immigrate to other countries, they bring their cultural norms and values with them. Within the context of different norms and values, the behavior and philosophy of immigrant women toward domestic violence are differently expressed (Raj & Silverman, 2002). Unlike Western culture, which encourages women to preserve equality and be independent, some other cultures may expect women to be subordinate and obedient to their husbands (Ahmad, Driver, McNally, & Stewart, 2009; Liao, 2006; Orloff, 2001).

Data gaps in research on domestic violence include insufficient information on violence against women of color (Lee, Thompson, & Mechanic, 2002). Recent immigrants remain underrepresented in survey samples: Reasons such as cultural and language barriers, fears of deportation, and fears of affecting relatives' applications for immigration have been cited for this oversight. There is a paucity of research on the effects of acculturation on domestic violence risk factors for women in similar immigrant populations (Lee et al., 2002).

A study examined the connection between initmate partner violence (IPV) and suicidality in a sample of 173 young adult 1.5 and second-generation Chinese, Korean, and Vietnamese American women found that 70% of them experienced lifetime suicidal ideation/intent. Additionally, after controlling for demographic factors and childhood abuse, a history of physical and/or sexual partner violence had the strongest connection to lifetime suicidal ideation/intent. Finally, the most commonly reported form of IPV was psychological aggression in the last 6 months, and then sexual coercion (Maru et al., 2018).

A study of 300 South Asian adults in the United States in 2015 found that almost a quarter of South Asian adults experienced relationship violence (24%); more than a quarter experienced some form of sexual abuse in childhood (exposure, touching, attempted penetration, and penetration); 41.2% reported witnessing violence against their mother; and those who reported any relationship violence were significantly more likely to have experienced child sexual abuse and suicide attempt (Nagaraj, Vyas, & McDonnell, 2018).

Scientific data on the impact of domestic violence experienced in childhood among South Asian people living in America are very rare (Nagaraj et al., 2018). A study examining 535 South Asian adult women living in the United States to get information on the connection between childhood exposure to violence and health behavior in adulthood found significant relations between verbal abuse in childhood and body esteem and subjective well-being in adulthood; childhood physical abuse and subjective well-being in adulthood; and having a battered mother and subjective well-being in adulthood (Nagaraj et al., 2018).

Tabibi, Ahmad, Baker, and Lalonde (2018) countered common misconceptions related to IPV by examining the experiences of IPV among immigrant women, including risk factors and vulnerabilities for IPV. This study highlights barriers faced by immigrant women when seeking safety and accessing services and supports and shares recommendation for violence prevention initiatives. While prevalence is not known, cultures that delegate subservient roles to women make those women particularly vulnerable to violence, abuse, and even femicide. Other barriers like fear of losing children, fear of breach of confidentiality, and fear of authority can mitigate against immigrant women victims of domestic violence receiving needed help.

Du Mont and Forte (2012) conducted an exploratory study on the consequences and contextual factors of IPV among immigrant and Canadian-born women. This exploratory study compared immigrant and Canadian-born women on the physical and psychological consequences of IPV found no differences. However, immigrant women's lower levels of trust and experiences of discrimination may have implications for help-seeking for IPV and suggests the need for culturally sensitive IPV-related intervention and prevention services.

The importance of culturally competent practice by social workers to assist battered immigrant women is noted by Ely (2004). Oppressive immigration laws affecting Latinx women who accompany abusive partners to the United States can serve as barriers to help-seeking. Unique challenges face South Asian and Islamic women immigrants, as they come from highly patriarchal cultures where women face burning, honor and dowry killings, and other atrocities. Grassroots agencies that provide culturally sensitive services to targeted populations of battered women can help to create opportunities for immigrant battered women to exit abusive relationships and obtain language skills and job training outside their abusive relationships. A human rights perspective requires social workers to serve each woman within the context of her own culture and expressed needs and desires, and to educate policymakers of the need for enlightened social welfare policies.

While not specifically addressing immigrant women and domestic violence, Postman (2015) uses an exploratory research design to examine differences among Caucasian, African American, and Latinx women related to victimization prevalence, if and to whom they disclose their victimization, and to whom they turned for services and support.

## Nondocumented Battered Women

Many nondocumented battered women may refuse to seek help for fear of being deported, according to Erez and Hartley (2003). This may be because their country of origin has laws protecting husbands who beat their wives and deportation may place an undocumented battered woman at risk of further abuse by family members on whom she would be dependent for support. It may also be because of the felt need of the victim to protect the interests of her family.

Inez married an American citizen and left an impoverished life in South America to live with her husband in the United States. She and her husband had three children, who were provided with material advantages they would not have had in her country of origin. Her husband never applied for citizenship status for her, and continually abused her. Inez refused to press charges or leave him, however, for fear that she would either lose her children to him or be forced to return to her country of origin, where they would live the same impoverished life she had escaped.

In this case, the fact that Inez's husband never petitioned for her green card permits him to keep her in virtual slavery. She is in a vulnerable position if she tries to leave her husband and he reports her to the BCIS. Her status also precludes her from receiving public assistance and creates barriers to her obtaining a job that could enable her to support herself and her children.

Some options exist for social workers who service immigrant women who are domestic violence victims. They include working collaboratively with agencies that provide information and access to benefits and services to special ethnic populations in their language as well as English; legal service agencies that specialize in immigration law and advocacy; and domestic violence shelters and nonresidential domestic violence programs. Most shelters and domestic violence programs, even if they receive government funding, will provide crisis services to domestic violence victims and their children regardless of citizenship status.

Undocumented battered women are among the most difficult to assist. In addition to the psychological problems such women may have to address, formidable social problems can create practical difficulties as well. Resources like the National Center for Immigrants' Rights are available to provide information for social workers who are assisting undocumented women address issues of domestic abuse. Social interventions, in addition to clinical interventions and education, are critical to the success of undocumented women in freeing themselves from battering situations. According to Warrier and Rose (2009), however, racial and cultural factors are concerns in social work practice with domestic violence victims. It is important for social workers to understand how immigrant women from different cultural backgrounds may experience domestic violence and face different barriers to ensuring their safety.

## Latinx Battered Women

Rios, in her paper titled "Double Jeopardy: Cultural and Systemic Barriers Faced by the Latinx Battered Woman" (n.d.), stresses the need for domestic violence workers to understand and respect the cultural differences presented by Latinx battered women, and—at the community level—to advocate against those institutional factors, such as lack of social justice, that negatively impact on the Latinx community, as well as other communities of color. A comparison of Anglo and Latinx family values and structure reveal major differences that have important implications for effectively serving Latinx battered women (Rios, n.d.).

In the Latinx culture, individuals are seen first and primarily as members of the family, and family members are expected to actively work toward its unity and preservation. However, the Latinx culture is also characterized by a patriarchal family structure and the expectation that traditional gender roles will be strictly adhered to. Consequently, the Latinx woman is expected to be family identified: Her sense of identity and self-esteem is linked to her perceived ability to fulfill the ideal of the self-sacrificing mother and wife. These factors, according to Rios, make it difficult for the Latinx battered woman to act against abuse by seeking judicial or police protection, or assistance through a shelter or family service agency. She is accustomed to subordinating her needs on behalf of her family, even at the risk of her own personal safety. Also, her sense of identity is so linked with her role of wife and mother that she may consider herself a failure if she takes action to break up her family.

These concerns may be supported and reinforced by family, friends, and community, and the victim may be urged to give the relationship another chance. Religious beliefs in the sanctity of marriage can provide another barrier. Service providers must acknowledge the conflicts engendered by a Latinx woman's decision to confront the battering situation. This is compounded by Latinxs' historical experience of oppression by the police and criminal justice system, which are viewed with suspicion. The lack of bilingual and culturally sensitive social workers can further alienate the Latinx victim of family violence, should she choose to reach out for assistance in spite of the internal and structural barriers she faces in doing so.

Bonilla-Santiago (2002) provides an overview of cultural barriers and social service and legal needs of Latinx battered women. A study conducted with Latinx women demonstrated that most receive little or no assistance or protection from police, legal aid, welfare, mental health, or counseling services due to cultural and language barriers. Also, because Latinx women are women from Latin America, Cuba, Mexico, the Dominican Republic, Central America, and South America, their differing immigration statuses complicate policy and practice issues. Many Latinx women are isolated and trapped in violent homes (34% experience some form of violence). Their perceptions of physical and psychological abuse also differ from Anglo and other women.

Studies on domestic violence among immigrant populations have found a high incidence of abuse against immigrant women by spouses and partners. In one study, 48% of Latinx women reported increased violence by a partner since immigrating to the United States (Dutton et al., 2000). Cultural, social, and structural explanations are proposed for this. Language barriers may limit an immigrant domestic violence victim's ability to understand and negotiate service and immigration systems, question social expectations and community pressures, and access financial resources independent of their partner or spouse (Warrier & Rose, 2009). IPV among Hispanic women has been reported as related to economic problems, acculturation stress, alcohol use, impulsivity, and trauma (Zarza et al., 2009).

Reina, Lohman, and Maldonado (2014) explored Latinx immigrant victims' experiences with domestic violence service outreach in the Midwest, using interviews and a focus group. Findings demonstrated that immigration status and the inability to understand domestic violence within given cultural norms are major barriers keeping Latinx women from seeking help from formal advocacy agencies. Other barriers include shame, isolation, lack of bilingual services, and lack of knowledge about resources.

## Asian Battered Women

Asian and Asia Pacific Americans may respond differently to domestic violence based on the meaning they assign to their experiences of abuse (Tjaden & Thoennes, 2000). Asian women are often taught that in their roles as wives and mothers, they are responsible for keeping the family unit together under all circumstances (Kwong, 2002). In a domestically violent situation, women are often blamed for causing instability in their family by not conforming to the social norms and their native culture (Orloff, 2001). One study of Korean American families found that male-dominant couples were four times more likely to engage in wife abuse (Kim & Sung, 2000). Wife abuse in Asian cultures seems to be compounded by economic stress (Kurst-Swanger & Petcosky, 2003).

There is a need to address lack of knowledge about female victims from diverse ethnic/racial backgrounds as well as men who batter them. Prevalence of spouse abuse in the Chinese community is not available. Within the Chinese immigrant population, there is an unfounded myth that abuse doesn't occur, because Chinese women underutilize formal services. In fact, there are culturally specific influences on spouse abuse in the Chinese community. For example, Confucianism suggests that the traditional Chinese sense of self is rooted in relationships with significant others in the family, primarily, and there is a de-emphasis on independence from the traditional family system (Yick, 2000). Women are encouraged to internalize values about endurance and submission to maintain the collective existence and family harmony. As a result, women face tremendous pressures in trying to break abusive cycles in their families. The family name is expected to be protected at all costs. Contextual factors, including immigration status, exacerbate these pressures.

Chinese men may use immigration status to psychologically threaten their female partners and keep them subservient in an abusive situation. Undocumented Chinese women are a vulnerable group as they are new immigrants without language, social skills, financial independence, and knowledge of American culture. Lacking refugee status creates an additional barrier. Women may get jobs more easily (such as low paying garment work), and men may resent this: Redistribution of power within the family can cause tension. Social isolation and immigration status further limit women's help-seeking behavior. They may need culturally sensitive social services and shelter, and access to language translation. Most choose to stay with their abusers, so access to couple therapy is also important. Community education, especially for the men, is another important intervention strategy.

Religious practices are often brought by immigrant women from their countries of origin and can be a source of support or censure for women dealing with domestic violence. Choi (2015) examined Korean clergy's response to domestic violence in their congregations, given the reliance of Korean immigrants on their churches for assistance in domestic violence situations. Results showed that Korean clergy's cultural values, ages, and length of residence in the United States influenced their responses to domestic violence. Recommendations include developing collaborative working relationships between Korean clergy and domestic violence advocates, as well as providing training, targeting their knowledge, beliefs/attitudes, and skills related to promoting safety of battered Korean immigrant women (Choi, 2015).

## Russian Battered Women

Russian Jewish immigrants were granted asylum in large numbers during and after the Cold War. This recent large-scale immigration parallels that of the 19th century and has resulted in newly created ethnic enclaves in large urban centers like New York. Judaism teaches that the Jewish home is a Mikdash Me'at, a holy space, and traditionally, Jewish women are responsible for domestic tranquility. One identified barrier to battered immigrant Jewish women seeking help is a deep sense of shame, leading them to minimize or redefine the abuse to avoid humiliation. Another is the lack of services that meet the specific needs of Jewish battered women: shelters with kosher facilities and arrangements with Jewish educational institutions where children can continue their education and observance of non-Christian holidays.

Lack of multilingual staff and fear of anti-Semitism by non-Jewish staff may also create reluctance on the part of Jewish women to seek services in battered women's shelters. Alternatively, they may also feel constrained in seeking services from a Jewish agency, out of fear that their community will find out they have been battered. Effective service delivery to this population includes some provision for kosher cooking utensils, access to a rabbi, and the opportunity to select a Jewish or non-Jewish counselor, if desired. Advertising services for victims of domestic violence through temples, sisterhoods, or women's organizations in temples, Hadassah, B'nai B'rith, rabbis, Hillel, and Jewish community centers can be useful for outreach.

It is important to recognize that the actual dynamics of battering in Jewish families are the same as in non-Jewish families, although there is some evidence that Jewish women tend to stay in battering relations longer than non-Jewish women and those seeking shelter may be older than non-Jewish women. The stress of migration and shifting roles in the household may contribute to domestic violence in the Russian immigrant family (Chazin & Ushakova, 2005). Key factors in serving Jewish victims of domestic violence are understanding the meaning of family in Jewish life and the deep humiliation Jewish women often feel about being battered.

## Indian and South Asian Battered Women

Domestic violence against women is an issue that many Indian Americans refuse to acknowledge as a problem within their community by contending it only occurs within poor, uneducated families (Bhandari, 2008; Liao, 2006). Women advocates within the Indian immigrant community suggest that this is not the case. The story of Sita, heroine of the Indian epic *Ramayana*, mythologizes the self-immolating woman who becomes the "ideal woman" through her continuous efforts to prove herself worthy of her husband, Ram. It is this feminine model of subjugation that female Indian children are taught to emulate.

While the dynamics of domestic violence are not unique in the Indian immigrant community, Indian battered women face additional problems due to immigration status, level of acculturation, and culturally insensitive mainstream organizations that create barriers to obtaining needed assistance (Bhandari, 2008). Traditional arranged marriages create patrilocal joint family households that make Indian women vulnerable to abuse by extended family members as well as spouses. Often the Indian woman's family of origin will not extend assistance once she is married as she is not considered their concern anymore.

According to Bhandari (2008), social stigma and pressure from the larger Indian community not to break up the family constitute significant deterrents to women reaching out for assistance through the formal service network. In recent years, a number of Indian and South Asian women have organized their own service network, including shelter services, to assist battered women in their communities. SAKHI, a New York based women's support group, is one of a number of organizations that have formed out of the Indian and South Asian communities to assist battered women and their families.

After examining the literature on vulnerability of South Asian women immigrants to domestic violence, Chaze and Medhekar (2017) find that language, gender, race, class, and immigration policy intersect to increase the vulnerability of Canadian South Asian immigrant women to domestic violence. Highlighted are the need for information and social support networks for vulnerable newcomer immigrant women and settlement needs as articulated by victims themselves.

A literature review of studies of South Asian domestic violence victims conducted by Kapur and Zajicek (2018) found subjects were framed within with several categories: manipulated and dependent victim, unaware victim, and empowered victim. Excerpts from selected studies illustrated with examples how subjects were depicted in each frame. The examples of scholarship showed how domestic violence is depicted for women on the margins of society and subtly distorts their reality, according to the authors.

## Arab and Middle Eastern Battered Women

Like other immigrant groups, Arab women bring the traditions, values, and cultures of their home countries. Arab immigrants represent multiple countries: Palestine, Lebanon, Egypt, Syria, Iraq, Jordon, Saudi Arabia, Sudan, Kuwait, Morocco, and the United Arab Emirates (Abu-Ras, 2007). Generally speaking, Arab families remain very traditional in their views of gender, marital expectations, views on marriage and conflict, divorce, honor, and never brining shame to the family (Abu-Ras, 2007; Kulwicki, Aswad, Carmona, & Ballout, 2010). The study examines the relationship between cultural beliefs and the utilization of services among Arab immigrant women. The results of the study found that their use of available services is affected by their cultural beliefs and attitudes toward wife beating and the anti-Arab political climate.

A study by Abu-Ras (2007) on Arab immigrant women and their perception of domestic violence and help-seeking behaviors found that women with more traditional beliefs and attitudes toward women and wife beating are less likely to take advantage of formal services to address partner violence. Other barriers to help-seeking behavior include immigration status, personal resources, culture, language, cultural beliefs in resolving domestic problems, religious leaders, discrimination, and fear of authorities especially after 9/11 (Abu-Ras, 2007; Kulwicki et al., 2010).

One of the obstacles for people of Middle Eastern descent to access mental health services is that many view Western psychotherapy as self-serving and culturally incompatible, due to it being developed in individualistic societies

(Balice et al., 2019). Islamic principles are often used as manuals for mental health, where the overall family health is of greater importance than the individual's (Balice et al., 2019).

Maintaining the family unit and stability are of the utmost importance for Arab families. If a domestic conflict arises, women will turn to their family for support and assistance. Some are reluctant to approach law enforcement and would rather stay in abusive relationships. A study by Kulwicki et al. (2010) found that utilization of support services for survivors of domestic violence are limited, and cited that greater outreach was needed to educate community members about available services for survivors of domestic violenc;, more attention and better treatment of domestic violence cases within the emergency room visits; language barriers and cultural competence of medical staff in emergency departments; cultural competence and language barriers from staff at domestic violence shelters; cultural sensitivity and confidentiality; services for batters; free or low cost legal services; and working with religious leaders. Removing these barriers would make it easier for survivors of domestic violence to receive the services they need.

Barkho, Fakhouri, and Arnetz (2011) examined the prevalence of IPV among immigrant Iraqi women in Detroit, Michigan, and explored the association between IPV and self-rated health. The study found that in this community, incidence of IPV was very high, and that there was an association between exposure to IPV and women's physical health and psychosomatic symptoms.

## Sub-Sahara African Battered Women

The number of immigrants from Sub-Sahara Africa living in the United States is relatively small, but that is slowly changing (Gambino, Trevelyan, & Fitzwater, 2014). Immigration from Africa is starting to increase due to political, social, and economic challenges experienced in those countries. African immigrants experience many of the same challenges as other immigrant groups, adjusting to a new country, finding a well-paying job to support a family, familiarizing themselves with the its laws, culture, learning a new language, negotiating new gender roles, and a new way of life. All of these changes have a stressful impact on the family. African women are at a risk for IPV because of religious and cultural barriers, and because of this they are less likely to seek outside assistance for IPV; instead many will rely on family members or religious leaders to find solutions to their marriages (Akinsulure-Smith, Chu, Keatley, & Rasmussen, 2013; Mose & Gillum, 2015).

The African family not only consists of the immediate family, but extended family members. The family is interdependent, and everyone is there to support each other. The husband is the head of the household. Mose and Gillum (2015) indicate that in Africa, bride wealth or dowry is practiced among families. This practice was a way for a husband's family to show appreciation to the family of the woman who will be his bride. This practice has now become a way to purchase women for marriage, and this in turn has made men feel that they own their wives, their labor, and sexuality. Bride price has been linked to IPV (Mose & Gillum, 2015). Both men and women are socialized to accept wife beating as a form of tradition, culture, and maintaining discipline. In the United States many women are afraid of reporting domestic violence to law enforcement or community-based organizations, partly because of lack of trust in law enforcement and the fear of being ostracized by their community in the United States and back home. If they need to seek help, assistance is sought from family members and religious leaders. IPV is considered a private family matter.

Akinsulure-Smith et al. (2013) conducted a study on how African men and women understand, cope, and seek assistance for IPV. Results from the study found that cultural expectations influence their coping strategies. West African men and women face difficult realities, with women reporting multiple instances of abuse and a sense of frustration.

### Adolescent Immigrants and Family Abuse

Literature on teen dating violence (TDV) states that relations to violence may differ along gender, culture, and acculturation. A recent study on 23 male Latinx American teens found that while they emphasized respect toward dating partners and the damaging impacts of TDV, they also described the pressure to demonstrate masculinity, which may point some male teens toward TDV (Haglund et al., 2018). Another TDV research project studied 25 South Asian American (76% had Indian origin) female teens and concluded that South Asian culture may provide some protection for youth experiencing TDV; however, the stigma against dating and generational differences may create unique challenges (Ragavan, Syed-Swift, Elwy, Fikre, & Bair-Merritt, 2018).

Literature on adolescent risky sexual behaviors (RSB) refers to inconsistent condom use, having multiple partners, having sex at a young age, and having sex while intoxicated or high, resulting in an elevated risk of sexually transmitted diseases (STDs) and unplanned pregnancy. The Centers for Disease Control and Prevention (CDC, 2019) presents that, although with less than 200,000 teen pregnancies, which was a national low record in 2017, the United States still has higher teen pregnancy rates than other Western industrialized countries. Additionally, in 2017 birth rates (number of births per 1,000 females aged 15–19) of American Indian/Alaska Native teens (32.9 %) was the highest, followed by Hispanic teens (28.9 %) and non-Hispanic Black teens (27.5), all of which were more than twice the rate for non-Hispanic White teens (13.2%) (CDC, 2019). Examining immigrant youth, researchers found that acculturation can be a protective (academic achievement, sexual knowledge, and sexual intention) or a risk-enhancing factor for RSBs among adolescents (Tsai et al., 2017).

While there is limited research on adolescent immigrants and family abuse, Perreira and Ornelas (2013), studied traumatic exposure and posttraumatic stress among immigrant Latinx adolescents and their caregivers. Using data from a random sample of 281 foreign-born adolescents and their parents, the study provides data on migration-related trauma exposures and how the migration process influences risk of experiencing trauma and developing posttraumatic stress disorder. While not specific to domestic violence, this is mentioned as one of the problems that migrating adolescents and their caregiving parents may experience before, during, and after migration (Perreira & Ornelas, 2013).

### Older Immigrants and Family Abuse

The changing demographics of migration, including more female migrants and the increased risks they face, suggests that women of all ages are subject to risk associated with domestic violence, including IPV as well as abuse perpetrated by adult children and grandchildren. As a result, a life course perspective is needed as a framework to discuss the differential impact of migration on girls and women of all ages. Specific to older women migrants, limited information is available on their experiences other than to note that older migrants are more likely to be women and may be subjected to various forms of neglect and abuse by a broader range of family members other than spouses (Dako-Gyeke, 2013).

Focus groups and individual interviews with a group of older immigrant women from the Sri Lankan Tamil community in Toronto (Guruge et al., 2010) found that women experienced various forms of neglect and abuse and the primary abusers were their husbands, children, and children-in-law. Their community and the Canadian society at large were also implicated. Women's responses to abuse were shaped by micro, mezzo, and macro level forces. Strategies needed to better support immigrant older women's attempts to cope with abuses and promote resilience are needed.

Guruge and Kanthasamy (2010) also queried subjects of focus groups and individuals through interviews about financial, physical, and emotional abuse and neglect along with other forms of power and control. Some determinants included children's and grandchildren's welfare, community expectations, unfamiliarity with the ways of the new country, financial and immigration concerns, and limitations in accessing health, social, and settlement services. Recommendations for assistance to older women immigrants experiencing domestic abuse included addressing family and community expectations of older women that lead to abusive situations, establishing language training and community expectations for older women, offering linguistically and culturally appropriate service supports and care, and removing immigration sponsorship criteria.

To better understand elder abuse and neglect among aging Chinese immigrants, Lai, Daoust, and Li (2014) reviewed the existing literature and available research findings related to understanding elder abuse and neglect in culturally diverse communities, specifically the Chinese immigrant community in Canada. The influence of race, ethnicity, immigration status, and cultural norms on the recognition, identification, prevention and intervention of elder abuse and neglect were found to be important to consider. Professionals serving this population must understand the social cultural context in which abuse emerges, as well as barriers to seeking and utilizing helping services.

Lee (2014) explored and compared the relevant sociocultural characteristics that influence elder mistreatment and help-seeking behavior among older Chinese and Korean immigrants. Older Korean immigrants compared with their Chinese counterparts demonstrated stronger influence of hierarchy and cultural beliefs in exclusive family ties and gender norms and were less likely to disclose abuse. Programs that maintain strict confidentiality, facilitate relationships and communication among family members, were sensitive to the prominent role played by religion and spirituality, and provide accessible linguistic and culturally appropriate services were most likely to be utilized by victims and their families.

Matsouka et al. (2012) evaluated a project intended to increase understanding of abused older immigrant women in Canada. Two significant themes emerged from the project, which consisted of a literature review, local meetings with key stakeholders in seven provinces, a public event in Toronto, and a 2-day interdisciplinary symposium with provincial stakeholders. Themes that emerged included the value of bringing professionals together representing multiple disciplines as well as service sectors and older immigrant women, and the need for changes in social policies to reduce older women's vulnerability to abuse and support their resilience. Importantly it focused attention on implications of familism within policies concerning prevention of abuse and the value of intersectoral collaboration.

A narrative review of 45 studies exploring IPV in older women focusing on prevalence, associated factors, impact, responses to IPV, interventions and key populations was conducted by Pathak, Dairying, and Tariq (2019). Data suggest that IPV is commonly experienced by older women, but their age and life transitions suggest they may experience abuse differently than younger women. They also face unique barriers to accessing help and need services specifically targeted to their needs. This article does not focus specifically on immigrant women.

Patterson and Malley-Morrison (2006) conducted a cross-cultural study of four groups of women vulnerable to abuse, one being older women. Using an ecological frame, the authors argue that variation in actual abuse practices may vary across cultures. For example, in Japan blaming elderly parents for personal failures was uniquely and relatively mentioned. Respect was often mentioned in Israel. Placing elders in nursing homes is considered unacceptable in Brazil. Elder abuse by daughters-in-law is reported in South Asian countries where older parents generally live with sons. In Israel, older Arabic women are reported to be particularly vulnerable to abuse. While not specific to immigrant women in the United States, this may have implications for immigrant communities reflecting specific cultures.

Recent changes in Canadian immigration policies have made intra-family adaptation and interaction more restrictive and stressful, which in turn has implications for intergenerational relations in post-migration contexts. Petosic et al. (2015) reviewed the literature on intergenerational violence using an intersectional approach and presented definitions of violence, risk and protective factors, and barriers to help-seeking. This analysis revealed that gender and gendered manifestations of violence intersect with ageism, racism, sexism and other factors leading to a complex understanding and nuanced solutions to addressing intergenerational violence in the post-migration context.

## INTERNATIONAL PERSPECTIVES ON DOMESTIC VIOLENCE: IMPLICATIONS FOR SOCIAL WORK WITH IMMIGRANTS IN THE UNITED STATES

Summers and Hoffman (2002) provide a cross-cultural comparison of domestic violence, which the authors state is a global problem. This includes overviews of domestic violence in 13 countries, including the United States. Studies of women who are domestic violence victims in native countries of origin can provide insight into cultural barriers faced by women from these countries who have immigrated to the United States.

Yoshihama (1998) reports that a Japanese nationwide study raised consciousness about physical and psychological abuse. A link between spouse abuse, child abuse, and abuse during pregnancy is reported with some frequency. Battered women in Japan sought help through women's centers and the health system. However, they didn't always seek help through formal systems, as they considered domestic violence a private and shameful matter. The belief that battered women caused their abuse limits access to services. Japanese women interpreted abuse somewhat differently than in other cultures (overturning the dinner table; having liquid thrown at them to "purify" them—considered psychological abuse). One-third of female murder victims in Japan are killed by intimate partners. Findings from focus groups with battered women in Japan suggest that they experience a web of entrapment with little hope of escape. Victim blaming by family, friends, and professionals, and lack of assistance programs and police protection exacerbate the feeling of entrapment.

## REMEDIES

According to ACS, foreign-born immigrants peaked in 2016 at 1.46 million and, by 2018, declined by a quarter of a million (Knapp, 2019). It further estimates that by the year 2050 more than half the people in the United States will be from a non-Western European background. This dramatic increase in immigrants from developing countries has spurred an interest on the part of the social work profession in developing assessment tools and intervention techniques to facilitate their ethnicity-sensitive practice.

A notable example is the *culturagram* developed by Congress (1994, 2002, 2008; Brownell, 1998; Congress & Brownell, 1998), a family assessment tool developed for use by social workers to individualize families from diverse cultures, assess the impact of those cultures on family members, and facilitate empathy and ability to empower culturally diverse clients. More information on the culturagram can be found in Chapter 1, Using the Culturagram and an Intersectional Approach in Practice With Culturally Diverse Families. While professional social workers have increasingly acknowledged the growing cultural diversity of the client population (Harper-Dorton & Lantz, 2007), this has not always translated into the development of specialized interventions for clients with socially stigmatizing problems such as domestic violence.

Four categories of remedies are discussed here, including three categories of remedies or interventions that have evolved out of social work practice with victims of domestic violence: social interventions, clinical interventions, and empowerment-oriented interventions that often utilize the criminal justice system as part of an intervention strategy. Legislative remedies are discussed as a fourth category in relation to access to needed benefits and services for immigrant domestic violence victims. Each presents opportunities and challenges for immigrant women and their social workers.

### Social Interventions

Social interventions for victims of domestic violence focus on practical problem-solving for battered women and their families. While short-term interventions are crisis-oriented, longer-term interventions are intended to assist the victim to live independently apart from the abuser. Examples include both residential and nonresidential services.

Mrs. L, who emigrated from China a year ago, was kept a virtual prisoner in the home by her husband and her mother-in-law, who forced her to do housework and care for all the family members as well as her children. She was beaten by her mother-in-law as well as her husband if she refused to comply with their demands. The victim experienced both physical and emotional abuse, and may be eligible for crisis counseling and case management services that include linkage and referrals to language-appropriate social and health services. Mrs. L may also require assistance in relocating to a shelter residence that provides safety and transitional housing services.

Residential services encompass all the shelter service models that have evolved to provide temporary safe havens for victims of domestic violence and their families fleeing a battering situation. They are considered the most extreme of the victim-centered interventions: Victims entering a shelter system must not disclose their whereabouts to anyone, not even their closest relatives. Shelters are also considered to be the most effective in protecting women and their children who are threatened by harm from their batterers. Currently, specialized shelters are primary resources for women and children seeking protection from domestic violence (Roberts, 2007).

Case management services are available for domestic violence victims through the shelters, which provide a maximum amount of time-limited security for residents, or in the community. Nonresidential services for victims of domestic violence may include emergency hotline services, assistance with relocation, accessing emergency cash and other resources, and crisis counseling (Roberts, 2007). Longer-term social interventions may include income support for battered women and their children, rehousing, and job training. Public assistance is an important resource for some battered women and their families; it remains to be seen whether welfare reform initiatives that include block grants to states will eliminate this important safety net.

Most social interventions have built-in barriers for domestic violence victims from nondominant cultures. Shelters may not include multilingual staff. Those that are funded by public dollars may exclude nondocumented immigrants. Nonresidential programs may not offer culturally sensitive services or hire workers who are multilingual, although this is deemed essential for effective shelter-based interventions (Erez & Hartley, 2003). Victims of domestic violence from immigrant communities may not know about available services or understand how to obtain access to them.

Nondocumented immigrants could have an even more difficult time using long-term social interventions. Public assistance is not an option for them, housing may be too expensive to afford, and employment is difficult to obtain without exploitation. Social workers who work with immigrant women may find it useful to know how to make referrals to any organizations serving discrete immigrant communities. For example, in New York City, the New York Agency for New Americans (NYANA) serves Russian and Central European immigrants, Sakhi for South Asian Women specializes in working with South Asian and Indian Women, and the New York Asian Women's Center serves the Chinese community. One dimension of multicultural practice with victims of domestic violence is an in-depth knowledge of resources available to immigrants of all ethnic groups in the geographic area served.

Many cultures do not recognize domestic violence, and immigrants' countries of origin may not have laws that define and set criminal and civil penalties for domestic violence. As a result, women and their children from these cultures may face abusive situations alone without adequate support or knowledge of legal protections. Stressful living conditions in the United States, including language barriers and economic hardship, foster violence and discourage battered immigrant women from leaving their abusive partners (Orloff, 2001).

Fear of deportation also impacts the help-seeking behavior of domestic violence victims. If the battered women are undocumented immigrants, they are less likely to contact the police than victims who are U.S. citizens or permanent residents (Orloff, 2003). Legal protection and accessibility to public assistance are essential in order for battered immigrant women to escape from domestic violence situations (Dutton et al., 2000; Orloff & Kaguyutan, 2001). While immigrant domestic violence victims have access to fewer remedies than citizens, some services and interventions exist that are targeted specifically to immigrants and refugees. All immigrants regardless of status are eligible for emergency medical services reimbursable under the federal Medicaid program. Other remedies include clinical or counseling services, legal and law enforcement strategies, and information and referral services.

Advocacy groups provide extensive information on social and legal services available for immigrant battered women on the Internet. Manuals with information on services and benefits offer information on all aspects of service provisions to immigrant battered women. These include overviews of domestic violence and immigrant women; cross-cultural issues; legal and policy issues in immigration cases and domestic violence; access to public benefits; and model programs. Other web-based information sources examine various immigration statuses of newcomers to the United States and discuss influences on service provision, access, and use, including service needs, and immigration legislation and its implication for services (National Organization of Women [NOW], 2012).

Intervention research by Cesario, Nava, Bianchi, McFarlane, and Maddoux (2014) measured the impact of shelter intervention and protective orders on the mental health, functioning, resiliency and further abuse of documented and undocumented immigrant women and their children in Houston, Texas. Improvements were observed in abused immigrant women's mental health, resiliency, and safety regardless of whether the intervention was safe shelter or justice services. Global policy for improved access and acceptability of shelter and justice services is essential to promote immigrant women's safety and to maximize functioning of women and children.

Ely (2004) noted the importance of culturally competent practice by social workers to assist battered immigrant women. Oppressive immigration laws affecting Latinx women who accompany abusive partners to the United States can serve as barriers to help-seeking. Unique challenges face South Asian and Islamic women immigrants, as they come from highly patriarchal cultures where women face burning, honor and dowry killings, and other atrocities. Grassroots agencies that provide culturally sensitive services to targeted populations of battered women can help to create opportunities for immigrant battered women to exit abusive relationships and obtain language skills and job training outside their abusive relationships. A human rights perspective requires social workers to serve each woman within the context of her own culture and expressed needs and desires, and to educate policymakers of the need for enlightened social welfare policies.

According to Gwinn and Strack (2019), an innovative program in San Diego increased legal services to domestic violence victims. The authors profiled a mother who fled Mexico for the United States with her infant son to escape an abusive husband and who was able to utilize services of an innovative justice program to fight a civil action filed in a Mexican court ordering the return of her son. This represents a new type of legal aid, and specifically the legal "incubator" developed by a non-profit agency in partnership with a law school in San Diego. This particular incubator model specializes in serving the legal needs of IPV survivors.

Nixon and Humphreys (2010) reframed domestic violence as one aspect of violence against women, making space for a recognition of culturally specific experiences while highlighting the imbalance of power and control that runs through women's experiences. While not specifically focused on immigrant women, they argue that the domestic violence movement must take account of and effectively integrate the experiences and narratives of women from ethnic minorities, indigenous women, women living in poverty and disabled women. It argues that a human rights framework should be used to encompass the diverse experiences of women living with domestic violence.

## Clinical Interventions

Clinical interventions, developed as part of family service agencies by social workers influenced by the medical profession and psychiatry, moved social workers away from the activist tradition of Jane Addams and Florence Kelley. However, the women's movement of the 1970s began to influence clinical social workers to move away from traditional clinical interventions and begin to incorporate empowerment strategies into their practice (Gondolf, 1997) Practice with immigrant battered women brings new challenges to professionals to develop culturally competent practice modalities. As the case example of Mr. and Mrs. D illustrates, immigrants engage in acculturation at different rates. This can cause tension to develop within families and between couples.

Mr. and Mrs. D sought counseling from an Indian therapist in their community. Mrs. D complained Mr. D had become abusive, both emotionally and physically, since they emigrated from India. Mr. D countered that Mrs. D had changed since coming to the United States. In India, she had been compliant and a good and respectful wife. In America, she began to become more independent and to demand greater freedom and autonomy.

This speaks to the need for a family therapist who is culturally sensitive. Traditional psychoanalytic interventions have not been found to be effective with victims of domestic violence. Classical psychoanalysis defines victims of domestic violence as masochistic: They are assumed to be receiving some gratification from the battering situation. Critics suggest that the traditional psychoanalytic approach to treatment of domestic violence victims promotes a "blame the victim" approach that encourages self-blame in victims.

While some feminist practitioners (Shainess, 1984) have reframed it to be more applicable to women who are victims of domestic violence, psychoanalytic thinking is also grounded in Western European culture and thought. As such, it may have little meaning for domestic violence victims from developing countries, Eastern cultures, or communities of color. Family therapy is a controversial treatment modality for couples experiencing domestic violence. According to the American Medical Association, couples counseling or family intervention is generally contraindicated in the presence of domestic violence and may increase the risk of serious harm (American Congress of Obstetricians and Gynecologists, 2012).

Family systems theory has been criticized as inappropriate for use with couples where there is active battering (Murray, 2006). In this approach, the family is looked upon as a system, and battering as a symptom of a dysfunctional system. No member is assigned blame: The victim is viewed as an active participant in the abusive situation. The abuser, in this model, can avoid responsibility for the abusive actions by claiming provocation or a desire to maintain the homeostasis of the family system. For immigrant families from cultures that emphasize the responsibility of the woman to maintain family stability at all cost, this approach could reinforce internalized cultural values encouraging her to remain in the abusive situation for the good of the family.

Previously, some therapists have claimed success in using conjoint family therapy to treat couples together where domestic violence results from marital conflict. The premise for this is that when a couple is seen together, they are treated "as a dynamic unit whose patterns of reactions are interdependent" (Geller & Wasserstrom, 1984, p. 35). Further, cultural background and ethnic identity can create barriers to help-seeking, particularly for immigrant couples experiencing domestic violence, and once a decision to seek help has been made, conjoint family therapy may be the only form of intervention the couple is willing to accept. While some practitioners support couples therapy for families where domestic violence is a factor, many therapists are adamantly opposed to couples being treated together when there is active battering. Reasons include the danger posed to both victim and therapist, and the concern that the hope of a "cure" will dissuade the victim from heeding danger signs or seeking protection when necessary.

Crisis intervention models of treatment are utilized both in domestic violence shelter settings as well as in community-based treatment for victims of domestic violence (Dziegielewski & Schwarz, 2007). In a crisis, people respond to traumatic events according to their individual personality traits, coping mechanisms, and cultural values. The crisis intervention model suggests that in the face of emotional and physical abuse, victims can learn new coping mechanisms and problem-solving skills.

Cognitive and behavioral approaches have been identified as effective short-term treatment modalities for victims of domestic violence (Dziegielewski & Swartz, 2007). They can also be utilized to assist the victim in addressing the abusive situation within the preferred cultural context. One example of a cognitive-behavioral approach is rational emotive therapy (RET), which seeks to assist clients to address emotional disturbances and improve life situations by targeting irrational belief systems.

According to Lega and Ellis (2001), RET is the treatment modality of choice when doing cross-cultural therapy or counseling. RET encourages the client to maintain their cultural reality and provides a basis for examining and challenging long cherished cultural assumptions only when they lead to dysfunctional emotions, behaviors, and consequences. It also provides clients with the tools to comprehend the link among beliefs, emotions, and behaviors but does not force clients to think, feel, or behave like members of the dominant culture in order to change (Lega & Ellis, 2001).

Feminist therapy models have been developed specifically to address the empowerment of women (Bricker-Jenkins & Hooyman, 1986; Peled, Eisikovits, Enosh, & Winstok, 2000). For example, survivor therapy, developed by Walker (2017), is an example of an intervention model intended to respond to the problems of battered women. It is based on the treatment approaches of both feminist therapy theory and trauma theory. By analyzing power and control factors in an abusive relationship, survivor therapy treats victims of violence by focusing on their strengths, a practice known as strengths-based therapy by social workers.

This model considers the woman's sociopolitical, cultural, and economic context, reflecting the dimensions of the nested ecological theory proposed by Dutton (2006). It also explores victims' coping strategies and assists them in building new ones, using many techniques from cognitive and behavioral therapeutic models. As a feminist model of psychotherapy, it explicitly incorporates the feminist therapist's goal of uncovering and respecting each client's cultural and experiential differences as an ethical guideline.

Objectives of feminist therapeutic intervention models include the empowerment of clients using strategies to assist the abused partner to redefine herself or himself as a survivor (not a victim). They also seek to enhance feelings of competence, strength, self-worth, and independence from the abuser (Walker, 2017). The feminist therapeutic models, as well as crisis intervention and cognitive-behavioral models like RET, seek to assist victims of domestic violence with the immediate crisis, as defined by the client, as well as to develop a new life philosophy that is based on empowerment and strength, not victimization.

Even feminist therapists may sometimes work with immigrant couples, particularly those who are self-referred. According to Lipchik (1994), if the identified problem is a lack of understanding of the laws governing family violence and both members of the couple are willing, the abusive husband may be referred to a batterers group as a way to learn about male–female relations in American culture and the legal ramifications of spouse abuse. This may be included as part of an intervention strategy if an assessment finds the couple is not knowledgeable about this country's laws against physical abuse. This represents part of a solution-focused approach that can assist the special needs of some immigrant families whose members are in different stages of assimilation and acculturation. For other family violence situations and particularly for those involving an undocumented partner who is the victim of abuse, the issues are much more problematic.

Recognizing the impact of cultural variables on battered women's responses to battering as well as other situational factors is essential to effective assessment and intervention. In addition, the effectiveness of clinical interventions depends in part on the ability of social workers and clients to verbally communicate. Even if clients can understand English, misinterpretations of meanings—mediated by cultural values—can result in the failure of the social worker to assist a client with whom they do not share a common culture.

> Most currently, trauma focused treatment for victims of domestic violence of all ages has moved to the forefront. Based on the theoretical work of Judith Herman (2015), it assumes that domestic violence

victims are traumatized by abuse perpetrated by loved ones and trusted others, and this trauma may extend into childhood. The Adverse Childhood Experiences Study (ACES) shows a link between non-validating childhood experiences and domestic violence in adulthood and even later life. (Vaughn et al., 2017)

Herman (2015) described that repeated trauma in childhood may (de)form the personality. This is due to the fact that in an abusive environment a child is faced with formidable tasks of adaptation and development, such as persevering to trust untrustworthy people; controlling terrifyingly uncontrollable situations; finding safety in unsafe situations and power in helplessness situations; bodily self-regulation and self-soothing; and developing a sense of self in relation to others who are helpless or cruel.

Abused children cannot develop a cohesive self-image and/or inner representation of others (Herman, 2015). As a reaction to several abuse experiences, children may develop dissociation or trance states as coping mechanisms. Developing self-blame is part of normal childhood; however, children unprotected to repeated, severe trauma may develop a "malignant sense of inner badness, which is often camouflaged by the abused child's persistent attempt to be good, for example becoming a superb performer" (Herman, 2015). Teicher and Samson (2016) stated that the maltreatment of children is the most important preventable cause of psychopathology accounting for nearly half (45%) of the attributable risk for childhood onset psychiatric disorders and that maltreatment changes the trajectories of brain development. A research study found that exposure to caregiver trauma caused indirect effects via deficits in cognitive control such as executive function (EF) between caregiver trauma and posttraumatic stress symptoms (PTSS), and externalizing problems; and its authors advise of the need for screening traumatized youth for executive dysfunction (Hodgdon et al., 2018).

Abuse also affects the body, as children are unable to regulate their basic biological functions (sleeping or eating, for example) and many abused children develop chronic hyperarousal, chronic sleep disturbance, eating disorders, gastrointestinal problems, and other bodily distress symptoms (Herman, 2015). Childhood traumatic stress may increase the likelihood of hospitalization with a diagnosed autoimmune disease decades later in adulthood (Dube et al., 2009). Dube et al. (2009) findings are consistent with recent biological studies on the impact of early life stress on subsequent inflammatory responses. Van der Kolk (2006) also reported that research reflecting on the impact of extreme stress on brain functions, such as people who experienced extreme trauma in the past may have "irrelevant or even harmful subcortically initiated reactions to sensory information in the present." This is explained by brain region activations due to reminders of traumatic experiences that facilitate intense emotions and inhibit central nervous system areas responsible for (a) integrating sensory input and motor output, (b) physiological arousal modulation functions, and (c) verbal expressions of experiences. In PTSD memory and attention fail also and interfere with the individual engaging in the present. According to a leading expert on trauma, traumatized individuals "lose their way in the world" (Van der Kolk, 2006). He recommended clinical interventions that boost interoception via (a) learning to tolerate sensations and feelings, (b) learning to modulate arousal, and

(c) learning to take effective actions to battle past physical helplessness. While the relationship between repeated childhood trauma and development of complex trauma in adulthood has not been studied for an immigrant population, witnessing intimate and interpersonal violence as children growing up in countries, communities, and households with significant violence and fear may have risk factors for trauma-related personality changes and fears (Herman, 2015).

## Legal Remedies and the Criminal Justice System

The criminal justice system was perceived by domestic violence advocates in the 1970s as not demonstrating responsiveness to the abuse of women. Increasingly, domestic violence advocates seek stronger protection for victims and punishment for perpetrators of abuse. Laws were passed to increase protections and sanctions in domestic violence situations. Again, however, many immigrant domestic violence victims were unable or unwilling to utilize these protections due to their ambiguous relationship with immigration and the law. This is another reason why social workers serving immigrant domestic violence victims need to work closely with immigrant lawyers or in an interdisciplinary social work and law setting.

Since the 1960s, the family court system has provided some protection and redress for victims of domestic violence through orders of protection and adjudication of family disputes. In addition, federal, state, and local funding has been appropriated for services to domestic violence victims and their families, obtained through the criminal justice system. While to date, most domestic violence service dollars have targeted victims and their families, attention is increasingly focusing on treatment for batterers as well. These treatment modalities range from mandatory arrest and court-ordered counseling to peer group support similar to the Alcoholics Anonymous (AA) model. Success with any of the available modalities for batterers has been intermittent, at best, and subject to mitigating circumstances (National Institute of Justice, 2003).

Remedies available through the criminal justice system may not be useful for battered immigrant women. In immigrant communities, both husband and wife may be unaware of laws that prohibit abuse of one spouse by another. The nondocumented domestic violence victim may not want to utilize the criminal justice system out of concern for exposure to BCIS. The court system may be intimidating or confusing to new immigrants, who may have difficulty communicating in English.

Domestic violence situations involving immigrant domestic violence victims present special challenges for social workers and advocates. The immigration issues at stake may require the services of an immigration attorney knowledgeable about domestic violence and immigration.

Social workers and immigration attorneys collaborating on cases involving the court system should make every effort to ensure that translators, if used in the court proceedings, are unbiased and knowledgeable about the domestic abuse situation. Translators should also be familiar with language dialects used by the victims, if applicable. Victims and their children may be especially vulnerable to efforts on the part of the abusers to seek deportation of victims as a way of gaining custody of their children and using the court system to assert their power and control.

## Legislative Remedies

Most of the social, legal, medical, and income services and benefits available to immigrant domestic violence victims in the United States are defined by federal and state laws and regulations, and funded through legislative appropriations at the federal, state, and local levels of government. Social workers who serve immigrant women in social service, legal, medical, and other settings must be knowledgeable about these laws and regulations to undertake effective assessments and work with victims to plan and implement effective safety strategies. Social workers must know how to work collaboratively with attorneys who specialize in immigration law and domestic violence. Finally, social workers are in excellent positions to identify service gaps and unmet needs of battered immigrant women, and their consequences on the well-being of battered immigrant women and their children. By providing legislative testimony and sharing the stories of their clients in a manner that protects confidentiality while highlighting needs for policy change, social workers can influence policy changes that improve and even save lives.

Social welfare policies can affect access to services and benefits in the United States for immigrant women who are domestic violence victims. These include the Violence Against Women's Act (VAWA I) of 1994; the Personal Responsibility and Work Opportunity Reconciliation Act (PRWORA) of 1996; the Illegal Immigrant Reform and Immigrant Responsibility Act (IIRIRA) of 1996; and the VAWA II of 2000. Each of these federal laws changed conditions under which battered immigrant women may be able to leave a battering situation and obtain social welfare services and benefits without facing deportation and separation from their families.

## Violence Against Women Act 1994

As a first systematic attempt to address the issue of domestic violence, the Violence Against Women's Act (VAWA) (Title IV of the Violent Crime Control and Law Enforcement Act of 1994—P. L. 103–322) was passed in 1994 with bipartisan support recognizing the significance of domestic violence as a serious problem (Murshid & Bowen, 2018).

VAWA created new legal penalties to address domestic violence and other forms of violence against women. The law provides grants to fund programs that encourage states to address violence against women. Program that are funded by the law include: grants for law enforcement and prosecution, grants to encourage arrest of perpetrators, funding against rural domestic violence, child abuse enforcement funding, funding for the National Domestic Violence Hotline, and shelters to house survivors of domestic violence (Murshid & Bowen, 2018).

Congress also recognized that many U.S. citizens or lawful permanent resident spouses abuse their battered spouses and use their immigration status as a weapon to control them (Kwong, 2002; Orloff, 2001). In 2000, Congress renewed VAWA together with the Victims of Trafficking and Violence Protection Act of 2000. The reauthorization of VAWA in 2000 included expansion of protections for immigrant victims of domestic violence, sexual assault, and human trafficking. The VAWA reauthorization also included the U-Visa. The U-Visa offers protection to immigrant victims of domestic violence, sexual assault, and other forms of violence (Murshid & Bowen, 2018).

Again in 2005, VAWA was expanded to include immigrant victims of IPV and other forms of gender based violence by including protections against deportations, improving access to immigration relief for immigrant victims of child abuse and elder abuse, improved confidentially protections, and expanding legal services including U-Visa (Murshid & Bowen, 2018). As stated earlier, VAWA in 1994, 2000, and 2005 were passed by strong bipartisan support in both the House and the Senate; however, in 2010, Republicans displayed significant challenges to reauthorizing VAWA. Republicans in the Senate were opposed to providing protections for three subgroups—Native Americans, LGBTQ individuals, and immigrants; this included undermining the U-Visa (Murshid & Bowen, 2018; Villalon, 2015). Ultimately, the Democrats prevailed and VAWA was reauthorized with the protections for the subgroups. Democrats accused the Republicans as being anti-women, while Republicans accused the Democrats as using VAWA to expand their electoral support (Villalon, 2015).

In the end, when VAWA was reauthorized in 2013, it included new regulations and definitions to increase availability, accountability, and transparency of funding for anti-violence programs; provide support for community-based responses and direct services to victims of domestic violence, dating violence, sexual assault, and stalking; improve judicial and law enforcement tools to combat gender violence; improve housing protections, economic security, and healthcare system responses for victims; and improve response to violence against underserved populations (Villalon, 2015). The one item that advocates were seeking that was not included in the reauthorization of VAWA that year, was increasing the number of U-Visas. In 2013, Congress authorized that only 10,000 U-Visas would be issued annually. According to Warren (2016), more than double the number of U-Visa requests are made each year. VAWA is again up for reauthorization and unfortunately because of political gridlock in Congress, VAWA has not be reauthorized this year.

## U-Visas

The U-Visa was enacted under P.L. 106-386, Victims of Trafficking and Violence Protection Act of 2000, which includes three categories the U-Visa is a provision under Division B: VAWA of 2000, providing temporary immigration benefits to immigrant victims of certain crimes, and providing benefits to their qualifying family members (Warren, 2016).

The U-Visa provides an opportunity for undocumented women to obtain U.S. citizenship if they cooperate with law enforcement. The law was created because there was a recognition in Congress that victims of domestic violence might not seek assistance from law enforcement officials because of immigration status.

The purpose of the law was to strengthen the ability of law enforcement officials, agencies (police department, sheriff, prosecutor, judge, or other government agency official authorized to sign a U-Visa application) to investigate and prosecute cases of domestic violence, sexual assault, trafficking, and other crimes while offering deportation protection to victims of domestic violence (Murshid & Bowen, 2018; Warren, 2016). Each year, Congress approves 10,000 U-Visas, the number of U-Visas approved for each year has not changed since 2000. To qualify for a U-Visa, the applicant is encouraged to complete the application with an attorney or an advocate. Once the U.S. Citizen and Immigration

Services (USCIS) receives the application it is considered pending. If the application is approved by USCIS, the victim then receives a Notice of Action letter, protecting the victim from deportation (Warren, 2016).

If the petition is accepted, a U-Visa is issued which then allows the person experiencing domestic violence or other forms of violence to obtain a work authorization from Social Security. After 3 years, the victim can apply for a green card. The U-Visa requires certification from law enforcement that proves that the victim is being helpful in the investigation, detection, prosecution, conviction, or sentencing of the criminal activity. Crimes that are eligible for the U-Visa are: abduction, abusive sexual contact, blackmail, domestic violence, extortion, false imprisonment, female genital mutilation, felonious assault, incest, involuntary servitude, kidnapping, manslaughter, murder, obstruction of justice, peonage, perjury, prostitution, rape, sexual assault and/or exploitation, torture, trafficking, witness tampering, unlawful criminal restraint, and other related crimes (Murshid & Bowen, 2018; Warren, 2016).

There are, however, limitation to the U-Visa. Besides the limited number of U-Visas available each year, other limitations exist. Law enforcement agencies are not required to provide information about the U-Visa, and, since the forms need to be certified by law enforcement, law enforcement may refuse to sign the U-Visa application (Warren, 2016). Another limitation is the immigrant victim has to come forward and report the criminal activity to law enforcement agencies to qualify for a U-Visa. This action can pose safety risks and concerns about economic loss and support (Murshid & Bowen, 2018). The length of time to receive a Green Card or become a permanent resident is lengthy—it could take up to 8 years. It could also be expensive to complete the application including obtaining and submitting supporting documents, though parts of the application may have fees waived. Since the application could be complicated, it is recommended that the form be completed with the assistance of an attorney, social workers or other advocates

The process of obtaining the visa is very difficult and requires assistance from attorneys and advocates. Social workers are advised to become familiar with the U-Visa and become advocates to change the rules and procedures for obtaining the U-Visa (Warren, 2016). Murshid and Bowen (2018) use a trauma informed policy analysis framework to the VAWA immigration protections to demonstrate how the Act's U-Visa provisions and implementation practices could be improved by incorporating trauma-informed principles of trustworthiness and transparency, empowerment, choice, safety, collaboration, and intersectionality.

### Personal Responsibility and Work Opportunity Reconciliation Act (1996)

The PRWORA (P. L. 104–193), Title I, created the Temporary Assistance to Needy Families program, a block grant program that replaced Aid to Families and Dependent Children, which was a federal cash grant entitlement program for poor families with dependent children enacted originally as part of the Social Security Act of 1935. In Title I and other titles of the PRWORA, immigrant eligibility was narrowed for federal and state welfare benefits, food stamps, Medicaid, and cash grant public assistance. Welfare reform initially affected more than 500,000 legal immigrants who received federal benefits including supplemental security income (SSI) and food stamps (Orloff & Little, 1999).

With the leadership of the late Senator Paul Wellstone (D-MN) and Senator Patty Murray (D-WA), an amendment to ease eligibility requirements for domestic violence victims was passed and incorporated into the Act as the Family Violence Option (FVO). The FVO eases or partially eases Temporary Assistance for Needy Families (TANF) requirements such as child support cooperation, work requirements, and the 60-month lifetime limit (Kogan, 2019). FVO could be a great instrument to use to help victims of domestic violence leave their abusers and become self-sufficient as TANF requires.

Sadly, as the names states, the FVO is only optional; not all states have adopted FVO. Some states have adopted their own version of FVO, while othershave not implemented the policy at all. Holcomb et al. (2017) in reviewing the literature found that not all state social service offices screen for domestic violence—rates for screening are as low as 2% to as high as 28%. Knowledge of the FVO among frontline workers is also limited, thereby limiting an important resource for victims of domestic violence (Holcomb et al., 2017). Depending on the state, information about FVO for clients is provided in brochures clients receive while meeting with their TANF worker or posters in the waiting room; other states provide a combination of posters and brochures, while other states do not provide any information about FVO at all.

Resources and easing of TANF requirements also vary by state and by employee knowledge. It is estimated that the current rate of abuse for TANF recipients ranges from 20% to 30%; despite this, states only grant .1% to 3% of waivers out of total enrollees. A literature review of state TANF policies suggests seeing if they include the FVO. The authors found that variations existed in the implementation and practice of FVO from the decision to adapt to the procedure in granting waivers (Holcomb et al., 2017).

PRWORA does allow certain categories of qualified immigrants to receive public assistance, assuming they also meet other categorical and financial requirements. The categories of qualified immigrants include lawful permanent residents, refugees, and asylees; persons granted conditional entry into the United States; aliens paroled into the United States for at least 1 year; and women and children who have been battered or subjected to extreme cruelty by a U.S. citizen or lawful permanent resident and have a VAWA approved pending a family-based petition on file with the INS (now BCIS).

## Illegal Immigrant Reform and Immigrant Responsibility Act (1996)

After the enactment of the PRWORA, Congress recognized the double jeopardy for battered immigrant women receiving financial assistance (Kwong, 2002; Orloff, 2001; Orloff & Kaguyutan, 2001). Previously undocumented battered immigrant women were not able to access public benefits because they were not "qualified immigrants."

Under the (IIRIRA (P. L. 104–208), Congress enacted a remedy by granting immigrant women access to the welfare safety net by enabling them to apply for qualified immigrant status. This was based on the recognition of the crucial role that economic independence plays in enabling battered immigrant women to extricate themselves from domestic violence (Orloff, 2001; Orloff & Little, 1999).

Despite the Trump Administration's changes to public assistance programs such the public charge rule or instilling work requirements on recipients of public assistance, populations protected from these changes include: refugees, asylees, survivors of domestic violence, individuals who have or are applying for a U- or T-Visa, children seeking Special Immigrant Juvenile Status, and active duty members (National Conference of State Legislators, 2018)

The poor implementation of the FVO of the PRWORA has hampered full realization of its intent: to enable survivors of domestic violence to achieve safety and self-sufficiency. The purpose of the law is to allow survivors of domestic violence using TANF to be exempt or partially exempt from the work requirements, child support cooperation, and the 60-month time limit. Unfortunately, FVO has not been implemented in all the states, some states have their own version of the FVO, while some states do not have any provision at all to protect and support survivors of domestic violence (Kogan, 2019).

## Implications for Social Work Practice

The cultural diversity of American society has stimulated the growth of social work models of practice since the inception of the profession in the 19th century. Service delivery to victims of domestic violence was an integral part of family services among the profession's forerunners in the charity organization and settlement house movement. Charity organization agents serving the urban immigrant communities addressed problems of domestic violence, although in the early days of social work, this was done as part of the prevailing "child saving" mission.

Early social work reformers were also maternalists and advocated against domestic abuse and for prohibition and women's pensions in order to achieve their (White middle-class) goal of assisting women to remain in the home caring for their children (Skocpol, 1992). Their clients were immigrant women, often from rural areas in their countries of origin, who were forced to cope with the harshness and uncertainties of urban industrial life. Early social workers rarely attempted to empathize with the subjects of their ministrations, instead projecting values that were often quite alien to their female clients and advice that was often counterproductive

However myopic these early reformers were regarding the problems facing immigrant families of the progressive era, they fought hard for solutions to social problems that affected all women. As social work began to turn inward in the 1920s, it began to look for solutions to social problems in psychotherapeutic techniques. The civil rights era and the women's movement of the 1960s and 1970s brought social workers back to a politicized and structural perspective in relation to social problems, including that of domestic violence.

At the beginning of the 21st century, the social work profession is responding to the globalization of social issues and the widespread immigration of families from cultures significantly different from the dominant European American culture, by developing multicultural approaches to working with clients. To address the problem of domestic violence within a multicultural context, social workers must develop a multidimensional understanding of the victim in relation to her family, community, and culture of origin, as well as intrapsychic processes. The ecological model of social work practice suggests intervention strategies that represent a synthesis of social and psychological techniques. It also requires a broad knowledge base and understanding of domestic violence victims from different cultures and their responses to new and existing service systems and modalities. Since the 1960s, social work has been struggling toward a multicultural model of service delivery that better reflects the basic tenet of social work practice: Begin where the client is. The 20th century feminist movement—although begun by White middle-class professionals—has also reached immigrant communities of color.

Research by social workers into domestic violence as a multicultural phenomenon can yield important information about characteristics of abuse in immigrant communities, barriers to service utilization, and successful practice models. This is a recognized gap in knowledge about domestic violence and how it affects immigrant women in the United States. Lack of access to study subjects has made this a difficult area of study. However, researchers are beginning to learn more about immigrant domestic violence victims through targeted surveys (Yick, 2000; Yoshihama, 2000) and in-depth interviews (Yoshioko, Gilbert, El-Bassel, & Baig-Amin, 2003).

The elimination of domestic violence by one adult family member against another—a key issue in the 20th-century women's movement—has challenged activists and social workers alike to evolve culturally sensitive models of service delivery. This reflects a new respect for diversity, as well as the commitment to reach underserved populations that have been isolated by language and culture. In doing so, social work is challenged to continually incorporate culturally sensitive values and techniques, in order to remain vital, relevant, and effective into the 21st century.

Culturally competent social work practice with immigrant victims of domestic violence requires professional social workers to be knowledgeable about social welfare and immigration policies, including federal and state laws and regulations. The ability of an immigrant domestic violence victim to ensure safety for herself and her children, as well as avoid deportation and possible separation from her children, rests on the informed application of existing policies by her service providers and advocates in her community.

The highly technical nature of many of these processes as defined by law and regulation require interdisciplinary collaboration between social workers and attorneys experienced in welfare and immigration law. Often, however, a social worker will be the first professional contact for an immigrant battered woman who seeks assistance through a medical facility, family service agency, or victims service program. This makes it essential that social workers have sufficient understanding of social welfare and immigration laws to enable them to provide support and empowerment, as well as interdisciplinary referrals as needed for legal counsel and advocacy, to immigrant clients who are victims of domestic violence.

The gaps and flaws in existing social welfare and immigration laws and regulations can mean continued danger and hardship for many immigrant battered women and their families. Section 6.04 of the NASW Code of Ethics states that "social workers should be aware of the impact of the political arena on practice and should advocate for changes in policy and legislation to improve social conditions in order to meet basic human needs and promote social justice" (NASW, 2008, p. 27). Social workers can use clinical interventions to assess, treat, and empower clients who are victims of domestic violence to leave an abusive relationship and seek safety for themselves and their children. However, as long as legal barriers remain, clients will have difficulty achieving the safety and stability essential to their well-being. By engaging in social action and change through political advocacy, social workers can enable and empower their clients to achieve their treatment goals through access to needed benefits, services, and legal protections.

Social workers need to understand social welfare policies and the implications for practice so that they can empower clients to access needed services for themselves and their families, and to learn how to influence and shape relevant policies to better serve their clients. Policy practice is an important dimension of social work practice (Jansson, 2010). The ethical responsibility for professional policy practice is stated in the NASW Code of Ethics under Section 6: Social Workers Ethical Responsibility for the Broader Society. This section emphasizes the social worker's responsibility not only to promote the general welfare of society and advocate for the fulfillment of basic human needs, but also to engage in social and political acts to promote social justice for all (NASW, 2008).

According to Jansson (2010), policy practice is defined as efforts to influence social policy development, enactment, implementation, and assessment. Policy advocacy is defined as a form of policy practice that is focused on assisting populations lacking power to effect social and political change on their own. Policy practice and advocacy on behalf of immigrant domestic violence victims transcend controversies within social work about whether the profession should focus on the needs of individuals or the larger society. Social work practitioners who engage in clinical or administrative practice or research with this population must become effective policy practitioners to ensure the best possible service outcomes for their clients.

## CONCLUSION

New immigrants remain as vulnerable today as they were over a century ago. In spite of the growing interest and understanding of the need to ensure culturally competent and sensitive social work practice, there is still a dearth of knowledge about the incidence and prevalence of domestic violence among immigrant women and communities of color. Even more essential is a systematic study of the impact of existing services and interventions on victims of domestic violence from cultures other than the dominant European American culture, and the need for changes in the service delivery system.

Many immigrants are from developing countries with cultures and languages significantly different from mainstream America. The influx of immigrants from Asia, South Asia, and Spanish-speaking countries in Central and South America, represent communities of color that are often marginalized in American society. Case examples of battered women from Asia, Eastern Europe, and India, as well as the nondocumented in general, illustrate the difficulties of their obtaining needed services in the United States. An understanding of how different immigrant communities view domestic violence can help social workers begin to reformulate their practice, advocate for policy changes, and formulate effective responses to assist battered immigrant women.

## REFERENCES

Abu-Ras, W. (2007) Cultural beliefs and service utilization by battered Arab immigrant women. *Violence Against Women, 13*(10), 1002–1028. doi:10.1177/1077801207306019

Ahmad, F., Driver, N., McNally, M. J., & Stewart, D. E. (2009). "Why doesn't she seek help for partner abuse?": An exploratory study with South Asian immigrant women. *Social Science and Medicine, 69*(4), 613–622. doi:10.1016/j.socscimed.2009.06.011

Akinsulure-Smith, A., Chu, T., Keatley, E., & Rasmussen, A. (2013) Intimate partner violence among West African immigrants. *Journal of Aggression, Maltreatment & Treatment, 22*, 109–126. doi:10.1080/10926771.2013.719592

American Congress of Obstetricians and Gynecologists. (2012). *Intimate partner violence*. Retrieved from http://www.acog.org

Balice, G., Aquino, S., Baer, S., Behar, M., Belur, A., Flitter, J., . . . Placencia, L. (2019). A review of barriers to treating domestic violence for Middle Eastern women living in the United States. *Psychology Cognitive Science Open Journal, 5*(1), 30–36. doi:10.17140/PCSOJ-5-146

Barker, R. L. (2003). *The social work dictionary*. Silver Springs, MD: National Association of Social Workers.

Barkho, E., Fakhouri, M., & Arnetz, J. (2011). Intimate partner violence among Iraqi women in metro Detroit: A pilot study. *Journal of Minority Health, 13*, 725–731. doi:10.1007/s10903-010-9399-4

Bhandari, S. (2008). Analysis of Violence Against Women Act and the South Asian immigrants in the United State. *Advances in Social Work, 9*(1), 44–50. doi:10.18060/170

Bonilla-Santiago, G. (2002). Latina battered women: Barriers to service delivery and cultural considerations. In A. R. Roberts (Ed.), *Handbook of domestic violence intervention strategies: Policies, programs, and legal remedies* (pp. 464–471). New York, NY: Oxford University Press.

Brace, C. L. (1872). *The dangerous classes of New York, and twenty years' work among them*. Silver Springs, MD: National Association of Social Workers.

Bricker-Jenkins, M., & Hooyman, N. (1986). *Not for women only: Social work practice for a feminist future*. Silver Springs, MD: National Association of Social Workers.

Brownell, P. (1998). The application of the culturagram in cross-cultural practice with elder abuse victims. *Journal of Elder Abuse & Neglect, 9*(2), 19–33. doi:10.1300/J084v09n02_03

Carey, C. (2003). *Immigration assistance for battered immigrant women: Self-petitions and battered spouse waivers*. New York, NY: Asian Women's Center.

Centers for Disease Control and Prevention. (2019). Reproductive Health: Teen Pregnancy. *CDC, Teen Pregnancy*. Retrieved from https://www.cdc.gov/teenpregnancy/about/index.htm

Cesario, S. K., Nava, A., Bianchi, A., McFarlane, J., & Maddoux, J. (2014). Functioning outcomes for abused immigrant women and their children 4 months after initiating intervention. *Revista Panamericana de Salud Pública, 35*(1), 8–14.

Chang-Muy, F. (2009). Legal classifications of immigrants. In F. Chang-Muy & E. Congress (Eds.), *Social work with immigrants and refugees: Legal issues, clinical skills, and advocacy* (pp. 39–62) New York, NY: Springer Publishing Company.

Chaze, F., & Medhekar, A. (2017). The intersectional oppressions of South Asian immigrant women and vulnerability in relation to domestic violence: A case study. *Faculty Publications and Scholarship, 21*. Retrieved from Semanticscholar.org/paper/The-Intersectional-Oppression-of-South-Asian-Women-Chaze-Medhekar/6ce5d420ab45sec327671cZde10de10d2550702289417

Chazin, R., & Ushakova, T. (2005). Working with Russian-speaking Jewish immigrants. In E. Congress & M. Gonzalez (Eds.), *Multicultural perspectives in working with families* (pp. 167–198). New York, NY: Springer Publishing Company.

Choi, Y. J. (2015). Determinants of clergy behaviors promoting safety of battered Korean immigrant women. *Violence Against Women, 21*(3), 394–415. doi:10.1177/1077801214568029

Congress, E. (1994). The use of culturagrams to assess and empower culturally diverse families. *Families in Society: The Journal of Contemporary Human Services, 75,* 531–540. doi:10.1177/104438949407500901

Congress, E. (2002). Using culturagrams with culturally diverse families. In A. Robert & G. Greene (Eds.), *Social work desk reference* (pp. 57–61). New York, NY: Oxford University Press.

Congress, E. (2008). The culturagram. In A. Roberts (Ed.), *Social work desk reference* (2nd ed., pp. 969–975). New York, NY: Oxford University Press.

Congress, E. P., & Brownell, P. (1998). The use of the culturagram in understanding immigrant women affected by domestic violence. In E. P. Congress (Ed.), *Battered women and their families: Intervention strategies and treatment programs* (2nd ed., pp. 387–404). New York, NY: Springer Publishing Company.

Connor, P., & Budiman, A. (2019). *Immigrant share in U.S. nears record high but remains below that of many other countries.* Pew Research Center: Fact Tank. Retrieved from https://www.pewresearch.org/fact-tank/2019/01/30/immigrant-share-in-u-s-nears-record-high-but-remains-below-that-of-many-other-countries

Dako-Gyeke, M. (2013). Conceptualization of female migrants' experiences across the lifespan. *Academic Journal of Interdisciplinary Studies, 2*(1), 259–266. doi:10.5901/ajis.2013.v2n3p259

Danis, F. (2003). Social work response to domestic violence: Encouraging news from a new look. *Affiliate, 18*(2), 177–191. doi:10.1177/0886109903018002007

Davies, J. A., Todahl, J., & Reichard, A. E. (2017). Creating a trauma-sensitive practice: A health care response to interpersonal violence. *American Journal of Lifestyle Medicine, 11*(6), 451–465.

Du Mont, J., & Forte, T. (2012). An exploratory study on the consequences and contextual factors of intimate partner violence among immigrant and Canadian-born women. *BMJ Open, 2,* e001728. doi:10.1136/bmjopen-2012-111728

Dube, S. R., Fairweather, D., Pearson, W. S., Felitti, V. J., Anda, R. F., & Croft, J. B. (2009). Cumulative childhood stress and autoimmune diseases in adults. *Psychosomatic Medicine, 71*(2), 243. doi:10.1097/PSY.0b013e3181907888

Dutton, M. (2006). *The abusive personality* (3rd ed.). New York, NY: Guilford Press.

Dutton, M. A., Orloff, L., & Hass, G. A. (2000). Symposium Briefing Papers; Characteristics of help-seeking behaviors, resources and service needs of battered immigrant Latinas: Legal and policy implications. *Georgetown Journal on Poverty Law & Policy, 7*(2), 245–305.

Dziegielewski, S., & Swartz. M. (2007). Social work's role with domestic violence: Women and the criminal justice system. In A. Roberts & D. Springer (Eds.), *Social work in juvenile and criminal justice settings* (3rd ed., pp. 269–284). Springfield, IL: Charles Thomas.

Ely, G. E. (2004). Domestic violence and immigrant communities in the United States: A review of women's unique needs and recommendations for social work practice and research. *Stress, Trauma and Crisis, 7*(4), 223–241. doi:10.1080/15434610490888027

Erez, E., Adelman, M., & Gregory, C. (2009). Intersections of immigration and domestic violence: Voices of battered immigrant women. *Feminist Criminology, 4*(1), 32–56. doi:10.1177/1557085108325413

Erez, E., & Globokar, J. (2009). Compounding vulnerabilities: The impact of immigration status and circumstances on battered immigrant women. *Sociology of Crime, Law and Deviance, 13,* 129–145. doi:10.1108/S1521-6136(2009)0000013011

Erez, E., & Hartley, C. C. (2003) Battered immigrant women and the legal system: A therapeutic jurisprudence perspective. *Western Criminology Review, 4*(2), 155–169.

Fong, R., McRoy, R., & Ortiz Hendricks, C. (Eds.). (2006). *Intersecting child welfare, substance abuse, and family violence: Culturally competent approaches.* Washington, DC: Council of Social Work Education.

Gambino, C., Trevelyan, E., & Fitzwater, J. (2014). *The foreign-born population from Africa 2008-2012.* United States Census Bureau. Retrieved from https://www2.census.gov/library/publications/2014/acs/acsbr12-16.pdf

Geller, J. A., & Wasserstrom, J. (1984). Cojoint therapy for the treatment of domestic violence. In A. R. Roberts (Ed.), *Battered women and their families* (pp. 33–48). New York, NY: Springer Publishing Company.

Gondolf, E. W. (1997). *Assessing women battering in mental health services.* Thousand Oaks: CA: Sage.

Gordon, L. (1988). *Heroes of their own lives: The politics and history of family violence.* New York, NY: Viking.

Guruge, S., & Kanthasamy, P. (2010). *Older women's perceptions of and responses to abuse and neglect in the post-migration context.* Toronto, Ontario: Wellesley Institute and Centre for Urban Health Initiatives.

Guruge, S., Kanthasamy, P., Jokarasa, J., Wan, T. Y. W., Chinichian, M., Shirpak, K. R., . . . Sathananthan, S. (2010). Older women speak about abuse and neglect in the post-migration context. *Women's Health and Urban Life, 9*(2), 15–41.

Gwinn, C., & Strack, G. (2019). Innovative program increases legal services to domestic violence victims. *Domestic Violence Report, 24*(5), 71–74.

Haglund, K., Belknap, R. A., Edwards, L. M., Tassara, M., Hoven, J. V., & Woda, A. (2018). The influence of masculinity on male Latino adolescents' perceptions regarding dating relationships and dating violence. *Violence Against Women, 25,* 1039–1052. doi:10.1177/1077801218808395

Harper-Dorton, K., & Lantz, J. (2007). *Cross-cultural practice: Social work with diverse populations.* (2nd ed.) Chicago, IL: Lyceum.

Herman, J. (2015). *Trauma and recovery: The aftermath of violence – from domestic violence to political terror.* New York, NY: Basic Books.

Hodgdon, H. B., Liebman, R., Martin, L., Suvak, M., Beserra, K., Rosenblum, W., & Spinazzola, J. (2018). The effects of trauma type and executive dysfunction on symptom expression of polyvictimized youth in residential care. *Journal of Traumatic Stress, 31*(2), 255–264. doi:10.1002/jts.22267

Holcomb, S., Johnson, L., Hetling, A., Postmus, J., Steiner, J., Braasch, L., & Riordan, A. (2017) Implementation of the family violence option 20 years later: A review of the state welfare rules for domestic violence survivors. *Journal of Policy Practice, 16*(4), 415–431. doi:10.1080/15588742.2017.1311820

Ibrahim, D. (2018). Violent victimization, discrimination and perceptions of safety: An immigrant perspective. Statistics Canada: Canadian Centre for Justice Statistics. Retrieved from www150.statcan.gc.ca/nt/pub/85-002-x/2018001/article/54911-eng.pdf

Jansson, B. S. (2010). *Becoming health care advocate.* Pacific Grove, CA: Brooks/Cole.

Kapur, S., & Zajicek, A. (2018). Constructions of battered Asian Indian marriage migrants: The narratives of domestic violence advocates. *Violence Against Women, 24*(16), 1928–1948. doi:10.1177/1077801218757373

Kim, J. Y., & Sung, K. (2000). Conjugal violence in Korean-American families: A residue of cultural tradition. *Journal of Family Violence, 15*(4), 331–345. doi:10.1023/A:1007502212754

Knapp, A. (2019). Net migration between U.S. and abroad added 595,000 to National Population Between 2018 and 2019. United States Census Bureau. Retrieved from https://www.census.gov/library/stories/2019/12/net-international-migration-projected-to-fall-lowest levels-this-decade.html

Kogan, J. (2019). The failure of the Wellstone-Murray family violence option to provide meaningful assistance to survivors of domestic violence. *Journal of Student Social Workers, 4,* 36–43.

Kulwicki, A., Aswad, B., Carmona, T., & Ballout, S. (2010). Barriers in the utilization of domestic violence services among Arab immigrant women: Perceptions of professionals, service providers and community leaders. *Journal of Family Violence, 25,* 727–735. doi:10.1007/s10896-010-9330-8

Kurst-Swanger, K., & Petcosky, J. L. (2003). *Violence in the home: Multi-disciplinary perspectives.* New York, NY: Oxford University Press.

Kwong, D. (2002). Removing barriers for battered immigrant women: A comparison of immigrant protections under VAWA I and II. *Berkeley Women's Law Journal, 17,* 137–152.

Lai, D. W. L., Daoust, G. D., & Li, L. (2014). Understanding elder abuse and neglect in aging Chinese immigrants in Canada. *The Journal of Adult Protection, 16*(5), 322–334. doi:10.1108/JAP-03-2014-0006

Lee, Y. (2014). Elder mistreatment, culture, and help-seeking: A cross-cultural comparison of older Chinese and Korean immigrants. *Journal of Elder Abuse & Neglect, 26*(3), 244–269. doi:10.1080/08946566.2013.820656

Lee, R., Thompson, V., & Mechanic, M. (2002). Intimate partner violence and women of color: A call for innovations. *American Journal of Public Health, 92*(4), 530–534. doi:10.2105/AJPH.92.4.530

Lega, L., & Ellis, A. (2001). Rational emotive behavior therapy (REBT) in the new millennium: A cross-cultural approach. *Journal of Rational Emotive Behavior Cognitive Behavioral Therapy, 19*(4), 201–222. doi:10.1023/A:1012537814117

Liao, M. S. (2006). Domestic violence among Asian Indian immigrant women: Risk factors, acculturation, and intervention. *Women and Therapy, 29*(1–2), 23–39. doi:10.1300/J015v29n01_02

Lipchik, E. (1994). Therapy for couples can reduce domestic violence. In K. Swisher & C. Wekesser (Eds.), *Violence against women* (pp. 154–163). San Diego, CA: Greenhaven Press.

Maru, M., Saraiya, T., Lee, C. S., Meghani, O., Hien, D., & Hahm, H. C. (2018). The relationship between intimate partner violence and suicidal ideation among young Chinese, Korean, and Vietnamese American women. *Women & Therapy, 41*(3–4), 339–355. doi:10.1080/02703149.2018.1430381

Matsouka, A., Guruge, S., Koehn, S., Beaulieu, M., Ploeg, J., Manuel, L., . . . Gomes, F. (2012). Prevention of abuse of older women in the post-migration context in Canada. *Canadian Review of Social Policy, 2,* 68–69, 107–120.

McDonald, R., Jouriles, E. N., Ramisetty-Mikler, S., Caetano, R., & Green, C. E. (2006). Estimating the number of American children living in partner-violent families. *Journal of Family Psychology, 20*(1), 137–142. doi:10.1037/0893-3200.20.1.137

Mills, L. G. (1998). *The heart of intimate abuse: New interventions in child welfare, criminal justice, and health settings.* New York, NY: Springer Publishing Company.

Mose, G., & Gillum, T. (2015) Intimate partner violence in African immigrant communities in the United States: Reflections from the IDVAAC African Women's Roundtable on domestic violence. *Journal of Aggression, Maltreatment & Trauma, 25*(1), 50–62. doi:10.1080/10926771.2016.1090517

Murray, C. E. (2006). Controversy, constraints and context: understanding family violence through family systems theory. *The Family Journal: Counseling and therapy for Couples and Families, 14*(3), 234–239. doi:10.1177/1066480706287277

Murshid, N., & Bowen, E. (2018). A trauma-informed analysis of the Violence Against Women's Act's provision for undocumented women. *Violence Against Women, 24*(13), 1540–1556. doi:10.1177/1077801217741991

Nagaraj, N. C., Vyas, A. N., & McDonnell, K. A. (2018). Is there a link between childhood family violence and adult health? Understanding family violence amongst South Asian American women. *Journal of Immigrant and Minority Health, 21*(5), 978–1003.

National Association of Social Workers. (2008). *NASW code of ethics.* Washington, DC: Author.

National Conference of State Legislators. (2018). *Immigration and public charge: DHS proposes new definition.* Retrieved from http://www.ncsl.org/research/immigration/immigration-and-public-charge-dhs-proposes-new-definition.aspx

National Institute of Justice. (2003). *Do batterers programs work? Two studies*. Washington, DC: United States Department of Justice.
National Organization of Women. (2012). *NOW and violence against women*. Retrieved from http://www.now.org/issues/ violence
Nixon, J., & Humphreys, C. (2010). Marshalling the evidence: Using intersectionality in the domestic violence frame. *Social Politics: International Studies in Gender, State & Society, 17*(2), 137–158. doi:10.1093/sp/jxq003
Orloff, L. (2001). Lifesaving welfare safety net access for battered immigrant women and children. *William & Mary Journal of Women and Law, 7*(3), 597–657.
Orloff, L. (2003). *Concerning New York City executive order*. Federal Document Clearing House Congressional Testimony.
Orloff, L. E., & Kaguyutan, J. V. (2001). Offering a helping hand: Legal protections for battered immigrant women: A history of legislative responses. *American University Journal of Gender, Social Policy and the Law, 10*(1), 95–183.
Orloff, L., & Little, R. (1999). Public benefits access for battered immigrant women and children. In L. E. Orloff (Ed.), *Somewhere to turn: Making domestic violence services accessible to battered immigrant women* (Chapter 11). Retrieved from library.niwap.org/wp-content/uploads/2015/Somewhere-to-Turn-2011.pdf
Pathak, N., Dairying, R., & Tariq, S. (2019). The experience of intimate partner violence among older women: A narrative review. *Maturitas, 121*, 63–75. doi:10.1016/j.maturitas.2018.12.011
Patterson, M., & Malley-Morrison, K. (2006). A cognitive-ecological approach to elder abuse in five cultures: Human rights and education. *Educational Gerontology, 32*(1), 73–84. doi:10.1080/03601270500338666
Peled, E., Eisikovits, Z, Enosh, G., & Winstok, Z. (2000). Choice and empowerment for battered women who stay: Toward a constructivist model. *Social Work, 45*(1), 9–25. doi:10.1093/sw/45.1.9
Perreira, K. M., & Ornelas, I. (2013). Painful passages: Traumatic experiences and post-traumatic stress among immigrant Latino adolescents and their primary caregivers. *International Migration Review, 47*(4), 976–1005. doi:10.1111/imre.12050
Petosic, T., Guruge, S., Wilson-Mitchell, K., Tandon, R., Gunraj, A., Robertson, A., . . . Bauder, H. (2015). *Intergenerational violence: The post-migration context in Canada*. RCIS Working Paper No. 2015/2. Toronto, Ontario: Ryerson Centre for Immigration and Settlement.
Postman, J. L. (2015). Women from different ethnic groups and their experiences with victimization and seeking help. *Violence Against Women, 21*(3), 376–393. doi:10.1177/1077801214568254
Radford, Y. (2019). *Key findings about U.S. immigrants*. Pew Research Center: Fact Tank. Retrieved from https://www.pewresearch.org/fact-tank/2019/06/17/key-findings-about-u-s-immigrants
Ragavan, M., Syed-Swift, Y., Elwy, A. R., Fikre, T., & Bair-Merritt, M. (2018). The influence of culture on healthy relationship formation and teen dating violence: A qualitative analysis of South Asian female youth residing in the United States. *Journal of Interpersonal Violence*. [ePub ahead of print] doi:10.1177/0886260518787815
Raj, A., & Silverman, J. (2002). A violence against immigrant women: The roles of culture, context and legal immigrant status on intimate partner violence. *Violence Against Women, 8*(3), 367–398. doi:10.1177/10778010222183107
Reina, A. S., Lohman, B. J., & Maldonado, M. M. (2014). He said they'd deport me. *Journal of Interpersonal Violence, 29*(4), 593–615. doi:10.1177/0886260513505214
Rios, E. A. (n.d.). *Double jeopardy: Cultural and systemic barriers faced by the Latina battered woman*. Unpublished paper.
Roberts, A. (2007). *Battered women and their families: Intervention strategies and treatment programs* (3rd ed.). New York, NY: Oxford University Press.

Romkens, R. (2001). Law as a Trojan horse: Unintended consequences of rights-based interventions to support battered women. *Yale Journal of Law and Feminism, 13*(2), 265–290.

Rothwell, L. (2001). VAWA 2000's retention of the "Extreme Hardship" standard for battered women in cancellation of removal cases: Not your typical deportation case. *Hawaii Law Review, 23,* 555.

Shainess, N. (1984). *Sweet suffering: Woman as victim.* New York, NY: Bobbs-Merrill.

Sitowski, L. R. (2001). Congress giveth, congress taketh away, congress fixeth its mistake? Assessing the potential impact of the battered immigrant Women Protection Act of 2000. *Law and Inequality Journal, 19*(2), 259–305.

Skocpol, T. (1992). *Protecting soldiers and mothers: The political origins of social policy in the United States.* Cambridge, MA: Harvard University Press.

Smith, S. G., Zhang, X., Basile, K. C., Merrick, M. T., Wang, J., Kresnow, M., & Chen, J. (2018). The *National Intimate Partner and Sexual Violence Survey (NISVS): 2015 Data Brief – Updated Release.* Atlanta, GA: National Center for Injury Prevention and Control, Centers for Disease Control and Prevention. Retrieved from https://www.cdc.gov/violenceprevention/pdf/2015data-brief508.pdf

Sue, D. W. (2006). *Multicultural social work practice.* Hoboken, NJ: Wiley.

Summers, R. W., & Hoffman, A. M. (2002). Introduction. In R. W. Summers & A. M. Hoffman (Eds.), *Domestic violence: A global view* (pp. xi–xvi). Westport, CT: Greenwood Press.

Tabibi, J., Ahmad, S., Baker, L., & Lalonde, D. (2018). Intimate partner violence against immigrant and refugee women. *Learning Network, Issue 26.* London, Ontario: Centre for Research & Education on Violence against Women & Children.

Teicher, M. H., & Samson, J. A. (2016). Annual research review: enduring neurobiological effects of childhood abuse and neglect. *Journal of Child Psychology and Psychiatry, 57*(3), 241–266. doi:10.1111/jcpp.12507

Tjaden, P., & Thoennes, N. (2000). *Full report of the prevalence, incidence, and consequences of intimate partner violence against women. Findings from the National Violence Against Women Survey.* Washington, DC: National Institute of Justice, Grant 93-IJ-0012.

U.S. Census Bureau. (2002). *Number of foreign-born up 57 percent since 1990, according to Census 2000.* Retrieved from https://www.census.gov/newsroom/releases/archives/census_2000/cb02-cn117.html

U.S. Department of Homeland Security. (2019). *Refugees and Asylees.* DHS, News. Retrieved from https://www.dhs.gov/immigration-statistics/refugees-asylees

van der Kolk, B. A. (2006). Clinical implications of neuroscience research in PTSD. *Annals of the New York Academy of Sciences, 1071,* 277–293. doi:10.1196/annals.1364.022

Vaughn, M. G., Salas-Wright, C. P., Huang, J., Qian, Z., Terzis, L., & Heton, J. J. (2017). Adverse childhood experiences among immigrants to the United States. *Journal of Interpersonal Violence, 32*(10), 1543–1564. doi:10.1177/0886260515589568

Villalon, R. (2015) Violence against immigrants in a context of crisis: A critical migration feminist of color analysis. *Journal of Social Distress and Homeless, 24*(3), 116–139. doi:10.1179/1053078915Z.00000000017

Walker, L. E. A. (2017). *The battered woman syndrome* (4th ed.). New York, NY: Springer Publishing Company.

Warren, S. (2016). The U-Visa for immigrant victims of violent crime: What social workers need to know. *Journal of Ethnic and Cultural Diversity in Social Work.* 25(4), 320–324. doi: 10.1080/15313204.2016.1187102

Warrier, S., & Rose, J. (2009). Women, gender-based violence, and immigration. In F. Chang-Muy & E. P. Congress (Eds.), *Social work with immigrants and refugees* (pp. 235–256). New York, NY: Springer Publishing Company.

Yick, A. G. (2000). Domestic violence beliefs and attitudes in the Chinese American community. *Journal of Social Service Research, 27*(1), 29–51. doi:10.1300/J079v27n01_02

Yoshihama, M. (1998). Domestic violence in Japan: Research, program development, and emerging movements. In A. R. Roberts (Ed.), *Battered women and their families: Intervention strategies and treatment programs* (2nd ed., pp. 405–447). New York, NY: Oxford University Press.

Yoshihama, M. (2000). Reinterpreting strength and safety in a socio-cultural context: dynamics of domestic violence and experiences of women of Japanese descent. *Children and Youth Services Review, 22*(3–4), 207–229. doi:10.1016/S0190-7409(00)00076-1

Yoshioko, M. R., Gilbert, L., El-Bassel, N., & Baig-Amin, M. (2003). Social support and disclosure of abuse: Comparing South Asian, African-American, and Hispanic battered women. *Journal of Family Violence, 18*(3), 171–180. doi:10.1023/A:1023568505682

Zarza, M. J., Ponsoda, V., & Carrillo, R. O. A. (2009). Predictors of violence and lethality among Latina immigrants: Implications for assessment and treatment. *Journal of Aggression, Maltreatment and Trauma, 18*(1), 1–16. doi:10.1080/10926770802616423

# 22

# Culture, Intersectionality, and Suicide

DANA ALONZO AND ROBIN EDWARD GEARING

## INTRODUCTION

Across the world, suicide rates are rising despite increased education; greater awareness, larger numbers of prevention and intervention programs such as suicide help phone and text lines; community and school programs; more effective medications to treat underlying risk factors such as depression, anxiety, and substance use; and increased access to empirically supported psychological treatments such as cognitive behavioral therapy (CBT) and dialectical behavioral therapy. Each suicide initiative is important, but the rising rates continue and are impacting people from every demographic. There is no suicide type; suicide affects us all. Traditionally, suicidology has examined the similarities, but investigating differences across cultures and groups may further strengthen our understanding and tools to combat this epidemic.

Global suicide rates have been steadily increasing across countries, regions, and the world. Research tends to focus on a country, ethnicity, or specific subgroup. In 2016, 800,000 deaths occurred by suicide globally (Global Health Estimates 2016, 2018). Differences and availability in national and regional reporting standards vary significantly. There are scarce or no data on suicide for more than half of the countries in the world (Khan, 2005). Clearly demonstrated in the research is that race and ethnicity have consistently been shown to be related to suicidal ideation and behavior (Beck-Cross & Cooper, 2015; Castle, Conner, & Kaukeinen, 2011; Eaton et al., 2011).

The world is changing, so too is the United States. It is estimated that by 2050, Caucasians will no longer be the majority population in the United States (Department of Health and Human Services, 2002). In 2017, the Latinx[1] population

---
[1] The term Latinx is increasingly being used in place of Hispanic/Latino since it denotes greater inclusion. As such, we use Latinx in this chapter.

was 18.1% of the U.S. population, but will comprise 24% to 29% of the population by 2050 (Alegria et al., 2008; Caplan et al., 2013; Pew Hispanic Center, 2017). It is also recognized that in the United States, minorities, particularly those who are depressed and suicidal, experience greater difficulty accessing mental health services (Bustamante et al., 2012; DuBard & Gizlice, 2008; Hines-Martin, Malone, Kim, & Brown-Piper, 2003; Rhodes et al., 2015), remaining engaged in treatment (Gearing, Townsend, Elkins, El-Bassel, & Osterberg, 2014; Kouyoumdjian, Zamboanga, & Hansen, 2003; Polo, Alegría, & Sirkin, 2012), and underutilize mental health services (Hough et al., 1987; Wells, Hough, Golding, Burnam, & Karno, 1987; Vega & Lopez, 2001; Wielen et al., 2015). The importance of mental health service utilization is concerning as approximately 90% of individuals who complete suicide have a mental illness, with depression being the most commonly diagnosed mental disorder (Alonzo & Gearing, 2018; Brent, Baugher, Bridge, Chen, & Chiappetta, 1999; Shaffer et al., 1996).

Consequently, accurate identification and assessment of suicide risk requires an understanding of the influence of culture, ethnicity, and race in relation to suicidality. If culture, race, and ethnicity are overlooked and it is assumed that individuals from all backgrounds experience the world in the same way, intervention and prevention efforts will remain largely unsuccessful at reducing suicide rates (Alonzo & Gearing, 2018). It is essential to understand the unique risk and protective factors for suicide among diverse populations and to adapt prevention and intervention efforts for each specific population in order for such efforts to be more effectively focused (Alonzo & Gearing, 2018). This chapter explores the diverse demographic and ethnic profile of suicidal behavior in the United States and reviews known psychosocial risk factors for suicide within these cultural groups. Critical factors related to culture to be considered when conducting a risk assessment with suicidal clients are reviewed. Treatment of suicidal individuals from culturally competent and evidence-based practice (EBP) perspectives is also explored.

## EPIDEMIOLOGY AND TRENDS IN SUICIDE RATES ACROSS CULTURE, RACE, AND ETHNICITY

Research demonstrates that rates of suicidal ideation, attempts, and completions vary across cultural and ethnic groups. The largest ethnic groups in the United States include Caucasians, Latinxs, African Americans, and Asians, while American Indian and Alaska Natives (AIANs) comprise the smallest ethnic group. All are important to consider.

### Caucasians

Caucasians currently comprise the largest ethnic group in the United States at approximately 63% of the U.S. population (U.S. Census Bureau, 2018). However, this percentage has decreased significantly over the past few decades from about 80% in the 1980s (U.S. Census Bureau, 2018). In 2017, the highest U.S. age-adjusted suicide rate was among Whites (15.85%; Centers for Disease Control and Prevention [CDC], 2017). Many groups comprise the larger Caucasian populations, and rates of suicide vary greatly within the Caucasian population across age and gender. Caucasian males have a higher rate of suicide than Caucasian females or males from other ethnic groups including Blacks, Asians, Latinxs, and AIAN (CDC, 2017). White males accounted for 69.67% of suicide deaths in 2017 (CDC, 2017). Caucasian middle-aged males, aged 45 to 65 years, who historically have had a low suicide rate, currently have the highest suicide rate followed by older adult White males aged 85 or more years (CDC, 2017). Male and female Caucasians have a higher rate of suicide than their African American and Latinx counterparts. In both 2015 and 2016, for example, the suicide rate among Caucasians was nearly 3 times the rate among African Americans and 2.5 times the rate of the Latinx population (CDC, 2016). This trend is more pronounced with age, with elderly Caucasian male suicide rates exceeding elderly Black male suicide rates by more than 2 to 1 (Joe, Baser, Breeden, Neighbors, & Jackson, 2006). The trend is even more pronounced with gender; Caucasian male suicide rates exceed African American female suicide rates 18 to 1 (Joe et al., 2006). Rates of suicide among non-Hispanic Whites continue to rise. Non-Hispanic White males, for example, had higher suicide rates in 2014 than in 1999 for all age groups under 75, with the greatest percentage increase in the 45 to 64 (59%) and 10 to 14 (57%) age groups (Curtin, Warner, & Hedegaard, 2016). Among non-Hispanic White females, the suicide rate for those aged 45 to 64 in 2014 increased 80% from 1999 and was three to four times higher than for females in other racial or ethnic groups (Curtin et al., 2016).

Among Caucasian adolescents, suicide is the third leading cause of death (CDC, 2017). The suicide rate in 2014 for non-Hispanic White females aged 10 to 14 more than tripled from 1999 (Curtin et al., 2016). Caucasian adolescents have a higher rate of completed suicide than their African American and Latinx peers (Lorenzo-Luaces & Phillips, 2014; Rutter & Behrendt, 2004). In 2017, among males, Caucasian adolescents reported greater rates of suicidal ideation than their African American and Latinx peers (13%, 7%, and 11%, respectively); however, they were less likely to report attempting suicide (5%, 6%, and 7%, respectively) (see CDC, 2017). Caucasian female adolescents were also less likely to report attempting suicide than their Latinx and African American peers (7%, 11%, and 13%, respectively) despite similar levels of ideation (CDC, 2017).

## Latinxs

In 2017, Latinxs represented the largest minority group in the United States, comprising 18.1% of the population (U.S. Bureau of the Census, 2011). Only Mexico has a larger Latinx population than the United States (CDC, 2014). As a group, Latinxs have a lower rate of suicide than Caucasians and a slightly lower rate than African Americans (CDC, 2014). Evidence shows that Latinxs report less suicidal ideation and make lower lethality attempts than non-Latinxs even when reporting similar degrees of suicide intent (Alonzo & Gearing, 2018; Oquendo et al., 2005). The lifetime prevalence of suicidal ideation for Latinxs was 11.35%, with the suicide attempt rate of 5.11% (Borges, Orozco, Rafful, Miller, & Breslau, 2012).

Suicide rates vary greatly among Latinx ethnic subgroups (Alonzo & Gearing, 2018). Facility of English language use, length of time in the United States, and attitudes toward mental health problems and help-seeking vary across cultures and may help to explain, in part, these differences. Cuban Americans have the lowest rate of lifetime suicide attempts (2%) followed by Mexican Americans (3%) (see Oquendo et al., 2004). Puerto Ricans have the highest rate of suicide attempts (9.1%) (see Baca-Garcia et al., 2011; Oquendo et al., 2004; Ungemack & Guarnaccia, 1998). Yet, the completed suicide rate for Puerto Ricans is lower than the completed suicide rates for other Latinx ethnic subgroups and for Caucasians (Oquendo et al., 2001). Mexican Americans also have a lower rate of completed suicide than Caucasians (Baca-Garcia et al., 2011; Oquendo et al., 2001). Among Latinxs, Latina adolescents have the highest rate of suicide attempts of all age groups (Alonzo & Gearing, 2018; Zayas, Aguilar-Gaxiola, Yoon, & Rey, 2015; Zayas, Lester, Cabassa, & Fortuna, 2005). Despite similar levels of psychopathology, Latina adolescents have a higher rate of suicide attempts than adolescent females from other ethnic groups (Kuhlberg, Pena, & Zayas, 2010; Zayas & Gulbas, 2012; Zayas et al., 2005).

## African Americans

At 13.4% of the population, African Americans are the second largest minority group in the United States (U.S. Census Bureau, 2018). The lifetime prevalences of suicidal ideation and suicide attempts of Blacks have been placed at 11.82% and 4.15%, respectively (Borges et al., 2012). Among African Americans, females have a lower rate of suicide than African American males (1 to 3; Bridge et al., 2018; Joe et al., 2006). African American females also have a lower rate of suicide than Caucasian females (1 to 2; Joe et al., 2006). According to the CDC (2017), African American females have the lowest suicide rate. In sociological literature, female African Americans have been referred to as a "protected group" due to their historically, consistently low suicide rate (Spates & Slatton, 2017). The low rates of suicide among African American women compared to Caucasian males and females are also referred to in suicide literature as the "Black–White suicide paradox" (Rockett, Samora, & Coben, 2006; Spates & Slatton, 2017).

Although suicide rates among African Americans are lower than overall U.S. rates, suicide affects African American youth at a much higher rate than adults (CDC, 2017). African Americans die by suicide a full decade earlier than Caucasian Americans (Substance Abuse and Mental Health Services Administration [SAMHSA], 2012). The average age of Black suicide decedents, people who have died, is 32 years of age and that of White decedents is 44 years of age. Historically, African American adolescents aged 13 to 17 have had lower suicide rates than have Caucasians with Caucasian teens continuing to have on average a 50% higher rate of completed suicide than Black teens (CDC, 2017). However, a recent study among Black youth aged 5 to 11 has found that suicide rates have increased during the periods of 1993 to 1997 and 2008 to 2012 (from 1.36 to 2.54 per million), whereas they decreased among Caucasian children of the same age (Bridge et al., 2018). This result was consistent across male and female children. In terms of suicide attempts, African American adolescents report the highest rate (9.8%). Additionally, among attempts that required treatment, rates are also highest for African American adolescents (3.4%; CDC, 2017). Further, the percentage of African American female adolescents reporting suicidal thoughts and plans was similar to that of Caucasian female adolescents but higher than that of African American male and Caucasian male adolescents (CDC, 2017).

## Asians

Asians are the third largest minority group in the United States, representing 5.6% of the population (U.S. Census Bureau, 2018). The suicide rate for Asian Americans (6.10 per 10,000) is about half that of the national rate (11.5 per 10,000); see Heron (2011). Suicide is the eighth leading cause of death for Asian Americans, whereas it is the 11th leading cause of death for all racial groups combined (Heron, 2011). Suicide is the second leading cause of death for Asian Americans aged 15 to 34, which is consistent with the national average (i.e., the second leading cause for 15- to 24-year-olds and the third leading cause for 25- to 34-year-olds). Among Asian Americans, those in the 20 to 24 age group have the highest suicide rate. Asian American males have a lower suicide rate compared to Caucasians and AIAN males for almost all age groups. Asian American females, however, aged 65 to 84 have the highest suicide rate of females from any other racial group in that age range (Heron, 2011).

Overall, Asian Americans report lower rates of suicidal ideation (8.6%) and attempts (2.5%) than the national average (13.5% for thoughts, 4.6% for attempts). Among Asian Americans, those aged 18 to 34 reported the highest rates of suicidal thoughts (11.9%), intent (4.4%), and attempts (3.8%) compared to other age groups (Duldulao, Takeuchi, & Seunghye, 2009).

However, results have been shown to vary based on the place of birth. Specifically, U.S.-born Asian American women have been shown to have a higher prevalence of suicidal ideation and suicide plan than U.S.-born Asian American men and immigrant Asian American men and women, and higher rates of suicidal thoughts (15.9%) compared to that of the general U.S. population (13.5%) (see Alonzo and Gearing, 2018; Duldulao et al. 2009).

## American Indian and Alaska Natives

Although the smallest ethnic group in the United States, AIANs had the sharpest rise of all racial and ethnic groups, with suicide rates rising by 89% for women and 38% for men. In 2017, the rates of suicide were highest for AIAN, non-Hispanic males (33.6 per 100,000) and females (11.0 per 100,000), followed by non-Hispanic Caucasian males (28.2 per 100,000) and females (7.9 per 100,000) (see CDC, 2017). Among young adults aged 18 to 24, the suicide rate is highest in the AIAN population for both males and females (34.3 and 9.9 deaths per 100,000 population, respectively). AIAN males were more than twice as likely to commit suicide as most other gender and racial and ethnic subgroups. It is important to note that deaths by suicide in the AIAN population are thought to be underreported by as much as 30% (Kochanek, Murphy, & Xu, 2015). Among AIAN groups, suicide rates have been shown to peak during adolescence and young adulthood and then decline with age. This pattern is in sharp contrast to that of the general U.S. population in which suicide rates peak midlife (CDC, 2017). AIAN individuals had among the highest age-adjusted suicide rates in 2014 (along with non-Hispanic Caucasians) and the highest suicide rates for females and males aged 15 to 24 and 25 to 44, respectively (Curtin et al., 2016). AIAN females had the greatest increase in suicide rates between 1999 and 2014 (89%; Curtin et al., 2016).

## PSYCHOSOCIAL RISK AND PROTECTIVE FACTORS

### Transcultural Risk Factors and Protective Factors

Research has attempted to identify risk and protective factors that are generalizable across cultures and ethnicities, which may be used to inform assessment of suicide risk; however, such research is limited. Overall across ethnicities, any individual with a history of prior suicide attempts is the most consistent risk factor for further attempts (Latinx, African American, and Caucasians), particularly for males (Borowsky, Ireland, & Resnick, 2001; Colucci & Martin, 2007). Exposure to family or friend suicide appears to be another risk factor for suicide shared across cultures (Colucci & Martin, 2007; Rew, Thomas, Horner, Resnick, & Beuhring, 2001). Other cross-cultural risk factors tend to include adolescence, old age, low socioeconomic status (SES), substance use, and recent stressful life events (Colucci & Martin, 2007; Rew et al., 2001). Conversely, general protective factors against suicidal behavior across different ethnicities include parent–family connectedness (Arango et al., 2018; Czyz, Liu, & King, 2012; Whitlock, Wyman, & Moore, 2014), social network and social connectedness (Alonzo & Gearing, 2018), and religiosity (Gearing & Alonzo, 2018; Gearing & Lizardi, 2009). Research in this area is challenging due to the significant influence of social factors (such as attitudes toward suicide, religiosity, gender norms and roles, etc.) and interpersonal factors (such as the nature of familial functioning, peer and social support, etc.) on risk of suicidality and how greatly these factors are affected and vary by culture, race, and ethnicity; it is unlikely that many universal risk factors exist (Alonzo & Gearing, 2018). Nor it is likely that prevention or intervention efforts based solely on transcultural risk factors can effectively reduce suicidal behavior.

Research examining the protective and risk factors across the dominant U.S. ethnic groups has identified some important differences and similarities. Although this field of research is growing, it is important to recognize that the larger ethnic groups in the United States are composed of various and often distinct subgroups. For example among Latinxs, Cuban American suicide rate is very low whereas Puerto Rican suicide rates are much higher. At times, the differences within ethnic subgroups can be larger than across ethnic groups. Research on specific ethnic subgroups is emerging slowly yet still is lacking; interpreting data from the dominant ethnic groups can prove helpful in the meantime but should be applied with caution.

### Culture-Specific Risk Factors and Protective Factors

To ensure that assessment, prevention, and intervention efforts target the most prevalent and significant issues for each individual, it is essential to consider the distinctive risk and protective factors among the individual's specific ethnic and cultural group(s). The following summarizes the current state of evidence regarding the main risk and protective factors for the dominant ethnic/cultural groups in the United States.

#### Caucasians

More often than other ethnic groups, Caucasians who engage in suicidal behavior are older and are more likely to have an anxiety disorder (Garlow, Purselle,

& Heninger, 2005; Vanderwerker et al., 2007). A major risk factor for suicide among Caucasians is disrupted family environment (Beghi, Rosenbaum, Cerri, & Cornaggia, 2013). Caucasians are also more likely to use alcohol prior to a suicide attempt (Groves, Stanley, & Sher, 2007; Vanderwerker et al., 2007). Loss of a family member or friend to suicide (Borowsky et al., 2001; Brent, Bridge, Johnson, & Connolly, 1996; Brent, Perper, Moritz, Baugher et al., 1993), access to firearms (Brent, Perper, Moritz, Baugher et al., 1993), and female gender (Grossman, Milligan, & Deyo, 1991; Lefebvre, Lesage, Cyr, & Toupin, 1998; Moscicki et al., 1988; Pirkis, Burgess, & Dunt, 2000; Schmidtke et al., 1996; Suominen, Isometsa, Haukka, & Lonnqvist, 2004; Woods et al., 1997) have also been identified as risk factors among Caucasians. Particularly among elderly Caucasians, physical illness has also been shown to be associated with increased risk of suicidality (Vanderwerker et al., 2007). Further, low income has been demonstrated to be associated with increased risk of suicidal ideation and behavior among non-Hispanic Whites (McMillan, Enns, Asmundson, & Sareen, 2010; Purselle, Heninger, Hanzlick, & Garlow, 2009).

Major protective factors against suicide for Caucasians include marriage, female gender, low levels of aggression and impulsivity, and religiosity (Oquendo et al., 2004, 2005). Among Caucasian youth, family cohesion has been identified as a major protective factor against suicidality (Borowsky et al., 2001).

### African Americans

Among African Americans, male gender, interpersonal conflict, and younger age have been demonstrated to be consistent predictors of suicide risk (Gibbs, 1997; Groves et al., 2007). Additionally, negative family interaction has been found to be associated with increased odds of suicide attempts among African Americans (Lincoln, Taylor, Chatters, & Joe, 2012). For example, African American youth who experience parental conflict are approximately seven times more likely to engage in suicidal behavior than those who do not experience parental conflict (Groves et al., 2007). Overall, African Americans are twice as likely as Caucasians to choose a violent method of suicide (Stack & Wasserman, 2005). For example, African Americans aged 15 and older are twice as likely as Caucasians to complete suicide via the use of firearms (Joe, Marcus, & Kaplan, 2007). Increased risk of suicidal ideation and behavior among African Americans has also been shown to be associated with substance use, specifically alcohol, marijuana, and cocaine (Garlow, 2002; Lorenzo-Luaces & Phillips, 2014).

Strong religious ties and family cohesiveness have been identified as protective factors (Ali & Maharajh, 2005; Hirsch, Nsamenang, Chang, & Kaslow, 2014; June, Segal, Coolidge, & Klebe, 2009; Walker, 2007) among African Americans. Further, African Americans also report greater reasons for living that serve as protector factors against suicide than their non-Latinx White counterparts, particularly moral objections to suicide and survival and coping related beliefs (Molock & Barksdale, 2013; Wang, Lightsey, Tran, & Bonaparte, 2013; Yip, Callanan, & Yuen, 2000). Receiving emotional and psychological support from family and friends has also been identified as a protective factor, particularly for African American females (Compton, Thompson, & Kaslow, 2005; Kaslow et al., 2002). Rural versus urban residency and higher level of educational attainment have also been found to protect against suicide among African Americans (Willis et al., 2003).

### Latinxs

Acculturative stress has been found to be a risk factor for suicide ideation and behavior among Latinxs, specifically adolescents (Cervantes, Goldbach, Varela, & Santisteban, 2014; Humensky et al., 2013; Smokowski, David-Ferdon, & Stroupe, 2009; Vega, Gil, Warheit, Apospori, & Zimmerman, 1993). The impact of acculturative stress on suicide risk is further increased when substance use is involved (Vega et al., 1993). Young age has also been identified as a risk factor for suicide among Puerto Ricans and Mexicans. Fatalism, or the belief that life is predetermined by fate, is a risk factor for suicide among Latinxs as it places the locus of control outside of the individual and reduces an individual's desire to cope with and manage stressors (Hoppe & Martin, 1986; Hovey & King, 1997; Sorenson & Golding, 1988). Among Latinx adolescent males, acculturative stress is associated with suicidal thoughts, while discrimination stress is associated with both suicidal thoughts and self-harm behavior. Among Latinas, acculturation stress and immigration stress are associated with self-harm behaviors (Cervantes et al., 2014).

Among Latina adolescents, research has examined the relationship between their notably high rate of suicide attempts and the quality/nature of the mother–daughter relationship. It has been proposed that a cultural discontinuity in which Latina adolescents struggle to reconcile traditional Latina gender role expectations with their own modern Western societal values and beliefs underlies their elevated rates (Zayas et al., 2015). This discontinuity often results in tension and conflict between daughter and mother that lead to escalating stress, which triggers a suicide attempt (Zayas & Gulbas, 2012; Zayas, Gulbas, Fedoravicius, & Cabassa, 2010; Zayas et al., 2015).

Familism, described as the close relationships with immediate family and extended family networks, serves as a protective factor against suicide for Latinxs (Hovey & King, 1997; Kuhlberg et al., 2010; Oquendo et al., 2005; Polanco-Roman & Miranda, 2013), and Latinxs have been shown to endorse greater responsibility toward family than their non-Hispanic counterparts (Oquendo et al., 2005). Moral objections to suicide, and survival and coping beliefs are also stronger among Latinxs than non-Latinxs (Oquendo et al., 2005). Among Latinxs, greater religiosity has been found to be a protective factor against suicide (Oquendo et al., 2005; Robinson, Bolton, Rasic, & Sareen, 2012).

### Asian Americans

Among Asian Americans, psychiatric illness, particularly a diagnosis of depression or anxiety, is associated with an increase in suicidality (Groves et al., 2007; Kuroki & Tilley, 2012). High parental conflict increases suicide risk by as much as 30-fold as compared to low parental conflict (Groves et al., 2007; Kuroki & Tilley, 2012; Lau, Jernewall, Zane, & Myers, 2002). A lower level of acculturation is an additional risk factor for suicidality among Asian Americans, particularly in the presence of parental conflict (Duldulao et al., 2009; Lau et al., 2002; Wong & Maffini, 2011).

Risk factors for suicide among Asian ethnic subgroups have been identified. Risk factors for suicide in South Asians have been found to include domestic violence, negative family environment, and depression (Ahmed & Mohan, 2007; Hicks & Bhugra, 2003). Academic stress has been found to be a strong risk factor for suicide among Koreans (Dawkins, 1996). Among the Chinese, research indicates that risk factors are primarily related to psychiatric illness (Zhang, Conwell, Zhou, & Jiang, 2004), poor health (Zhang et al., 2004), and hopelessness (Chen, Chien-Chang Wu, Yousuf, & Yip, 2011; Stewart et al., 2005). Secondary predictors include lack of social support, negative life events, lower SES, religious affiliation, and family conflict (Zhang et al., 2004). Impulsivity is also a risk factor for suicide (Huang et al., 2017; Pearson, Phillip, He, & Ji, 2002).

Traditional values of obedience and respect have been found to be protective against suicide attempts among Asian populations, independent of the quality of family relationships (Lam et al., 2004). Similarly, endorsing a strong ethnic group identification has been found to be protective among Asian Americans (Cheng et al., 2010). Research has also identified social support and higher degrees of hope as protective factors against suicide among the Chinese (Chen et al., 2011; Cho & Haslam, 2010).

### American Indian and Alaska Natives

Suicide rates among AIAN populations vary across individual tribes as a result of geographic location, historical experiences, and access to clinical and community service programs, making it difficult to generalize findings regarding risk and protective factors for suicide in these groups (Herne, Bartholomew, & Weahkee, 2014). Nevertheless, limited research has identified some consistent risk and protective factors. Among AIAN youth, the risk factors most strongly associated with suicide are substance use, a family history of drug or alcohol abuse, having an arrest record, depression, a history of physical or sexual abuse, exposure to the suicide of a family member or peer, and racial discrimination (Freedenthal & Stiffman, 2004; Olson & Wahab, 2006).

Connectedness to family has been identified as a key protective factor for AIAN youth (Alcántara & Gone, 2007). Perceived social support has been associated with decreased risk of depression, and may then indirectly serve as a protective factor against suicide (Burnette et al., 2017). Indigenous spiritual beliefs and activities, once positioned to serve as protective factors, now show some inconsistency and have been found in some Indigenous groups to be associated with poorer psychological outcomes, including increased depression, anger, anxiety, and interpersonal difficulties, which may serve to increase suicide risk (Walls, Whitbeck, & Armenta, 2016)

## CULTURAL AND INTERSECTIONAL ISSUES

### Cultural Affiliation and Suicide Risk

To more fully understand the role that culture plays as a potential risk or protective factor for suicide, it is essential to ascertain a client's degree of cultural affiliation. Simply having awareness of a client's culture does not provide an accurate understanding of the relevant risk or protective factors that need to be considered during risk assessment. Culture influences suicide in a number of ways: There may be culture-specific patterns in regard to the precipitants of suicidal behavior; the risk and protective factors for suicidal behavior themselves may be influenced by one's cultural context; the characteristics of suicidal behaviors may differ from culture to culture; individuals will view, understand, and respond to suicidal behaviors in different ways across cultures; and culture will impact help-seeking behaviors. However, the degree to which these factors will be relevant to an individual client will vary based on their degree of cultural affiliation. This suggests, then, that merely providing a cultural label for your client (e.g., Italian, Puerto Rican, Russian) will not suffice. A thorough assessment of risk will require that a clinician explore how a client defines their culture and the degree to which a client identifies and affiliates with their culture.

### The Influence of Immigration on Suicide

Immigration has been found to be associated with increased levels of stress, mental illnesses, and suicide risk (Kushner, 1991; Lester, 1997. 1998; Shoval, Schoen, Vardi, & Zalsman, 2007). A number of factors related to immigration are positively correlated with depression and anxiety (Arbona et al., 2010; Cervantes, Padilla, Napper, & Goldbach, 2013; Hiott, Grzywacz, Arcury, & Quandt, 2006). Generally acknowledged as a stressful life event, the process of immigrating often represents a crisis event (Ponizovsky & Ritsner, 1999). Immigrating individuals are forced to deal with the process of acculturation while simultaneously having to deal with the loss of previously established protective factors, particularly one's social support network (Sorenson & Shen, 1996). Immigrants also tend to experience heightened prejudice and discrimination (Shoval et al., 2007). In addition, immigrants often earn less money (Sorenson & Shen, 1996), and a lower SES is associated with increased risk of suicidal behavior (Alonzo & Gearing, 2018). They experience greater difficulty accessing or seeking out mental health services (Bustamante et al., 2012; DuBard & Gizlice, 2008; Rhodes et al., 2015) and remaining engaged in treatment (Gearing et al., 2014; Kouyoumdjian et al., 2003; Polo et al., 2012), which may potentially support the individual through the difficult transitions resulting from immigrating (Sorenson & Shen, 1996).

However, research is inconsistent (Shoval et al., 2007). A seminal work by Kushner (1991) found that during the mid-20th century, migration increased the risk of suicide. Findings specifically demonstrated that foreign-born persons had nearly twice the suicide rate of native-born persons (Kushner, 1991). Kushner (1991) proposed that foreign-born persons from countries with higher suicide rates maintained a higher suicide risk after immigration. This association between suicide rates of immigrants and rates of suicide in their country of origin has received further support from other studies (Lester, 1997, 1998; Spallek & Razum, 2015). Another study found immigrant adolescents had a lower suicide rate than nonimmigrant peers (Greenfield et al., 2006). Yet another study found a significant association between the length of residency in the United States and negative suicide attitudes, and also between psychological acculturation and negative suicide attitudes (Eshun, 2006). Other research has found that the overall suicide risk is lower among immigrants prior to migration compared to U.S.-born natives, but that such differences equalize over time after migration (Borges et al., 2012).

Others have similarly found that foreign-born persons are generally at lower risk of suicide than U.S.-born persons (Sorenson & Shen, 1996). However, that risk varied by ethnicity in that there was a higher risk for foreign-born Caucasians than for native-born Caucasians, while foreign-born Latinxs had lower risk and foreign-born Blacks and Asians shared similar risks with native-born persons (Sorenson & Shen, 1996). Research has found that recent immigrants retain some protective health effects acquired from their country of origin, which often extend 5 years post immigration (Jasso, Massey, Rosenzweig, & Smith, 2004). Yet, as time in the United States increases, these protective effects have been found to diminish (Alegria, 2008; Gonzalez et al., 2009). This phenomenon for Latinxs immigrating from Mexico, known as the Hispanic health paradox, has been generally consistent over the past 30 years (Franzini, Ribble, & Keddie, 2001; Markides & Eschbach, 2005; Palloni & Morenoff, 2001; Teruya & Bazargan-Hejazi, 2013). Recent research, however, has found the effects of the Hispanic health paradox significantly eroding, possibly due to the amount and intensity of anti-immigration rhetoric during the past few years in the political and social arenas (Gearing et al., under review).

Four potential hypotheses regarding factors that may mediate any suicide risk were proposed:

1. Culture of origin effects are protective factors derived from individuals' culture of origin that they carry with them to their culture of destination. Catholicism's belief regarding suicide (values life, views suicide as a sin) and Confucianism's belief regarding suicide (values self-sacrifice, potentially views suicide as a virtue), for example, may mitigate suicide risk among immigrants whose culture of origin endorses these beliefs.
2. Country of destination factors speak to the nature of the environment to which one has immigrated. Conditions such as crowded housing arrangements, which may lead to discovering suicide attempts sooner, or availability of suicide method (e.g., firearms) may be protective or risk factors.
3. Personal characteristics of immigrants may also serve as protective factors; for example, immigrants are often healthier and less depressed than the U.S.-born population (Stephen, Foote, Hendershot, & Schoenborn, 1994).
4. Migration selectivity theory recognizes that migration is a process in which only certain people elect or are selected to immigrate. This theory posits that only healthy individuals, who have a good chance of succeeding in the new country and may be able to bring over the rest of the family and/or send money back to their country of origin, are supported or encouraged to migrate (Sorenson & Shen, 1996). Conversely, individuals who are not likely to succeed may not be selected by the new country as candidates for immigration (Marmot, Adelstein, & Bulusu, 1984). Consequently, individuals prone to suicidality are less likely to immigrate and more likely to return to their country of origin (Sorenson & Shen, 1996).

Conversely, other research identified that being foreign-born instead of native-born was a significant risk factor for suicide. These results held true across genders and across all age groups except for males aged 30 to 49 (Johansson et al.,

1997). Similarly, a study found an overrepresentation of foreign-born suicide among psychiatric patients. However, it was recognized that unemployment and poor social integration may have been confounding factors (Chandrasena, Beddage, & Fernando, 1991). Overall, these findings indicate that the risk of suicide as related to immigration is culture-specific. Further, they suggest that other factors may mediate to confound the relationship between immigration and suicide risk.

### The Influence of Acculturation and Assimilation on Suicide

Acculturation is defined as the process that immigrants experience as they adjust to their host culture. Acculturative stress and subsequent depression are related, which can also be linked to increased suicidal ideation and suicidal risk (Cervantes et al., 2013; Hovey, 2000). It has been defined as the struggle to maintain one's identity, traditions, values, and customs associated with one's culture of origin, while adapting to the mainstream culture to which one has emigrated (Alonzo & Gearing, 2018). This period is often associated with increased feelings of depression, anxiety, isolation, and suicidality (Hovey & King, 1997), referred to as acculturative stress (Berry & Kim, 1988; Hovey & King, 1996, 1997; Padilla, Cervantes, Maldonado, & Garcia, 1988; Williams & Berry, 1991).

Research regarding the association between suicide risk and acculturation has found that, counterintuitively, for many cultural groups in the United States, individuals with higher levels of acculturation are at more risk for engaging in suicidal behavior than those with lower levels of acculturation. Among Native Americans, for example, acculturative stress is a strong predictor of suicide (Gray & McCullagh, 2014; Lester, 1999). Similar results have been found for native Hawaiians (Yuen, Nahulu, Hishinuma, & Miyamoto, 2000) and Latinxs (Gutierrez, Osman, Kopper, & Barrios, 2000; Vega et al., 1993). Additionally, Mexican Americans born in the United States have been found to have higher rates of suicide and suicidal ideation than Mexican Americans born in Mexico (Sorenson, & Golding, 1988; Swanson, Linskey, Quintero-Salinas, Pumariega, & Holzer, 1992). High levels of acculturative stress have also been found to be a risk factor for suicide among Central Americans (Hovey, 2000) and Puerto Ricans (Monk & Warshauer, 1974; Oquendo et al., 2004). Further, greater acculturation has also been found to be associated with increased risk of suicidal ideation among African Americans (Eaton et al., 2011). Gomez, Miranda, and Polanco (2011) also found acculturative stress to be related to increased odds of lifetime suicide attempt, with African Americans at the highest risk and Asian Americans at the lowest risk (Gomez et al., 2011).

However, research suggests the relationship between acculturation and suicidality is more nuanced. For example, some studies have found that acculturation is related to suicidal ideation but not to suicidal behavior (Kennedy, Parhar, Samra, & Gorzalka, 2005; Lessenger, 1997). Kennedy et al. (2005) found that suicidal ideation, plans, and attempts did not vary by generational level or overall ethnic group among Europeans, Chinese, and Indo-Asians.

Risk or protective factors for suicide risk related to acculturation have been identified and should be assessed when attempting to evaluate suicide risk (Alonzo & Gearing, 2018). These factors include availability of social supports in the new community; level of familial support from both immediate and extended family networks; religiosity; SES, including changes in work status, education, and employment; language ability; expectations for the future; and pre-immigration level of cognitive functioning and quality of coping skills (Hovey & King, 1997; Williams & Berry, 1991).

It is essential to consider not only the rates and trends in suicide among various ethnic groups but equally important to consider the level of acculturation and degree of cultural affiliation of each client and how these might impact his or her suicide risk. When evaluating and treating suicidal individuals, a comprehensive assessment should be conducted concerning the process of immigration for the individuals and their families, the acculturation process, signs of acculturative stress, their degree of cultural affiliation to their culture of origin, and their level of connection to their host culture.

## INTERNATIONAL PERSPECTIVES AND ATTITUDES ON SUICIDE

Lay theories are commonly held beliefs by a community in general (Walker, Lester, & Sean, 2006). Lay beliefs and the acceptability of suicide vary across cultural, ethnic, and societal groups (Angermeyer & Matschinger, 1999; Knight, Furnham, & Lester, 2000). In some cultures, under certain conditions, suicide may be seen as a positive, moral act, while in other cultures, suicide is considered unaccepted and forbidden under all circumstances and is equated with a mental illness (Alonzo & Gearing, 2018).

Within-group cultural differences also exert influence on beliefs about and attitudes toward suicide (Pridmore & Walter, 2013). For example, in the Indian subcontinent, female suicide rates are among the highest in the world (Bhugra, 2005; Thompson & Bhugra, 2000). Traditional and cultural beliefs regarding rigid gender roles and the positionality of women contribute to their increased suicide risk. Limited access to mental health services; high rates of domestic violence; deference to males; arranged marriages; women being viewed as the property of males; limited opportunities for choice regarding employment, education, and family; and the ritual act Sati or burning oneself on the funeral pyre of one's husband influence the acceptability of or viewing of suicide as a reasonable option (Bhugra, 2005; Thompson & Bhugra, 2000).

In Japan, where being part of society is valued more than being an individual, the traditional act of suicide (jisatsu) is viewed as an acceptable and appropriate behavior in certain circumstances (Pfeffer, 1991). Further, suicide may be considered an affirmation of the value of one's moral duty to others (giri) (Young, 2002). There is also less traditional sanctioning for double suicide (shinju; e.g., parent–child or husband–wife suicide) and youth suicide (Pfeffer, 1991). The collectivist values of Japan are distinctly different from the autonomous values held in North America, thereby influencing the respective cultures' attitudes toward suicide.

Ethnic and cultural groups within the United States hold different beliefs regarding who has greater influence and control over their lives (e.g., God, individual, the government) and for what circumstances suicide is a viable option (e.g., intrapsychic, interpersonal, or societal difficulties) (see Walker et al., 2006). According to Walker et al. (2006), European Americans are more likely than African Americans to attribute suicidal thoughts to interpersonal problems (e.g., conflict, work stress, broken home). In addition, European Americans attribute ownership of life to the individual or government. Conversely, African Americans attribute ownership of life to God.

This provides yet further support for the importance of understanding one's culture in order to assess for life-affirming beliefs and values or potentially attitudes that are more accepting and understanding of suicidal behaviors. The process of assessing for this information may not only facilitate and strengthen a social worker's engagement and therapeutic alliance with the client, but will also provide valuable information on potential protective and/or risk factors that may be incorporated into treatment strategies (Alonzo & Gearing, 2018).

## CLINICAL ASSESSMENT

### Models of Cultural Influences on Suicidal Behavior

It may be useful to frame a suicide risk assessment within a model of suicidal behavior that allows for the examination of culturally relevant factors. Although no one universal model exists as an explanation for suicidality, a stress–diathesis model of suicidal behavior has been proposed (Goldney, 2002; Mann, Waternaux, Haas, & Malone, 1999) and has gained acceptance as a means to understand suicidal behavior (Grunebaum et al., 2006).

According to this model, environmental factors (referred to as triggers or stressors) exist at certain times that can be considered state-dependent (Mann et al., 1999). In addition, genetic and/or biochemical factors or mechanisms (referred to as a threshold or diathesis) exist that are considered trait-dependent. When risk factors from only one of these domains is present (state *or* trait), it is not sufficient to elicit suicidal behavior (Mann et al., 1999). However, when factors from both domains are present (state *and* trait), the likelihood of suicidal behavior occurring is increased (Malone, Haas, Sweeny, & Mann, 1995). Individuals who engage in suicidal behavior are considered to have a vulnerability for suicide. This vulnerability may be innate, as a result of genetic or familial factors, such as having a first-degree relative with a history of suicide attempts (Malone et al., 2000; Mann et al., 1999; Pfeffer, Normandin, & Kakuma, 1994; Roy, 1983; Roy, 1986; Roy, Segal, Centerwall, & Robinette, 1991), or it may be the result of traumatic experiences such as parental loss, childhood physical and/or sexual abuse (Adam, Bouckoms, & Streiner, 1982; Briere & Runtz, 1990; Farber, Herbert, & Reviere, 1996; Levi, Fales, Stein, & Sharp, 1966), and alcoholism or substance abuse (Malone et al., 1995).

The stress–diathesis model allows for variance in several areas that may account for the differential rates of suicidal behavior that exist across cultures and ethnicities in that state factors are subject to cultural influences. For example, substance abuse, physical abuse, sexual abuse, unemployment, undereducation, immigration status, migration experiences, and acculturation experiences occur in varying rates across cultures and have a direct influence on an individual's vulnerability toward suicidal acts (Alonzo & Gearing, 2018).

The Cultural Theory and Model of Suicide forwarded by Chu et al. (2013) was presented to explain the variance in suicidal behavior that is seen across cultures. This model, drawn from an empirical literature analysis of research across 20 years, examined the beliefs, values, norms, practices, and customs that have been found to be associated with the suicidal behavior of Latinx Americans; African Americans; Asian Americans; and LGBTQ individuals. Chu et al. (2013) found that culture influences suicide through four key distinct constructs:

1. Cultural sanctions: Cultural messages regarding the acceptability of triggers for suicide and of suicidal behavior itself, including the amount of shame incurred associated with it.
2. Idioms of distress: Culturally influenced expressions of psychological distress that influence the way in which suicidal behavior is expressed and one's method or means for engaging in suicidal behavior.
3. Minority stress: The added stress that individuals in stigmatized minority groups experience that influences the way experiences are perceived and makes it more difficult to cope.
4. Social discord: The interpersonal conflict in one's social support system.

The Cultural Theory and Model of Suicide provides an explanation of how culture impacts each step of an individual's decision to attempt suicide (Chu et al., 2013). This model posits that an individual's culture influences not only the way in which one interprets life events, but the ways in which one expresses suicidal ideation or suicidal intent, as well as the meaning of suicide as a response to extreme life stress (Chu et al., 2013). As an example, life stressors, such as minority stress and social discord, may be interpreted through the lens of cultural sanctions, through which one's cultural identity sends messages about the acceptability of these stressors (Chu et al., 2013). If the life stressors are considered to be culturally unacceptable, the individual may express suicidal ideation through his or her culturally specific idioms of distress. At this point, one's cultural sanctions may indicate that suicide is an acceptable response to the life stressors and, if he or she is unable to tolerate stressors, may then attempt suicide (Chu et al., 2013).

Multiple empirical studies delineate a specific cultural risk and protective factors that should be incorporated into the risk assessment of specific cultural groups. For example, Kaslow et al. (2004), emphasize assessing for aggression as a key risk factor for suicide among African Americans, whereas Cheng et al. (2010) suggest that family conflict and perceived discrimination are key factors for identifying risk among Asian Americans. However, more general guidelines to be used across cultures are less fully developed. Further, although a few models for incorporating information regarding cultural factors into current suicide risk assessment practices have been presented, no guidelines have been universally accepted. Others further question the efficacy of existing cultural competence guidelines to reduce mental health disparities, given the lack of operationalization, guidance, resources, and/or support for their implementation (Vega & Lopez, 2001).

Alonzo and Gearing (2018) propose that culturally competent suicide assessment requires careful and active consideration of culture-specific risk and protective factors as well as attitudes regarding suicide acceptability. Similarly, the American Psychiatric Association Work Group on Suicidal Behaviors (2003) recognizes that views of death and cultural beliefs regarding suicide vary greatly, even among members of apparently homogeneous racial, ethnic, or cultural groups. As such, it proposes that part of an effective risk assessment must include exploration of the client's beliefs about death and suicide and the role of cultural and family dynamics in these beliefs.

## TREATMENT

### Mental Health Service Utilization and Ethnicity

Racial and ethnic disparities in mental health service utilization have consistently been reported in research. Several historical and contemporary factors likely contribute to these disparities. For example, historical abuses (e.g., the Tuskegee experiment) have contributed to a culture of mistrust that likely impacts the level of health and mental health service utilization among minorities (Breland-Noble, 2004; Goldston et al., 2008; Nickerson, Helms, & Terrell, 1994). Further, racial/ethnic minorities, especially those who are less acculturated, are more likely to seek help from traditional/alternative venues (e.g., faith healers, religious providers) than from formal mental health services (Snowden & Yamada, 2005). Although there is stigma surrounding mental health in general, it is even more pronounced in the case of suicidal ideation and behaviors (Goldston et al., 2008) and even more so among racial/ethnic minorities (Freedenthal & Stiffman, 2004; Novins et al., 2004), furthering increasing disparities in mental health service utilization.

Racial/ethnic minorities in the United States have lower mental health service utilization rates compared to Caucasians, with 22.4% of Latinxs and 25% of African Americans receiving treatment for a diagnosed mental illness compared to 37.6% of Whites (Gearing et al., 2014; Hough et al., 1987; Vega & Lopez, 2001; Wells et al., 1987; Wells, Lagomasino, Palinkas, Green, & Gonzalez, 2001; Wielen et al., 2015). In addition, failure to make initial treatment contact and delayed treatment contact have also been found to be associated with racial/ethnic minority status (Bustamante et al., 2012; DuBard & Gizlice, 2008; Hines-Martin et al., 2003; Kouyoumdjian et al., 2003; Polo et al., 2012; Rhodes et al., 2015; Wang et al., 2005). Furthermore, mental healthcare among individuals with suicidal thoughts and behaviors mirrors these general trends of racial/ethnic disparity. Among adults who attempted suicide in the past year, receipt of mental health treatment over the same time period was lower among non-Hispanic Blacks (39.7%) and Latinxs (44.4%) than among non-Hispanic Whites (65.8%) (see Han, Compton, Gfroerer, and McKeon, 2014; Wang et al., 2005).

### Culturally Responsive Practice

Suicidal individuals are an extremely difficult population to engage in treatment, with low rates of initial entry into treatment and even lower rates of ongoing treatment adherence (Alonzo, 2016; Lizardi & Stanley, 2010). Efforts to improve treatment engagement and adherence of culturally diverse clients will be unsuccessful if they fail to consider the treatment expectations of clients and how such expectations are influenced by one's culture. At present, there is a lack of ethnocultural comparative studies needed to develop culturally responsive prevention and intervention strategies for suicidality (Colucci & Martin, 2007). Researchers in the field of suicidality have established that each culture exerts positive and negative influences on suicidality, and intervention efforts need to incorporate and account for these cultural differences (Bhugra & Mastrogianni, 2004).

It is essential that clinicians are aware of and sensitive to the cultural expectations and issues of clients and of the cultural differences between clients and themselves (Dalton, 2005). According to Sue and colleagues (Sue, Arredondo, & McDavis, 1992; Sue et al., 1982; Sue & Sue, 2003), cultural competence is often more recently referred to as cultural responsiveness, acknowledging that one is never fully competent but that the process of understanding and awareness is ongoing. Sue and Sue (2003) describe this process as requiring clinicians to work toward several specific goals including:

1. Actively and continually seeking to become aware of their own assumptions, bias, values, and personal limitations
2. Recognizing that their worldview is different than their clients
3. Being in the process of actively trying to practice appropriate, sensitive, and relevant intervention strategies and skills in working with culturally diverse clients (Sue & Sue, 2003)

Research indicates that the ability to work from a culturally responsive perspective remains an area of concern in the field of suicidality. For example, research demonstrates that stereotypes are often taken as facts, potentially resulting in misdiagnosis and treatment (Burr, 2002). Cultural responsiveness is an active process in which the practitioner remains engaged with the individual in front of him or her and does not presume an understanding of the client based solely on an awareness of his or her culture. At the same time, it is important to acknowledge that research has demonstrated that by emphasizing cultural differences, a clinician may run the risk of increasing prejudice toward different cultures and reinforcing overgeneralizations (Takahashi, 1997). The lesson, then, is that practicing cultural responsiveness requires the clinician to take the time to engage the client in a discussion of what culture means to the client, how the client defines his or her culture, and the client's self-identified degree of cultural affiliation.

## EVIDENCE-BASED APPROACH TO PRACTICE WITH DIVERSE POPULATIONS

Although EBPs for the treatment of suicidal behavior have been developed in recent years, there remains a dearth of research regarding the cultural relevance of such treatments for minority populations. Most EBPs determine the effectiveness of a given intervention within an ethnic majority population first and then test for generalizability to diverse populations. Some argue that to maximize cultural responsiveness, EBPs would ideally be developed in a bottom-up manner in collaboration with cultural groups and tested among diverse populations in their local treatment settings (Whitley; 2007). Others further argue that an overemphasis on the development, testing, and implementation of EBPs may lead to decreased attention to cultural variations in service delivery and may serve to invalidate and/or exclude culture-specific interventions and/or traditional healing practices often used by minority groups (Isaacs, Huang, Hernandez, & Echo-Hawk, 2005). Having an adequate representation of ethnic/racial populations in data gathered on the feasibility, acceptability, and effectiveness of an intervention is essential for determining the translatability of clinical efficacy trials to real-world settings and diverse populations.

Practice-based evidence (PBE) has been developed to address this concern. PBE is considered a set of unique, inherent cultural practices that have nontraditional evidence based on and derived from community consensus (Martinez, 2008). PBE approaches the treatment needs of individuals from a culture-specific framework. Although PBE interventions lack an empirical evidence base, they are responsive to and respectful of diverse communities and their respective unique cultures and traditions (Martinez, 2007). This kind of cultural foundation of PBEs is in contrast to the scientific basis of EBPs. Together, however, the two have the potential to effectively address the treatment needs of diverse communities (Isaacs et al., 2005). Further, such a dually informed approach to research would infuse cultural responsiveness into EBPs.

Notwithstanding the limitations of existing EBPs, CBT is among the most widely researched psychosocial intervention. While there is significant research on this approach as a psychotherapeutic treatment model in general, research specifically examining the treatment of suicidal behavior using CBT is more limited (Alonzo & Gearing, 2018). Nevertheless, it has gained more support for the treatment of suicidal thoughts and behaviors in recent years.

CBT attributes suicidal behavior to vulnerabilities that result from certain cognitive characteristics including rigidity, poor problem-solving skills, and poor coping skills (Brown et al., 2005; Coleman & Casey, 2007; Freeman & Reinecke, 1994; Hetrick et al., 2014; Joiner, 2006; Pollock & Williams, 1998. Suicidal individuals, therefore, have difficulty generating solutions when faced with emotional problems (Brown et al., 2005; Freeman & Reinecke, 1994; Joiner, 2006; Pollock & Williams, 1998). They tend to have a negative attributional style, including negative views of themselves and of their future. Suicidal individuals will typically have experiences based on distortions, irrational beliefs, or pathological ways of viewing oneself and the world leading to hopelessness and a of lack positive expectations. Suicidal behavior is seen as the result of erroneous or faulty logic (Beck, Rush, Shaw, & Emery, 1979). Such behavior is seen as an ineffective effort to resolve a problem (Rotheram-Borus, Piacentini, Miller, Graae, & Castro-Blanco, 1994).

Tarrier, Haddock, Lewis, Drake, and Gregg (2006) conducted a meta-analysis comparing 28 studies treating suicidal behavior with CBT. Overall findings indicated that CBT can reduce suicidal behavior in the immediate, short term and maintains significant, albeit less, reduction in suicidal behavior for the medium term. This review also found that CBT was highly effective in the treatment of adults with suicidality. However, findings were nonsignificant for adolescents (Tarrier et al., 2006) although the authors recognize that there were limited studies focusing solely on adolescents, which may have contributed to this finding. In addition, findings suggested that CBT was more effective when it directly focused on specific aspects of suicidal behavior, rather than when it primarily focused on other symptoms (e.g., depression) with a secondary focus on suicidality (Tarrier et al., 2006). A more recent systematic review on the effectiveness of CBT in reducing suicidal thoughts and behavior found similar results. Among adults, CBT focused on suicidal cognitions and behaviors was more effective than CBT focused on general symptoms of mental illness (Mewton & Andrews, 2016).

Models of CBT that focus on building and developing problem-solving skills have also yielded some encouraging findings relating to reduced suicidality (Eskin, Ertekin, & Demir, 2008; Salkovskis, Atha, & Storer, 1990). In a systematic review, a CBT-based approach composed of cognitive behavioral and problem-solving therapy was associated with fewer participants repeating self-harming behavior at the 6-month and 12-month follow-ups as well as significant improvements in depression, hopelessness, suicidal ideation, and problem-solving (Hawton et al., 2016).

CBT has been found to be effective when delivered face to face as well as online (Guille et al., 2015; Lai, Maniam, Chan, & Ravindran, 2014; Mewton & Andrews, 2015; Morris et al., 2016; Robinson et al., 2014; Wagner et al., 2016; Wagner, Horn, & Maercker, 2014); as a model of crisis intervention (Asarnow, Berk, & Baraff, 2009; Bilsker & Forster, 2003); as a form of family-based intervention for suicidal adolescents (Asarnow, Berk, Hughes, & Anderson, 2015; Stanley et al., 2009); and as a treatment for use specifically with adolescents with co-occurring substance abuse and suicidality (Donaldson, Spirito, & Esposito-Smythers, 2005; Esposito-Smythers, Spirito, Uth, & LaChance, 2006).

Given the focus on the nature of one's thoughts, CBT may be able to incorporate an examination of the cultural context of the individual. That is, the model requires examination of one's thoughts and how these thoughts are formed. A culturally responsive clinician practicing CBT should consider how the individual's culture is influencing the way he or she interprets events and the meanings they are assigned. In this respect, CBT has the potential to be effective across a variety of cultures. Research has begun to examine culturally adapted models of CBT. For example, a culturally adapted model of CBT for Puerto Rican adolescents with depression demonstrated efficacy in reducing depressive symptoms (Rosselló & Bernal, 1999; Rosselló, Bernal, & Rivera-Medina, 2012) and was also shown to decrease suicidal ideation at the posttreatment assessment (Rosselló, Duarté-Vélez, Bernal, & Zualaga, 2013). Future research, however, is needed to provide greater support for the application of CBT for the treatment of suicidal thoughts and behaviors across diverse cultures.

## Family Therapy

Given the important role of families in mental health help-seeking among minority populations, treatment approaches that emphasize family involvement would likely have a high chance of success. Brief strategic family therapy (BSFT) is an evidence-based treatment model that was originally developed to target acculturation conflicts between Cuban American adolescents and their parents (Szapocznik, Schwartz, Muir, & Brown, 2012) and has been shown to improve treatment engagement and reduce behavioral problems and drug use in adolescents by changing patterns of family relationship (Santisteban, Suarez-Morales, Robbins, & Szapocznik, 2006; Szapocznik et al., 2012). BSFT has been widely used with a diverse group of Latinx, African American, and Caucasian adolescents (Robbins et al., 2011). BSFT is a short-term, structured intervention typically delivered in 12 to 15 sessions over a 3-month period.

Based on the structural approach of Minuchin (1974) and the strategic approaches of Haley (1976) and Madanes (1981), BSFT is grounded in the idea that family relationships play a critical role in the development of behavior problems and, thus, are the main target for intervention. BSFT proposes that a family is part of and is influenced by a larger social system (Szapocznik & Kurtines, 1993). Sensitivity to this larger social system and contextual factors, including an understanding of the influence of peers, schools, and neighborhoods on the development of children's behavior problems, is a core component of the model (Szapocznik & Kurtines, 1993). Understanding the impact of immigration, SES, and acculturation on family processes is central to BSFT (Szapocznik, Santisteban, Kurtines, Perez-Vidal, & Hervis, 1984). As such, BSFT incorporates a focus on several of the core cultural issues found to be associated with increased risk of suicide.

BSFT suggests that the behavior of one family member can only be understood by examining the family in which it occurs and that for treatment to be successful, it must be implemented at the family level and must account for complex relationships within the family system. It is equally important to understand the structure of the family and the repetitive patterns of interactions that occur among family members that either serve to meet the family's goals or to trigger and maintain behavior problems (Szapocznik & Kurtines, 1993).

BSFT is focused on process (patterns of interactions) rather than on content (what is being said) and utilizes a strategic approach that employs practical, problem-focused, and planned interventions that are tailored to individual families. These interventions identify and modify patterns of interaction within the family system that are considered to be directly related to the negative behavioral symptoms of the youth. Change occurs by modifying the process (Szapocznik & Kurtines, 1993).

Given the short-term nature of the intervention, the family involvement, and the consideration of culturally based contextual factors affecting families, specifically immigration and acculturation, this intervention has the potential to serve as an effective intervention for the treatment of suicidal behavior among culturally diverse youth populations. Limited research, however, has examined the effectiveness of BSFT at reducing suicide risk across cultures. Future research should focus on assessing the effectiveness of this intervention specifically for suicidal behavior.

## CONCLUSION

Suicide is a problem that knows no cultural boundaries. As the minority population in the United States continues to grow, it is essential for health and mental health providers to develop culturally relevant prevention and intervention efforts to address these at-risk populations. Risk and protective factors vary across culture and ethnicities, as do attitudes and perspectives regarding suicide acceptability. Intervention and prevention efforts should be guided by culturally relevant risk and protective factors for suicide and an understanding of attitudes toward suicide among the target population.

A culturally responsiveness approach requires that one refrain from making assumptions based on a client's culture. Also, how a clinician understands and views his or her own culture(s) does not necessarily translate into awareness and understanding of clients from the same culture group, as their experience can be distinctly different than the clinician's. However, a fine line exists between lending too much importance to cultural distinctions and overlooking culturally significant factors that may better inform practice. Emphasizing cultural nuances may lead to increasing prejudice toward different cultures and the reinforcement of overgeneralizations (Alonzo & Gearing, 2018; Takahashi, 1997). Thus, a model that allows for a tailored, personalized assessment is critical. Future research focused on further development and testing of culturally responsive models of suicide assessment and treatment is needed.

## REFERENCES

Adam, K. S., Bouckoms, A., & Streiner, D. (1982). Parental loss and family stability in attempted suicide. *Archives of General Psychiatry, 39,* 1081–1085. doi:10.1001/archpsyc.1982.04290090065013

Ahmed, K., & Mohan, R. A. (2007). Self-harm in South Asian women: A literature review informed approach to assessment and formulation. *American Journal of Psychotherapy, 61*(1), 71–81. doi:10.1176/appi.psychotherapy.2007.61.1.71

Alcántara, C., & Gone, J. P. (2007). Reviewing suicide in Native American communities: Situating risk and protective factors within a transactional–ecological framework. *Death Studies, 31*(5), 457–477. doi:10.1080/07481180701244587

Alegría, M., Canino, G., Shrout, P. E., Woo, M., Duan, N., Vila., & Meng, X. L. (2008). Prevalence of mental illness in immigrant and non-immigrant U.S. Latino groups. *American Journal of Psychiatry, 165*(3), 359–369. doi:10.1176/appi.ajp.2007.07040704

Ali, A., & Maharajh, H. D. (2005). Social predictors of suicidal behaviour in adolescents in Trinidad and Tobago. *Social Psychiatry & Psychiatric Epidemiology, 40*(3), 186–191. doi:10.1007/s00127-005-0846-9

Alonzo, D. (2016). Suicidal individuals and mental health treatment: A novel approach to engagement. *Community Mental Health, 52*(5), 527–533.

Alonzo, D., & Gearing, R. E. (2018). *Suicide assessment and treatment: Empirical and evidence-based practices (2 ed.).* New York, NY: Springer Publishing Company.

Angermeyer, M. C., & Matschinger, H. (1999). Lay beliefs about mental disorders: A comparison between the western and the eastern parts of Germany. *Social Psychiatry and Psychiatric Epidemiology, 34*(5), 275–281. doi:10.1007/s001270050144

Arango, A., Cole-Lewis, Y., Lindsay, R., Yeguez, C. E., Clark, M., & King, C. (2018). The protective role of connectedness on depression and suicidal ideation among bully victimized youth. *Journal of Clinical Child & Adolescent Psychology, 48*(5), 728–739. doi:10.1080/15374416.2018.1443456

Arbona, C., Olvera, N., Rodriguez, N., Hagan, J., Linares, A., & Wiesner, M. (2010). Acculturative stress among documented and undocumented Latino immigrants in the United States. *Hispanic Journal of Behavioral Sciences, 32*(3), 362–384. doi:10.1177/0739986310373210

Asarnow, J. R., Berk, M. S., & Baraff, L. J. (2009). Family Intervention for suicide prevention: A specialized emergency department intervention for suicidal youths. *Professional Psychology: Research and Practice, 40*(2), 118. doi:10.1037/a0012599

Asarnow, J. R., Berk, M., Hughes, J. L., & Anderson, N. L. (2015). The SAFETY program: A treatment-development trial of a cognitive-behavioral family treatment for adolescent suicide attempters. *Journal of Clinical Child & Adolescent Psychology, 44*(1), 194–203. doi: 10.1080/15374416.2014.940624

Baca-Garcia, E., Perez-Rodriguez, M. M., Keyes, K. M., Oquendo, M. A., Hasin, D. S., Grant, B. F., & Blanco, C. (2011). Suicidal ideation and suicide attempts among Hispanic subgroups in the United States: 1991-1992 and 2001-2002. *Journal of Psychiatric Research, 45*(4), 512–518. doi:10.1016/j.jpsychires.2010.09.004

Beck, A. T., Rush, A. J., Shaw, B. F., & Emery, G. (1979). *Cognitive therapy of depression: A treatment manual.* New York, NY: Guilford Press.

Beck-Cross, C., & Cooper, R. (2015). Micro- and macrosystem predictors of high school male suicidal behaviors. *Children and Schools, 37*(4), 231–239. doi:10.1093/cs/cdv028

Beghi, M., Rosenbaum, J. F., Cerri, C., & Cornaggia, C. M. (2013). Risk factors for fatal and nonfatal repetition of suicide attempts: A literature review. *Neuropsychiatric Disease and Treatment, 9*, 1725. doi:10.2147/NDT.S40213

Berry, J. W., & Kim, U. (1988). *Acculturation and mental health*. London, UK Sage.

Bhugra, D. (2005). Sati: A type of non-psychiatric suicide. *Crisis: The Journal of Crisis Intervention and Suicide Prevention, 26*(2), 73–77. doi:10.1027/0227-5910.26.2.73

Bhugra, D., & Mastrogianni, A. (2004). Globalization and mental disorders: Overview with relation to depression. *British Journal of Psychiatry, 184*, 10–20. doi:10.1192/bjp.184.1.10

Bilsker, D., & Forster, P. (2003). Problem-solving intervention for suicidal crises in the psychiatric emergency service. *Crisis: The Journal of Crisis Intervention and Suicide Prevention, 24*(3), 134. doi:10.1027//0227-5910.24.3.134

Borges, G., Orozco, R., Rafful, C., Miller, E., & Breslau, J. (2012). Suicidality, ethnicity and immigration in the USA. *Psychological Medicine, 42*(6), 1175–1184. doi:10.1017/S0033291711002340

Borowsky, I. W., Ireland, M., & Resnick, M. D. (2001). Adolescent suicide attempts: Risks and protectors. *Pediatrics, 107*, 485–493. doi:10.1542/peds.107.3.485

Breland-Noble, A. M. (2004). Mental healthcare disparities affect treatment of Black adolescents. *Psychiatric Annals, 34*(7), 534–538. doi:10.3928/0048-5713-20040701-14

Brent, D. A., Baugher, M., Bridge, J., Chen, T., & Chiappetta, L. (1999). Age- and sex-related risk factors for adolescent suicide. *Journal of the American Academy of Child & Adolescent Psychiatry, 38*(12), 1497–1505. doi:10.1097/00004583-199912000-00010

Brent, D., Bridge, J., Johnson, B. A., & Connolly, J. (1996). Suicidal behavior runs in families: A controlled family study of adolescent suicide victims. *Archives of General Psychiatry, 53*(12), 1145–1152. doi:10.1001/archpsyc.1996.01830120085015

Brent, D. A., Perper, J. A., & Moritz, G. (1993). Psychiatric sequelae to the loss of an adolescent peer to suicide. *Journal of the American Academy of Child & Adolescent Psychiatry, 32*, 509–517. doi:10.1097/00004583-199305000-00004

Brent, D., Perper, J., Moritz, G., Baugher, M., Schweers, J., & Roth, C. (1993). Firearms and adolescent suicide: A community case-control study. *American Journal of Disorders of Childhood, 147*, 1066–1071. doi:10.1001/archpedi.1993.02160340052013

Bridge, J. A., Horowitz, L. M., Fontanella, C. A., Sheftall, A. H., Greenhouse, J., Kelleher, K. J., & Campo, J. V. (2018). Age-related racial disparity in suicide rates among U.S. youths from 2001 through 2015. *JAMA Pediatrics, 172*(7), 697–699. doi:10.1001/jamapediatrics.2018.0399

Briere, J., & Runtz, M. (1990). Differential adult symptomatology associated with three types of child abuse histories. *Child Abuse and Neglect, 14*, 357–364. doi:10.1016/0145-2134(90)90007-G

Brown, G. K., Have, T. T., Henriques, G. R., Xie, S. X., Hollander, J. E., & Beck, A. T. (2005). Cognitive Therapy for the prevention of suicide attempts: A randomized controlled trial. *Journal of the American Medical Association, 294*, 563–570. doi:10.1001/jama.294.5.563

Burnette, C. E., Roh, S., Lee, K. H., Lee, Y. S., Newland, L. A., & Jun, J. S. (2017). A comparison of risk and protective factors related to depressive symptoms among American Indian and Caucasian older adults. *Health & Social Work, 42*(1), e15–e23. doi:10.1093/hsw/hlw055

Burr, J. (2002). Cultural stereotypes of women from South Asian communities: Mental health care professionals' explanations for patterns of suicide and depression. *Social Science & Medicine, 55*(5), 835–845. doi:10.1016/S0277-9536(01)00220-9

Bustamante, A. V., Fang, H., Garza, J., Carter-Pokras, O., Wallace, S. P., Rizzo, J. A., & Ortega, A. N. (2012). Variations in healthcare access and utilization among Mexican immigrants: the role of documentation status. *Journal of Immigrant and Minority Health, 14*(1), 146–155. doi:10.1007/s10903-010-9406-9

Caplan, S., Escobar, J., Paris, M., Alvidrez, J., Dixon, J. K., Desai, M. M., . . . Whittemore, R. (2013). Cultural influences on casual beliefs about depression among Latino immigrants. *Journal of Transcultural Nursing, 24*(1), 68–77. doi:10.1177/1043659612453745

Castle, K., Conner, K., Kaukeinen, K., & Tu, X. (2011). Perceived racism, discrimination, and acculturation in suicidal ideation and suicide attempts among Black young adults. *Suicide and Life-Threatening Behavior, 41*(3), 342–351. doi:10.1111/j.1943-278X.2011.00033.x

Centers for Disease Control and Prevention. (2014). *Fatal injury reports, national and regional, 1999–2014.* Retrieved from http://webappa.cdc.gov/sasweb/ncipc/mortrate10_us.html

Centers for Disease Control and Prevention. (2016). *About underlying cause of death, 1999–2018.* Retrieved from https://wonder.cdc.gov/ucd-icd10.html

Centers for Disease Control and Prevention. (2017). *Data & Statistics Fatal Injury Report for 2017.* Retrieved from https://webappa.cdc.gov/sasweb/ncipc/mortrate.html

Cervantes, R., Goldbach, J. T., Varela, A., & Santisteban, D. A. (2014). Self-harm among Hispanic adolescents: Investigating the role of culture-related stressors. *Journal of Adolescent Health, 55*(5), 633–639. doi:10.1016/j.jadohealth.2014.05.017

Cervantes, R. C., Padilla, A. M., Napper, L. E., & Goldbach, J. T. (2013). Acculturation-related stress and mental health outcomes among three generations of Hispanic adolescents. *Hispanic Journal of Behavioral Sciences, 35*(4), 451–468. doi:10.1177/0739986313500924

Chandrasena, R., Beddage, V., & Fernando, M. L. (1991). Suicide among immigrant psychiatric patients in Canada. *British Journal of Psychiatry, 159,* 707–709. doi:10.1192/bjp.159.5.707

Chen, Y. Y., Chien-Chang Wu, K., Yousuf, S., & Yip, P. S. (2011). Suicide in Asia: Opportunities and challenges. *Epidemiologic Reviews, 34*(1), 129–144. doi:10.1093/epirev/mxr025

Cheng, J. K. Y., Fancher, T. L., Ratanasen, M., Conner, K. R., Duberstein, P. R., Sue, S., & Takeuchi, D. (2010). Lifetime suicidal ideation and suicide attempts in Asian Americans. *Asian American Journal of Psychology, 1*(1), 18. doi:10.1037/a0018799

Cho, Y. B., & Haslam, N. (2010). Suicidal ideation and distress among immigrant adolescents: The role of acculturation, life stress, and social support. *Journal of Youth and Adolescence, 39*(4), 370–379. doi:10.1007/s10964-009-9415-y

Chu, J., Floyd, R., Diep, H., Pardo, S., Goldblum, P., & Bongar, B. (2013). A tool for the culturally competent assessment of suicide: The Cultural Assessment of Risk for Suicide (CARS) measure. *Psychological Assessment, 25,* 424–434. doi:10.1037/a0031264

Coleman, D., & Casey, J. T. (2007). Therapeutic mechanisms of suicidal ideation: The influence of changes in automatic thoughts and immature defenses. *Crisis, 28*(4), 198–203.

Colucci, E., & Martin, G. (2007). Ethnocultural aspects of suicide in young people: A systematic literature review part 2: Risk factors, precipitating agents, and attitudes toward suicide. *Suicide & Life Threatening Behavior, 37*(2), 222–237. doi:10.1521/suli.2007.37.2.222

Compton, M. T., Thompson, N. J., & Kaslow, N. J. (2005). Social environment factors associated with suicide attempt among low-income African Americans: The protective role of family relationships and social support. *Social Psychiatry and Psychiatric Epidemiology, 40*(3), 175–185. doi:10.1007/s00127-005-0865-6

Curtin, S. C., Warner, M., & Hedegaard, H. (2016). *Increase in suicide in the United States, 1999–2014.* NCHS data brief, no 241. Hyattsville, MD: National Center for Health Statistics.

Czyz, E. K., Liu, Z., & King, C. A. (2012). Social connectedness and one-year trajectories among suicidal adolescents following psychiatric hospitalization. *Journal of Clinical Child and Adolescent Psychology, 41,* 214–226. doi:10.1080/15374416.2012.651998

Dalton, B. (2005). Teaching cultural assessment. *Journal of Teaching in Social Work, 25*(3–4), 45–61. doi:10.1300/J067v25n03_04

Dawkins, K. (1996). The interaction of ethnicity, sociocultural factors, and gender in clinical psychopharmacology. *Psychopharmacology Bulletin, 32*(2), 283–289.

Department of Health and Human Services. (2002). Youth Risk Behavior Survey, Center for Disease Control.

Donaldson, D., Spirito, A., & Esposito-Smythers, C. (2005). Treatment for adolescents following a suicide attempt: Results of a pilot trial. *Journal of the American Academy of Child & Adolescent Psychiatry, 44*(2), 113–120. doi:10.1097/00004583-200502000-00003

DuBard, C. A., & Gizlice, Z. (2008). Language spoken and differences in health status, access to care, and receipt of preventive services among U.S. Latinxs. *American Journal of Public Health, 98*(11), 2021–2028. doi:10.2105/AJPH.2007.119008

Duldulao, A. A., Takeuchi, D. T., & Seunghye, H. (2009). Correlates of Suicidal Behaviors among Asian Americans. *Archives of Suicide Research, 13*(3), 277–290. doi:10.1080/13811110903044567

Eaton, D. K., Foti, K., Brener, N. D., Crosby, A. E., Flores, G., & Kann, L. (2011). Associations between risk behaviors and suicidal ideation and suicide attempts: Do racial/ethnic variations in associations account for increased risk of suicidal behaviors among Hispanic/Latina 9th- to 12th-grade female students? *Archives of Suicide Research, 15*(2), 113. doi:10.1080/13811118.2011.565268

Eshun, S. (2006). Acculturation and suicide attitudes: A study of perceptions about suicide among a sample of Ghanaian immigrants in the United States. *Psychological Reports, 99*(1), 295–304. doi:10.2466/pr0.99.1.295-304

Eskin, M., Ertekin, K., & Demir, H. (2008). Efficacy of a problem-solving therapy for depression and suicide potential in adolescents and young adults. *Cognitive Therapy and Research, 32*(2), 227–245. doi:10.1007/s10608-007-9172-8

Esposito-Smythers, C., Spirito, A., Uth, R., & LaChance, H. (2006). Cognitive behavioral treatment for suicidal alcohol abusing adolescents: Development and pilot testing. *The American Journal on Addictions, 15*, s126–s130.

Farber, E. W., Herbert, S. E., & Reviere, S. L. (1996). Child abuse and suicidality in obstetrics patients in a hospital-based urban pre-natal clinic. *General Hospital Psychiatry, 18*, 56–60. doi:10.1016/0163-8343(95)00098-4

Franzini, L., Ribble, J., & Keddie, A. (2001). Understanding the Hispanic paradox. *Ethnicity & Disease, 11*, 496–518.

Freedenthal, S., & Stiffman, A. R. (2004). Suicidal behavior in urban American Indian adolescents: A comparison with reservation youth in a southwestern state. *Suicide and Life-Threatening Behavior, 34*(2), 160–171. doi:10.1521/suli.34.2.160.32789

Freeman, A., & Reinecke, M. (Eds.). (1994). *Cognitive therapy of suicidal behavior.* New York, NY: Springer Publishing Company.

Garlow, S. J. (2002). Age, gender, and ethnicity differences in patterns of cocaine and ethanol use preceding suicide. *American Journal of Psychiatry, 159*, 615–619. doi:10.1176/appi.ajp.159.4.615

Garlow, S. J., Purselle, D., & Heninger, M. (2005). Ethnic differences in patterns of suicide across the life cycle. *American Journal of Psychiatry, 162*, 319–323. doi:10.1176/appi.ajp.162.2.319

Gearing, R. E., & Alonzo, D. (2018). Religion and suicide: New findings. *Journal of Religion & Health, 57*(6), 2478–2499. doi:10.1007/s10943-018-0629-8

Gearing, R. E., & Lizardi, D. (2009). Religion and suicide. *Journal of Religion & Health, 48*(3), 332–341. doi:10.1007/s10943-008-9181-2

Gearing, R. E., Townsend, L., Elkins, J., El-Bassel, N., & Osterberg, L. (2014). Strategies to predict, measure, and improve psychosocial treatment adherence. *Harvard Review of Psychiatry, 22*(1), 31–45. doi:10.1097/HRP.10.1097/HRP.0000000000000005

Gearing, R. E., Washburn, M., Torres, L. R., Carr, L. C., Cabrera, A., & Olivares, R. (under review). Immigration policy changes and the mental health of Mexican American immigrants. *Journal of Latinx Psychology.*

Gibbs, J. T. (1997). African-American suicide: A cultural paradox. *Suicide & Life-Threatening Behavior, 27*, 68–79.

Global Health Estimates 2016. (2018). *Deaths by cause, age, sex, by country and by region, 2000–2016.* Geneva: World Health Organization. Retrieved from http://www.who.int/healthinfo/global_burden_disease/estimates/en/index1.html

Goldney, R. D. (2002). A global view of suicidal behaviour. *Emergency Medicine, 14*, 24–34. doi:10.1046/j.1442-2026.2002.00282.x

Goldston, D. B., Molock, S. D., Whitbeck, L. B., Murakami, J. L., Zayas, L. H., & Hall, G. C. (2008). Cultural considerations in adolescent suicide prevention and psychosocial treatment. The *American Psychologist, 63*(1), 14–31. doi:10.1037/0003-066X.63.1.14

Gomez, J., Miranda, R., & Polanco, L. (2011). Acculturative stress, perceived discrimination, and vulnerability to suicide attempts among emerging adults. *Journal of Youth & Adolescence, 40*(11), 1465. doi:10.1007/s10964-011-9688-9

Gonzalez, H., Ceballos, M., Tarraf, W., West, B., Bowen, M., & Vega, W. (2009). The health of older Mexican Americans in the long run. *American Journal of Public Health, 99*, 1879–1885. doi:10.2105/AJPH.2008.133744

Gray, J. S., & McCullagh, J. A. (2014). Suicide in Indian country: The continuing epidemic in rural Native American communities. *Journal of Rural Mental Health, 38*(2), 79–86. doi:10.1037/rmh0000017

Greenfield, B., Rousseau, C., Slatkoff, J., Lewkowski, M., Davis, M., Dube, S., ... Harnden, B. (2006). Profile of a metropolitan North American immigrant suicidal adolescent population. *Canadian Journal of Psychiatry, 51*, 155–159. doi:10.1177/070674370605 100305

Grossman, D. C., Milligan, B. C., & Deyo, R. A. (1991). Risk factors for suicide attempts among Navajo adolescents. *American Journal of Public Health, 81*, 870–874. doi:10.2105/AJPH.81.7.870

Groves, S. A., Stanley, B., & Sher, L. (2007). Ethnicity and the relationship between adolescent alcohol use and suicidal behavior. *International Journal of Adolescent Medicine & Health, 19*(1), 19–25. doi:10.1515/IJAMH.2007.19.1.19

Grunebaum, M. F., Ramsay, S. R., Galfalvy, H. C., Ellis, S. P., Burke, A. K., Sher, L., ... Oquendo, M. A. (2006). Correlates of suicide attempt history in bipolar disorder: A stress-diathesis perspective. *Bipolar disorders, 8*(5p2), 551–557.

Guille, C., Zhao, Z., Krystal, J., Nichols, B., Brady, K., & Sen, S. (2015). Web-based cognitive behavioral therapy intervention for the prevention of suicidal ideation in medical interns: A randomized clinical trial. *JAMA Psychiatry, 72*(12), 1192–1198. doi:10.1001/jamapsychiatry.2015.1880

Gutierrez, P. M., Osman, A., Kopper, B. A., & Barrios, F. X. (2000). Why young people do not kill themselves: The Reasons for Living Inventory for Adolescents. *Journal of Clinical Child Psychology, 29*, 177–187. doi:10.1207/S15374424jccp2902_4

Haley, J. (1976). *Problem-solving therapy.* San Francisco, CA: Jossey-Bass.

Han, B., Compton, W. M., Gfroerer, J., & McKeon, R. (2014). Mental health treatment patterns among adults with recent suicide attempts in the United States. *American Journal of Public Health, 104*(12), 2359–2368. doi:10.2105/AJPH.2014.302163

Hawton, K., Witt, K. G., Salisbury, T. L. T., Arensman, E., Gunnell, D., Hazell, P., ... van Heeringen, K. (2016). Psychosocial interventions for self-harm in adults. *Cochrane Database of Systematic Reviews, 2016*(5). doi:10.1002/14651858.CD012189

Herne, M. A., Bartholomew, M. L., & Weahkee, R. L. (2014). Suicide mortality among American Indians and Alaska Natives, 1999–2009. *American Journal of Public Health, 104*(S3), S336–S342. doi:10.2105/AJPH.2014.301929

Heron, M. (2011). Deaths: Leading causes for 2007. *National Vital Statistics Reports, 59*, 8.

Hetrick, S., Yuen, H. P., Cox, G., Bendall, S., Yung, A., Pirkis, J., & Robinson, J. (2014). Does cognitive behavioural therapy have a role in improving problem solving and coping in adolescents with suicidal ideation? *The Cognitive Behaviour Therapist, e13.* doi:10.1017/S1754470X14000129

Hicks, M. H. R., & Bhugra, D. (2003). Perceived causes of suicide attempts by U.K. South Asian women. *American Journal of Orthopsychiatry, 73*(4), 455–462. doi:10.1037/0002-9432.73.4.455

Hines-Martin, V., Malone, M., Kim, S., & Brown-Piper, A. (2003). Barriers to mental health care access in an African American population. *Mental Health Nursing, 24*(3), 237–256. doi:10.1080/01612840305281

Hiott, A., Grzywacz, J. G., Arcury, T. A., & Quandt, S. A. (2006). Gender differences in anxiety and depression among immigrant Latinos. *Families, Systems, & Health, 24,* 137–146. doi:10.1037/1091-7527.24.2.137

Hirsch, J. K., Nsamenang, S. A., Chang, E. C., & Kaslow, N. J. (2014). Spiritual well-being and depressive symptoms in female African American suicide attempters: Mediating effects of optimism and pessimism. *Psychology of Religion and Spirituality, 6*(4), 276.

Hoppe, S. K., & Martin, H. W. (1986). Patterns of suicide among Mexican Americans and Anglos, 1960-1980. *Social Psychiatry, 21,* 83–88. doi:10.1007/BF00578747

Hough, R. L., Landsverk, J. A., Karno, M., Burnam, A., Timbers, D. M., Escobar, J. I., & Regier, D. A. (1987). Utilization of health and mental health services by Los Angeles Mexican Americans and non-Hispanic Whites. *Archives of General Psychiatry, 44,* 702–709.

Hovey, J. D. (2000). Acculturative stress, depression, and suicidal ideation in Mexican American immigrants. *Cultural Diversity & Ethnic Minority Psychology, 6,* 134–151. doi:10.1037/1099-9809.6.2.134

Hovey, J. D., & King, C. A. (1996). Acculturative stress, depression, and suicidal ideation among immigrant and second-generation Latino adolescents. *Journal of the American Academy of Child & Adolescent Psychiatry, 35*(9), 1183–1192.

Hovey, J. D., & King, C. A. (1997). Suicidality among acculturating Mexican Americans: Current knowledge and directions for research. *Suicide & Life Threatening Behavior, 27*(1), 92–103.

Huang, Y., Liu, H., Tsai, F., Sun, F. J., Huang, K. Y., Chiu, Y. C., ... Liu, S. I. (2017). Correlation of impulsivity with self-harm and suicidal attempt: A community study of adolescents in Taiwan *BMJ Open, 7*(12), e017949. doi:10.1136/bmjopen-2017-017949

Humensky, J. L., Gil, R., Coronel, B., Cifre, R., Mazzula, S., & Lewis-Fernandez, R. (2013). Life is precious: Reducing suicidal behavior in Latinas. *Ethnicity and Inequalities in Health and Social Care, 6*(2–3), 54–61. doi:10.1108/EIHSC-10-2013-0027

Isaacs, M. R., Huang, L. N., Hernandez, M., & Echo-Hawk, H. (2005). *The road to evidence: The intersection of evidence-based practices and cultural competence in children's mental health.* Washington, DC: The National Alliance of Multi-Ethnic Behavioral Health Associations.

Jasso, G., Massey, D. S., Rosenzweig, M. R., & Smith, J. P. (2004). Immigrant health: Selectivity and acculturation. In N. B. Anderson, R. A. Bulatao, & B. Cohen (Eds.), *Critical perspectives on racial and ethnic differences in health in late life* (pp. 227–266). Washington, DC: The National Academic Press.

Joe, S., Baser, R. E., Breeden, G., Neighbors, H. W., & Jackson, J. S. (2006). Prevalence of and risk factors for lifetime suicide attempts among Blacks in the United States. *Journal of the American Medical Academy, 296,* 2112–2123. doi:10.1001/jama.296.17.2112

Joe, S., Marcus, S. C., & Kaplan, M. S. (2007). Racial differences in the characteristics of firearm suicide decedents in the United States. *American Journal of Orthopsychiatry, 77*(1), 124–130.

Johansson, L. M., Sundquist, J., Johansson, S. E., Bergman, B., Qvist, J., & Traskman-Bendz, L. (1997). Suicide among foreign-born minorities and native Swedes: An epidemiological follow-up study of a defined population. *Social Science and Medicine, 44*(2), 181–187. doi:10.1016/S0277-9536(96)00142-6

Joiner, T. (Ed.). (2006). *Why people die by suicide.* Cambridge, MA: Harvard University Press.

June, A., Segal, D. L., Coolidge, F. L., & Klebe, K. (2009). Religiousness, social support and reasons for living in African American and European American older adults: An exploratory study. *Aging & Mental Health, 13*(5), 753–760. doi:10.1080/13607860902918215

Kaslow, N. J., Thompson, M. P., Okun, A., Price, A., Young, S., Bender, M., ... Parker, R. (2002). Risk and protective factors for suicidal behavior in abused African American women. *Journal of Consulting and Clinical Psychology, 70*(2), 311. doi:10.1037/0022-006X.70.2.311

Kaslow, N. J., Webb Price, A., Wyckoff, S., Bender Grall, M., Sherry, A., Young, S., ... Bethea, K. (2004). Person factors associated with suicidal behavior among African American women and men. *Cultural Diversity and Ethnic Minority Psychology, 10*(1), 5–22.

Kennedy, M. A., Parhar, K. K., Samra, J., & Gorzalka, B. (2005). Suicide ideation in different generations of immigrants. *Canadian Journal of Psychiatry, 50*(6), 353–356. doi:10.1177/070674370505000611

Khan, M. (2005). Suicide prevention and developing countries. *Journal of the Royal Society of Medicine, 98*, 459–463. doi:10.1177/014107680509801011

Knight, M. T. D., Furnham, A. F., & Lester, D. (2000). Lay theories of suicide. *Personality and Individual Differences, 29*(3), 453–457. doi:10.1016/S0191-8869(99)00205-6

Kochanek, K. D., Murphy, S. L., & Xu, J. Q. (2015). Deaths: Final data for 2011. *National Vital Statistics Reports, 63*(3). Hyattsville, MD: National Center for Health Statistics. Retrieved from http://www.cdc.gov/nchs/data/nvsr/nvsr63/nvsr63_03.pdf

Kouyoumdjian, H., Zamboanga, B. L., & Hansen, D. J. (2003). Barriers to community mental health services for Latinos: Treatment considerations. *Clinical Psychology: Science and Practice, 10*(4), 394–422. doi:10.1093/clipsy.bpg041

Kuhlberg, J. A., Pena, J. B., & Zayas, L. H. (2010). Familism, parent-adolescent conflict, self-esteem, internalizing behaviors and suicide attempts among adolescent Latinas. *Child Psychiatry and Human Development, 41*(4), 425–440. doi:10.1007/s10578-010-0179-0

Kuroki, Y., & Tilley, J. L. (2012). Recursive partitioning analysis of lifetime suicidal behaviors in Asian Americans. *Asian American Journal of Psychology, 3*(1), 17. doi:10.1037/a0026586

Kushner, H. I. (1991). *American suicide: A psychocultural exploration*. New Brunswick, NJ: Rutgers University Press.

Lai, M. H., Maniam, T., Chan, L. F., & Ravindran, A. V. (2014). Caught in the web: a review of web-based suicide prevention. *Journal of Medical Internet Research, 16*(1), e30. doi:10.2196/jmir.2973

Lam, T. H., Stewart, S. M., Yip, P. S., Leung, G. M., Ho, L. M., Ho, S. Y., & Lee, P. W. (2004). Suicidality and cultural values among Hong Kong adolescents. *Social Science & Medicine, 58*(3), 487–498. doi:10.1016/S0277-9536(03)00242-9

Lau, A. S., Jernewall, N. M., Zane, N., & Myers, H. F. (2002). Correlates of suicidal behaviors among Asian American outpatient youth. *Cultural Diversity & Ethnic Minority Psychology, 8*(3), 199–213. doi:10.1037/1099-9809.8.3.199

Lefebvre, F., Lesage, A., Cyr, M., & Toupin, J. (1998). Factors related to utilization of services for mental health reasons in Montreal, Canada. *Social Psychiatry and Psychiatric Epidemiology, 33*, 291–298. doi:10.1007/s001270050057

Lessenger, L. H. (1997). Use of acculturation rating scale for Mexican Americans-II with substance abuse patients. *Hispanic Journal of Behavioral Sciences, 19*(3), 387–399. doi:10.1177/07399863970193010

Lester, D. (1997). Suicide in America: A nation of immigrants. *Suicide & Life Threatening Behavior, 27*(1), 50–59. doi:10.1521/suli.2006.36.1.50

Lester, D. (1998). Suicide rates of immigrants. *Psychological Reports, 82*(1), 50. doi:10.2466/pr0.1998.82.1.50

Lester, D. (1999). Native American suicide rates, acculturation stress and traditional integration. *Psychological Reports, 84*(2), 398. doi:10.2466/pr0.1999.84.2.398

Levi, L. D., Fales, C. H., Stein, M., & Sharp, V. H. (1966). Separation and attempted suicide. *Archives of General Psychiatry, 15*, 158–164. doi:10.1001/archpsyc.1966.01730140046008

Lincoln, K. D., Taylor, R. J., Chatters, L. M., & Joe, S. (2012). Suicide, negative interaction and emotional support among black Americans. *Social Psychiatry and Psychiatric Epidemiology, 47*(12), 1947–1958.

Lizardi, D., & Stanley, B. (2010). Treatment engagement and suicide attempters: A review. *Psychiatric Services, 61*, 1183–1191.

Lorenzo-Luaces, L., & Phillips, J. (2014). Racial and ethnic differences in risk factors associated with suicidal behavior among young adults in the U.S.A. *Ethnicity and Health, 19*(4), 458–477. doi:10.1080/13557858.2013.846299

Madanes, C. (1981). *Strategic family therapy.* San Francisco, CA: Jossey-Bass.

Malone, K. M., Haas, G. L., Sweeny, J. A., & Mann, J. J. (1995). Major depression and the risk of attempted suicide. *Journal of Affective Disorders, 34,* 173–185. doi:10.1016/0165-0327(95)00015-F

Malone, K. M., Oquendo, M. A., Haas, G. L., Ellis, S. P., Li, S., & Mann, J. J. (2000). Protective factors against suicidal acts in major depression: reasons for living. *American Journal of Psychiatry, 157,* 1084–1088. doi:10.1176/appi.ajp.157.7.1084

Mann, J. J., Waternaux, C., Haas, G. L., & Malone, K. M. (1999). Towards a clinical model of suicidal behavior in psychiatric patients. *American Journal of Psychiatry, 156,* 181–189.

Markides, K., & Eschbach, K. (2005). Aging, migration, and mortality: Current status of research on the Hispanic paradox. *The Journals of Gerontology Series B: Psychological Sciences and Social Sciences, 60*(Special Issue 2), S68–S75. doi:10.1093/geronb/60.Special_Issue_2.S68

Marmot, M. G., Adelstein, A. M., & Bulusu, L. (1984). Lessons from the study of immigrant mortality. *Lancet, 1*(8392), 1455–1457. doi:10.1016/S0140-6736(84)91943-3

Martinez, K. (2007). *Mental Health and Systems of Care Frequently Asked Questions.* Technical Assistance Partnership for Child and Family Mental Health. Retrieved from http://www.tapartnership.org/advisors/mental_health/faq/sept07.asp

Martinez, K. (2008). *Evidence Based Practices, Practice Based Evidence and Community Defined Evidence in Multicultural Mental Health.* Presented at the 2008 NAMI Annual Convention in Orlando, FL.

McMillan, K. A., Enns, M. W., Asmundson, G. J. G., & Sareen, J. (2010). The association between income and distress, mental disorders, and suicidal ideation and attempts: Findings from the collaborative psychiatric epidemiology surveys. *The Journal of Clinical Psychiatry, 71*(9), 1168–1175. doi:10.4088/JCP.08m04986gry

Mewton, L., & Andrews, G. (2015). Cognitive behaviour therapy via the internet for depression: a useful strategy to reduce suicidal ideation. *Journal of Affective Disorders, 170,* 78–84.

Mewton, L., & Andrews, G. (2016). Cognitive behavioral therapy for suicidal behaviors: Improving patient outcomes. *Psychology Research and Behavior Management, 9,* 21. doi:10.2147/PRBM.S84589

Minuchin, S. (1974). *Families and family therapy.* Cambridge, MA: Harvard University Press.

Molock, S., & Barksdale, C. (2013). Relationship between religiosity and conduct problems among African American and Caucasian Adolescents. *Journal of Child & Family Studies, 22*(1), 4–14. doi:10.1007/s10826-012-9584-2

Monk, M., & Warshauer, M. E. (1974). Completed and attempted suicide in three ethnic groups. *American Journal of Epidemiology, 130,* 348–360. doi:10.1093/oxfordjournals.aje.a112042

Morris, J., Firkins, A., Millings, A., Mohr, C., Redford, P., & Rowe, A. (2016). Internet-delivered cognitive behavior therapy for anxiety and insomnia in a higher education context. *Anxiety, Stress, & Coping, 29*(4), 415–431. doi:10.1080/10615806.2015.1058924

Moscicki, E. K., O'Carroll, P., Rae, D. S., Locke, B. Z., Roy, A., & Regier, D. A. (1988). Suicide attempts in the Epidemiologic Catchment Area Study. *Yale Journal of Biology & Medicine, 61,* 259–268.

Nickerson, K. J., Helms, J. E., & Terrell, F. (1994). Cultural mistrust, opinions about mental illness, and Black students' attitudes toward seeking psychological help from White counselors. *Journal of Counseling Psychology, 41*(3), 378–385.

Novins, D. K., Beals, J., Moore, L. A., Spicer, P., Manson, S. M., & AI-SUPERPFR Team. (2004). Use of biomedical services and traditional healing options among American Indians: Sociodemographic correlates, spirituality, and ethnic identity. *Medical Care,* 670–679.

Olson, L. M., & Wahab, S. (2006). American Indians and suicide: A neglected area of research. *Trauma, Violence, & Abuse, 7*(1), 19–33. doi:10.1177/1524838005283005

Oquendo, M. A., Dragatsi, D., Harkavy-Friedman, J., Dervic, K., Currier, D., Burke, A. K., . . . Mann, J. J. (2005). Protective factors against suicidal behavior in Latinos. *Journal of Nervous & Mental Disease, 193,* 438–443. doi:10.1097/01.nmd.0000168262.06163.31

Oquendo, M. A., Ellis, S. P., Greenwald, S., Malone, K. M., Weissman, M. M., & Mann, J. J. (2001). Ethnic and sex differences in suicide rates relative to major depression in the United States. *American Journal of Psychiatry, 158*(10), 1652–1658. doi:10.1176/appi.ajp.158.10.1652

Oquendo, M. A., Lizardi, D., Greenwald, S., Weissman, M. M., & Mann, J. J. (2004). Rates of lifetime suicide attempt and rates of lifetime major depression in different ethnic groups in the United States. *Acta Psychiatrica Scandinavica, 110*(6), 446–451. doi:10.1111/j.1600-0447.2004.00404.x

Padilla, A. M., Cervantes, R. C., Maldonado, M., & Garcia, R. E. (1988). Coping responses to psychosocial stressors among Mexican and Central American immigrants. *Journal of Community Psychology, 16,* 418–427. doi:10.1002/1520-6629(198810)16:4<418::AID-JCOP2290160407>3.0.CO;2-R

Palloni, A., & Morenoff, J. (2001). Interpreting the paradoxical in the Hispanic paradox. *Annals of the New York Academy of Sciences, 954,* 140–174. doi:10.1111/j.1749-6632.2001.tb02751.x

Pearson, V., Phillip, M. R., He, F., & Ji, H. (2002). Attempted suicide among young rural women in the People's Republic of China: Possibilities for prevention. *Suicide & Life Threatening Behavior, 32*(4), 359–369. doi:10.1521/suli.32.4.359.22345

Pew Hispanic Center. (2017). *Facts on U.S. Latinos, 2015.* Retrieved from https://www.pewhispanic.org/2017/09/18/facts-on-u-s-latinos

Pfeffer, C. R. (1991). Suicide in Japan. *Journal of the American Academy of Child and Adolescent Psychiatry, 30*(5), 847–848. doi:10.1016/S0890-8567(10)80029-2

Pfeffer, C. R., Normandin, L., & Kakuma, T. (1994). Suicidal children grow up: Suicidal behavior and psychiatric disorders among relatives. *Journal of the American Academy of Child & Adolescent Psychiatry, 33*(8), 1087–1097. doi:10.1097/00004583-199410000-00004

Pirkis, J., Burgess, P., & Dunt, D. (2000). Suicidal ideation and suicide attempts among Australian adults. *Crisis: The Journal of Crisis Intervention & Suicide Prevention, 21*(1), 16–25. doi:10.1027//0227-5910.21.1.16

Polanco-Roman, L., & Miranda, R. (2013). Culturally related stress, hopelessness, and vulnerability to depressive symptoms and suicidal ideation in emerging adulthood. *Behavior Therapy, 44*(1). 75–87. doi:10.1016/j.beth.2012.07.002

Pollock, L. R., & Williams, M. G. (1998). Problem solving and suicidal behavior. *Suicide and Life-Threatening Behavior, 28*(4), 375–387.

Polo, A. J., Alegría, M., & Sirkin, J. T. (2012). Increasing the engagement of Latinos in services through community-derived programs: The right question project-mental health. *Professional Psychology: Research and Practice, 43*(3), 208–216. doi:10.1037/a0027730

Ponizovsky, A. M., & Ritsner, M. S. (1999). Suicidal ideation among recent immigrants to Israel from the former Soviet Union: An epidemiological survey of prevalence and risk factors. *Suicide and Life-Threatening Behavior, 29,* 376–392.

Pridmore, S., & Walter, G. (2013). Culture and suicide set points. *German Journal of Psychiatry, 16*(4), 143–151.

Purselle, D. C., Heninger, M., Hanzlick, R., & Garlow, S. J. (2009). Differential association of socioeconomic status in ethnic and age-defined suicides. *Psychiatry Research, 167,* 258–265. doi:10.1016/j.psychres.2008.02.003

Rew, L., Thomas, N., Horner, S. D., Resnick, M. D., & Beuhring, T. (2001). Correlates of recent suicide attempts in a triethnic group of adolescents. *Journal of Nursing Scholarship, 33,* 361–367. doi:10.1111/j.1547-5069.2001.00361.x

Rhodes, S. D., Mann, L., Simán, F. M., Song, E., Alonzo, J., Downs, M., . . . Hall, M. A. (2015). The impact of local immigration enforcement policies on the health of immigrant Latinxs/Latinos in the United States. *American Journal of Public Health, 105*(2), 329–337. doi:10.2105/AJPH.2014.302218

Robbins, M. S., Feaster, D. J., Horigian, V. E., Rohrbaugh, M., Shoham, V., Bachrach, K., . . . Szapocznik, J. (2011). Brief strategic family therapy versus treatment as usual: Results of a multisite randomized trial for substance using adolescents. Journal of consulting and clinical psychology, 79(6), 713. doi:10.1037/a0025477

Robinson, J. A., Bolton, J. M., Rasic, D., & Sareen, J. (2012). Exploring the relationship between religious service attendance, mental disorders, and suicidality among different ethnic groups: Results from a nationally representative survey. *Depression and Anxiety, 29*(11), 983–990. doi:10.1002/da.21978

Robinson, J., Hetrick, S., Cox, G., Bendall, S., Yung, A., Yuen, H. P., . . . Pirkis, J. (2014). The development of a randomised controlled trial testing the effects of an online intervention among school students at risk of suicide. *BMC Psychiatry, 14*(1), 155. doi:10.1186/1471-244X-14-155

Rockett, I. R., Samora, J. B., & Coben, J. H. (2006). The black–white suicide paradox: Possible effects of misclassification. *Social Science & Medicine, 63*(8), 2165–2175. doi:10.1016/j.socscimed.2006.05.017

Rosselló, J., & Bernal, G. (1999). The efficacy of cognitive-behavioral and interpersonal treatments for depression in Puerto Rican adolescents. *Journal of Consulting and clinical Psychology, 67*(5), 734. doi:10.1037/0022-006X.67.5.734

Rosselló, J., Bernal, G., & Rivera-Medina, C. (2012). Individual and group CBT and IPT for Puerto Rican adolescents with depressive symptoms. *Journal of Latina/o Psychology, 1*, 36–51. doi:10.1037/2168-1678.1.S.36

Rosselló, J., Duarté-Vélez, Y., Bernal, G., & Zuluaga, M. G. (2013). Ideación suicida y respuesta a la terapia cognitiva conductual en adolescentes puertorriqueños/as con depresión mayor. *Revista Interamericana de Psicologia/Interamerican Journal of Psychology, 45*(3), 321–329.

Rotheram-Borus, M. J., Piacentini, J., Miller, S., Graae, F., & Castro-Blanco, D. (1994). Brief cognitive-behavioral treatment for adolescent suicide attempters and their families. *Journal of the American Academy of Child & Adolescent Psychiatry, 33*(4), 508–517. doi:10.1097/00004583-199405000-00009

Roy, A. (1983). Family history of suicide. *Archives of General Psychiatry, 40*, 971–974. doi:10.1001/archpsyc.1983.01790080053007

Roy, A. (1986). Genetics of suicide. *Annals of the New York Academy of Science, 487*, 97–105. doi:10.1111/j.1749-6632.1986.tb27889.x

Roy, A., Segal, N. L., Centerwall, B. S., & Robinette, C. D. (1991). Suicide in twins. *Archives of General Psychiatry, 48*, 29–32. doi:10.1001/archpsyc.1991.01810250031003

Rutter, P. A., & Behrendt, A. E. (2004). Adolescent suicide risk: Four psychosocial factors. *Adolescence, 39*, 295–302.

Salkovskis, P. M., Atha, C., & Storer, D. (1990). Cognitive-behavioural problem solving in the treatment of patients who repeatedly attempt suicide a controlled trial. *The British Journal of Psychiatry, 157*(6), 871–876. doi:10.1192/bjp.157.6.871

Santisteban, D. A., Suarez-Morales, L., Robbins, M. S., & Szapocznik, J. (2006). Brief strategic family therapy: Lessons learned in efficacy research and challenges to blending research and practice. *Family Process, 45*(2), 259–271. doi:10.1111/j.1545-5300.2006.00094.x

Schmidtke, A., Bille-Brahe, U., DeLeo, D., Kerkhof, A., Bjerke, T., Crepet, P., . . . Sampaio-Faria, J. G. (1996). Attempted suicide in Europe: rates, trends and sociodemographic characteristics of suicide attempters during the period 1989-1992. Results of the WHO/EURO Multicentre Study on Parasuicide. *Acta Psychiatrica Scandinavica., 93*(5), 327–338. doi:10.1111/j.1600-0447.1996.tb10656.x

Shaffer, D., Gould, M., Fisher, P., Trautman, P., Moreau, D., & Kleinman, M. (1996). Psychiatric diagnosis in child and adolescent suicide. *Archives of General Psychiatry, 53*, 339–348. doi:10.1001/archpsyc.1996.01830040075012

Shoval, G., Schoen, G., Vardi, N., & Zalsman, G. (2007). Suicide in Ethiopian immigrants in Israel: A case for study of the genetic-environmental relation in suicide. *Archives of Suicide Research, 11*(3), 247–253. doi:10.1080/13811110701402603

Smokowski, P. R., David-Ferdon, C., & Stroupe, N. (2009). Acculturation and violence in minority adolescents: A review of the empirical literature. *The Journal of Primary Prevention, 30*(3–4), 215–263. doi:10.1007/s10935-009-0173-0

Snowden, L. R., & Yamada, A. M. (2005). Cultural differences in access to care. *Annual Review of Clinical Psychology, 1*, 143–166. doi:10.1146/annurev.clinpsy.1.102803.143846

Sorenson, S. B., & Golding, J. M. (1988). Prevalence of suicide attempts in a Mexican-American population: Prevention implications of immigration and cultural issues. *Suicide and Life-Threatening Behavior, 18*, 322–333. doi:10.1111/j.1943-278X.1988.tb00170.x

Sorenson, S. B., & Shen, H. (1996). Youth suicide trends in California: An examination of immigrant and ethnic group risk. *Suicide & Life Threatening Behavior, 26*(2), 143–154.

Spallek, J., & Razum, O. (2015). Migration and Gender. *Public Health Forum, 23*(2), 73–75. doi:10.1515/pubhef-2015-0027

Spates, K., & Slatton, B.C. (2017). I've Got My Family and My Faith: Black Women and the Suicide Paradox. *Socius: Sociological Research for a Dynamic World; 3*, 1–9. doi:10.1177/2378023117743908

Stack, S., & Wasserman, I. (2005). Race and method of suicide: Culture and opportunity. *Archives of Suicide Research, 9*(1), 57–68. doi:10.1080/13811110590512949

Stanley, B., Brown, G., Brent, D. A., Wells, K., Poling, K., Curry, J., . . . Hughes, J. (2009). Cognitive-behavioral therapy for suicide prevention (CBT-SP): treatment model, feasibility, and acceptability. *Journal of the American Academy of Child & Adolescent Psychiatry, 48*(10), 1005–1013. doi:10.1097/CHI.0b013e3181b5dbfe

Stephen, E. H., Foote, K., Hendershot, G. E., & Schoenborn, C. A. (1994). Health of the foreign-born population: United States, 1989-1990. *Advanced Data, 14*, 1–12.

Stewart, S. M., Kennard, B. D., Lee, P. W., Mayes, T., Hughes, C. W., & Emslie, G. (2005). Hopelessness and suicidal ideation among adolescents in two cultures. *Journal of Child Psychology & Psychiatry & Allied Disciplines, 46*(4), 364–372. doi:10.1111/j.1469-7610.2004.00364.x

Substance Abuse and Mental Health Services Administration. (2012). *Results from the 2011 National Survey on Drug Use and Health: Mental health findings.* Rockville, MD: Author.

Sue, D. W., Arredondo, P., & McDavis, R. J. (1992). Multicultural counseling competencies and standards: A call to the profession. *Journal of Counseling and Development, 70*(4), 477–486. doi:10.1002/j.1556-6676.1992.tb01642.x

Sue, D. W., Bernier, J. E., Durran, A., Feinberg, L., Pedersen, P., Smith, E. J., & Vasquez-Nuttall, E. (1982). Position paper: Cross-cultural counseling competencies. *Counseling Psychologist, 10*(2), 45. doi:10.1177/0011000082102008

Sue, D. W., & Sue, D. (2003). *Counseling the culturally diverse: Theory and practice.* New York, NY: John Wiley & Sons, Inc.

Suominen, K., Isometsa, E., Haukka, J., & Lonnqvist, J. (2004). Substance use and male gender as risk factors for deaths and suicide--a 5-year follow-up study after deliberate self-harm. *Social Psychiatry & Psychiatric Epidemiology, 39*(9), 720–724. doi:10.1007/s00127-004-0796-7

Swanson, J. W., Linskey, A. O., Quintero-Salinas, R., Pumariega, A. J., & Holzer, C. E. (1992). A binational school survey of depressive symptoms, drug use, and suicidal ideation. *Journal of the American Academy of Child and Adolescent Psychiatry, 31*, 669–678. doi:10.1097/00004583-199207000-00014

Szapocznik, J., & Kurtines, W. M. (1993). Family psychology and cultural diversity: Opportunities for theory, research and application. *American Psychologist, 48*(4), 400–407. doi:10.1037/0003-066X.48.4.400

Szapocznik, J., Santisteban, D., Kurtines, W. M., Perez-Vidal, A., & Hervis, O. E. (1984). Bicultural Effectiveness Training (BET): A treatment intervention for enhancing intercultural adjustment. *Hispanic Journal of Behavioral Sciences, 6*(4), 317–344. doi:10.1177/07399863840064001

Szapocznik, J., Schwartz, S. J., Muir, J. A., & Brown, C. H. (2012). Brief strategic family therapy: An intervention to reduce adolescent risk behavior. *Couple and Family Psychology: Research and Practice, 1*(2), 134. doi:10.1037/a0029002

Takahashi, Y. (1997). Culture and suicide: From a Japanese psychiatrist's perspective. *Suicide & Life Threatening Behavior, 27*(1), 137–145.

Tarrier, N., Haddock, G., Lewis, S., Drake, R., & Gregg, L. (2006). Suicide behaviour over 18 months in recent onset schizophrenic patients: The effects of CBT. *Schizophrenia Research, 83*(1), 15–27. doi:10.1016/j.schres.2005.12.846

Teruya, S. A., & Bazargan-Hejazi, S. (2013). The immigrant and Hispanic paradoxes: A systematic review of their predictions and effects. *Hispanic Journal of Behavioral Sciences, 35*(4), 486–509. doi:10.1177/0739986313499004

Thompson, N., & Bhugra, D. (2000). Rates of deliberate self-harm in Asians: Findings and models. *International Review of Psychiatry, 12*(1), 37–43. doi:10.1080/09540260074102

Ungemack, J. A., & Guarnaccia, P. J. (1998). Suicidal ideation and suicide attempts among Mexican Americans, Puerto Ricans and Cuban Americans. *Transcultural Psychiatry, 35*, 307–327. doi:10.1177/136346159803500208

U.S. Bureau of the Census. (2011). State and County QuickFacts.

U.S. Census Bureau. (2018). *Quick Facts*. Retrieved from https://www.census.gov/quickfacts/fact/table/US/PST045218

Vanderwerker, L. L., Chen, J. H., Charpentier, P., Paulk, M. E., Michalski, M., & Prigerson, H. G. (2007). Differences in risk factors for suicidality between African American and White patients vulnerable to suicide. *Suicide & Life Threatening Behavior, 37*(1), 1–9. doi:10.1521/suli.2007.37.1.1

Vega, W. A., Gil, A., Warheit, G., Apospori, E., & Zimmerman, R. (1993). The relationship of drug use to suicide ideation and attempts among African American, Hispanic, and white non-Hispanic male adolescents. *Suicide & Life Threatening Behavior, 23*(2), 110–119.

Vega, W. A., & Lopez, S. R. (2001). Priority issues in Latino mental health services research. *Mental Health Services Research, Special Issue, 3*(4), 189–200. doi:10.1023/a:1013125030718

Wagner, B., Horn, A. B., & Maercker, A. (2014). Internet-based versus face-to-face cognitive-behavioral intervention for depression: a randomized controlled non-inferiority trial. *Journal of Affective Disorders, 152*, 113–121. doi:10.1016/j.jad.2013.06.032

Wagner, S. L., Koehn, C., White, M. I., Harder, H. G., Schultz, I. Z., Williams-Whitt, K., . . . Wright, M. D. (2016). Mental health interventions in the workplace and work outcomes: A best-evidence synthesis of systematic reviews. *The International Journal of Occupational and Environmental Medicine, 7*, 607. doi:10.15171/ijoem.2016.607

Walker, R. L. (2007). Acculturation and acculturative stress as indicators for suicide risk among African Americans. *American Journal of Orthopsychiatry, 77*(3), 386–391. doi:10.1037/0002-9432.77.3.386

Walker, R. L., Lester, D., & Sean, J. (2006). Lay theories of suicide: An examination of culturally relevant suicide beliefs and attributions among African Americans and European Americans. *Journal of Black Psychology, 32*(3), 320–334. doi:10.1177/0095798406290467

Walls, M. L., Whitbeck, L., & Armenta, B. (2016). A cautionary tale: Examining the interplay of culturally specific risk and resilience factors in indigenous communities. *Clinical Psychological Science, 4*(4), 732–743. doi:10.1177/2167702616645795

Wang, P. S., Berglund, P., Olfson, M., Pincus, H. A., Wells, K. B., & Kessler, R. C. (2005). Failure and delay in initial treatment contact after first onset of mental disorders in the

National Comorbidity Survey Replication. *Archives of General Psychiatry, 62*(6), 603–613. doi:10.1001/archpsyc.62.6.603

Wang, M. C., Lightsey Jr, O. R., Tran, K. K., & Bonaparte, T. S. (2013). Examining suicide protective factors among black college students. *Death Studies, 37*(3), 228–247. doi:10.10 80/07481187.2011.623215

Wells, A., Lagomasino, I. T., Palinkas, L. A., Green, J. M., & Gonzalez, D. (2013). Barriers to depression treatment among low-income, Latino emergency department patients. *Community Mental Health Journal, 49*(4), 412–418.

Wells, K. B., Hough, R. L., Golding, J. M., Burnam, M. A., & Karno, M. (1987). Which Mexican-Americans underutilize health services? *American Journal of Psychiatry, 144*(7), 918–922. doi:10.1176/ajp.144.7.918

Whitley, R. (2007). Cultural competence, evidence-based medicine, and evidence-based practices. *Psychiatric Services, 58*(12), 1588–1590. doi:10.1176/ps.2007.58.12.1588

Whitlock, J., Wyman, P. A., & Moore, S. R. (2014), Connectedness and suicide prevention in adolescents: Pathways and implications. *Suicide Life Threatening Behavior, 44*, 246–272. doi:10.1111/sltb.12071

Wielen, L. M., Gilchrist, E. C., Nowels, M. A., Petterson, S. M., Rust. G., & Miller, B. F. (2015). Not near enough: Racial and ethnic disparities in access to nearby behavioral health care and primary care. *Journal of Health Care for the Poor and Underserved, 26*(3), 1032–1047. doi:10.1353/hpu.2015.0083

Williams, C. L., & Berry, J. W. (1991). Primary prevention of acculturative stress among refugees: application of psychological theory and practice. *American Psychologist, 46*, 632–641. doi:10.1037/0003-066X.46.6.632

Willis, L. A., Coombs, D. W., Drentea, P., & Cockerham, W. C. (2003). Uncovering the mystery: Factors of African American suicide. *Suicide and Life-Threatening Behavior, 33*(4), 412–429.

Wong, Y. J., & Maffini, C. S. (2011). Predictors of Asian American adolescents' suicide attempts: A latent class regression analysis. *Journal of Youth and Adolescence, 40*(11), 1453. doi:10.1007/s10964-011-9701-3

Woods, E. R., Lin, Y. G., Middleman, A., Beckford, P., Chase, L., & DuRant, R. H. (1997). The associations of suicide attempts in adolescents. *Pediatrics, 99*, 791–796. doi:10.1542/peds.99.6.791

Yip, P. S., Callanan, C., & Yuen, H. P. (2000). Urban/rural and gender differentials in suicide rates: east and west. *Journal of Affective Disorders, 57*(1–3), 99–106. doi:10.1016/S0165-0327(99)00058-0

Young, J. (2002). Morals, suicide, and psychiatry: A view from Japan. *Bioethics, 16*(5), 412–424. doi:10.1111/1467-8519.00299

Yuen, N. Y., Nahulu, L. B., Hishinuma, E. S., & Miyamoto, R. H. (2000). Cultural identification and attempted suicide in Native Hawaiian adolescents. *Journal of the American Academy of Child & Adolescent Psychiatry, 39*(3), 360–367. doi:10.1097/00004583-200003000-00019

Zayas, L. H., Aguilar-Gaxiola, S., Yoon, H., & Rey, G. N. (2015). The distress of citizen-children with detained and deported parents. *Journal of Child and Family Studies, 24*(11), 3213–3223. doi:10.1007/s10826-015-0124-8

Zayas, L. H., & Gulbas, L. E. (2012). Are suicide attempts by young Latinas a cultural idiom of distress? *Transcultural Psychiatry, 49*(5), 718–734. doi:10.1177/1363461512463262

Zayas, L., Gulbas, L. E., Fedoravicius, N., & Cabassa, L. J. (2010). Patterns of distress, precipitating events, and reflections on suicide attempts by young Latinas. *Social Science & Medicine, 70*(11), 1773–1779. doi:10.1016/j.socscimed.2010.02.013

Zayas, L. H., Lester, R. J., Cabassa, L. J., & Fortuna, L. R. (2005). Why do so many Latina teens attempt suicide? A conceptual model for research. *American Journal of Orthopsychiatry, 75*(2), 275–287. doi:10.1037/0002-9432.75.2.275

Zhang, J., Conwell, Y., Zhou, L., & Jiang, C. (2004). Culture, risk factors and suicide in rural China: a psychological autopsy case control study. *Acta Psychiatrica Scandinavica, 110*(6), 430–437. doi:10.1111/j.1600-0447.2004.00388.x

# Part VI

Ethical Issues and Future Directions

# 23

# Ethical Issues and Future Directions

ELAINE P. CONGRESS

## INTRODUCTION

Family therapy is often the most value-conflicted and ethically challenging of therapies because family therapy often evokes strong countertransference of feelings in the practitioner. Although professionals may not have had the same experiences as their individual clients, almost all family therapists share a similar experience with their clients as the former have also grown up in families. Often family therapists must guard against imposing their own values on families with whom they work. Practitioners' beliefs about families may be highly influenced by their own individual experiences and cultural backgrounds. Research suggests that even highly experienced clinicians may still be powerfully affected by their own cultural background (McGoldrick & Hardy, 2008). Ethical practice with culturally diverse families necessitates that clinicians understand their own cultural background before undertaking work with families from different cultures (Carteret, 2010; McGoldrick & Hardy, 2008).

The current National Association of Social Workers (NASW) Code of Ethics (2018) stresses the need for social workers to understand their clients and "to demonstrate competence in the provision of services that are sensitive to clients' cultures and to differences among people and cultural groups" (NASW, 2018, p. 9). The NASW Code of Ethics (2018) also advises social workers to oppose discrimination based on immigration status. The American Psychological Association (APA) also speaks to the importance of its members being aware of and respecting cultural differences (APA Code of Ethics Principle E).

In the past 25 years, clinicians have increasingly focused on values, ethical issues, and dilemmas in work with individual clients (Congress, 1999; Lowenberg, Dolgoff, & Harrington, 2000; Reamer, 1999). There has been some attention in the literature to family therapy from a multicultural perspective (Cole, 2008; Fallicov, 2009; Keeling & Piercy, 2007; Pakes & Roy-Chowdhury, 2007;

Shibusawa, 2009; Singh, 2009). Despite an attempt to integrate a social justice perspective into a family therapy program with a focus on cultural diversity (McGoldrick, Almeida, Preto, & Bibb, 1999), attention to ethical issues in work with families has been limited (Congress, 2005). A review of the literature indicates only one recent book on ethics in family therapy (Wilcoxon, Remley, & Gladding, 2011) and only a few articles on ethical practice with culturally diverse families (Bryan 2000; Cole, 2008; Donovan, 2003). The current NASW code (2018) includes only one reference to family work and that only in terms of confidentiality. It has been suggested that attention to ethical rules that one has learned as a family therapist may be contraindicated in family therapy with culturally diverse families (Cole, 2008).

Although most family therapists believe in self-determination and confidentiality, how are these values translated into ethical practice? How does family therapy affect self-determination? Are individual family members and the family as a whole able to freely determine their own behavior or is a certain type of behavior considered "bad" or "dysfunctional?" These questions may be particularly relevant for the family from a cultural background very different from that of the practitioner. The clinician often assumes the role of expert "knower," evaluating the family in terms of his or her perception rather than understanding the family through each member's perception (Laird, 1995). Narrative therapy emerges as a value-based model that requires the therapist to not begin family therapy with any preconceived understanding of the family and to permit each family member to tell his or her own story. Allowing families to tell their own cultural stories (McGill, 1992), using genograms in a multicultural perspective (Estrada & Haney, 1998), developing family culturagrams (Congress, 1994, 2002), and using postmodernist approaches (Donovan, 2003) seem to maximize self-determination. In 2008, the International Association of Applied Psychology (IAAP) and the International Union of Psychological Science (IUPsyS, 2008) adopted a Universal Declaration of Ethical Principles, which reaffirms the commitment of the psychology community to help build a better world where peace, freedom, responsibility, justice, humanity, and morality will prevail. Promoting the new universal declaration promises to be a contribution to the creation of a global society based on respect and caring for individuals and peoples (Gauthier, 2008).

The importance of family relationships to culturally diverse families has been stressed (McGoldrick, 2008). Family therapists from cultures that stress an individualist approach must guard against viewing a family from a culture that stresses family connectedness as too "enmeshed" if family members seem very close to each other. For example, a mother who must have her adolescent children accompany her shopping or is reluctant to allow her child to attend an out-of-state college may be described as not establishing appropriate boundaries by encouraging her adolescents to separate and individualize. A family in which older children are asked to care for younger children or to work in family businesses may be seen as exploitative of children. The family therapist must avoid labeling families from different cultures as dysfunctional because they favor a more collective modus operandi than the practitioner.

An important question is how much family therapy promotes individual self-determination. Often the family therapist is faced with a situation in which the goals of different family members conflict. For example, one spouse may see family therapy as a means to strengthen a marriage, while the other spouse envisions family therapy as helping them move toward separation and divorce. What goal does the family therapist promote? The family therapist may be asked to support one member's right to self-determination over the other, especially if there is conflict. How does a family therapist make decisions of this type?

Family therapists must struggle with maintaining their own objectivity. At times, family therapists may find themselves supporting what is familiar to them from their own background and experience. Family therapists who believe that families should stay together and that all areas of conflict can be resolved are more likely to support the spouse who wants to continue the relationship. Family therapists who see separation and divorce as valid options for seriously conflictual relationships may tend to support the spouse who wants to terminate the relationship.

Often ethical dilemmas arise in helping families reconcile conflicts. How should the family therapist intervene when family conflicts arise around acculturation differences? It is well known that children and adolescents, possibly because of their greater association with the American educational system and peer culture, often become acculturated faster than their parents. This may lead to family conflict, especially during adolescence. How does the family therapist support individual self-determination when adolescent clients seek more association with peers and activities outside the home, while parents maintain that adolescents should primarily pursue home and family responsibilities? This conflict may be challenging for family therapists raised and trained within an American culture that usually views peer contacts outside the home as part of normal adolescent development. These therapists must avoid allying themselves with adolescents in the family they see lest they lose the adults within the family. On the other hand, family therapists from a similar culture to the family often run the risk of supporting the parents and thus losing the children. Family therapists must strive to maintain a focus on the total family system and not ally with any one member or subgroup of the family.

Conflict of interest in family therapy is a concern for both psychologists and social workers. Both NASW and APA codes of ethics address this issue and advise their members from the beginning to clarify what their relationship is with each member and, if involved in a conflictual situation, to work on clarifying their roles and withdraw if needed.

The APA Standard 10.02 (Therapy Involving Couples or Families) states:

> (a) When psychologists agree to provide services to several persons who have a relationship (such as spouses, significant others, or parents and children), they take reasonable steps to clarify at the outset which of the individuals are clients/patients and the relationship the psychologist will have with each person.

Confidentiality is often a challenging issue for the family therapist. Practitioners often have differing opinions as to what information should be kept confidential and from whom. Some believe that whatever is discussed during individual sessions should be kept confidential, while others maintain that whatever is shared individually must be discussed by the family as a whole (Corey, Corey, & Callahan, 2002). Informing clients about their and the agency's policy in regard to handling individual communication in family work is considered an ethical practice (APA, 2017; NASW, 2018). Both professions in their most recent codes of ethics address current challenges in maintaining confidentiality in a technological world.

The NASW Code of Ethics addresses the importance of confidentiality in family work by stressing that the therapist "should seek agreement among [families] concerning each individual's right to confidentiality and obligation to preserve the confidentiality of information shared by others" (NASW, 2008, p. 11). Clients should be informed, however, that confidentiality cannot be guaranteed.

The handling of confidentially is especially challenging for those who work with families from cultures who have a very different understanding of confidentiality. In a previous article on culturally diverse children, this author noted that often children and parents from different cultures have a very different concept of confidentiality than the prevailing social work value of confidentiality (Congress & Lynn, 1994). Neither children nor adults believed that group leaders would keep confidential information shared in group sessions. Healy (2001) notes that in Africa often extended families and community networks are involved in working with families, which mitigates a strict definition of confidentiality. African families, as well as those from other countries who favor a more collective approach, may question the American concept of confidentiality. Meer and VandeCreek (2002) point out that the values about confidentiality promoted in our codes of ethics are based on our emphasis on individualism and autonomy while those from other countries may have a different view of confidentiality. Increasingly, social workers and psychologists work with families from many parts of the world that have a family community approach to problem-solving that contrasts with the prevailing American concept of maintaining individual confidentiality. The Universal Declaration of Ethical Principles for Psychologists (2008) developed by the IUPsyS speaks about the "protection of confidentiality of personal information, as culturally defined and relevant for individuals, families, groups, and communities" while the International Federation of Social Workers (IFSW) Global International Statement of Ethical Principles does not specifically address cultural differences in its statement: "6.1 Social workers respect and work in accordance with people's rights to confidentiality and privacy unless there is risk of harm to the self or to others or other statutory restrictions" (IFSW, 2018).

Since I wrote earlier editions of *Multicultural Perspectives in Working with Families*, I have become increasingly aware of how much our Code of Ethics is based on an Anglo-Saxon perspective. Even compared to the codes of other developed countries, the provisions about confidentiality in the U.S. NASW Code of Ethics are the most comprehensive and include the most specific practice situations (Congress & McAuliffe, 2006; Congress & Kim, 2007). The focus on strict confidentiality is particularly challenging at a time during which more and more families come from diverse backgrounds. Professionals must continually struggle with promoting confidentiality with families for whom the concept has limited meaning. Often a dilemma arises between enforcing American concepts of confidentiality and being sensitive to cultural differences in the use of confidentiality. The IFSW (2004) represents an attempt to develop ethical standards for social workers around the world. The standards make a general statement about confidentiality, that is, that social workers should maintain confidentiality about people who use their services except when there is "a greater ethical requirement" (such as the preservation of life; IFSW, 2004, 1.4 Respect for Privacy in Family and Community Life). It is interesting to note that this international standard uses an individualist approach to confidentiality and does not recognize a more collective perspective in providing social work services. There is a statement, however, that social workers should also adhere to the codes of their respective countries, which does provide for cultural differences in the use of confidentiality. The International Statement of Ethical Principles for Psychologists (2008) does mention that cultural differences may affect the way that confidentiality is used: "protection of confidentiality of personal information, as culturally defined and relevant for individuals, families, groups, and communities." In addition, the IFSW (2018) in its Global International Statement of Ethical Principles does not specifically address cultural differences: "6.1 Social workers respect and work in accordance with people's rights to confidentiality and privacy unless there is risk of harm to the self or to others or other statutory restrictions."

Although rights to privacy and confidentiality are stressed in American culture in general and psychology and social work practice in particular, these values may not have the same meaning for families from different cultures. For example, undocumented families may be reluctant to talk with family therapists. They may fear that practitioners, whom they view as unknown authority figures possibly associated with the government, may share information about them with immigration officials, thus leading to deportation. This may be particularly true now as subsequent to 9/11 and the passing of the Patriot Act, there is greater government scrutiny of those who are not American citizens. Even if the family has legal status, past oppression and discrimination experienced by family members may make them reluctant to share information with outsiders (family therapists) from different cultural backgrounds.

All families have different ways of communicating and sharing personal information. In some families, there is very open communication between family members. Other families have many secrets that are kept confidential and especially not shared with children. Not only do family therapists have different ways of handling confidentiality, but also different families handle confidentiality in different ways. Some families from a similar cultural background may handle confidentiality in a similar way; others may approach confidentiality in a way unique for the family. Similar to the therapy process, confidentiality may not be a one-size-fits-all concept. Results indicate that clients from non-Western cultures do not completely understand the concept of privileged communication or the limits to confidentiality (Mignone, Klostermann, Mahadeo, Papagni, & Jankie, 2017). It is necessary for the family therapist to explore a family's unique beliefs about privacy, confidentiality, and maintaining secrets. The family therapist must then be careful not to impose his or her own beliefs about maintaining secrets in family therapy. For example, a family therapist who insisted that there be no secrets in family therapy and then insisted that an unemployed father discuss his feelings of inadequacy in a family session alienated the father and the family never returned for additional sessions. More specific information is needed from non-Western clients regarding how to modify the confidentiality process in a way that is respectful, yet still provides the safeguards intended. Given that confidentiality is the cornerstone of the therapeutic process, it is imperative that clinicians find a culturally respectful way to make clients safe to reveal what may be embarrassing or personally sensitive information in treatment (Younggren & Harris, 2008).

Different family members may have different understandings about confidentiality. Parents from cultures that believe that adolescents should share openly their beliefs and behaviors and not maintain secrets may be in conflict with their adolescents influenced by American teenage culture, who may want to hide personal information from other family members. Recent court decisions that support adolescents' right to confidentiality for healthcare decisions may also affect family therapy with families from diverse backgrounds.

Informed consent is considered essential for ethical social work and psychology practice (NASW, 2008; APA, 2018) as well as for the psychology profession as stated in their Universal Declaration of Ethics Principles: "Psychologists respect the dignity and worth of all people, and the rights of individuals to privacy, confidentiality and self-determination. Respecting a client's right to self-determination both manifests a core value of the profession and plays a helpful and important role in providing services that will benefit clients" (Gauthier, 2008). Because of the vulnerability of many poor multicultural clients, the use of informed consent has been seen as strengthening and empowering to families from diverse backgrounds (Palmer & Kaufman, 2003). Furthermore, informed consent is a required component for evidence-based social work. Informed consent can occur, however, only if clients and families understand the nature of the treatment they will receive.

How can the family therapist facilitate informed consent with families from diverse cultural and linguistic backgrounds? Family therapists must be able to communicate with families in a language they can understand. This points to the need for family therapists to speak in the same language as the families whom they see. This is often challenging given the diversity of languages spoken by American immigrant families.

Using children as interpreters can be problematic as communication can be distorted and the parent's power within the family can be threatened. An example of distorted communication occurred when a student asked a 10-year-old daughter to inquire of her mother how she felt. The mother spoke for 10 minutes. At the end, the daughter interpreted her mother's response as, "She says she feels fine." Another, perhaps, more troubling communication problem occurred when a 15-year-old boy with behavior problems was asked to interpret for his parents when they came for a family session. By using the adolescent as an interpreter, the tenuous power relationships in a family were weakened even more.

Even if the therapist is able to communicate in the language of the family, ensuring informed consent can be problematic. Whereas informed consent can occur with parents, how much informed consent do children have? This is an issue in all family therapy, but may be more acute in families from cultures in which children are not seen as having rights. Family therapy can be affected by parents who have not explained to children why they are coming for therapy and furthermore do not see the need for family therapy. The ethical family therapist must strive to enable all members of a family to exercise informed consent. The purpose of family therapy may have to be explained in a way that children and those not familiar with family therapy can understand.

What new trends have influenced family therapy in the 21st century? Mental health treatment has already been greatly affected by the need for evidence-based models that can demonstrate positive results after a short number of sessions. The current focus on more short-term solution focused models of treatment may be very effective with immigrant families who have limited resources and want treatment that is time limited with very specific treatment objectives. The emphasis on evidence-based treatment also necessitates a specific focus on clear goals and objectives that will appeal to culturally diverse families who want to see clear results within a limited amount of time.

A concern has been raised that family therapy needs a major overhaul. This is seen essentially true for families with adolescents who seem to function in a world very different from the world their parents or therapists know (Taffel, 1996).

With current limits on covering mental health treatment, family therapy is not always reimbursable. There is no accepted diagnostic system for families comparable to the *Diagnostic and Statistical Manual of Mental Disorders, Fifth Edition* (*DSM-5*; American Psychiatric Association, 2013), which is used to measure individual dysfunction and symptomatology. A challenge is that mental health family treatment often involves billing at full rate for the primary client (identified patient) and billing for other family members as collaborative visits. Thirty-five percent of mental health treatment is paid by private insurance, while 44% is paid for by Medicaid and Medicare, a total of 80% (Substance Abuse and Mental Health Services Administration [SAMHSA], 2011). Thus immigrants, especially those who are undocumented and on limited income, may have difficulty in paying for family therapy.

Evidence-based practice is conducive to family therapy with diverse families. First, an exploration of client values is conducted. This is essential in work with families that may have a different value system from that of the therapist. A second major component is the need for informed consent so that the family may choose from different family therapy models. As stated previously, this is challenging given the diversity of cultural backgrounds and languages. Some culturally diverse families may rely on the therapist as the expert and not want to choose among different options. Also, the therapist may believe that he or she is the expert and knows what model would work best with the family. A third major component of evidence-based practice that is firmly supported by the Code of Ethics is that social workers should only rely on models that have proven to be effective. This is challenging as there has been limited research on the effectiveness of the different family models, and even less research on the effectiveness of different family therapy models with clients from different cultural backgrounds.

Practice wisdom suggests that family work would be advisable for people from diverse cultures that favor a collective approach to resolving problems. Family therapy seems particularly appropriate when families seek treatment as a group, in contrast to the many Americans who seek individual treatment. Certain treatment models such as narrative therapy that encourages families to tell their own stories may be particularly useful in working with culturally diverse families (Freeman & Couchonnal, 2006). One challenge, however, might be that those families from cultures in which there is a male-dominated hierarchy within the family may be resistant to therapy in which each member has an equal voice, and there is an expectation that each is open in discussing feelings and problems.

The rise of the Internet has greatly affected the field of family therapy. First, there is a new array of diagnoses for the family therapist including cybersex and cyber addiction (Delmonico & Griffin, 2008; Goldberg, Peterson, Rosen, & Sara, 2008). There may also be new forms of web-based treatment (Gilkey, Carey, & Wade, 2009) that may pose new ethical challenges.

The United States, similar to other countries around the world, is becoming increasingly culturally diverse. In New York City, 40% of the population is foreign-born; for the United States as a whole, the average percentage of foreign-born is 20% (U.S. Census Bureau, 2018). Because of increased poverty and violence, many communities where new immigrants live are currently under siege and can provide only limited support to their residents. One can predict that this situation will not improve very soon with cutbacks in financial and social service resources for poor people. Culturally competent family treatment that focuses on strengthening families provides much support for families in a challenging social environment.

Family therapists work more and more with families from many different cultural backgrounds. Also, as many people from diverse cultural backgrounds seek professional education, one can predict that family therapists will increasingly come from diverse cultural backgrounds. In the past, there was some evidence to suggest, however, that it has been difficult to attract and retain trainees of color, as "family therapy is not the world in which they are familiar . . . though their own values are very family oriented" (McGoldrick et al., 1999, p. 194). Other explanations that McGoldrick and colleagues offer for the limited number of trainees of color is that many from non-White backgrounds view the family therapy field as White-dominated, and second, therapists of color must contend with many life stresses that may prevent them from pursuing specialized training in family therapy. There is some evidence, however, that family therapists may be more receptive to complementary and alternative medical practice (Becvar, Caldwell, & Winek, 2006). Also the current focus on narrative therapy that encourages the family therapist to let the family tell their own story may build more connections between the therapist and the families from different cultural backgrounds. It has been suggested that family therapists from different countries and cultural backgrounds may work differently with issues of gender, culture, and power (Keeling & Piercy, 2007).

One anticipates that this will change as more people of color and immigrants move into the middle class and seek professional education. Many begin to work with families after pursuing a master's in social work. Currently, the Council on Social Work Education (CSWE) reports that approximately 20% of graduating MSW students are from other than Caucasian backgrounds (Lennon, 2002). The focus in social work education is to prepare students for culturally competent practice with families, as well as individuals, groups, and communities. In the years to come, an increasing number of families from diverse cultural backgrounds will be able to receive culturally competent family therapy from professional social workers. In 2015, 86% of psychologists in the U.S. workforce were White, 5% were Asian, 5% were Hispanic, 4% were Black/African American, and 1% were multiracial or from other racial/ethnic groups. This is less diverse than the U.S. population as a whole, which is 62% White and 38%

racial/ethnic minority (APA, 2018). Although members of racial/ethnic minority groups account for less than one-fifth of the psychology workforce, the profession has become more diverse over time. Between 2005 and 2013, the percentage of racial/ethnic minority groups within the psychology workforce grew from 8.9% to 16.4%, compared to 39.6% for the overall workforce and 25.8% for the general doctoral/professional workforce (APA, 2015).

This newly revised edition includes the most current knowledge and research to help practitioners work more effectively with culturally diverse families. In this book, there are four new chapters written by psychologists, which address important emerging issues in family therapy such as multiracial families. Furthermore, it adopts an intersectional approach to deepen the understanding of families from diverse backgrounds, a most necessary and important consideration as the number and combination of cultures expand. The culturagram, which is a family assessment tool, has been expanded to include this intersectional approach.

## REFERENCES

American Psychological Association. (2015, July). *2005-13: Demographics of the U.S. Psychology Workforce.* Retrieved from https://www.apa.org/workforce/publications/13-demographics

American Psychological Association. (2017). *Ethical principles of psychologists and code of conduct.* Washington, DC: Author.

American Psychological Association. (2018). *How Diverse is the Psychology Workforce.* Retrieved from https://www.apa.org/monitor/2018/02/datapoint

Becvar, D. S., Caldwell, K. L., & Winek, J. L. (2006). The relationship between marriage and family therapists and complementary and alternative medicine approaches: A qualitative study. *Journal of Marital and Family Therapy, 32*(1), 115–126. doi:10.1111/j.1752-0606.2006.tb01592.x

Bryan, L. (2000). Neither mask nor mirror: One therapist's journey to ethically integrate feminist family therapy and multiculturalism. *Journal of Feminist Family Therapy and Multiculturalism, 12*(2/3), 105–121. doi:10.1300/J086v12n02_04

Carteret, M. (2010). Cultural differences in family dynamics. Retrieved from https://www.dimensionsofculture.com/2010/11/culture-and-family-dynamics/

Cole, E. (2008). Navigating the dialectic: Following ethical rules versus cultural appropriate practice. *The American Journal of Family Therapy, 36,* 425–436. doi:10.1080/01926180701804642

Congress, E. (1994). The use of culturagrams to assess and empower culturally diverse families. *Families in Society, 75*(9), 531–540. doi:10.1177/104438949407500901

Congress, E. (1999). *Social work values and ethics: Identifying and resolving professional dilemmas.* Belmont, CA: Wadsworth.

Congress, E. (2002). Using culturagrams with culturally diverse families. In A. Roberts & G. Greene (Eds.), *Social work desk reference* (pp. 57–61). New York, NY: Oxford University Press.

Congress, E. (2005). Ethical issues and future directions. In E. Congress & M. Gonzalez (Eds.), *Multicultural perspectives in working with families* (2nd ed., pp. 442–452). New York, NY: Springer Publishing Company.

Congress, E., & Lynn, M. (1994). Group work programs in public schools: Ethical dilemmas and cultural diversity. *Social Work in Education, 16*(2), 107–114. doi:10.1093/cs/16.2.107

Congress, E., & McAuliffe, D. (2006). Social work ethics: Professional codes in Australia and the United States. *International Social Work, 49*(2), 165–176. doi:10.1177/0020872806061211

Congress, E., & Kim, W. (2007). A comparative study on social work ethical codes in Korea and the United States. *Korean Journal of Clinical Social Work, 4*(2), 175–192.

Corey, G., Corey, M., & Callahan, P. (2002). *Issues and ethics in the helping professions.* Pacific Grove, CA: Wadsworth Publishing Company.

Delmonico, D. L., & Griffin, E. J. (2008). Cybersex and the e-teen: What marriage and family therapists should know. *Journal of Marital and Family Therapy, 34*(4), 431–444. doi:10.1111/j.1752-0606.2008.00086.x

Donovan, M. (2003). Family therapy beyond post modernism: Some consideration on the ethical orientation of contemporary practice. *Journal of Family Therapy, 25,* 285–306. doi:10.1111/1467-6427.00249

Estrada, A., & Haney, P. (1998). Genograms in a multicultural perspective. *Journal of Family Psychotherapy, 9*(2), 55–62. doi:10.1300/J085V09N02_05

Fallicov, C. (2009). Commentary: On the wisdom and challenges of culturally attuned treatments for Latinos. *Family Process, 48*(2), 292–309. doi:10.1111/j.1545-5300.2009.01282.x

Freeman, E. M., & Couchonnal, G. (2006). Narrative and culturally based approaches in practice with families. *Families in Society: The Journal of Contemporary Social Services, 87*(2), 198–208. doi:10.1606/1044-3894.3513

Gauthier, J. (2008, October). *The Universal Declaration of Ethical Principles for Psychologists.* Retrieved from https://www.apa.org/international/pi/2008/10/gauthier

Gilkey, S. L., Carey, J., & Wade, S. L. (2009). Families in crisis: Considerations for the use of Web-based treatment models in family therapy. *Families in Society: The Journal of Contemporary Social Services, 90*(1), 37–45. doi:10.1606/1044-3894.3843

Goldberg, P. D., Peterson, B. D., Rosen, K. H., & Sara, M. L. (2008). Cybersex: The impact of a contemporary problem on the practices of marriage and family therapists. *Journal of Marital and Family Therapy, 34*(4), 469–480. doi:10.1111/j.1752-0606.2008.00089.x

Healy, L. (2001). *International social work: Professional action in an interdependent world.* New York, NY: Oxford University Press.

International Union of Psychological Science. (2008). *Declaration of Ethical Principles for Psychologists.* Retrieved from http://www.iupsys.net/about/governance/universal-declaration-of-ethical-principles-for-psychologists.html

International Federation of Social Workers. (2004). *What Is Social Work?* Retrieved from https://www.ifsw.org/what-is-social-work/global-definition-of-social-work

International Federation of Social Workers. (2018). *Global Social Work Statement of Ethical Principles.* Retrieved from https://www.ifsw.org/global-social-work-statement-of-ethical-principles/?hub=main

Keeling, M. L., & Piercy, F. P. (2007). A careful balance: Multinational perspectives on culture, gender, and power in marriage and family therapy practice. *Journal of Marital and Family Therapy, 33*(4), 443–463. doi:10.1111/j.1752-0606.2007.00044.x

Laird, J. (1995). Family centered practice in postmodern era. *Families in Society, 76*(3), 150–160. doi:10.1177/104438949507600303

Lennon, T. (2002). *Statistics on social work education in the United States: 2000.* Silver Springs, MD: Council on Social Work Education.

Lowenberg, F., Dolgoff, R., & Harrington, D. (2000). *Ethical decisions for social work practice.* Itasca, IL: F. E. Peacock Publishers.

McGill, D. W. (1992). The cultural story in multicultural family therapy. *Families in Society, 73*(6), 339–349. doi:10.1177/104438949207300602

McGoldrick, M., & Hardy, K. V. (2008). *Re-visioning family therapy: Race, culture, and gender in clinical practice.* New York, NY: Guilford Press.

McGoldrick, M., Almeida, R., Preto, N. G., & Bibb, A. (1999). Efforts to incorporate social justice perspectives into a family training program. *Journal of Marital and Family Therapy, 25*(2), 191–210. doi:10.1111/j.1752-0606.1999.tb01122.x

Meer, D., & VandeCreek, L. (2002) Cultural consideration in release of information. *Ethics Behavior, 12*(2), 143–156. doi:10.1207/S15327019EB1202_2

Mignone, T., Klostermann, K., Mahadeo, M., Papagni, P., & Jankie, J. (2017). Confidentiality and family therapy: Cultural considerations. *ARC Journal of Psychiatry, 2*(1), 9–16.

National Association of Social Workers. (2008). *Code of ethics.* Washington, DC: NASW Press.

Pakes, K., & Roy-Chowdhury, S. (2007). Culturally sensitive therapy? Examining the practice of cross-cultural family therapy. *Journal of Family Therapy, 29,* 267–283. doi:10.1111/j.1467-6427.2007.00386.x

Palmer, N., & Kaufman, M. (2003). The ethics of informed consent: Implications for multicultural practice. *Journal of Ethnic and Cultural Diversity in Social Work, 12*(1), 1–26. doi:10.1300/J051v12n01_01

Reamer, F. (1999). *Social work values and ethics.* New York, NY: Columbia University Press.

Shibusawa, T. (2009). A commentary on "Gender perspectives in cross-cultural couples." *Clinical Social Work Journal, 37*(3), 230–233. doi:10.1007/s10615-009-0199-z

Singh, R. (2009). Constructing the family across culture. *Journal of Family Therapy, 31*(4), 359–383. doi:10.1111/j.1467-6427.2009.00473.x

Substance Abuse and Mental Health Services Administration. (2011). *The NSDUH Report.* Retrieved from http://store.samhsa.gov/product/Sources-of-Payment-for-Mental-Health-Treatment-for-Adults/NSDUH11–0707

Taffel, R. (1996). *Family Therapy as We Know It Needs to Change.* Retrieved from https://www.psychotherapynetworker.org/blog/details/1408/family-therapy-as-we-know-it-needs-to-change

U.S. Census Bureau. (2018). The foreign-born population in the United States: 2010. Retrieved from https://www.census.gov/library/publications/2012/acs/acs-19.html

Wilcoxon, A., Remley, T., & Gladding, S. (2011). *Legal, and professional issues in the practice of marriage and family ethical therapy* (5th ed.). New York, NY: Prentice Hall.

Younggren, J. N., & Harris, E. A. (2008). Can you keep a secret? Confidentiality in Psychotherapy. *Journal of Clinical Psychology, 64,* 589–600. doi:10.1002/jclp.20480

# Index

ACA. *See* Patient Protection and Affordable Care Act
acculturation, 65
  Asian immigrant families, 197–198
  bi-dimensional model, 60
  globalization, 60–61
  Latinx social identity, 59
  suicide risk, 396–397
  tri-dimensional acculturation measure, 60
  unidimensional models, 60
adolescents, cross-cultural perspectives
  bicultural identity, 140–141
  case vignette, 141–142
  culturagram, 143–145
  culturally informed models, 137
  Erikson's psychosocial stage theory, 137, 138
  ethnic/racial identity models, 139–140
  gender and sexual identity models, 141
  Hays's ADDRESSING framework, 144–146
  individualistic vs. collectivistic cultures, 138
  tight and loose cultures, 138–139
adoption
  adoptees naming process, 47
  African American children, 41–42
  African Intercountry adoptees, 43–44
  birth culture, 47–48
  case vignette, 48–50
  Central and South America, 43
  Chinese adoptees, 43
  cultural socialization, 44
  domestic adoption, 39–42
  East, Southeast, and South Asian Intercountry Adoptees, 42
  ethnic socialization, 45–46
  Holt Adoption Program, 42
  Indian Adoption Project, 41
  intercountry adoptions, 40
  intercountry and international, 40–44
  Korean adoptees, 42–43
  Native American children, 40–41
  racial identity development, 47
  racial socialization, 44–45
  transracial socialization, 46
  White adoptive parents, 47
African Americans families
  historical overview, 170
  intersectionality, 173–174
  relational and narrative family therapy, 174–175
  skin color dynamics, 172, 178
  slave trauma syndrome, 170–172
  treatment implications, 177–178
African Intercountry adoptees, 43–44
Afrocentricity
  Black psychology, 173
  Eurocentric paradigms, 172–173
  family treatment, 169
  historical overview, 170
  Mazama's argument, 173
  Nguzu Saba, 176–177
  social science framework, 169
AIANs. *See* American Indian and Alaska Natives
Alaska Native Claims Settlement Act, 213
alcohol use, 334
Alcohol Use Disorders Identification Test (AUDIT), 338
Alzheimer's disease, 155
ambivalent approach, 45
American Civil Liberties Union (ACLU), 28
American Indian and Alaska Natives (AIANs), 389, 393
American Psychiatric Association Work Group on Suicidal Behaviors, 399
American Psychological Association (APA) Presidential Task Force, 70
anti-miscegenation, 28
antiretroviral medication, 316
appreciation stage, Poston's model, 140

Arab American families
  asylees and refugees, 229
  average length of residency, 229
  empowerment approaches, 239–240
  faith-based coping, 240–241
  family support and family therapy, 241–242
  mental health services access, 231–237
  Ottoman Empire, 228
  post-9/11 government surveillance policies, 230
  protective factors, 227
  psychoeducational interventions, 238–239
  psychosocial risks and needs, 229–231
  sexuality, 237
  sociodemographics, 228–229
  subcultures, 227
  Sunni Muslims, 228
Asian American Identity Development Model, 140
Asian clansmen's groups, 11
Asian immigrant families
  acculturation and intergenerational family conflicts, 197–200
  case vignette, 204–206
  collectivism, 196
  communication styles, 197
  cultural brokers and allies, 202–203
  cultural values, 196
  culturally responsive interventions, 201–204
  diversity and history, 195–196
  interdependent self-construal, 196
  mental health support, 200
  mental healthcare access and disparity, 201
  parentification, 198
  parenting styles, 198–199, 201–202
  psychosocial experiences, 196
  separation and individuation issues, 199–200
  socialeconomic status variables, 196
astronaut families, 8
asylee, 350
asylum interview, 109–110
ataque de nervios, 188
AUDIT. *See* Alcohol Use Disorders Identification Test
autonomy, Helms's model, 139
avoidant approach, 45
awakening stage, Kim's model, 140

BCIS. *See* Bureau of Citizenship and Immigration Services
BDI. *See* Beck Depression Inventory
Beck Depression Inventory (BDI), 76
Berry's acculturation model, 140
bicultural identity, 60, 140–141
bicultural/bilingual children, 123
bi-dimensional model, 60
bilingual social workers, 8
binge drinking, 334
Biracial Identity Development Model, 140
biracial identity paradigm, 30
Black psychosocial functioning, 173
Black Racial Identity Model, 139
brief strategic family therapy (BSFT), 340, 403–404
BSFT. *See* brief strategic family therapy
Bureau of Citizenship and Immigration Services (BCIS), 350

CAIR. *See* Council on American-Islamic Relations
Cass's Identity Model, 141
casual stage, Ruiz's model, 140
CBT. *See* cognitive behavioral therapy
CCSWP. *See* culturally competent social work practice
Central and South American intercountry adoptees, 43
CFI. *See* Cultural Formulation Interview
CHAT. *See* Cultural Health Assessment Tool
child abuse, 11
Child Welfare League of America, 41
child/family/school triangle, 119
Children of Lesbian and Gay Parents Everywhere (COLAGE), 267
Chinese adoptees, 43
Chinese Exclusion Act, 195
CHIP. *See* Medicaid and Children's Health Insurance Program
choice of group stage, Poston's model, 140
Circle of Wellness model, 220
citizens and immigrants
  family sponsorship, 104–105
  refugee protection, 107–111
  Special Juvenile Immigrant Status Act, 106–107
  U.S. citizenship, 110–111
  Violence Against Women Act, 105–106
classical psychoanalysis, 365
client empowerment, 91

# INDEX 435

clinical interventions, domestic violence victims
  case example, 365
  childhood traumatic stress, 368
  cognitive-behavioral approach, 366
  conjoint family therapy, 366
  crisis intervention model, 366
  family intervention, 366
  family systems theory, 366
  feminist therapy models, 367
  legislative remedies, 370
  psychoanalysis, 365
  rational emotive therapy, 366
  self-blame, 368
  solution-focused approach, 367
  trauma focused treatment, 367–368
cognitive behavioral therapy (CBT), 366
  cultural competence principles, 75–76
  depressive feelings, 75
  Hispanics, 76
  Native Americans families, 220
  short-term therapy approach, 75
  substance abuse, 340
  suicide risk, 402–403
  16-week intervention, 76
cognitive stage, Ruiz's model, 140
COLAGE. *See* Children of Lesbian and Gay Parents Everywhere
collateral relationship patterns, 305
collectivistic communities, 138
colorblindness, 45
communication, 8, 197
community domain, DRF, 63
community-specific clinical assessment, Arab American families
  counseling, 235
  gender roles, 235
  less structured orientation to time, 236
  somatic presentation, 234
  stable support system, 234
competent leadership and human resources
  diversity research, 88
  factors affecting, 88
  job satisfaction, 88
  policy compliance and organizational morale, 93
  racial affinity group meetings, 88
  socialization opportunities, 93
conditioning theories, 61
confianza, 185
conflict theory, 61

conjoint family therapy, 366
consequence stage, Ruiz's model, 140
constructivism, 175
contact, Helms's model, 139
corporal punishment, 10
Council of Social Work Education (CSWE) reports, 84, 428
Council on American-Islamic Relations (CAIR), 232
Crenshaw's conceptualization of intersectionality, 34
crisis intervention model, 366
Cross's model of African American racial identity development, 30
CSWE reports. *See* Council of Social Work Education reports
culturagram, 3, 5
  case example, 16–18
  crisis events, 10–11
  cultural institutions, 11
  culturally competent practice, 4
  discrimination and racism, 11–12
  family structure values, 13–15
  health beliefs and access, 9–10
  holidays and special events, 11
  immigrant domestic violence victims, 362
  immigrant family, case vignette, 18–21
  Indigenous peoples, 4
  language, 8–9
  legal status, 6–7
  length of time, community, 7–8
  oppression, 11
  reasons for relocation, 6
  work and education values, 12
cultural adaptation, evidence-based treatments
  conceptual frameworks, 73
  definition, 73
  Ecological Validity and Culturally Sensitive Framework, 73–74
  mental health research, 73
  psychosocial treatments, 73
  Psychotherapy Adaptation and Modification Framework, 74
cultural awareness, 348
cultural competence, 62, 71–72
  barriers, 94–95
  cultural humility, 85
  ethical and legal social work practice, 85
  HIV/AIDS, 326–327
  intersectionality, 86

cultural competence (cont.)
  leadership and human resources management, 87–88, 91–93
  organizational culture, 85
  school social workers and psychologists, 127–131
  service delivery, 86–87, 89–91
cultural, definition, 44
Cultural Formulation Interview (CFI), 62, 65–66
cultural genocide, 41
Cultural Health Assessment Tool (CHAT)
  Healthy Immigrant Effect, 285
  immigrants' health, 284
  inadequate income, 284
  pre-migration experience, 283
  transit experience, 284
cultural humility, 62, 85, 203–204
cultural identity, 219
cultural risk factors and protective factors
  African Americans, 391–392
  AIAN populations, 393
  Asian Americans, 392–393
  Caucasians, 390–391
  Latinxs, 392
cultural sanctions, 399
cultural socialization, 44
Cultural Theory and Model of Suicide, 398–399
cultural worldviews
  anthropologists and social psychologist, 303
  harmony-with-nature orientation, 306
  innate human nature, 306
  interpersonal relationships, 304–305
  mastery-over-nature orientation, 306
  orientation stresses activity, 304
  Papajohn and Spiegel's model, 303–304
  subjugation-to-nature orientation, 305–306
culturally competent social work practice (CCSWP), 130
culturally diverse families
  culturagram (see culturagram)
  cultural and ethnic differences, 4
  generic cultural identity, 4
  intersectional design tool, 16–21
  social workers, 3
  United States, 3
culturally sensitive psychotherapy, 72
culture and diagnosis, 85
  client's language, 62–63
  Cultural Formulation Interview, 62

  diversity/resilience formulation, 63, 65
  individual's subjective experience, 62
  intersectionality, 63
  LGBTQ immigrant clients, 63

DACA. See Deferred Action for Childhood Arrivals
DAST. See Drug Abuse Screening Test
DAWN. See Drug Abuse Warning Network
Deferred Action for Childhood Arrivals (DACA), 283
depression, 156
developmental crises, 10
DHS. See U.S. Department of Homeland Security
diabetes, Native Americans families, 215
*Diagnostic and Statistical Manual of Mental Disorders*, Fifth Edition (*DSM-5*)
  acculturation, 59–61
  case vignette, 63
  culturally competent practice, 62
  culture, 62–63
  disorder criteria, 55
  globalization, 57
  immigration, 57–58
  intersectionality, 58–59
  Latinx population, 55–57
  Pew Research Center analysis, 56
  U.S. Census Bureau project, 55
didactic level adaptation, CBT group intervention, 76
disability, 121
disintegration, Helms's model, 139
diversity domain, DRF, 63
diversity/resilience formulation (DRF), 56, 63
domain-based psychosocial developmental model, 140
domestic violence, 6, 348. See also immigrant domestic violence victims
  abusive relationships, 350
  battering, 350
  categories, 350
  definition, 349
  and immigration, 350
  impressive social and legal remedies, 347
  legislative and regulatory changes, 347
Don't Forget Us program, 220
DRF. See diversity/resilience formulation
Drug Abuse Screening Test (DAST), 338

Drug Abuse Warning Network (DAWN), 335
DSM-5. *See* Diagnostic and Statistical Manual of Mental Disorders, Fifth Edition

EBP. *See* evidence-based practice
Ecological validity and Culturally Sensitivity framework, 73–74
ecologically informed treatment, Hispanics
  ecological-structural family treatment, 191–192
  ego-supportive treatment, 190–191
  life model approach, 189
  social/environmental change agent role model, 191
ecological-structural family treatment, 191–192
ecomap, 4
ego-supportive treatment, 190–191
emotional parentification, 198
empowerment approaches, 239–240
English as a second language (ESL), 17, 125
enmeshment/denial stage, Poston's model, 140
enslavement, 170
ESL. *See* English as a second language
espiritismo, 327
ethnic awareness stage, Kim's model, 140
ethnic, definition, 44
ethnic identities, 31
ethnic socialization, 45–46
ethnically diverse clients. *See* evidence-based practice
ethnic/racial identity models, 139–140
  Asian American Identity Development Model, 140
  Black Racial Identity Model, 139
  Latin American Identity Development Model, 140
  White Racial Identity Development Model, 139
Evangelical Christians, 300
Evangelical Lutheran Church in American (ELCA), 309
evidence-based practice (EBP)
  APA Presidential Task Force, 70
  cultural adaptation, 73–75
  cultural competence, 71–72
  culturally adapted cognitive-behavioral therapy, 75–77
  culture and socioethnographic variables, 70
  ethnocultural patient populations, 69–70
  family therapy, 427
  intersectionality, 72
  mental health treatment, 72–73
  psychosocial therapies, 69
  suicide risk, 401–404
experiential meditative exercise, 16-week CBT group intervention, 76

faith-based coping, 240–241
familism, 321–322, 326
familismo, 184
family abuse
  and adolescent immigrants, 359
  and older immigrants, 359–361
Family and Medical Leave Act (FMLA), 158
family court system, 369
family identity, 124
family loyalty, 305
family sponsorship, 104–105
family structure
  Asian cultures, 14
  Chinese culture, 13
  generational hierarchy, 13
  male-female relationships, 13
  socioeconomic status, 13
  subsystems, 13–14
family systems theory, 366
family therapy, 421
  Arab American families, 241–242
  communication problem, 426
  confidentiality, 423–426
  cultural backgrounds, 428
  ethical dilemmas, 423
  ethical practice, 421
  evidence-based practice, 427
  family relationships, 422
  informed consent, 426
  mental health treatment, 427
  narrative therapy, 422, 427
  NASW Code of Ethics, 421
  practitioners' beliefs, 421
  self-determination, 422–423
  social justice perspective, 422
Family Violence option (FVo), 373
fatalismo, 322
Feminist Identity Development Model, 141
feminist therapy models, 367
financial abuse, 350
FMAPF. *See* Formative Method for Adapting Psychotherapy Framework

FMLA. *See* Family and Medical Leave Act
Formative Method for Adapting Psychotherapy Framework (FMAPF), 75
FVo. *See* Family Violence option

Gay Identity Acquisition Model, 141
gender and sexual identity models, 141
gender scripts, 320–321
gender violence, 319
generic cultural identity, 4
genogram, 4
globalization, 57
globalization-based acculturation
    classroom interaction, 61
    cultural challenges, 61
    diversity, 61
    internal migration, 60
    multicultural experiences, 61
    psychological consequences, 60
    risks, 60–61
green card holders, 7

harmony-with-nature orientation, 306
health beliefs and access
    cultural beliefs, 9
    health beliefs, 9
    holistic mind-body-spirit conceptualization, 9
    mental illness, 9
    physical illness, 9
    undocumented immigrants, 10
Health Care Reform Act, 10
health issues and care
    case vignette, 288–290
    Healthy People 2020, 282
    heart disease, 282
    HIV/AIDS, 282
    immigrant status, 282–283
    immigrants and refugees, 279
    life expectancy, 281
    maternal mortality, United States, 280–281
    mental health/behavioral health, 287–288
    Patient Protection and Affordable Care Act, 282
    prevention, 286
    spiritualist, 287
Healthy Immigrant Effect, 285
Healthy Living in Two Worlds project, 221
Hispanic individuals and families
    cultural characteristics, 183–188

    ecologically informed treatment, 188–192
    elements, 181
    gender-specific roles, 185–186
    nervios, 188
    religion and spirituality, 186–188
    in United States, 181–183
historical trauma, 219, 321
HIV/AIDS and Latinx families
    antiretroviral medication, 316
    assessment, 325–326
    case vignette, 327–328
    challenges, 317
    cultural competence, 326–327
    diagnosis, 317
    familism, 321–322
    fatalismo, 322
    gender scripts, 320–321
    gender violence, 319
    historical trauma, 321
    immigration and trauma, 321
    incidence, 317
    intersectionality, 317–323
    intersectionality perspective, 323
    language barriers, 319
    macro-structural factors, 318
    maternal disclosure, 323
    meso-institutional factor, 318
    micro-interpersonal factors, 318
    poverty, 318, 323–324
    prevention, 316–317
    risk factors, 324
    social and environmental inequality, 317–319
    social workers, 315
    stigma and confidentiality, 322–325
    viral load, 316
    virus types, 316
holistic mind-body-spirit conceptualization, 9
Holt Adoption Program, 42
human services organizational leadership, 84–85
humanitarianism, 45

IAAP. *See* International Association of Applied Psychology
ICE. *See* Immigration and Customs Enforcement
ICWA. *See* Indian Child Welfare Act
idealism, 302
identity, performance, and policy triangle, 120
IDT. *See* intersectional design tool

IHS. *See* Indian Health Service
IIRIRA. *See* Illegal Immigrant Reform and Immigrant Responsibility Act
Illegal Immigrant Reform and Immigrant Responsibility Act (IIRIRA), 373–374
Imani, 176
immersion/emersion, Helms's model, 139
immigrant domestic violence victims
   adolescent immigrants and family abuse, 359
   Arab and Middle Eastern battered women, 357–358
   Asian battered women, 355
   clinical interventions, 365–369
   culturagram, 362
   culturally competent practice, 352
   exploratory study, 352
   immigrant battered women, 349
   immigration profile, United States, 348–349
   Indian and South Asian battered women, 356–357
   intimate partner violence and suicidality, 351, 352
   Japanese nationwide study, 361–362
   Latinx battered women, 353–354
   lawful permanent residents, 348
   legal remedies and criminal justice system, 369
   legislative remedies, 370–374
   nondocumented battered women, 352–353
   older immigrants and family abuse, 359–361
   Pew Research Center analysis, 348
   research data gaps, 351
   risks and needs, 351–361
   Russian battered women, 356
   social interventions, 362–365
   social work practice, 370–374
   Sub-Saharan African battered women, 358–359
   trauma-sensitive services, 348
immigrant status, healthcare access
   age differences, 286
   cultural factors, 285
   Healthy Immigrant Effect, 285
   healthy practices, 285–286
immigrants and refugees
   immigrants and citizens, 104–111
   nonimmigrant and undocumented, 102–104
   social service providers, 111–112
Immigration Act, 102

Immigration and Customs Enforcement (ICE), 103
immigration status, 349–350
incorporation stage, Kim's model, 140
Indian Adoption Project, 41
Indian Child Welfare Act (ICWA), 41, 211
Indian Child Welfare Crisis, 41
Indian Health Service (IHS), 211
Indian orphanages, 41
individualism, 305
individualistic societies, 138
informed consent, 426
instrumental parentification, 198
integration stage, Poston's model, 140
interdependent self-construal, 196
intergenerational conflicts, 8
internalized oppression, 177
International Association of Applied Psychology (IAAP), 422
International Federation of Social Workers (IFSW) Global International Statement of Ethical Principles, 424–425
International Union of Psychological Science (IUPsyS), 422
interpersonal domain, DRF, 63
interracial marriages, 28
intersectional design tool (IDT), 14
   case example, 16–18
   immigrant family, case vignette, 18–21
intersectionality
   African Americans families, 173–174
   cultural competence, 86
   evidence-based practice, 72
   HIV/AIDS and Latinx families, 317–323
   intimate partner violence victims, 58–59
   multicultural triangle, 118
   older adults, 154
   substance abuse, 335–336
intimate partner violence (IPV)
   Black women, 174
   victims, 58–59
intrapersonal domain, DRF, 63
IPV. *See* intimate partner violence
IUPsyS. *See* International Union of Psychological Science

Kujuchagulia, 176, 178
Kuumba, 176, 178
Kwanzaa principles, 176

Latin American Identity Development Model, 140

lawful permanent residency
  family sponsorship, 104–105
  refugee protection, 107–111
  Special Juvenile Immigrant Status Act, 106–107
  U.S. Citizenship, 110–111
  Violence Against Women Act, 105–106
lay theories, 397
leadership and human resources management
  board directors recruitment, 92
  mentoring, 92–93
  socialization opportunities, 93
  training, 92
  written policies, 92
legal remedies and criminal justice system, 369
legal status, family, 6–7
legislative remedies, domestic violence victims
  IIRIRA, 373–374
  PRWORA, 372–373
  social workers, 370
  U-Visa, 371–372
  Violence Against Women's Act, 370–371
LEP. *See* limited English proficiency
lesbian, gay, bisexual, and transgender (LGBT)
  adolescents coming out process, 259–261
  behavior modeling, 267–268
  cultural factors, 257–258
  demographic profile, 253
  direct instruction, 266–267
  disclosure management, 259
  ecological perspective of work practice, 252
  emotional factors, 258–259
  in family, 256–257
  family-centered approach, 264
  family-centered practice, 252
  gender identity expression, 254–256
  HIV/AIDS and Latinx families, 325
  identity, 251
  initial meeting, 265
  initial preparations, 264–265
  intervention, 264
  mental health illness, 254
  parent coming out process, 262–264
  problem-solving strategies, 268
  psychosocial risks/psychosocial needs, 253–254
  racism, 254
  religious factors, 257
  sexual orientation, 254–256
  stigmatizing status, 251
  strengths and problems assessment, 266
  subsequent contacts, 265
  substance abuse, 254
  trauma, 254
LGBT. *See* lesbian, gay, bisexual, and transgender
life span approach, 31
limited English proficiency (LEP), 125
loose societies, 139

machismo, 184, 186, 320
macro advocacy competencies, 112
male immigrants, 349
male-dominant hierarchical family structure, 13
marginality, 30
marianismo, 184, 320
masochism, 186
mastery-over-nature orientation, 306
maternal mortality, United States, 280–281
Medicaid and Children's Health Insurance Program (CHIP), 10
memory loss, 155
mental health care, evidence-based, 72–73
mental health services access, Arab American families
  anti-Arab and anti-Muslim sentiments, 233, 234
  community-specific clinical assessment, 234–236
  cultural stigma, 231
  discrimination, 232
  imams, 231
  strengths and resources, 236–237
mental illness, 9
  lesbian, gay, bisexual, and transgender, 254
mezzo advocacy competencies, 112
MI. *See* motivational interviewing
Michigan Alcoholism Screening Test-geriatric version (MAST-G), 338–339
micro advocacy competencies, 111
microaggression, 31–32, 94–95
microassaults, 95
microinvalidations, 95
minority stress, 399
Monitoring the Future (MTF) survey, 334
monoracial identity paradigm, 30
monoracial parents, 28–29
motivational interviewing (MI), 339
multicultural triangle, child

bicultural/bilingual children, 123
case vignettes, 121–122
child/family/school triangle, 119
culturally based and biased criteria, 123
culturally competent school social workers and psychologists, 127–131
disability, 121
educational policies and practices, 126
family identity, 124
identity, performance, and policy triangle, 120
intersectionality approach, 118
learning difficulties, 121, 122
mental health perspective, 117
overburdened parents, 120
school performance, 125–126
school performance assessment, 119–120
school setting, 118
multiculturalism, 85
multiracial individuals and families
anti-miscegenation, 28
case vignette, 32–33
experiences, 29–30
identity development, 30–31
interracial marriages, 28
intersectionality, 34–35
monoracial parents, 28–29
quantitative analyses, 28
racism and colorism, 34–35
therapists' competence, 35–36
U.S. Census surveys, 27

narrative therapy, 422
National Association of Social Workers (NASW) Code of Ethics, 348
National Family Caregiver Support Program, 158
National Indian Child Welfare Association, 220
National Security Entry-Exit Registration System (NSEERS), 232
Native Americans families
assessment, 217–219
average age, 210
balance concept, 218
case vignette, 221
clan systems, 217
demographic profile, 210–211
discrimination, 212
generations, 217
group cohesiveness, 218
health, 214–215
Indigenous populations, 210
legal and policy context, 210–211
medicine wheel, 218–219
mental health, 215
poverty, 210, 215
psychosocial risks and needs, 213–217
reservation-based populations, 212–213
resilience, 218
service access, 211–213
sovereignty vs. colonization, 210–211
substance misuse, 215
trauma, 213–214
treatment approaches, 219–221
urbanization, 215
violent crime rate, 216
naturalism, 302
nervios, 188
New York Agency for New Americans (NYANA), 363
Nguzu Saba, 176–177
nonimmigrant and undocumented newcomers, 349
crime victims, 103–104
Immigration Act, 102
Latin American countries, 102
Mexicans, 102
social service providers, 103
trafficking victims, 103
U.S. Visa Waiver Program, 102
visa, 103
NSEERS. See National Security Entry-Exit Registration System
NYANA. See New York Agency for New Americans

older adults
age-adjusted death rate, 153
case vignette, 161–162
economics, 156–157
education, 157–158
health and healthcare, 155–156
intersectionality, 154
life expectancy, 153
multicultural practice, 158–161
palliative care, 161
screening and assessment, 160
social connections, 158
social determinants of health, 154–158
older immigrants and family abuse
Canada, 360–361
Chinese immigrant community, 360
cross-cultural study, 361
determinants, 360

older immigrants and family abuse (*cont.*)
  elder mistreatment and help-seeking behavior, 360
  focus groups and individual interviews, 360
  intimate partner violence, 361
  life course perspective, 360
  migration demographics, 359–360
oppressive immigration laws, 352
organizational culture, 93–94
orientation stresses activity, 304
outrageous punishment, 10

PAMF. *See* Psychotherapy Adaptation and Modification Framework
parental subsystem, 13
parentification, Asian American families, 198
passive acceptance, 141
Patient Protection and Affordable Care Act (ACA), 155, 212, 282
personal identity stage, Poston's model, 140
Personal Responsibility and Work opportunity Reconciliation Act (PRWORA), 372–373
personalismo, 184, 327
pharmacology, substance abuse, 341
policy advocacy, 376
positivism, 302
posttraumatic stress disorder (PTSD), 214
poverty
  HIV/AIDS and Latinx families, 323–324
  Native Americans families, 210
practice-based evidence (PBE), suicide risk, 401–402
PRWORA. *See* Personal Responsibility and Work opportunity Reconciliation Act
pseudo-independence, Helms's model, 139
psychoanalysis, 365
psychoeducation
  Arab American families, 238–239
  substance abuse, 337
Psychotherapy Adaptation and Modification Framework (PAMF), 75

racial, definition, 44
racial domain, culturally sensitive psychotherapy, 72
racial identity development
  Cross's model, 30
  ecological perspective, 31
  life span approach, 31
  marginality, 30

microaggression, 31–32
Poston's stages, 31
theory of biracial identity, 30
racial microaggressions, 94
racial socialization, 28–29
  ambivalent approach, 45
  avoidant approach, 45
  colorblindness, 45
  microaggressions, 44
  racial discrimination, 44
  White adoptive parents, 44
racism and colorism, 34–35
rational emotive therapy (RET), 366
rationalism, 302
redirection stage, Kim's model, 140
refugee, 349–350
reintegration, Helms's model, 139
religious faith, 11
religious trends
  case study, 307–308
  Christians, 296–297
  cultural worldviews, 303–307
  LGBT individuals, 299
  mixed religion marriages, 297
  race and ethnicity, 297–298
  vs. spirituality, 300–301
  in United States, 296–297
  worldviews, 302–303
reservation-based populations, 212–213
respeto, 184–185, 327
RET. *See* rational emotive therapy
reward pathway, 338
risky sexual behaviors (RSB), 359

SBIRT. *See* Screening, Brief Intervention, and Referral to Treatment
schizophrenia, 7
school social workers and psychologists
  competent cross-cultural practice, 128
  comprehensive data and evaluation, 128
  constructivist approach, 127
  cultural competence, 127
  cultural self-awareness, 128–129
  culturally competent social work practice, 130
  diversity, 129–130
  holistic approach, 127
  indicators, 129
  multicultural framework, 130–131
Screening, Brief Intervention, and Referral to Treatment (SBIRT), 338
self-acceptance, 178
service access, Native Americans families Alaska, 213

federal studies, 212
Indian Health Service, 211–212
Violence Against Women Act, 212
service delivery, cultural competence
community health center clients, 86–87
consumer advisory group setup, 91
cultivating leaders and peer mentors, 91
evidence-based interventions, 86, 90–91
immigrants and refugees, 87
intersectionality and power, 87
marginalization, 87
recruitment and outreach, 91
sexual identity and orientation, 87
spiritual interventions, 87
staff and manager training, 90
staff profile and consumer diversity, 89–90
SFBT. *See* solution-focused brief therapy
simpatía, 184
16-week cognitive-behavioral group therapy intervention, 76
SJIS Act. *See* Special Juvenile Immigrant Status Act
slave trauma syndrome (STS)
consequences, 171
ever-present anger, 172
PTSS, 171
racial oppression, 171
racist socialization, 172
traumatic conditions, 171
vacant self-esteem, 172
SNAP. *See* Supplemental Nutritional Assistance Program
social discord, 399
social identity, 86
social interventions, domestic violence victims
advocacy groups, 364
case management services, 363
culturally competent practice, 364
fear of deportation, 364
incubator model, 365
longer-term social interventions, 363
nondocumented immigrants, 363
nonresidential services, 363
public assistance, 363
shelter intervention and protective orders, 364
shelter service models, 363
stressful living conditions, 364
social work agencies
challenges, 83–84
cultural competence, 85–86
demographics, 83

human services organizational leadership, 84–85
U.S. workforce, 84
social work practice
advocacy, 376
charity organization agents, 374
culturally competent, 375
ecological model, 374–375
interdisciplinary collaboration, 375
social welfare policies, 376
social/environmental change agent role model, 191
solution-focused brief therapy (SFBT), 203
sovereignty, 210–211
Special Juvenile Immigrant Status (SJIS) Act, 106–107
spirituality. *See also* religious trends
definition, 300
DRF, 63
spousal subsystem, 13
stress-diathesis model, 398
structural level adaptation, CBT group intervention, 76
STS. *See* slave trauma syndrome
subjective spirituality, 301
subjugation-to-nature orientation, 305–306
substance abuse
adolescence, 334
alcohol use, 334, 335
AUDIT and DAST, 338
case vignette, 341
family-based approaches, 337
intersectionality, 335–336
lesbian, gay, bisexual, and transgender, 254
Michigan Alcoholism Screening Test, 338–339
Monitoring the Future survey, 334
multicultural practice, 336–338
older adults, 156
opioids, 334
SBIRT and CAGE, 338
screening and assessment, 338–339
substance use disorders, 333
treatment approaches, 339–341
substance misuse, Native Americans families, 215
substance use disorders (SUDs), 333–334
successful resolution stage, Ruiz's model, 140
SUDs. *See* substance use disorders
suicide risk
acculturation, 396–397
African Americans, 388

suicide risk (*cont.*)
  American Indian and Alaska Natives, 389
  Asians, 389
  Caucasians, 386–387
  and cultural affiliation, 393–394
  cultural influences, 398–399
  cultural risk factors and protective factors, 390–393
  culturally responsive practice, 400–401
  evidence-based approach, 401–404
  family therapy, 403–404
  global suicide rates, 385
  and immigration, 394–396
  international perspectives and attitudes, 397–398
  Latinxs, 387–388
  mental health service utilization and ethnicity, 400
  transcultural risk factors and protective factors, 390
Supplemental Nutritional Assistance Program (SNAP), 15

TDV. *See* teen dating violence
teen dating violence (TDV), 359
Temporary Assistance for Needy Families (TANF) requirements, 373
theory of biracial identity, 30
tight societies, 138–139
traditional psychoanalytic interventions, 365
tradition-oriented religiousness, 301
transnationalism, 327
transracial adoption
  adoptees naming process, 47
  birth culture, 47–48
  case vignette, 48–50
  cultural socialization, 44
  domestic adoption, 39
  ethnic socialization, 45–46
  intercountry adoptions, 40
  intercountry and international adoption, 42–44
  international adoptions, 40
  racial identity development, 47
  racial socialization, 44–45
  research, 39–40
  transracial socialization, 46
  White adoptive parents, 47
transracial socialization, 46
trauma
  lesbian, gay, bisexual, and transgender, 254

Native Americans families, 213–214
tri-dimensional acculturation measure, 60
two-person psychological model, 175

Ujamma, 176
Ujima, 176, 177
UNAIDS. *See* United nations Joint Program on HIV/AIDS
undocumented immigrants, 7, 10
UNESCO. *See* United Nations, Educational Scientific and Cultural Organization
unexpected events and crises, 10
unidimensional models, 60
United Nations, Educational Scientific and Cultural Organization (UNESCO), 61
United Nation's International Migration Report, 57
United Nations Joint Program on HIV/AIDS (UNAIDS), 318
Unoja, 176
U.S. Census Bureau Educational Attainment data, 58–59
U.S. Citizen and Immigration Services (USCIS), 371–372
U.S. citizenship, 110–111
U.S. Department of Homeland Security (DHS), 103, 349
U.S. immigration legal classifications
  immigrants and citizens, 104–111
  nonimmigrant and undocumented, 102–103
U.S. Refugee Act, 108
U.S. Visa Waiver Program (VWP), 102
USCIS. *See* U.S. Citizen and Immigration Services
U-Visa, 371–372

vacant self-esteem, 172
VAWA. *See* Violence Against Women Act
Violence Against Women Act (VAWA), 105–106, 212
  gender based violence, 371
  legal penalties, 370
  reauthorization, 370, 371
VWP. *See* U.S. Visa Waiver Program

White identification stage, Kim's model, 140
White Racial Identity Development Model, 139
working through stage, Ruiz's model, 140
workplace challenges
  leadership and human resources management, 87–88, 91–93
  service delivery, 86–87, 89–91

CPSIA information can be obtained
at www.ICGtesting.com
Printed in the USA
BVHW092259180122
626547BV00004B/14